a LANGE me

Thoracic Anesthesia

Notice

Medicine is an ever-changing science. As new research and clinical experience broaden our knowledge, changes in treatment and drug therapy are required. The authors and the publisher of this work have checked with sources believed to be reliable in their efforts to provide information that is complete and generally in accord with the standards accepted at the time of publication. However, in view of the possibility of human error or changes in medical sciences, neither the authors nor the publisher nor any other party who has been involved in the preparation or publication of this work warrants that the information contained herein is in every respect accurate or complete, and they disclaim all responsibility for any errors or omissions or for the results obtained from use of the information contained in this work. Readers are encouraged to confirm the information contained herein with other sources. For example and in particular, readers are advised to check the product information sheet included in the package of each drug they plan to administer to be certain that the information contained in this work is accurate and that changes have not been made in the recommended dose or in the contraindications for administration. This recommendation is of particular importance in connection with new or infrequently used drugs.

a LANGE medical book

Thoracic Anesthesia

Atilio Barbeito, MD
Assistant Professor
Department of Anesthesiology
Duke University Medical Center
Durham, North Carolina

Andrew D. Shaw, MB, FRCA, FCCM
Associate Professor
Department of Anesthesiology
Duke University Medical Center
Durham, North Carolina

Katherine Grichnik, MD, MS, FASE
Professor
Department of Anesthesiology
Duke University Medical Center
Durham, North Carolina

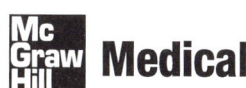

New York   Chicago   San Francisco   Lisbon   London   Madrid   Mexico City
Milan   New Delhi   San Juan   Seoul   Singapore   Sydney   Toronto

The McGraw-Hill Companies

Thoracic Anesthesia

Copyright © 2012 by The McGraw-Hill Companies, Inc. All rights reserved. Printed in the United States of America. Except as permitted under the United States Copyright Act of 1976, no part of this publication may be reproduced or distributed in any form or by any means, or stored in a data base or retrieval system, without the prior written permission of the publisher.

1 2 3 4 5 6 7 8 9 0   DOC/DOC   17 16 15 14 13 12

ISBN 978-0-07-162566-1
MHID 0-07-162566-6

This book was set in Adobe Garamond by Cenveo Publisher Services.
The editors were Brian Belval and Christie Naglieri.
The production supervisor was Catherine Saggese.
Project management was provided by Manisha Singh.
The cover image of an anterolateral view (right side) of the larynx, trachea, and bronchial tree is from Medical RF.
RR Donnelley was printer and binder.

This book is printed on acid-free paper.

Library of Congress Cataloging-in-Publication Data

Thoracic anesthesia / [edited by] Atilio Barbeito,
   Andrew D. Shaw, Katherine Grichnik.—1st ed.
       p. ; cm.
   Includes bibliographical references and index.
   ISBN-13: 978-0-07-162566-1 (hardcover : alk. paper)
   ISBN-10: 0-07-162566-6 (hardcover : alk. paper)
   [etc.]
   I. Barbeito, Atilio.   II. Shaw, Andrew D.   III. Grichnik, Katherine.
   [DNLM: 1. Anesthesia—methods.   2. Thoracic Diseases—surgery.
   3. Postoperative Care.   4. Thoracic Surgical Procedures—methods.   WF 980]
   617.96754—dc23   2011040084

McGraw-Hill books are available at special quantity discounts to use as premiums and sales promotions, or for use in corporate training programs. To contact a representative please e-mail us at bulksales@mcgraw-hill.com.

*I dedicate this book to my wife Luz María and our dear children
(José María, Francisca, Solano, Benjamín and Santiago).
They make my work light, coming home a joy, and life a blessing.
I would also like to dedicate this work to my father—my first
and best Anesthesiology teacher.*

Atilio Barbeito, MD

*To my wife Kate for putting up with the long days and missed dinners,
and my children Maddie and Tom, whose unwavering love and support
remind me how lucky I am to be their Dad.*

Andrew D. Shaw, MB, FRCA, FCCM

*To my husband Jim, and my children Matthew and Sarah,
for their endless love, support and confidence.*

Katherine Grichnik, MD, MS, FASE

Contents

Contributors   xiii
Preface   xvii

PART 1 THE PRINCIPLES OF THORACIC ANESTHESIA

Chapter 1 History and Scope of Anesthesia for Thoracic Surgery   2
The Early Years of Thoracic Surgery / 2
Endotracheal Intubation and Anesthesia / 6
Advances in Thoracic Surgery / 11
Alternatives to General Anesthesia / 11
Early One-Lung Ventilation / 12
Development of Intraoperative Mechanical Ventilation / 16
Advances in Intraoperative Monitoring / 17
Improvements in Oxygenation for One-Lung Ventilation / 18
Improvements in Postoperative Analgesia / 19
Current Scope of Anesthesia for Thoracic Surgery / 20

Chapter 2 Practice Improvement and Patient Safety in Thoracic Anesthesia: A Human Factors Perspective   25
Prospective Memory Enhancement:
    Checklists, Guidelines, Protocols, and Cognitive Aids / 28
Teamwork / 32
Monitoring and Alarms / 35
Medication Errors / 37
Respiratory Events / 38

Chapter 3 Physiology of One-Lung Ventilation   45
Pulmonary Ventilation / 45
Normal Lung Volumes and Effects of Anesthesia, Positioning,
    and Positive Pressure Ventilation / 48
Ventilation and Pulmonary Gas Exchange / 49
Pulmonary Circulation / 50
Pulmonary Circulation Pressure-Flow Relationships / 51
Pulmonary Vasodilation and Vasoconstriction / 52
Apneic Oxygenation / 53
Physiology of One-Lung Ventilation (OLV) / 53
Hemodynamic Changes During OLV / 55
Oxygenation During OLV / 55
Effects of Drugs and Anesthesia on Blood Flow Distribution / 57
Summary / 61

Chapter 4 Perioperative Management of the Patient with Pulmonary Hypertension — 63
Normal Pulmonary Physiology and Hypoxic Pulmonary Vasoconstriction / 63
Pulmonary Hypertension / 65
Effects of Pulmonary Resection on Right Ventricular and Pulmonary Vascular Dynamics / 66
Preoperative Medical Management of Patients with Pulmonary Hypertension / 67
Preoperative Preparation / 68
Perioperative Care / 70
Intraoperative Hypotension / 72
Initial Management of Intraoperative Pulmonary Hypertension / 74
Selective Pulmonary Vasodilators / 75
Supportive Medications / 77
Postoperative Recovery / 77

Chapter 5 Lung Separation Techniques — 82
Double-Lumen Endotracheal Tubes / 82
Bronchial Blockers / 90
Arndt Blocker / 90
Cohen Flexitip Endobronchial Blocker / 92
Fuji Uniblocker / 94
Comparison of Independent Bronchial Blockers / 94
Univent Endotracheal Tube / 94
Complications with the use of Bronchial Blockers / 95
Lung Separation in the Tracheostomized Patient / 96
Lung Collapse Following Lung Separation / 97
Summary / 98

Chapter 6 Mechanisms of Pain in Thoracic Surgery — 102
Overview of Pain Pathways and Neurochemistry / 103
The Development of Hyperalgesia and Central Sensitization / 109
Mechanisms of Neuropathic Pain / 110
Analgesia / 111

Chapter 7 The Biology of Lung and Esophageal Cancer — 116
Oncogenes / 116
Tumor Suppressors / 117
Genomics and Proteomics / 120
Mouse Models / 121
Cancer Stem Cells / 123
Conclusion / 123

Chapter 8 Anatomy, Imaging and Practical Management of Selected Thoracic Surgical Procedures   127

Anatomy / 127
Airway and Lungs / 128
Esophagus / 130
Mediastinum / 131
Diagnostic Imaging Modalities / 131
Practical Management of Thoracic Surgical Procedures / 137
Summary / 145

PART 2 THORACIC ANESTHESIA PRACTICE

Chapter 9 Preoperative Risk Stratification of the Thoracic Surgical Patient   150

Evaluation of Respiratory Function / 151
Cardiac Evaluation / 156
Chemotherapy and Radiation / 161
Radiation Therapy / 163
Pulmonary Rehabilitation / 164
Smoking Cessation / 164
Perioperative Respiratory Medications / 165
Metastatic Disease / 165
Metabolic and Paraneoplastic Effects of Cancer / 166
Lung Isolation and Postoperative Pain Control / 167
Conclusion and Recommendations / 167

Chapter 10 Bronchoscopy, Mediastinoscopy, and Chamberlain Procedure   173

Flexible Fiberoptic Bronchoscopy / 174
Rigid Bronchoscopy / 178
Mediastinoscopy / 181

Chapter 11 Therapeutic Bronchoscopy, Airway Stents, and Other Closed Thorax Procedures   191

Rigid Bronchoscopy / 192
Anesthetic Management for Rigid Bronchoscopy / 196
Therapeutic Procedures / 201
Therapies with Delayed Effect / 206
Airway Stenting / 207
Case Reports / 212
Conclusion / 214

Chapter 12 Mediastinal Masses: Implications for Anesthesiologists   217

Clinical Aspects of Mediastinal Masses / 218
Anterior Mediastinal Masses—Anesthetic Aspects / 221

Anesthetic Management   /   228
Superior Vena Cava Syndrome   /   233

Chapter 13 Lung Resections for Cancer and Benign Chest Tumors   237
Types of Lung Tumors   /   238
Lung Resection—Procedure Planning   /   239
Preoperative Assessment   /   240
Anesthetic Plan   243

Chapter 14 Extrapleural Pneumonectomy   255
Malignant Pleural Mesothelioma   /   256
Technique of Extrapleural Pneumonectomy   /   259
Patient Selection   /   261
Anesthetic Management   /   262
Complications after Extrapleural Pneumonectomy   /   264
Trimodality Therapy for Mesothelioma   /   269
Conclusion   /   270

Chapter 15 Lung Volume Reduction Surgery   274
Pathophysiology of COPD   /   275
Surgical Techniques for Lung Volume Reduction Surgery   /   279
Preoperative Assessment and Patient Selection   /   285
Perioperative Management   /   293
Pain Management in Lung Volume Reduction Surgery   /   301
Summary   /   302

Chapter 16 Pericardial Window Procedures   308
Pathophysiology of Cardiac Tamponade   /   310
Diagnosis of Pericardial Effusion and Tamponade   /   312
Surgical Management   /   316
Anesthetic Considerations   /   316
Summary   /   319

Chapter 17 Esophageal Cancer Operations   322
Esophageal Cancer   /   323

Chapter 18 Bronchopleural Fistula: Anesthetic Management   342
Clinical Presentation   /   345
Management   /   350
Prognosis   /   355
Prevention   /   355
Summary   /   356

Chapter 19 Anesthesia for Lung Transplantation — 358
Background / 359
Preoperative Evaluation and Preparation / 364
Intraoperative Management / 367
Postoperative Management / 372
Anesthesia after Lung Transplantation / 375

Chapter 20 Thoracic Trauma Management — 378
Blunt Versus Penetrating Trauma / 379
Triage and Initial Management / 381
Pulmonary Contusion / 389
Pulmonary Laceration / 390
Diaphragmatic Injury / 390
Laryngeal and Tracheobronchial Trauma / 391
Cardiac Trauma / 393
Great Vessel Trauma / 397

Chapter 21 Anesthesia for Pediatric Thoracic Surgery — 403
Overview / 404
Specific Conditions / 411
Congenital Cystic Adenomatous Malformations / 411
Foreign Body in the Airway / 415
Pediatric Anterior Mediastinal Mass / 417
Summary / 420

PART 3 POSTOPERATIVE MANAGEMENT OF THORACIC SURGICAL PATIENTS

Chapter 22 Routine Postoperative Care of the Thoracic Surgical Patient — 426
Risk Stratification / 427
Assessment Upon Admission / 427
Postoperative Ventilatory Support / 428
Pulmonary Physiotherapy and Early Ambulation / 428
Pneumonia Prevention / 428
Chest Tube Management / 429
Fluid Management / 433
Prophylactic Antibiotics / 434
Nutrition / 435
Glycemic Control / 435
Venous Thromboembolism Prophylaxis / 436
Summary / 436

Chapter 23 Respiratory, Renal, and Cardiovascular Postoperative Complications — **440**

Respiratory Complications / 441
Postpneumonectomy Pulmonary Edema / 441
Pneumonia / 445
Bronchopleural Fistula / 446
Acute Lung Injury / 447
Prolonged Mechanical Ventilation and the Need for Tracheostomy / 449
Renal Complications / 450
Cardiac Complications / 454
Conclusion / 461

Chapter 24 Acute and Chronic Post-Thoracotomy Pain — **467**

Mechanisms of Pain / 468
Management of Acute Post-Thoracotomy Pain / 469
Chronic Post-Thoracotomy Pain / 480
Conclusion / 483

Index — **491**

Contributors

David Amar, MD
Professor
Department of Anesthesiology
Weill Medical College of Cornell University
Anesthesiology and Critical Care Medicine
Memorial Sloan-Kettering Cancer Center
New York, New York

Atilio Barbeito, MD
Assistant Professor
Department of Anesthesiology
Duke University Medical Center
Durham, North Carolina

Raquel R. Bartz, MD
Assistant Professor
Department of Anesthesiology
Duke University Medical Center
Durham, North Carolina

Shahar Bar-Yosef, MD
Assistant Consulting Professor
Department of Anesthesiology
Duke University Medical Center
Durham, North Carolina

Mark F. Berry, MD
Assistant Professor
Department of Surgery
Duke University Medical Center
Durham, North Carolina

Marcelle Blessing, MD
Assistant Professor
Department of Anesthesiology
Yale University School of Medicine
New Haven, Connecticut

Jessica A. Boyette-Davis, PhD
Assistant Professor
Department of Behavioral Sciences, Psychology
York College of Pennsylvania
York, Pennsylvania

Thomas Buchheit, MD
Associate Professor
Department of Anesthesiology
Duke University Medical Center
Durham, North Carolina

Javier Campos, MD
Professor
Department of Anesthesia
University of Iowa Healthcare
Iowa City, Iowa

Edmond Cohen, MD
Professor
Department of Anesthesiology
Mount Sinai School of Medicine
New York, New York

Thomas A. D'Amico, MD
Professor
Department of Surgery
Duke University Medical Center
Durham, North Carolina

Laura K. Diaz, MD
Assistant Professor
Department of Anesthesiology and Critical Care Medicine
Perelman School of Medicine
University of Pennsylvania
Philadelphia, Pennsylvania

Patrick M. Dougherty, PhD
Professor
Department of Anesthesia and Pain Medicine
The University of Texas M.D. Anderson Cancer Center
Houston, Texas

John B. Eck, MD
Associate Professor
Department of Anesthesiology and Pediatrics
Duke University Medical Center
Durham, North Carolina

Contributors

David J. Ficke, MD
Cardiothoracic Anesthesiologist
United Hospital System
Kenosha, Wisconsin

Arjunan Ganesh, MBBS
Assistant Professor
Department of Anesthesia and
  Critical Care
The Children's Hospital of Philadelphia
Perelman School of Medicine at the
  University of Pennsylvania
Philadelphia, Pennsylvania

Katherine Grichnik, MD, MS, FASE
Professor
Department of Anesthesiology
Duke University Medical Center
Durham, North Carolina

Hilary P. Grocott, MD, FRCPC, FASE
Professor
Department of Anesthesia and Surgery
University of Manitoba
Cardiac Anesthesia Fellowship Director
I.H. Asper Clinical Research Institute
Winnipeg, Canada

Harleena Gulati, MD, FRCPC
Assistant Professor
Department of Anesthesia and
  Perioperative Medicine
University of Manitoba
Winnipeg, Canada

David H. Harpole, MD
Professor
Department of Surgery
Duke University Medical Center
Durham, North Carolina

Steven E. Hill, MD
Professor
Department of Anesthesiology
Duke University Medical Center
Durham, North Carolina

Brendan L. Howes, MD
Anesthesiologist
American Anesthesiology of North Carolina
  WakeMed Health and Hospitals
Raleigh, North Carolina

Christopher C. C. Hudson, MD, FRCPC
Assistant Professor
Division of Cardiac Anesthesia and Critical
  Care Medicine
University of Ottawa Heart Institute
Ottawa, Canada

Jordan K. C. Hudson, MD, FRCPC
Assistant Professor
Department of Anesthesiology
The Ottawa Hospital-Civic Campus
University of Ottawa
Ottawa, Canada

Jorn Karhausen, MD
Assistant Professor
Department of Anesthesiology
Duke University Medical Center
Durham, North Carolina

Jerome M. Klafta, MD
Professor
Department of Anesthesia and Critical Care
University of Chicago Medical Center
Chicago, Illinois

David R. Lindsay, MD
Assistant Professor
Department of Anesthesiology
Duke University Medical Center
Durham, North Carolina

Frederick W. Lombard, MBChB, FANZCA
Assistant Professor
Department of Anesthesiology
Duke University Medical Center
Durham, North Carolina

G. Burkhard Mackensen, MD, PhD, FASE
Professor and Chief
UW Medicine Research and Education
 Endowed Professor in Anesthesiology
Department of Anesthesiology and
 Pain Medicine
UW Medicine Regional Heart Center (RHC)
University of Washington
Seattle, Washington

Jonathan B. Mark, MD
Professor
Department of Anesthesiology
Duke University Medical Center
Durham, North Carolina

Joseph P. Mathew, MD, MHSc
Professor
Department of Anesthesiology
Duke University Medical Center
Durham, North Carolina

Timothy E. Miller, MB ChB, FRCA
Assistant Professor
Department of Anesthesiology
Duke University Medical Center
Durham, North Carolina

Richard E. Moon, MD, FACP, FCCP, FRCPC
Professor
Department of Anesthesiology
Department of Medicine
Medical Director
Center for Hyperbaric Medicineand
 Environmental Physiology
Duke University Medical Center
Durham, North Carolina

Alina Nicoara, MD
Assistant Professor
Department of Anesthesiology
Duke University Medical Center
Durham, North Carolina

E. Andrew Ochroch, MD, MSCE
Associate Professor
Department of Anesthesiology, Critical Care
 and Surgery
University of Pennsylvania
Philadelphia, Pennsylvania

Mark W. Onaitis, MD
Assistant Professor
Department of Surgery
Duke University Medical Center
Durham, North Carolina

Wendy L. Pabich, MD
Staff Anesthesiologist
Physicians Anesthesia Service
Swedish Medical Center
Physicians Anesthesia Service
Seattle, Washington

Alessia Pedoto, MD
Assistant Attending
Department of Anesthesiology and Critical
 Care Medicine
Memorial Sloan Kettering Cancer Center
New York, New York

Srinivas Pyati, MD, DA, MRCA, FCARCS
Assistant Professor
Department of Anesthesiology
Duke University Medical Center
Durham, North Carolina

Mihai V. Podgoreanu, MD, FASE
Associate Professor with Tenure
Division of Cardiothoracic Anesthesia and
 Critical Care
Division of Basic Sciences
Director
Perioperative Genomics Program
Duke University Medical Center
Durham, North Carolina

Bernhard Riedel, MD, MBA, PhD
Director
Department of Anaesthetics
Cancer Anaesthetics and Pain Management
Peter MacCallum Cancer Center
Melbourne, Australia

Rebecca A. Schroeder, MD, MMCi
Associate Professor
Department of Anesthesiology
Duke University Medical Center
Durham, North Carolina

Noa Segall, PhD
Assistant Professor
Department of Anesthesiology
Duke University Medical Center
Durham, North Carolina

Mark L. Shapiro, MD
Associate Professor
Department of Surgery
Associate Director
Trauma Services
Department of Surgery
Duke University Medical Center
Durham, North Carolina

Andrew D. Shaw, MB, FRCA, FCCM
Associate Professor
Department of Anesthesiology
Duke University Medical Center
Durham, North Carolina

Scott Shofer, MD, PhD
Assistant Professor
Department of Medicine
Duke University Medical Center
Durham, North Carolina

Mark Stafford-Smith, MD, CM, FRCPC, FASE
Professor
Department of Anesthesiology
Duke University Medical Center
Durham, North Carolina

Dilip Thakar, MD
Professor
Department of Anesthesiology and
   Perioperative Medicine
The University of Texas MD Anderson
   Cancer Center
Houston, Texas

Betty C. Tong, MD, MHS
Assistant Professor
Department of Surgery
Duke University Medical Center
Durham, North Carolina

Angela Truong, MD
Associate Professor
Department of Anesthesiology and
   Perioperative Medicine
University of Texas MD Anderson
   Cancer Center
Houston, Texas

Dam-Thuy Truong, MD
Professor
Anesthesiology and Perioperative Medicine
University of Texas MD Anderson
   Cancer Center
Houston, Texas

Momen M. Wahidi, MD, MBA
Associate Professor
Department of Medicine
Duke University Medical Center
Durham, North Carolina

Ian J. Welsby, MBBS, FRCA
Associate Professor
Department of Anesthesiology
Duke University Medical Center
Durham, North Carolina

Preface

One hundred years have passed since the first report by Charles Elsberg on the use of tracheal insufflation anesthesia for thoracic surgical procedures. The progress that has been made in the delivery of anesthesia for thoracic surgery over the past century has been remarkable. In fact, it may be argued that no other surgical subspecialty has depended so heavily on the progress of anesthesia practice to evolve. The field of thoracic anesthesiology has grown dramatically: our understanding on the mechanisms of thoracic pain, the biology of the different diseases of the chest such as lung and esophageal cancer, the physiology of one lung ventilation and the development of multiple lung isolation techniques are but a few examples of the expanding scope of this fascinating discipline.

The goal of this textbook is to provide the reader with an updated review on the core concepts of thoracic anesthesia practice, together with some very practical management suggestions for the most commonly encountered problems. The work is intended for physicians in training and for those who do not practice thoracic anesthesia exclusively. Each chapter, written by specialists in the topic, provides a review of the key concepts needed to understand the disease at hand and summarizes the different anesthetic management strategies that will allow the delivery of safe, high quality perioperative care to thoracic surgical patients.

Our work is not an exhaustive review of the literature on thoracic anesthesiology, but a practical handbook designed for everyday use. Despite this, we include a chapter on the history of thoracic anesthesia practice. We share GK Chesterton's view that "history is a hill or high point of vantage, from which alone men see the town in which they live or the age in which they are living." We felt we could not tell the reader where we are without describing how we got here. We also include a chapter on practice improvement and patient safety, which contains important concepts for the delivery of modern, high-quality thoracic surgical care using a multidisciplinary, team approach. The remainder of the first section includes chapters on the scientific principles of the subspecialty of thoracic anesthesiology: chest physiology, mechanisms of pain, biology of chest malignancies and lung separation techniques.

The second section includes chapters on the most commonly performed invasive thoracic procedures, with up to date information on pathophysiology and management. Each chapter begins with a short clinical vignette, aimed at providing the reader with a concrete example of the application of the contents of the particular chapter.

The last section in the book pertains to routine and complicated post-operative care of the thoracic surgical patient. We hope the reader finds this material of practical use in their occasional thoracic anesthetic practice.

This book is the result of the dedication and hard work of our many contributors; it represents their accomplishment more than ours, and we are grateful to every one of them. We would also like to thank Melinda Macalino for her logistical and administrative assistance. Lastly, we extend our gratitude to the Department of Anesthesiology at Duke University, our chairman Dr. Mark Newman, and our teachers and trainees for their unwavering support to this project.

Atilio Barbeito, MD
Andrew D. Shaw, MB, FRCA, FCCM
Katherine Grichnik, MD, MS, FASE

PART 1

The Principles of Thoracic Anesthesia

CHAPTERS

1. History and Scope of Anesthesia for Thoracic Surgery — 2
2. Practice Improvement and Patient Safety in Thoracic Anesthesia: A Human Factors Perspective — 25
3. Physiology of One-Lung Ventilation — 45
4. Perioperative Management of the Patient with Pulmonary Hypertension — 63
5. Lung Separation Techniques — 82
6. Mechanisms of Pain in Thoracic Surgery — 102
7. The Biology of Lung and Esophageal Cancer — 116
8. Anatomy, Imaging and Practical Management of Selected Thoracic Surgical Procedures — 127

History and Scope of Anesthesia for Thoracic Surgery

Marcelle Blessing
Edmond Cohen

The history of anesthesia for thoracic surgery encompasses much of the history of anesthesia because the modern practice of thoracic anesthesia relies on major advances in preoperative evaluation, airway management, intraoperative monitoring, pharmacological agents, and improvements in postoperative pain management and intensive care management. These advances equip the modern thoracic anesthesiologist with the tools and techniques to care for even the frailest patients undergoing complex surgical operations. Many patients who would have been deemed inoperable in the past are operative candidates today, because of improvements in both anesthetic and surgical techniques that have augmented safety for all patients undergoing thoracic surgery. The current practice of anesthesia for thoracic surgery represents a culmination of 100 years of advances in anesthesia techniques, and these techniques continue to evolve.

THE EARLY YEARS OF THORACIC SURGERY

The safe delivery of anesthesia for thoracic surgery is a relatively late development in the history of anesthesia because of the ingenuity needed to overcome the unique challenges of safely performing surgery in the thorax. It is easy to forget today that prior to advances in general anesthesia techniques, specifically positive pressure ventilation and controlled respiration with endotracheal intubation, surgery that trespassed the chest wall posed grave risks to patients. Although inhalational anesthesia was introduced in the 1840s, it took another 100 years before anesthesiologists made significant headway in providing safe care for patients undergoing operations in the chest. Improvements in anesthetic practice permitted thoracic surgery to flourish as a specialty; the growth of no other surgical subspecialty depended so heavily on the progress of anesthesia. Although intrathoracic procedures have become routine, thoracic surgeons and anesthesiologists retain a unique relationship; few areas of surgery require as much communication and cooperation between surgeon and anesthesiologist.

As the scope of thoracic surgery has increased greatly, so has the scope of anesthetic practice for it. Today, knowledge of anesthesia techniques for thoracic surgery has become more important than ever. Greater numbers of and types of procedures for lung, esophageal, mediastinal, anterior and posterior spinal, thoracic aortic and cardiac surgery rely on thoracic approaches that require use of one-lung ventilation (OLV). Also, more intrathoracic procedures are being performed with minimally invasive approaches that rely on OLV for adequate surgical exposure. To safely provide the OLV that is universally favored by thoracic surgeons, anesthesiologists must be knowledgeable about the physiology of OLV, be familiar with the range of tools available for providing it, and be aware of techniques for preventing hypoxemia. A variety of double lumen endotracheal tubes and modern endobronchial blockers are now available to provide safe and reliable OLV for most patients.

The Pneumothorax Problem

The inherent danger of performing surgery within the thorax has been known since antiquity. Almost 2000 years ago, the Roman encyclopedia author Celsus, in *De Medicina,* described the problem succinctly by noting that when a knife penetrates the chest death ensues at once, even though the belly can be opened safely with the patient breathing spontaneously.[1] Celsus was describing the so-called "pneumothorax problem": When the chest is opened and the lung is exposed to atmospheric pressure, the operative lung suddenly collapses because of the loss of the normally negative intrapleural pressure. The collapsed lung would paradoxically expand during expiration and collapse again during inspiration, as air was transferred from healthy to collapsed lung by the patient struggling to breathe. The transfer of air between the two lungs became known as "pendelluft." A surgeon brave enough to open the chest wall of a spontaneously breathing patient would also face vigorous side-to-side movement of the mediastinum with respiration known as "mediastinal flapping" that would cause compression of the contralateral lung. The patient would quickly become tachypneic and cyanotic while struggling to breathe spontaneously. Only the briefest intrathoracic procedures could be performed under these circumstances, and for this reason thoracic surgery was mostly limited to procedures of the extrathoracic chest wall in the first third of the 20th century. John W. Strieder, an eminent thoracic surgeon, gave a colorful description of operating in the "good old days" where "the period of operation was, with dismaying frequency, a race between the surgeon and the impending asphyxia of the patient."[2]

After the advent of inhalational anesthesia in the 1840s, the delivery of general anesthesia became routine and permitted the rapid growth of most areas of surgery. However, the techniques favored for delivering inhalational anesthesia until the 1930s remained mask or open drop administration of ether or chloroform, with or without nitrous oxide. Muscle relaxants did not yet exist, and endotracheal intubation was considered an invasive procedure that was used only by a few experts. Typically, patients would breathe spontaneously, and thus could control the depth of anesthesia with their depth and rate of respirations. Also, long before the use of cuffed endotracheal tubes, an intact cough reflex was valued during general anesthesia for protecting the lungs from gastric aspiration, so relatively light planes of anesthesia were the norm. Prior to the introduction of antibiotics in the 1930s, patients frequently presented with empyema, pulmonary abscess or tuberculosis, and often had copious secretions and formidable coughs. Clearly, operating conditions were poor for the early 20th century thoracic surgeon facing a lightly-anesthetized patient asphyxiating and coughing with an unprotected airway. With this in mind, it is no surprise that thoracic surgery remained in its infancy well into the 20th century, until anesthetic techniques progressed sufficiently to provide improved operating conditions.

Prior to the development of antibiotics, the main indication for thoracic surgery was infection. Opening the pleural cavity did not necessarily pose a significant danger to these patients because long-standing infections often resulted in adhesions that formed between the lung and chest wall, preventing the formation of a significant open pneumothorax or mediastinal shift. In fact, repeated aspirations were often attempted to promote the formation of adhesions so that subsequently the pleural cavity could be opened safely, or substances such as air or water were injected into the pleural space as irritants, also to encourage adhesions, in preparation for surgery.[3,4] Another brutal technique to cope with the open pneumothorax, "Muller's handgrip," was also woefully inadequate: The surgeon would grab the lung while the chest was open and pull it into the wound to plug the thoracotomy incision.[5] Pulmonary resection was usually performed using a snare or tourniquet technique, and reoperation would be necessary to remove necrotic tissue. Not surprisingly, such staged procedures could result in sepsis from remaining necrotic tissue. Complications were common and mortality from thoracic surgery was astonishingly high. In a review from 1922 by Howard Lillienthal, the mortality rate for lobectomy performed for chronic pus formation was 42%, and in the 10 cases where more than one lobe was involved, mortality was 70%.[6]

Differential Pressure Breathing

Better anesthetic techniques were sought to meet the demands of thoracic surgeries. The first promising solution to prevent the development of an open pneumothorax was developed in Germany by the surgeon Ernst Ferdinand Sauerbruch.[7] In 1893, Sauerbruch's mentor Johann von Mikulicz-Radecki asked him to tackle the "pneumothorax problem," and his solution, differential pressure breathing, became the prevailing method for anesthetic management in thoracic surgery until World War II. Sauerbruch performed thoracotomies on dogs and found that spontaneous ventilations were sustained without lung collapse if the exposed lung was kept at a pressure 10 cm H_2O below atmospheric pressure, and later used this technique during thoracotomies on humans (Figure 1–1). To provide the negative pressure, the patient and surgical team had to work within a negative pressure chamber constructed of steel, and the patient's head extended outside the cabinet and was exposed to ambient pressure. Throughout the surgery, the patient would breathe spontaneously and the lungs would remain inflated from the negative pressure within the chamber. The surgeon within the chamber was separated from the anesthetist by a thick wall so that communication was only possible by telephone, and then only with difficulty due to the loud noise in the chamber created by the pump that created the negative pressure. Although impractical, Sauerbruch's method was considered a triumph and differential pressure breathing was adapted throughout Europe and America; Sauerbruch became a very influential figure in the history of thoracic anesthesia.

Chapter 1 / History and Scope of Anesthesia for Thoracic Surgery

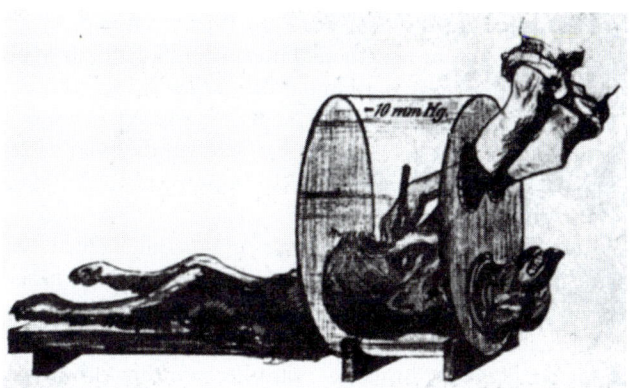

Figure 1-1. Sauerbruch's experimental negative pressure box for performing thoracotomies on dogs. The dog's chest is enclosed in the box in which the pressure is −10 mm Hg (1904). (From: Mushin WW, Rendell-Baker L, eds. *The Principles of Thoracic Anesthesia.* Springfield, IL: Charles C Thomas; 1953, with permission. Copyright Wiley-Blackwell.)

Even though Sauerbruch's methods were highly commended, his negative pressure technique did not gain many followers because it required investment in an expensive and cumbersome negative pressure chamber. However, another option became popular that was based on essentially the same principle. Ludolph Brauer, a colleague of Sauerbruch's, conducted his own experiments and developed a different solution simultaneously. In fact, his description of the use of a positive pressure chamber was initially presented in the same issue of the same journal as Sauerbruch's initial presentation of his research. Instead of applying negative pressure to the open chest, Brauer increased the intrapulmonary pressure by placing his subject's head in a positive pressure chamber. His original apparatus was simply a large box into which the head of the patient was placed after induction of anesthesia. Anesthesia was maintained using oxygen and chloroform, and the patient would breathe spontaneously without assistance. Prior to the opening of the chest, the pressure inside the box would be raised by adding compressed air. Brauer found that if the pressure were raised 10 mm Hg above the atmospheric pressure applied to the open lung, no pneumothorax developed. An obvious limitation and challenge of Brauer's apparatus was that the anesthetist had no access to the patient's head during surgery.[7] Brauer's device bears a striking resemblance to the helmets used for delivering noninvasive continuous positive airway pressure (CPAP), a tool for treating acute respiratory failure outside of the operating room (OR).[8]

Brauer's positive pressure technique was the favored method for preventing pneumothorax because the equipment involved was simpler, less bulky, and inexpensive compared with negative pressure chambers. At the same time, even more complicated versions of Sauerbruch's negative pressure chamber were developed. The American surgeon Willy Meyer modified the Sauerbruch device to create his "universal differential pressure chamber" that included both a positive and negative pressure chamber so that the patient's head, an anesthetist and assistant could be enclosed in a positive pressure chamber.[9] He constructed the only negative pressure chamber for such a use in the United States. By using both chambers, the pressure gradient could be maintained by applying positive pressure to the head, negative pressure to the open chest, or both. The chamber was used not only to support respiration during surgery, but also to improve wound drainage and lung expansion postoperatively.[10]

Both the positive-pressure and negative-pressure methods relied on maintaining a pressure gradient between the air inside and outside the lungs, otherwise known as differential pressure anesthesia. Both methods were successful at preventing the formerly inevitable open pneumothorax after thoracotomy, but both were ultimately doomed to become historical relics because they provided dangerously inadequate ventilation. Hypoventilation, hypercarbia, hypoxemia, and impaired venous return were significant problems during prolonged cases. Clinical deterioration was not unusual after long cases using these techniques, even though the lungs never collapsed. Meyer recognized that carbon dioxide accumulation was probably the culprit in such cases of unexplained shock, and recommended periodically deflating the lungs by applying rhythmic variations in pressure coinciding with spontaneous respirations to assist ventilation.[10]

ENDOTRACHEAL INTUBATION AND ANESTHESIA

While the debate continued regarding the merits of positive versus negative pressure application, an alternative anesthetic method for preventing the development of the open pneumothorax evolved from earlier discoveries in tracheal intubation and mechanical ventilation and became popular in America. This new method, called tracheal insufflation anesthesia, was the clear precursor to the endotracheal anesthesia that is universally used for thoracic surgery today.

Endotracheal Intubation

Tracheal intubation and mechanical ventilation were by no means new discoveries. Because of widespread reluctance to accept tracheal intubation for common use, the course of its development did not follow a smooth path. Andreas Vesalius described tracheal intubation and positive pressure ventilation of a pig in 1543. He performed a tracheotomy and passed a reed into the trachea of a pig and blew into the tube to provide artificial ventilation during a thoracotomy and was able to prevent a potentially lethal pneumothorax. However, his findings went unnoticed and had to be rediscovered. In the 18th century, interest in artificial ventilation for resuscitation grew. In 1788, Charles Kite resuscitated victims of drowning from the Thames using curved metal cannulas that he placed blindly in the trachea. Application of these resuscitation techniques to anesthesia delivery began soon after the discovery of inhalational anesthetics in the 1840s. In 1869, Friedrich Trendelenburg used a tracheostomy tube with an inflatable cuff to administer chloroform during head and neck procedures. William MacEwen, a Scottish surgeon, is credited with the first use of oral tracheal intubation for an anesthetic. On July 5, 1878, MacEwen placed a flexible metal tube in the larynx of an awake patient who was to have an oral tumor removed at the Glasgow Royal Infirmary.[11] Unaware of earlier uses of intubation, Joseph O'Dwyer, a pediatrician, performed blind oral tracheal intubations on children suffering from diphtheria in 1885.[12] O'Dwyer later developed a rigid tube with a conical tip that occluded the larynx sufficiently to facilitate positive pressure ventilation. In 1893, George Fell attached O'Dwyer's metal tube to a bellows and T-piece, creating the Fell-O'Dwyer apparatus. Fell used the apparatus to provide ventilatory support for opioid-induced respiratory depression (Figure 1–2).

By the 1890s, there was interest in the application of endotracheal anesthesia to thoracic surgery as a possible solution to the pneumothorax problem. Two French surgeons, Tuffier and Hallion, reported on their use of tracheal intubation and artificial ventilation for thoracotomies on animals in 1896.[11] Their device also incorporated a bellows that was used for rhythmic inflation of the lungs, and a water valve that could control the degree of resistance to expiration, a precursor of the modern use of positive end-expiratory pressure (PEEP). Rudolph Matas,

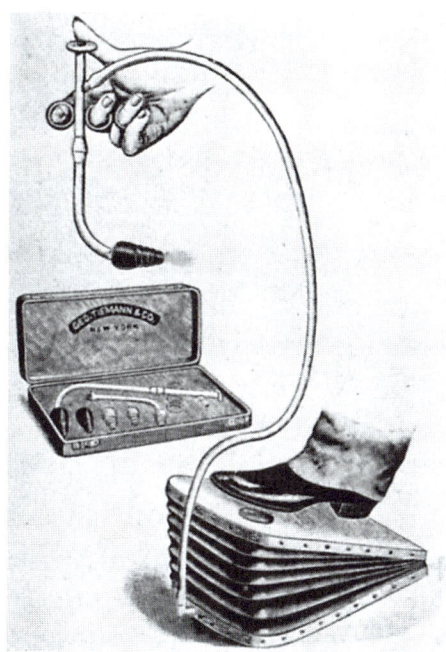

Figure 1–2. The Fell-O'Dwyer apparatus (c. 1888). O'Dwyer's laryngeal tube has a curved right angle and uses fitted, interchangeable, conical heads of different sizes designed to fit securely into the larynx. Rings were provided for the operator's fingers and the operator's thumb was placed over the expiratory orifice during inflation.
(From: Mushin WW, Rendell-Baker L, eds. *The Principles of Thoracic Anesthesia*. Springfield, IL: Charles C Thomas; 1953, with permission. Copyright Wiley-Blackwell.)

among his many pioneering contributions to anesthesiology, made modifications to the Fell-O'Dwyer apparatus so it could be used for surgical purposes. He cited the research of Tuffier and Hallion as his inspiration, and was convinced that these methods were ideal for thoracic cases. His modifications to the Fell-O'Dwyer apparatus included a graduated cylinder for delivery of precise volumes of gases and a mercurial manometer for direct measurement of intrapulmonary pressures. He also added an intralaryngeal cannula connected by a stopcock to a rubber tube and funnel that could be used for administration of chloroform.[13]

Tracheal Insufflation

Until 1907, endotracheal techniques always involved an endotracheal tube that was similar in width to the trachea, through which inspiration and exhalation occurred. However, in 1907, a different method was introduced by Barthélemy and Dufour that became known as "tracheal insufflation".[11] Insufflation anesthesia consisted of placing a thin tube in the trachea and then continuously blowing gases under positive pressure into the lower portion of the trachea. Expired gases escaped between the tracheal tube and the tracheal wall. Meltzer and Auer, American physiologists, used this technique extensively in animal studies. They showed that curarized dogs could be anesthetized by blowing air and ether continuously into a tube inserted into the trachea, and that gas exchange would occur "without any normal or artificial rhythmical respiratory movements whatever" because expired gases could escape around the tracheal tube.[14] Because gas was insufflated continuously, and no rhythmic applications of pressure were used, the insufflation method was similar to Brauer's positive pressure method; however, efficiency of gas exchange was improved by the decrease in dead space achieved by placing the cannula in the trachea.

Charles Elsberg, a thoracic surgeon in New York City, was inspired by Meltzer and Auer's physiology research, and he utilized and modified their insufflation technique for application to thoracic surgery. His modifications included replacing the bellows of Meltzer and Auer's apparatus with an electric motor. He also favored placement of the tracheal cannula under direct vision using either a Killian bronchoscope or Chevalier Jackson's laryngoscope, after topicalization with cocaine.[15] Elsberg first used insufflation to resuscitate a myasthenic patient who had become cyanotic and pulseless. After initiation of insufflation, her color improved and pulse returned, but resuscitation was discontinued after 5 hours because she did not regain consciousness. Bolstered by his success, Elsberg presided over the first use of tracheal insufflation anesthesia for thoracotomy.[16] In February 1910, a 55-year-old butcher was admitted to the Mt. Sinai Hospital with a 13-month history of productive cough. A diagnosis of lung abscess was made, and the thoracic surgeon Howard Lilienthal sought a definitive operative cure, so he enlisted Elsberg for his expertise with tracheal insufflation. When the pleura was opened, 15 mm Hg pressure was applied, and the lung was described as "two-thirds of its capacity, mottled, and rosy pink in color." Different pressures were applied and the lung readily collapsed and distended. He recommended the periodic interruption in the stream of insufflation every 2 or 3 minutes to allow the lungs to collapse and improve carbon dioxide elimination, bringing this method closer to modern positive pressure ventilation. The anesthetic was considered a great success, and Elsberg promoted tracheal insufflation for all types of surgery requiring general anesthesia. Just 1 year later, he published on his experiences anesthetizing over 200 patients with this technique.[17] Elsberg's method of tracheal insufflation strongly resembles the modern practice of oxygen insufflation used during rigid bronchoscopy that was introduced by Sanders in 1968.[18]

In the 1920s and 30s, tracheal insufflation anesthesia was the most popular anesthetic method for thoracic surgery in the United States. Insufflation anesthesia became popular in Europe for head and neck surgery because it gave the surgeon better access than mask or hand drop techniques. However, differential pressure anesthesia remained the preferred anesthetic technique for thoracic procedures in Europe for years to come. Reasons for this include the dominance of Sauerbruch and his refusal to endorse any other method. In 1916, Sauerbruch's own assistant, Giertz, conducted experiments on animals that showed that rhythmic inflation of the lungs was superior to either continuous negative or positive pressure anesthesia. Giertz's experiments demonstrated that differential pressure anesthesia resulted in inadequate ventilation, carbon dioxide retention, and impaired venous return causing circulatory depression.[7] Tracheal insufflation was far from perfect. Carbon dioxide accumulation frequently occurred if gas flow went uninterrupted, so modifications to Elsberg's apparatus were developed that periodically stopped airflow to permit lung collapse. Also, dangerously high-intrapulmonary pressure could occur when the return of gas was impeded. Cases of alveolar rupture and surgical emphysema referred to as "wind-tumor" occurred, probably as a result of vocal cord spasm around thin insufflation catheters interfering with the exit of expired gases.[11]

Advances in Laryngoscopy

Even though instruments for direct laryngoscopy existed by the 1920s, they were infrequently used. Blind placement of endotracheal tubes required considerable skill and could be a traumatic procedure. Prior to 1895, direct visual examination of the larynx was assumed to be impossible. Alfred Kirstein, a physician in Berlin, is credited with inventing the first direct laryngoscope in 1895.[19] Kirstein's "autoscope" was not used by anesthetists, but it was the prototype for most laryngoscopes to follow. In 1913, Chevalier Jackson developed his own laryngoscope and published a landmark paper on proper positioning and technique for laryngoscopy.[20] In the 1940s, there was a renewed interest in laryngoscope blade design. Robert Miller created the familiar Miller blade in 1941, but the origins of its design are evident in Kirstein's and Jackson's laryngoscopes. Only 2 years later, Sir Robert Macintosh released his familiar curved blade that would go on to become the most popular blade in the world.

Endotracheal Tubes

Alongside the development of direct laryngoscopy, came the development of improved endotracheal tubes. World War I produced many casualties with head and neck injuries requiring reconstructive plastic surgery. In 1919, the British anesthetists Ivan Magill and Stanley Rowbotham were assigned to work with the British army plastics unit, and they were forced to adapt endotracheal anesthesia to safely care for these patients. They became experts in blind nasal tracheal intubations to provide unhindered access to the face and airway. They were dissatisfied with the thin endotracheal catheters that were in use for insufflation anesthesia, so they progressed to using wide-bore tubes that more closely resemble what are in use today. By using larger tubes, they returned to the older inhalation method where respiration occurred in both directions through one tube. By doing this, they rejected the popular insufflation technique. Magill's wide-bore red rubber tubes resisted kinking and were better suited to the contours of the upper airway. "Magill tubes" remained the standard endotracheal tubes until plastic tubes were introduced.

In 1928, Arthur Guedel and Ralph Waters introduced an endotracheal tube with a detachable inflatable cuff (Figure 1–3).[21] Prior to Guedel and Waters, there were sporadic proponents of cuffed tubes. As early as 1871, Trendelenburg fitted a cuff on a tracheotomy cannula, followed by Eisenmenger in 1893, and Dorrance in 1910.[22] However, none of these early attempts to apply cuffs to endotracheal tubes attracted much interest. Guedel demonstrated the effectiveness of the cuff's seal with his colorful "dunked dog" demonstrations. He submerged his intubated and anesthetized dog, Airway, in an aquarium, from which he emerged unharmed.[23] Guedel's cuffed endotracheal tube could prevent the aspiration of gastric contents, so it was no longer necessary to keep the patient "light" so the cough reflex would remain intact. Also, since deeper planes of anesthesia could be used, suctioning the trachea without coughing was possible. Aside from aspiration prevention, cuffed endotracheal tubes enabled the most important advancement in anesthetic

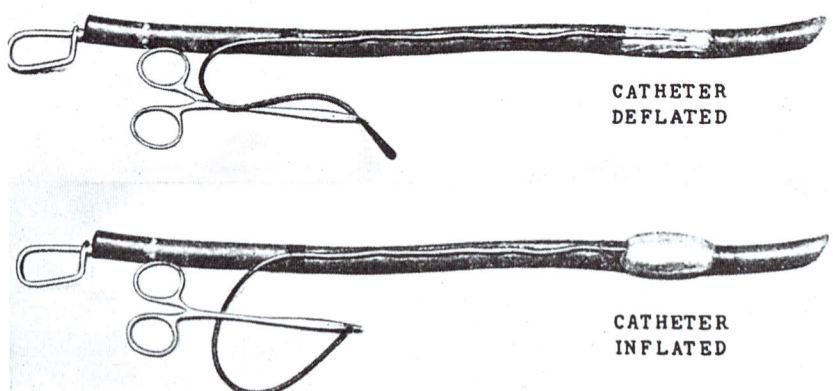

Figure 1–3. Guedel and Waters "new intratracheal catheter" (1928). The catheter is shown deflated and then inflated. The tube was 14 inches long and made of rubber.
(From: Mushin WW, Rendell-Baker L, eds. *The Principles of Thoracic Anesthesia*. Springfield, IL: Charles C Thomas; 1953, with permission. Copyright Wiley-Blackwell.)

management for thoracic surgery: the use of controlled positive pressure ventilation. By increasing the depth of anesthesia and delivering controlled breaths using a cuffed endotracheal tube, hyperventilation was now possible to suppress respiratory efforts.

By 1930, all aspects of airway management necessary to conquer the "pneumothorax problem" were well-described. However, these methods did not gain immediate acceptance. Sauerbruch's differential pressure method was still in wide use until World War II. Also, the advantage of cuffed tubes was not universally recognized. For example, in 1948, in a review of a series of 309 anesthetics for thoracic surgery, the authors still advocated placing the patient in steep Trendelenburg position to promote drainage of secretions through and around uncuffed tracheal tubes. Also, the authors of this review did not even recommend routine use of controlled ventilation.[24]

ADVANCES IN THORACIC SURGERY

As anesthetic techniques improved, pulmonary surgery made slow progress in the 1920s, leading to significant advances in the 1930s. The two-stage snare or tourniquet technique for lung resection was replaced by the individual-structure ligation technique that reduced complications such as air leak, tension pneumothorax, hemorrhage, and infection from necrotic residual lung tissue. Harold Brunn was the first to use this technique extensively in 1929.[25] Many landmark thoracic surgeries were preformed in the 1930s: Rudolph Nissen performed the first successful two-stage pneumonectomy in 1931 and Evarts Graham performed the first successful one-stage total pneumonectomy for a malignant tumor in 1933.[26,27] Graham's historic pneumonectomy anticipated the future of pulmonary surgery where cases of malignant disease would soon overshadow those of infection. Another critical development in thoracic surgery in the 1930s was the introduction of routine postoperative pleural drainage with closed-chest thoracostomy. Esophageal surgery also progressed in the 1930s. In 1933, the first successful transthoracic esophagectomy was performed in Japan.[28] Not long before, these surgeries were too perilous to be attempted, but anesthetic techniques had improved sufficiently to accommodate the surgical advances of the 1930s. With the introduction of OLV and mechanical ventilation in the 1930s and 40s, anesthesiologists were able to further assist the development of thoracic surgery.

ALTERNATIVES TO GENERAL ANESTHESIA

Before the 1940s, when general anesthesia using endotracheal intubation became routine for thoracic surgery, regional and spinal anesthesia for thoracic surgery were frequently used. Advocates of regional techniques believed that the cough reflex was preserved and that respiration was not detrimentally affected. According to Magill, spinal anesthesia was an excellent technique for thoracoplasty, lobectomy, and even pneumonectomy! He found that patients generally would breathe well and infrequently needed supplemental oxygen and that the cough reflex was well-maintained. He also found it helpful to have a cooperative patient who could participate in breath holding, an advantage at the time over general anesthesia that infrequently employed controlled ventilation.[29] Others did not have similar success with spinal anesthesia. Nosworthy declared, "I like my anaesthetic technique to be such that I have the whole situation under control. I do not feel that I am in a position to cope with any emergency when chest surgery is performed under spinal anaesthesia."[30] Nosworthy found the cough reflex to be inadequate and dyspnea to be frequent during procedures on the open thorax under spinal anesthesia.

EARLY ONE-LUNG VENTILATION

With the union of direct laryngoscopy, tracheal intubation, and controlled ventilation, interest in lung separation soon followed. Prior to the development of lung separation techniques, most thoracic surgeries were still performed for cases of infection, and spillage from the infected lung was a frequent problem. Patients frequently had copious secretions, requiring aggressive preoperative physiotherapy to reduce the risk of spillage in the OR. In 1931, Gale and Waters reported the first use of OLV for thoracic surgery.[31] Their technique was simply to intubate the healthy bronchus blindly with a long endotracheal tube. They used a standard rubber Guedel-Waters cuffed endotracheal tube. The tube was softened with hot water and molded to have a lateral curve. It was placed in the trachea and then blindly advanced into either bronchus, stopping as soon as resistance was felt. The cuff provided a seal for the intubated bronchus, while also occluding the bronchus of the diseased lung. Their desire was to prevent the "pneumothorax syndrome" by isolating the lung exposed to ambient pressure. Also, they acknowledged the advantages of an immobile lung, quiet surgical field, and the prevention of secretions from entering the trachea. Prevention of contamination from infection was not of paramount importance for them. Although the simplicity of their technique was admirable, it was not very stable and did not become widely used.

In 1936, Rovenstine attempted to improve upon Gale and Waters' technique by using a single-lumen endotracheal tube with two cuffs.[32] By having two cuffs, either one lung or both lungs could be ventilated. Rovenstine's endobronchial tube was made of woven silk and also would be molded in hot water to create a lateral curve and then be advanced blindly into either bronchus. The upper cuff was inflated first, above the carina. With the upper cuff alone inflated, both lungs could be ventilated. When the lower cuff was inflated, the trachea was occluded at the carina.

Bronchial Blockers

Bronchial blockade, another method of lung separation, was also first introduced into anesthetic practice in the 1930s. By placing an obstruction to ventilation in the bronchus to a lung or lobe, the unventilated lung distal to the obstruction will subsequently collapse. In 1935, Archibald gave the first description of the use of bronchial blockade. In order to control secretions during lobectomy, he used an inflatable balloon at the end of a rubber catheter to occlude the main bronchus of the diseased lung. He confirmed appropriate placement with x-ray films.[33]

He reported that this balloon was easy to place and that it prevented escape of pus from the diseased lobe. Although the use of x-ray made this technique cumbersome, the idea of using a balloon for bronchial blockade was promising and numerous refinements of this technique have been made and are still in current use.

In 1936, Magill improved on Archibald's design by designing a similar bronchial blocker (BB) that could be placed under direct vision using a device of his own called a tracheoscope, eliminating the need for x-ray guidance. The BB was a long tube with a balloon at its distal end that was inserted alongside an endotracheal tube. It also had a suction catheter for the blocked lung, and Magill recommended the use of the blocker for the control of secretions; however, he did also acknowledge its ability to promote atelectasis and thus improve surgical exposure. Magill recommended its placement after topicalizing the larynx, but prior to induction of general anesthesia, so secretions could be suctioned during anesthetic induction. Magill also performed lung separation using endobronchial intubation using a technique similar to Gale and Waters', but his endobronchial tube was made of rubber over fine metal tubing and was placed under direct vision with an endoscope through the lumen.[29] All of these techniques required considerable skill and experience, limiting their popularity. Thompson's BB, introduced in 1943, was modeled after Magill's, and is the prototype for all BBs to follow. Thompson's blocker consisted of two tubes fused together. One tube inflated a gauze-covered balloon and the other provided suction from the blocked bronchus. The blocker had a stylet and was placed through a rigid bronchoscope.[34] Many other devices were employed as BBs prior to the development of the plastic BBs that are in use today. In 1938, Crafoord described his bronchial tamponage technique that used a ribbon gauze tampon for the control of secretions. The tampon was inserted through a rigid bronchoscope into the selected bronchus while the healthy lung would be ventilated by an endotracheal tube in the carina.[35]

In the 1950s, multiple single-lumen endotracheal tubes were developed with incorporated BBs. In 1953, Stuertzbecher introduced an endotracheal tube with an incorporated styletted BB and suction catheter. Vellacott introduced a similar tube in 1954, as did Macintosh and Leatherdale in 1955 and Green in 1958.[36-38] These tubes are the clear predecessors of the Univent tube, the first modern endotracheal tube designed for bronchial blockade. First marketed in 1982, the Univent tube (Univent, Fuji Systems Corp., Tokyo, Japan) is a large endotracheal tube with a small internal lumen that contains a retractable, cuffed bronchial blocker.[39] Once a procedure requiring bronchial blockade is over, the blocker can be retracted to its internal lumen and the tube functions as a conventional single-lumen tube. Although this is a convenient method for providing OLV in patients who may require postoperative mechanical ventilation, the Univent tube is bulky and has a larger diameter than standard single-lumen endotracheal tubes of the same ID number, causing potentially increased airflow resistance.[40]

Balloon-tipped catheters designed for other uses, such as Fogarty embolectomy catheters, Swan-Ganz catheters, and Foley catheters have been used as bronchial blockers. Although the Fogarty embolectomy catheter was designed as a tool for vascular surgery, there are numerous reports of its successful use as a bronchial blocker.[41] Fogarty catheters have significant limitations because they were not designed for use as bronchial blockers. They have low-volume, high-pressure cuffs capable of damaging bronchial mucosa and there is no communicating channel for suction or oxygen insufflation. Positioning of Fogarty catheters is especially difficult in the left main bronchus because they were not designed with a mechanism to guide them. Recently, new balloon-tipped bronchial blockers have been designed that are specifically intended for bronchial blockade.[42-44] All use balloons with low-pressure cuffs to decrease bronchial trauma, and all are intended for placement with guidance by flexible fiber-optic bronchoscopy.

Double-Lumen Endobronchial Tubes

The origins of the double-lumen tube date back to 1889 when Head used a tube with two lumens to study respiratory physiology in dogs. In 1949, Bjork and Carlens designed the first double-lumen tube (DLT) used for thoracic surgery, although it was initially developed for differential bronchospirometry.[45] The tube was designed for intubation of the left main bronchus. Carlens' tube consisted of two cuffed tubes of unequal length fused together, a longer tube for intubating the left main bronchus and a shorter tube that ends in the trachea. Because the endobronchial intubation was performed blindly, a carinal hook was used to grip the carina and aid placement (Figure 1–4). In 1959, Bryce-Smith modified the Carlens tube by eliminating the carinal hook since it could cause damage to the trachea and it often hindered more than it helped in correct placement.[46] Both of these tubes were suitable for all types of intrathoracic procedures except for left pneumonectomy, where the left main bronchus is cut close to the carina. For this reason, effective means of intubating the right main bronchus were needed. Because it is difficult to intubate the right main bronchus without occluding the opening of the right upper lobe bronchus, most endobronchial and DLTs were initially designed for use on the left. In 1960, Bryce-Smith and Salt described a right-sided DLT that included a slit in the endobronchial cuff for ventilation of the right upper lobe, and White designed a right-sided version of the Carlens' tube that also used a slit in the endobronchial cuff.[47,48]

These early DLTs were fraught with problems. Occlusion by kinking, trauma from carinal hooks, high-airway resistance during OLV and simply difficult placement were not uncommon. In 1962, Robertshaw introduced a new DLT that had no carinal hook and novel cross-sectional D-shaped lumens (Figure 1-5).[49] The D-shaped lumens provided a larger cross-sectional area and reduced resistance to airflow compared with the older round lumens. Disposable plastic (polyvinyl chloride) DLTs have replaced these older red rubber tubes, but contemporary DLTs strongly resemble Robertshaw's original design. Advantages of plastic tubes include large lumens that reduce resistance to gas flow, suctioning, or bronchoscopy. Also, plastic tubes use high-volume, low-pressure cuffs, as opposed to the older low-volume, high-pressure cuffs that could potentially cause more airway trauma. However, red rubber reusable tubes are still used in parts of the world where resources are scarce.

Prior to the introduction of fiberoptic bronchoscopy in the 1970s, endobronchial placement of DLTs was essentially blind and confirmation of placement

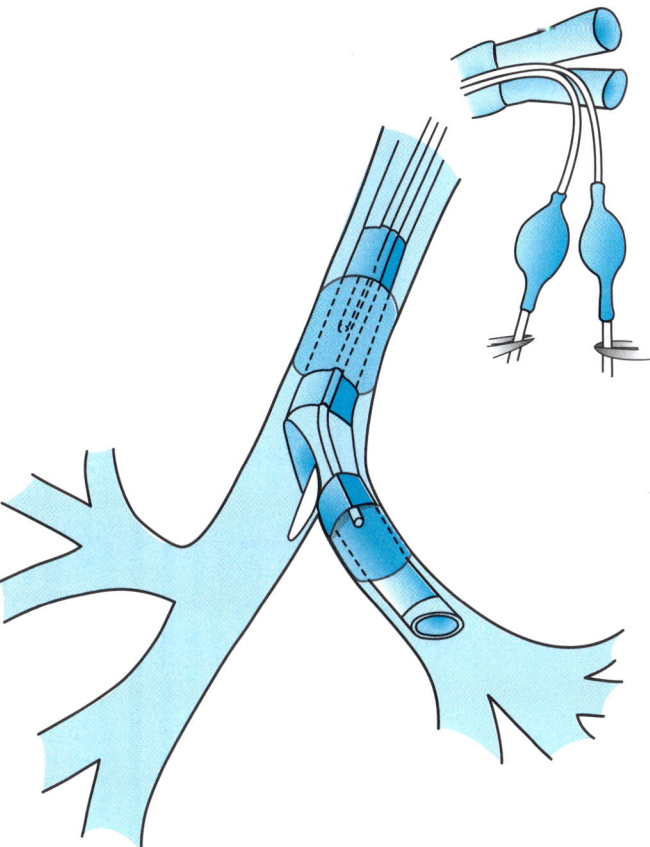

Figure 1-4. Bjork and Carlen's double-lumen catheter (1949). This is the first double-lumen endobroncheal tube intended for intubation of the left mainstem bronchus. Note the presence of the carinal hook. (From: Mushin WW, Rendell-Baker L, eds. *The Principles of Thoracic Anesthesia*. Springfield, IL: Charles C Thomas; 1953, with permission. Copyright Wiley-Blackwell.)

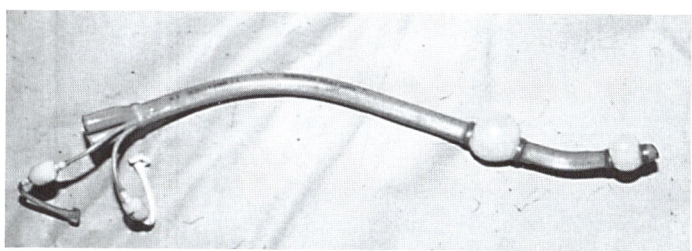

Figure 1-5. Robertshaw's red rubber (left-sided) double-lumen tube (1962).

relied on clinical examination. Small, flexible fiberoptic bronchoscopes permit precise evaluation of the positioning of DLTs, endobronchial tubes, and endobronchial blockers. In the 1980s, fiberoptic bronchoscopes were first used for positioning of DLTs in the OR, and this has now become a common practice. All catheter-guided BBs rely on fiberoptic bronchoscopy for positioning. Positioning can also easily be reconfirmed once patients are moved from supine to lateral decubitus position by using fiberoptic bronchoscopy, and positioning can also be easily reassessed mid-operation. In addition to its utility in precise placement of DLTs and bronchial blockers, fiberoptic bronchoscopy assists examination and identification of unusual airway anatomy and can guide tracheal toilet. Because of these advantages, many experts recommend its routine use for placement of DLTs.[50,51]

DEVELOPMENT OF INTRAOPERATIVE MECHANICAL VENTILATION

Although the "pneumothorax problem" was solved by the application of positive pressure ventilation to the lungs, the routine use of intermittent positive pressure ventilation was impractical before the development of muscle relaxants and mechanical ventilators. In 1909, Meltzer and Auer recommended the use of curare in their animal studies of tracheal insufflation; however, curare was only first used as part of a general anesthetic in 1942.[14,52] In 1946, Harroun used curare, nitrous oxide, and morphine for thoracic surgery, an important new technique because it included no flammable agents and permitted the use of electrocautery during surgery.[53] Muscle relaxation facilitated the use of controlled ventilation by suppressing spontaneous respiratory efforts with lighter planes of anesthesia and without hyperventilation. Safety problems with curare soon became evident, but numerous safer neuromuscular agents were introduced to replace curare, eventually making the administration of muscle relaxants a routine part of a general anesthetic.

Some early mechanical ventilators have already been described here, such as the Fell-O'Dwyer apparatus from 1892, and Matas' modification of the Fell-O'Dwyer apparatus that incorporated manometry and delivery of inhaled anesthetics. Giertz' experiments and writings advocating controlled ventilation had gone mostly ignored; however, Frenckner, a Swedish otolaryngologist, familiar with Giertz, developed the "Spiropulsator" in 1934 for rhythmic inflation of the lungs. In 1938, Crafoord, a colleague of Frenckner, modified the apparatus by including a reservoir bag from which the patient could take a breath, since spontaneous respirations were not uncommon because these early air-driven ventilators predated muscle relaxants.[54] The reservoir bag was intended to keep the patient from fighting the ventilator. Crafoord and Frenckner routinely intubated patients under topical anesthesia and then used their ventilator during thoracic surgery. The "Spiropulsator" became popular in Scandinavia, but in the 1930s and 40s there was very limited interest in controlled ventilation elsewhere, since continuous positive pressure delivered by mask and tracheal insufflation were widely used (Figure 1–6).

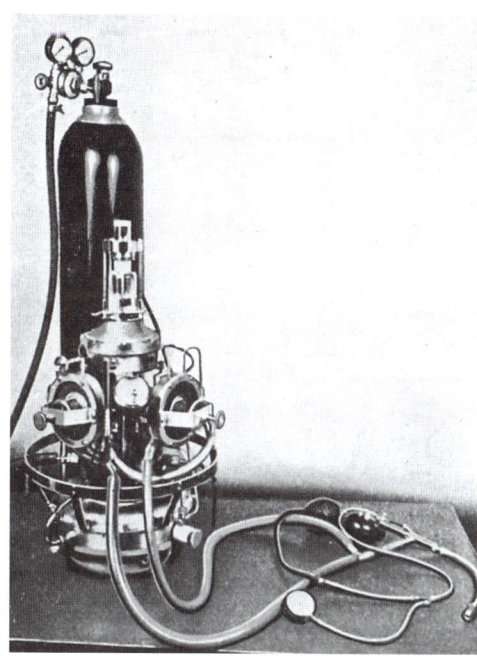

Figure 1-6. The Frenckner Spiropulsator (1934). Note the cuffed endotracheal tube lying to the right. (From: Mushin WW, Rendell-Baker L, eds. *The Principles of Thoracic Anesthesia.* Springfield, IL: Charles C Thomas; 1953, with permission. Copyright Wiley-Blackwell.)

Routine use of ventilators intraoperatively only occurred after they were routinely used outside of the OR. In 1952, an epidemic of poliomyelitis in Copenhagen overwhelmed Blegdam's hospital. Three thousand patients presented with polio, and one-third of these presented with paralysis. Faced with so many patients with respiratory insufficiency, the hospital turned to an anesthesiologist, Bjorn Ibsen, for help. Ibsen believed that performing tracheostomies and providing controlled ventilation for weak children would increase survival rates.[55] Initially, since the hospital had few mechanical ventilators, medical students squeezed breathing bags in shift, but toward the end of the epidemic they were replaced with mechanical ventilators. Ibsen proved correct, survival rates increased dramatically and the modern intensive care unit (ICU) was born and the iron lung was left behind. In 1955, Björk and Engstrom used their ventilator for postoperative ventilatory support for the frailest of their thoracic surgery patients.[56] After proving their safety and efficacy in the ICU, mechanical ventilators gained acceptance in OR in the 1960s and 70s.

ADVANCES IN INTRAOPERATIVE MONITORING

Use of complex intraoperative patient monitors is commonplace today; however, prior to the 1960s, intraoperative monitoring consisted of merely observation, palpation and auscultation with an anesthesiologist relying on a blood pressure cuff, electrocardiogram, and esophageal stethoscope. Hypoxemia was only detected by the presence of peripheral cyanosis, frequently a late and unreliable sign. The development of accurate invasive monitoring of peripheral arterial, central venous, and pulmonary arterial pressures improved monitoring, but noninvasive monitors of oxygenation and ventilation, specifically pulse oximetry and end-tidal capnography, have become crucial elements of safe anesthetics for all types of surgery, especially during OLV. Severinghaus declared, "Pulse oximetry is arguably the most important technological advance ever made in monitoring the well-being and safety of patients during anesthesia, recovery, and critical care."[57] In 1942, Millikan developed the first oximeter for the ear intended for use by pilots in World War II to warn them of hypoxia from an oxygen supply failure. Takuo Aoyagi, a Japanese engineer, refined the oximeter to measure pulse in addition to oxygen saturation, creating the first pulse oximeter.[58] Pulse oximetry was not used in the OR routinely until the 1980s, making it a relatively recent addition to the routine monitors available to anesthesiologists. The history of capnography also followed a similar course. The initial application of infrared absorption to measure expired carbon dioxide occurred in 1943; however, capnography did not appear routinely in ORs until the 1980s.[59] Pulse oximetry and capnography have decreased the need for direct measurement of arterial blood gases, but have not replaced it entirely. Both provide rapid and continuous guides to gas exchange, and serve as a guide when direct blood gas measurements are appropriate.

IMPROVEMENTS IN OXYGENATION FOR ONE-LUNG VENTILATION

In 1956, Halothane was introduced in England, and it quickly replaced ether and cyclopropane because of its favorable safety profile, high potency, less noxious odor, nonflammability, and kinetic properties that provided a more rapid induction and emergence.[60] Halothane's potency made nitrous oxide unnecessary during OLV, and it could be used safely with electrocautery because it is nonflammable. Although halothane has largely been replaced by isoflurane, sevoflurane, and desflurane because of its association with liver toxicity and cardiac arrhythmias, the practice of using potent inhalational agents without nitrous oxide for maintenance of anesthesia remains standard during OLV.

Even though potent inhaled anesthetics made delivery of 100% oxygen possible during OLV, hypoxemia was still frequently encountered due to blood shunted through the nonventilated lung. CPAP and PEEP are both ventilatory maneuvers that were developed for respiratory support outside of the OR, but have found their respective roles for improving oxygenation during OLV. In 1971, CPAP was first described for use in infants with idiopathic respiratory distress syndrome.[61] Since the 1980s, CPAP applied to the nonventilated lung has been used as an effective treatment for hypoxemia during OLV.[62] However, CPAP often cannot be used during thoracoscopic procedures because it may interfere with surgical exposure. PEEP applied to the ventilated lung is also frequently included to improve oxygenation during OLV.[63] High-frequency jet ventilation (HFJV) with oxygen to the nondependent lung has also been used during OLV to improve oxygenation.[64] HFJV uses a jet of fresh gas delivered from a high-pressure source directly into the airway through a small catheter at rates of approximately 100 to 400 breaths per minute. Because of the small tidal volumes delivered, the collapsed lung field remains quiet for the surgeon. HFJV has advantages in many situations, including ventilating patients with bronchopleural fistulas and in interrupted airways such as in patients with tracheal stenosis or those undergoing reconstructive surgery of the airway.

IMPROVEMENTS IN POSTOPERATIVE ANALGESIA

Advances in pain management have improved care for patients undergoing thoracic surgery. Very severe pain results from thoracotomy incisions, and post-thoracotomy pain has a profound impact on recovery after surgery by interfering with return of pulmonary function. Also, inadequate treatment of acute pain following thoracic surgery can contribute to the development of disabling chronic pain. Awareness by anesthesiologists and thoracic surgeons of the impact of inadequately managed acute pain on morbidity has sparked the development of multiple modalities of pain management. Prior to the 1980s, the only option for patients was systemic opioids, frequently administered intramuscularly. Today, options include systemic opioids, regional local anesthesia, epidural local anesthesia, and epidural opioids; and all can be delivered using patient-controlled analgesia (PCA). Between the variety of pharmacologic agents available and the possibility of combining modes of analgesia, the options for patients are numerous and analgesic regimens can be tailored on an individual basis.

The introduction of neuraxial opioids to the analgesic armamentarium has probably been the most significant improvement. Thoracic epidural analgesia had been attempted in the past for post-thoracotomy pain, but when limited to local anesthetics, hypotension was frequently encountered, so this method was not considered viable for routine use.[65] The first advocate for the use of neuraxial opioids was Rudolf Matas himself, who, in 1900, combined morphine with cocaine for spinal anesthesia, to reduce the excitatory effect on the central nervous system caused by cocaine.[66] Interest in neuraxial opioid use remained dormant until the 1970s. In 1979, Behar et al, first described the use of epidural morphine for the treatment of pain, and noted its long duration of action.[67] Numerous studies have demonstrated advantages of epidural over intravenous opioid analgesia, and epidural analgesia, usually combining dilute local anesthetics with lipophilic opioids, has become routine practice; some advocate it should be used for all post-thoracotomy patients.[68] The routine placement of epidural catheters for management of postoperative pain has contributed to the formation of acute pain services, and thus expanded the role of anesthesiologists.[69] Paravertebral blockade has also been advocated as an alternative to thoracic epidural analgesia. Many studies have demonstrated analgesic equivalence between the two techniques, while paravertebral blocks consistently have fewer side effects.[70] Whether paravertebral blockade will replace thoracic epidural analgesia as the gold standard technique remains to be determined. Intercostal blocks can also be performed before or after thoracic procedures for postoperative analgesia, and they can be performed by the surgeon from within the thorax.

CURRENT SCOPE OF ANESTHESIA FOR THORACIC SURGERY

Thoracic surgical procedures have increased in both numbers and complexity, and the increased quality and diversity of anesthetic methods for caring for these patients has contributed to this development. Lung cancer continues to be a major public health problem, with 219,440 estimated new cases of lung cancer in the United States in 2009.[71] Since the development of antibiotics, malignancy has been the most common indication for pulmonary surgery. However, important procedures for nonmalignant disease, such as lung transplantation and lung volume reduction surgery (LVRS), are now performed routinely at academic centers, thus making the frailest patients surgical candidates. Lung transplantation has increased from 33 transplants performed in the United States in 1988 to 1478 in 2008.[72] The most common indications for transplantation are severe chronic obstructive pulmonary disease (COPD), followed by idiopathic pulmonary fibrosis, cystic fibrosis, alpha1-antitrypsin deficiency and primary pulmonary hypertension. LVRS is an option for patients with severe upper lobe emphysema to improve quality of life; however, the surgery remains controversial because of the very high cost of the surgery and rehabilitation. Also, postoperative mortality is high and careful preoperative selection of patients is crucial for identifying those who will benefit. Alternative, nonsurgical, approaches to lung volume reduction surgery, specifically endobronchial insertion of bronchial valves or injection of tissue fibrin glue, are under investigation and being introduced into clinical practice.

Progress in surgically treating patients with such compromised pulmonary function has increased the need for anesthesiologists to be involved as perioperative physicians, in addition to their role intraoperatively. Careful preoperative evaluation of patients for thoracic surgery is crucial so that anesthetic management can be tailored appropriately, including making appropriate plans for postoperative management. Anesthesiologists are also involved in perioperative pain management as well as management of those patients requiring ICU care postoperatively. Because of the variety of roles anesthesiologists fill when caring for patients undergoing thoracic surgery, care for these patients exemplifies the expanded role of anesthesiologists as perioperative physicians.

Another major advance in thoracic surgery has been the development of minimally invasive techniques. The success of laparoscopy for minimally invasive abdominal surgery in the 1980s, as well as improvements in endoscopic video systems and instruments spurred thoracic surgeons to develop minimally invasive techniques of their own. Video-assisted thoracoscopic surgery (VATS) has been widely performed since the early 1990s, and is increasingly replacing traditional open approaches for more and more complex procedures. VATS requires lung separation with OLV for adequate surgical exposure because retraction of the operative lung by the surgeon is not possible. The benefits of VATS over open techniques include less postoperative pain and shorter hospital stays with faster recovery of preoperative function.[73] Patients are demanding minimally invasive surgery and forcing surgeons to become more agile with these techniques. There have been concerns, particularly in Europe, that VATS may be inferior treatment for early-stage malignancy; however, available data confirms that VATS lobectomy for early-stage lung cancer is equivalent to thoracotomy in terms of survival.[74] Minimally invasive esophagectomies and mediastinal procedures are also now frequently performed. Robotic-assisted techniques for thoracic procedures have also attracted interest, but the benefits and utility of the robot in the thorax still needs to be defined.

Modern thoracic anesthesia with the prevalence of VATS has increased the need for anesthesiologists to master OLV, and has spurred the development of new techniques for lung separation, especially the proliferation of bronchial blockers in recent years. The Arndt blocker (Cook Critical Care, Bloomington, IN), introduced in 1994, is wire-enabled and requires coaxial placement for fiber-opticbronchoscopic guided placement. In 2004, the Cohen tip deflecting endobronchial blocker (Cook Critical Care) was introduced. It possesses a rotating wheel for flexing the tip of the blocker and can be placed under either coaxial or parallel bronchoscopic guidance. Fuji Systems now also manufactures a bronchial blocker, the Uni-blocker that is essentially the bronchial blocker from the Univent tube sold separately. The newest bronchial blocker, the EZ blocker (EZ blocker BV, Rotterdam, The Netherlands) has a novel design featuring a bifurcated distal end.

Dual lumen endotracheal tubes (DLTs) also continue to be refined. At least five different manufacturers now produce DLTs for either the right or the left bronchus in a variety of sizes. A relatively new DLT, the Silbroncho, is a left-sided DLT made of silicone rubber with a wire-reinforced tip. Proposed advantages of the Silbroncho include a smaller cuff to prevent left upper lobe occlusion, and the flexible, reinforced tip is intended to prevent bronchial lumen compression.[75]

With the array of bronchial blockers and DLTs now available, OLV is easier, safer, and more versatile than ever. Today, single-lumen endotracheal tubes are only rarely used for OLV for adults because of the availability of DLTs and bronchial blockers that are better suited for lung separation. However, they are still used frequently for children because the relatively small airways of infants and small children cannot accommodate DLTs and placement of bronchial blockers can also be very challenging. The proliferation of tools and techniques for OLV has also been spurred by increased use of thoracic and minimally invasive approaches to spinal, cardiac, esophageal, and vascular procedures. Such a wide range of procedures requiring OLV has made facility with these techniques a necessity for most anesthesiologists because these surgical techniques must be aborted without adequate lung separation.

Anesthesiologists are also frequently involved in other types of thoracic procedures. Tumors of the bronchi and trachea are frequently treated with stents and or laser therapy. Airway stenting to palliate patients with severe airway obstructions, usually due to malignant causes, has become increasingly common. These procedures may require special ventilatory techniques, such as high-frequency jet ventilation or the Sanders injection system. Also, stents are now frequently placed by interventional pulmonologists outside of the OR, posing unique challenges to the anesthesiologist.

The variety and complexity of procedures now routinely performed by thoracic surgeons would not be possible without the improvements in anesthetic techniques described here. Anesthesiologists have refined methods of securing the airway, lung isolation, physiologic monitoring, and ventilatory techniques to the point where anesthetizing frail patients for complex procedures appears deceptively easy.

REFERENCES

1. Celsus A. *De Medicina.* Loeb Classical Library, 1938. http://penelope.uchicago.edu/Thayer/E/Roman/Texts/Celsus/home.html. Accessed September 12, 2009.
2. Strieder JW. Anesthesia from the viewpoint of the thoracic surgeon. *Anesthesiology.* 1950;11(1):60-64.
3. Souttar HS. A British Medical Association lecture on recent advances in the surgery of the chest. *Br Med J.* 1926;1(3413):933-936.
4. Matas R. On the management of acute traumatic pneumothorax. *Ann Surg.* 1899;29(4):409-434.
5. Barry JE, Adams AP. The development of thoracic anesthesia. In: Hurt R. *The History of Cardiothoracic Surgery from Early Times.* New York: Parthenon; 1996:131-152.
6. Lilienthal H. Resection of the lung for suppurative infections with a report based on 31 operative cases in which resection was done or intended. *Ann Surg.* 1922;75(3):257-320.
7. Mushin WM, Rendell-Baker L. *The Principles of Thoracic Anaesthesia: Past and Present.* Springfield, IL: Charles C Thomas; 1953:48-66.
8. Bellani G, Patroniti N, Greco M, Foti G, Pesenti A. The use of helmets to deliver non-invasive continuous positive airway pressure in hypoxemic respiratory failure. *Minerva Anestesiol.* 2008;74(11):651-656.
9. Meyer W. Pneumectomy with the aid of differential air pressure: an experimental study: the new type of apparatus used. *JAMA.* 1909;53(24):1978-1987.
10. Meyer W. Some observations regarding thoracic surgery on human beings. *Ann Surg.* 1910;52(1):34-58.
11. Gillespie NA. The evolution of endotracheal anaesthesia. *J Hist Med Allied Sci.* 1946;1(4):583-594.
12. O'Dwyer J. Fifty cases of croup in private practice treated by intubation of the larynx. *Med Rec.* 1887;(32):557-561.
13. Matas R. Intralaryngeal Insufflation. *JAMA.* 1900;34(23):1468-1473.
14. Meltzer SJ, Auer J. Continuous respiration without respiratory movements. *J Exp Med.* 1909;11(4):622-625.
15. Elsberg CA. Clinical experiences with intratracheal insufflation (Meltzer), with remarks upon the value of the method for thoracic surgery. *Ann Surg.* 1910; 52(1):23-29.
16. Lilienthal H. The first case of thoracotomy in a human being under anaesthesia by intratracheal insufflation. *Ann Surg.* 1910;52(1):58-66.
17. Elsberg CA. Experiences in thoracic surgery under anaesthesia by the intratracheal insufflation of air and ether. *Ann Surg.* 1911;54(6):749-757.
18. Mette PJ, Sanders RD. Ventilation bronchoscopy: a new technic. *Anaesthesist.* 1968;17(10):316-321.
19. Kirstein A. Autoskopie des Larynx und der Trachea. *Berl Klin Woch.* 1895;(32): 476-478.
20. Jackson C. The technique of insertion of intratracheal insufflation tubes. *Surg Gyn Obst.* 1913;(17):507-509.
21. Guedel AE, Waters RM. A new intratracheal catheter. *Current Researches in Anesth Analg.* 1928;(7):238-239.
22. White GM. Evolution of endotracheal and endobronchial intubation. *Brit J Anaesth.* 1960;32(5):235-246.

23. Waters RM, Arthur E Guedel. *Brit J Anaesth.* 1952;24(4):292-299.
24. Fisher K, Lee LD, Stegeman DE, et al. Anesthetic management for surgery within the thorax: a report of 309 cases. *Anesthesiology.* 1948;9(6):623-636.
25. Brunn H. Surgical priniciples underlying one-stage lobectomy. *Arch Surg.* 1929;18(1):490-515.
26. Herbsman H. Early history of pulmonary surgery. *J Hist Med Allied Sci.* 1958;13(3):329-348.
27. Graham AE, Singer JJ. Successful removal of an entire lung for carcinoma of the bronchus. *JAMA.* 1933;101(18):1371-1374.
28. Ohsawa T. Surgery of the esophagus. *Arch Jpn Chir.* 1933;(10):605-608.
29. Magill IW. Anaesthesia in thoracic surgery with special reference to lobectomy. *Proc Roy Soc Med.* 1936;29(6):643-653.
30. Nosworthy MD. Anesthesia in chest surgery. *Proc Roy Soc Med.* 1941;34(8):479-506.
31. Gale JW, Waters RM. Closed endobronchial anesthesia in thoracic surgery. *J Thorac Surg.* 1931;(1):432-437.
32. Rovenstine EA. Anaesthesia for intrathoracic surgery: the endotracheal and endobronchial techniques. *Surg Gyn Obst.* 1936;(63):325-330.
33. Archibald E. A consideration of the dangers of lobectomy. *J Thorac Surg.* 1935;(4):335-351.
34. Rusby NL, Thompson VC. Carcinoma of the lung: diagnosis and surgical treatment. *Postgrad Med J.* 1943;19(207):44-53.
35. Crafoord C. On the technique of pneumonectomy in man. *Acta Chir Scand.* 1938;(81):5-142.
36. Vellacott WN. A new endobronchial tube for broncho-pleural fistula repair. *Brit J Anaesth.* 1954;26(6):442-444.
37. Macintosh R, Leatherdale RA. Bronchus tube and bronchus blocker. *Brit J Anaesth.* 1955;27(11):556-557.
38. Gordon W, Green R. Right lung anaesthesia: anaesthesia for left lung surgery using a new right endobronchial tube. *Anaesthesia.* 1957;12(1):86-93.
39. Kamaya H, Krishna PR. New endotracheal tube (Univent tube) for selective blockade of one lung. *Anesthesiology.* 1985;63(3):342-343.
40. Slinger PD, Lesiuk L. Flow resistances of disposable double-lumen, single-lumen, and Univent tubes. *J Cardiothorac Vasc Anesth.* 1998;12(2):142-144.
41. Ginsberg RJ. New technique for one-lung anesthesia using an endobronchial blocker. *J Thorac Cardiovasc Surg.* 1981;82(4):542-546.
42. Arndt GA, Buchika S, Kranner PW, DeLessio ST. Wire-guided endobronchial blockade in a patient with a limited mouth opening. *Can J Anaesth.* 1999;46(1):87-89.
43. Cohen E. The Cohen flexitip endobronchial blocker: an alternative to a double lumen tube. *Anesth Analg.* 2005;101(6):1877-1879.
44. Mungroop HE, Mijzen L, Woltersom B, et al. Feasibility of a new Y shaped bronchial blocking device and comparison with a DLT: a Manikin Study. 2009 ASA meeting. Abstract A541.
45. Bjork VO, Carlens E. The prevention of spread during pulmonary resection by the use of a double lumen catheter. *J Thorac Surg.* 1950;20(1):151-157.
46. Bryce-Smith R. A double-lumen endobronchial tube. *Brit J Anaesth.* 1959;(31):274-275.
47. Bryce-Smith R, Salt R. A right-sided double lumen tube. *Brit J Anaesth.* 1960;(32):230-231.
48. White GM. A new double lumen tube. *Brit J Anaesth.* 1960;(32):232-234.
49. Robertshaw FL. Low resistance double-lumen endobronchial tubes. *Brit J Anaesth.* 1962;(34):576-579.
50. Ehrenwerth J. Pro: proper positioning of a double-lumen endobronchial tube can only be accomplished with endoscopy. *J Cardiothoracic Anesth.* 1988;2(1):101-104.
51. Campos JH. Current techniques for perioperative lung isolation in adults. *Anesthesiology.* 2002;97(5):1295-1301.
52. Griffith HR and Johnson GE. The use of curare in general anesthesia. *Anesthesiology.* 1942;3(4):418-420.
53. Harroun P, Beckert FE, Hathaway HR. Curare and nitrous oxide anesthesia for lengthy operations. *Anesthesiology.* 1946;7(1):24-28.
54. Anderson E, Crafoord C, Frenckner P. A new and practical method of producing rhythmic ventilation during positive pressure anaesthesia with description of apparatus. *Acta Oto-laryngologica.* 1940;28(1):95-102.

55. Ibsen B. The anaesthetist's viewpoint on the treatment of respiratory complications in poliomyelitis during the epidemic in Copenhagen, 1952. *Proc Roy Soc Med.* 1954;47(1):72-74.
56. Bjork VO, Engstrom CG. The treatment of ventilatory insufficiency after pulmonary resection with tracheotomy and prolonged artificial ventilation. *J Thorac Surg.* 1955;30(3):356-367.
57. Severinghaus JW, Honda Y. Pulse oximetry. *Int Anesthesiol Clin.* 1987;25(4):205-214.
58. Severinghaus JW. Takuo Aoyagi: discovery of pulse oximetry. *Anesth Analg.* 2007;105(supp 6):S1-4.
59. Luft K. Method der registrieren gas analyse mit hilfe der absorption ultraroten Strahlen ohne spectrale Zerlegung. *Z Tech Phys.* 1943;(24)97.
60. Raventos J. The action of fluothane-a new volatile anaesthetic. *Br J Pharmacol.* 1956;11(4):394-410.
61. Gregory GA, Kitterman JA, Phibbs RH, et al. Treatment of the idiopathic respiratory distress syndrome with continuous positive airway pressure. *NEJM.* 1971;284(24):1333-1340.
62. Capan LM, Turndorf H, Patel C, Ramanathan S, Acinapura A, Chalon J. Optimization of arterial oxygenation during one-lung anesthesia. *Anesth Analg.* 1980;59(11):847-851.
63. Cohen E, Eisenkraft JB. Positive end-expiratory pressure during one-lung ventilation improves oxygenation in patients with low arterial oxygen tensions. *J Cardiothorac Vasc Anesth.* 1996;10(5):578-582.
64. Godet G, Bertrand M, Ben Ammeur M, et al. Comparison of HFJV vs CPAP for separate lung ventilation in patients surgically treated aneurysm of the thoracic aorta. *Ann Fr Anesth Reanim.* 1989; (supp8): R266.
65. Shuman RL, Peters RM. Epidural anesthesia following thoracotomy in patients with chronic obstructive airway disease. *J Thorac Cardiovasc Surg.* 1976;71(1)82-88.
66. Matas R. Local and regional anesthesia with cocaine and other analgesic drugs, including the subarachnoid method, as applied in general surgical practice. *Philadelph Med J.* 1900;(6):820-843.
67. Behar M, Magora F, Olshwang D, Davidson JT: Epidural morphine in treatment of pain. *Lancet.* 1979;1(8115):527-529.
68. Slinger PD. Pro: every postthoracotomy patient deserves thoracic epidural analgesia. *J Cardiothorac Vasc Anesth.* 1999;13(3):350-354.
69. Ready LB, Oden R, Chadwick HS, et al. Development of an anesthesiology-based postoperative pain management service. *Anesthesiology.* 1988;68(1):100-106.
70. Joshi GP, Bonnet F, Shah R, et al. A systematic review of randomized trials evaluating regional techniques for postthoracotomy analgesia. *Anesth Analg.* 2008;107(3):1026-1040.
71. National Cancer Institute. Surveillance epidemiology and end results. http://seer.cancer.gov/statfacts/html/lungb.html. Accessed October 12, 2009.
72. Organ procurement and transplant network data reports. http://optn.transplant.hrsa.gov/latestData/viewDataReports.asp. Accessed October 12 2009.
73. Demmy TL and Nwogu C. Is video-assisted thoracic surgery lobectomy better? Quality of life considerations. *Ann Thorac Surg.* 2008;85(2):S719-728.
74. Flores RM and Alam N. Video-assisted thoracic surgery lobectomy (VATS), open thoracotomy, and the robot for lung cancer. *Ann Thorac Surg.* 2008;85(2):S710-715.
75. Lohser J, Brodsky JB. Silbroncho double-lumen tube *J Cardiothorac Vasc Anesth.* 2006;20(1):129-131.

Practice Improvement and Patient Safety in Thoracic Anesthesia: A Human Factors Perspective

Noa Segall
Jonathan B. Mark

Clinical Vignette

A 46-year-old woman was scheduled for bronchoscopy and mediastinoscopy. Following uneventful induction of general anesthesia and tracheal intubation with an 8.0 mm endotracheal tube, bronchoscopy was performed. The upper thorax and neck were then prepped for mediastinoscopy using a standard iodine/alcohol surgical preparation solution (Iodine Povacrylex [0.7% available Iodine] and Isopropyl Alcohol, 74% w/w). The endotracheal tube was moved and secured to the right side of the patient's mouth, and the breathing circuit was secured to the side of the patient's head. Surgical incision and dissection were assisted with a standard electrosurgical unit. Approximately 10 minutes into the procedure, the anesthesiologist detected a breathing circuit leak. She checked all external connections and determined that the endotracheal tube pilot balloon was defective. To maintain effective ventilation, the endotracheal tube position was adjusted, additional air was added to the pilot balloon, and the circuit fresh gas flow was increased from 1 to 6 L/min. When the procedure was finished and the drapes removed, the anesthesiologist noted that the surgical drape on the right side of the patient's neck, near the endotracheal tube, was charred, and there was a 6 cm^2 2nd and 3rd degree burn on the patient's right shoulder. In retrospect, an unusual smell was noted during the case by the operating room scrub nurse, but he attributed this to the leaking anesthetic gas and did not mention this to the rest of the surgical team.

Anesthesia practice is becoming progressively safer,[1] and anesthesiology is recognized as the leading medical specialty in addressing patient safety.[2] Nonetheless, patients are still harmed by their anesthesia care, mostly due to preventable human error.[3] Thoracic anesthesia presents special risks to patients, owing to patient comorbidities and the complexity of both the surgical and anesthesia care required. Airway and ventilation management are shared anesthesiology and surgery concerns, requiring tight coordination of care through good communication. Issues such as monitoring and positioning, airway management and ventilation—important considerations in any case requiring general anesthesia—are complicated by the nature of the thoracic surgical intervention. Patients undergoing thoracic surgery often have

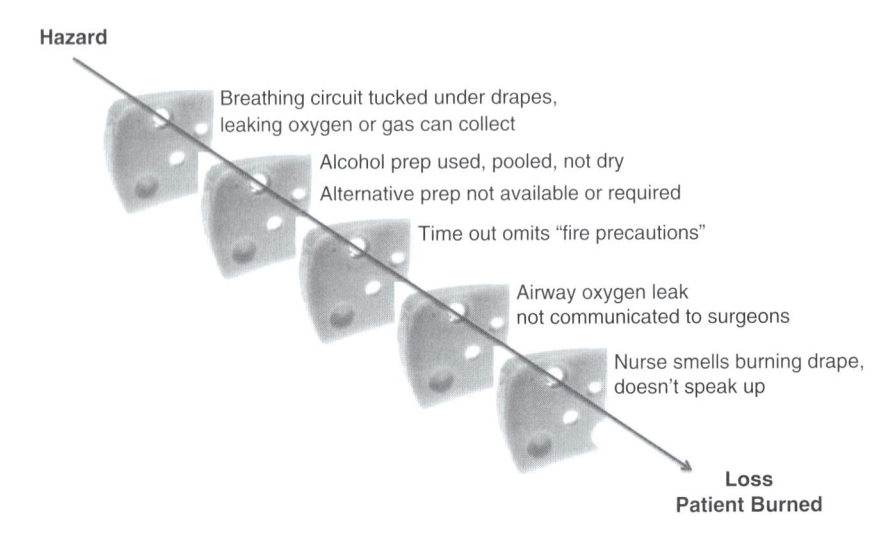

Figure 2–1. "Swiss cheese" model of system accidents. (From: Reason J. Human error: models and management. *British Medical Journal*. 2000;320(7237):768-770; Adapted to vignette.)

preexisting pulmonary disease, cardiac disease, and other major medical problems. Indeed, thoracic surgical procedures are performed on sicker patients than in the past.[4] These and other factors make the management of thoracic cases particularly challenging and can contribute to the likelihood of medical errors.

One of the most widely accepted paradigms for describing system failures is the Swiss cheese model put forth by James Reason.[5] When adapted to the healthcare domain, this model stipulates that medical errors resulting in patient injury are seldom caused by a single mistake and rarely are they only the result of an individual provider's negligence. When an adverse event occurs, it is often a consequence of the alignment of "holes" in the different defensive layers (depicted as Swiss cheese slices) developed by healthcare organizations to prevent errors (Figure 2–1). These holes, or system weaknesses, arise for two reasons: **active failures** and **latent conditions**. Active failures are committed by providers and can include, for example, **slips**, **mistakes**, and **procedure violations**. Distraction, momentary inattention, fixation, and other contributors to active failures are natural human behaviors in a working environment that is characterized by long periods of routine activity interrupted by moments of intense stress. Latent conditions originate from decisions made by system designers, managers, and procedure writers and, unlike active failures, can be anticipated and remedied before an adverse event occurs.[5,6]

Latent conditions that contribute to errors in anesthesia care can be grouped into provider, teamwork, technology, and organization-level issues (Table 2–1). Providers are more likely to make mistakes when they are tired, frequently interrupted in their work, or lack experience.[7] Teamwork errors often center around communication failures, which are cited in over 60% of sentinel events.[8] In the

Table 2-1. Examples of Latent Conditions in Healthcare Systems that Can Contribute to Errors in Anesthesia Care

Provider issues
  Fatigue
  Lack of experience
  Distractions
  Stress
  Low motivation

Teamwork issues
  Incomplete transfer of information
  Incorrect transfer of information
  Lack of assertion

Technology-related issues
  Equipment failure
  Poor design
  High rates of false alarms
  Insufficient training

Organization-level issues
  Production pressure
  Cost cutting
  Regulation
  Fear of litigation

operating room (OR), these errors include communication that is too late to be effective, content that is not complete or accurate, exclusion of key individuals from a discussion, and issues that are left unresolved until the point of urgency.[9] Technology-related errors may stem from equipment that is poorly designed, fails to work under required clinical conditions, or creates high false alarm rates that clinicians ignore or routinely silence.[10] Lastly, organizational issues such as cost cutting, regulation, fear of litigation, and production pressure are additional latent conditions that can increase error rates and compromise patient care. For example, placement of a thoracic epidural catheter may improve perioperative pain control and reduce pulmonary complications, but providers may feel pressured to avoid placing catheters for thoracic surgical patients in order to maintain high patient turnover or to reduce expenses. Decisions made at the organizational level can also affect provider, teamwork, and technology issues. Over-scheduling providers, implicitly discouraging preoperative OR team briefings to reduce turnover time, purchasing medical equipment without considering its usability, and many other management decisions may contribute to errors in the perioperative setting and compromise the safety of the OR environment.

In most healthcare organizations, rather than focusing on system changes to reduce latent errors, there is a disproportionate emphasis on prevention of active failures committed by individual care providers. In an effort to prevent these failures from recurring, management responses may include sanctions, exhortations, stricter procedures, training, and similar interventions. These measures are only appropriate, however, if the providers who committed the errors are particularly error-prone, inexperienced, undermotivated, or ill trained. Since this is rarely the case in anesthesia practice, efforts and resources should be directed at preventing latent conditions rather than active failures.[6]

A human factors approach to patient safety involves addressing all levels of latent conditions in order to reduce the likelihood of medical errors. **Human factors engineering** is the application of a body of knowledge about human capabilities and limitations to the design of tools, machines, systems, tasks, jobs, and environments for safe, comfortable, and effective human use.[11] For example, an understanding of human information processing strengths and weaknesses can be applied to health information technology design. Tasks at which humans excel, such as decision making or noticing changes in patterns, can be allocated to clinical users, while tasks for which computers are better designed, such as making rapid calculations or filtering data streams, can be automated, thereby leaving clinicians more time to devote to their patient care tasks. In this chapter, we will discuss patient safety topics that are relevant to thoracic anesthesia (and anesthesia in general) and human factors tools that can be used to address them.

PROSPECTIVE MEMORY ENHANCEMENT: CHECKLISTS, GUIDELINES, PROTOCOLS, AND COGNITIVE AIDS

The term **prospective memory** refers to the human ability to remember to perform an intended action following some delay. **Deferred tasks** can be classified as event-based or time-based. Event-based tasks are to be executed when a certain external event occurs (eg, "If high peak inspiratory pressure develops, check the position of the double lumen tube."). Time-based tasks are to be executed at a certain time (eg, "Check CK… at 6-hour intervals until returning to normal.")[12] and are more difficult to recall, since no environmental cue exists to prompt task execution.[13,14] Failures of prospective memory may be the most common form of human fallibility.[15] In thoracic anesthesia, prospective memory errors may result from the demanding work environment, which often requires dynamic multitasking and is fraught with interruptions, delays, and other distractions. At least 12% of critical anesthesia incidents may be attributable to factors associated with inadvertent neglect of future tasks, including haste, distractions, and failure to follow personal routine or institutional practice.[7,16]

In addition to individual efforts (eg, anticipating triggering cues or avoiding busy conditions and interruptions), experts recommend the use of external prompts such as **checklists** to assist in the recall of delayed intentions.[15,17] In addition to their utility as reminders, checklists are useful in standardizing clinical practice, allowing providers to deliver evidence-based care consistently.[18] They can also assist providers when confronted by novel, urgent, or rare situations. Checklists have been shown to reduce prospective memory errors, decrease risk, and improve outcomes in safety-critical industries such as aviation and manufacturing.[19] Their more widespread use has been recommended in healthcare,[20] and several researchers have begun to explore their utility in anesthesiology.

Checklists have been developed for several perioperative tasks. In an attempt to prevent incomplete checkouts of anesthesia equipment, which have been shown to lead to anesthetic mishaps,[21] the Food and Drug Administration developed a comprehensive anesthesia equipment checklist. However, this checklist was neither well-understood nor reliably utilized by anesthesia providers[22] and did not promote better checks than when providers used their own checkout methods.[23] More recently, the American Society of Anesthesiologists published a template for developing an equipment checklist tailored to individual anesthesia machines and practice settings.[22] Although it has not been evaluated formally, it is hoped that the ability to adapt it to each institution's requirements will make it useful and effective.

Standardized preoperative briefings and OR "time outs" have been mandated by the Joint Commission as part of its Universal Protocol.[24] Time outs are to be conducted before each surgical procedure to verify that the correct patient, positioning, surgical site, and procedure are identified. A Surgical Safety Checklist developed by the World Health Organization[25] (Figure 2–2) has been shown to reduce patient morbidity and mortality worldwide.[26] The checklist begins during a preoperative team briefing (Sign In) conducted before induction of anesthesia and includes verification of patient identity, allergies, surgical site, and needed supplies. Before incision, a formal Time Out is used to introduce team members, confirm patient identity, operative site, and procedure correctness, review anesthesia, surgery, and nursing concerns, and verify that prophylactic antibiotics have been

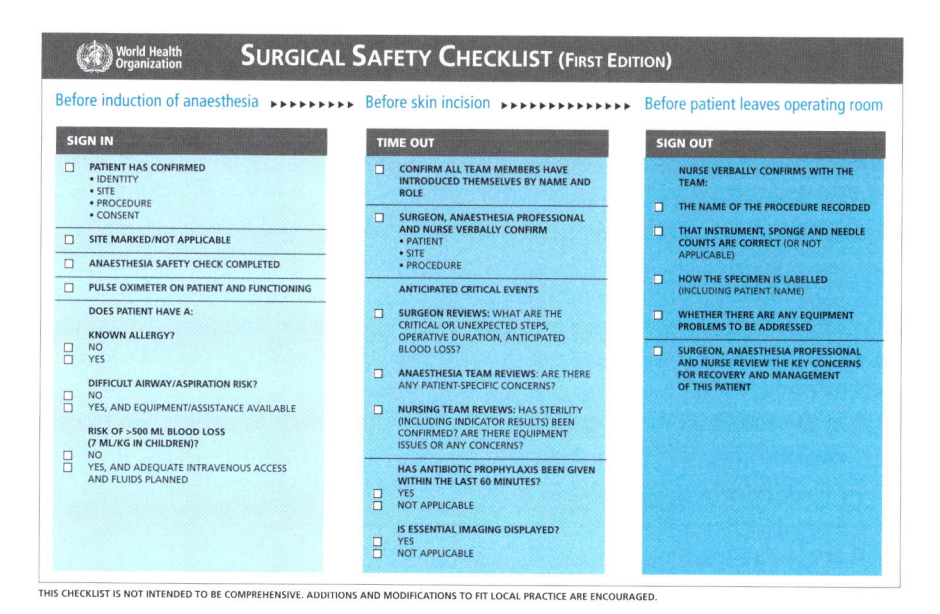

Figure 2–2. World Health Organization Surgical Safety Checklist. (Reproduced with permission from World Health Organization. Surgical Safety Checklist 2008; http://www.who.int/entity/patientsafety/safesurgery/tools_resources/SSSL_Checklist_finalJun08.pdf. Accessed August 27, 2009.)

given and relevant imaging displayed. Finally, after surgery is completed, the nurse leads a debriefing or Sign Out and confirms the name of the surgical procedure performed, instrument and sponge counts, correct specimen labeling, and equipment or other problems that need to be followed up. The Sign Out concludes with a team discussion of patient recovery and management concerns.

In addition to checklists, other memory aids that have been advocated to improve patient safety include the use of written treatment algorithms, or cognitive aids, that may be very useful for crisis management. It has been estimated that 5% of anesthesia cases develop into critical situations.[27] During a crisis, the anesthesia provider must perform multiple complex, dynamic tasks involving high workload and information load, such as hypothesizing the source of the problem, testing different assumptions, monitoring changes in patient state, administering drugs, ventilating the patient, communicating with the surgical staff, etc. Given this task complexity, suboptimal communication and teamwork, and often coexisting fatigue and stress, it is not surprising that errors occur during the management of these incidents. Algorithms have been created to improve decision making and reduce errors during these critical events,[27-29] and they include guidelines for managing many different events, ranging from malignant hyperthermia to OR fires.

Although there are only a few treatment algorithms that have been developed specifically for crisis management during thoracic anesthesia care, other general anesthesia crisis management algorithms are highly relevant. One example of an evidence-based thoracic anesthesia algorithm focuses on determining the need for intensive care unit (ICU) admission following lung resection.[30] Several general crisis management protocols that are particularly relevant for thoracic anesthesia include those developed for treating high-peak inspiratory pressure or hypoxemia during mechanical ventilation[27,29] (see Table 2–2). Although checklists used for healthcare in general[19] and in anesthesiology in particular[31] have been shown to improve clinical outcomes, these memory aids have not yet found the same acceptance in medicine that they have in other high-risk industries, such as aviation.[19] An opportunity exists for developing specific checklists, algorithms, and cognitive aids that are unique to the practice of thoracic anesthesia. For instance, management of hypoxemia or high peak inspiratory pressure arising during one-lung ventilation (OLV) can be summarized in a checklist useful for troubleshooting these common thoracic anesthesia problems. This complex domain would profit from systematic protocol development and evaluation for both routine care and crisis management.

Despite evidence of the benefits of checklists, their implementation in healthcare has been limited[19,32,33] due to both operational and cultural barriers. It is difficult to standardize medical procedures because of variations in patient physiology, individual practice preferences, and institutional policies. Care providers often resist the adoption of checklists for various reasons, such as concern that clinical innovation may be stifled, their role as decision makers will be reduced,[32] or that using a checklist would be perceived as a show of weakness or lack of professional expertise.[33,34] In addition, the checklist itself may be unclear or difficult to apply.[34] For these reasons, it is important to assess the utility and acceptance of checklists before they are implemented in the OR.

Table 2-2. Hypoxemia Treatment Cognitive Aid Developed by the VA National Center for Patient Safety.

Manifestations
  Decreased or low O_2 saturation measured by pulse oximetry
  Decreased or low PaO_2 via arterial blood gas
  Cyanosis or dark blood in the surgical field
  Cyanotic mucus membrane or skin color
  Late signs of hypoxemia include:
    Tachycardia or hypertension
    Bradycardia or hypotension
    Arrhythmias
    MYOCARDIAL ISCHEMIA
    CARDIAC ARREST

Immediate action
  Quickly check oximeter function or try alternate probe site
  Assume that low O_2 saturation indicates actual hypoxemia until proven otherwise
  Increase FiO_2 to 100%, with high O_2 flow
    Verify that FiO_2 approaches 100% (LOW F_{IO_2})
  Check that ventilation is adequate
    Check end-tidal CO_2
    Check tidal volume and rate of ventilation and check for leaks
    Check for absence of full excursion of the bellows (not filling = leak, not emptying = high resistance to flow)
    Check PIP (HIGH PIP)
    Auscultate the breath sounds bilaterally, assess the adequacy and symmetry of chest movement, listen for rales or wheezing
  Check the patency, position of, and insertion depth of the ETT
    If necessary use fiber-optic bronchoscopy or chest x-ray
    Adjust the position of the ETT if necessary
    Give several large breaths and suction
  Switch to hand ventilation to assess pulmonary compliance
  Give several large breaths and/or Valsalva maneuver to open collapsed airways and suction
  If hypoxemia does not resolve, confirm with a blood gas
    Check thoroughly for conditions that increase venous admixture
      Atelectasis
      BRONCHOSPASM
      Increased intracardiac shunting in congenital heart disease
      PNEUMOTHORAX
      Pulmonary aspiration of gastric contents
      Pulmonary emboli

Secondary management
  Terminate surgery as soon as possible
  Consider adding PEEP and maintain large tidal volumes (12-15 mL/kg)
  Use aggressive pulmonary toilet
    Suction ETT
    Consider bronchoscopy

(Continued)

Table 2–2. Hypoxemia Treatment Cognitive Aid Developed by the VA National Center for Patient Safety. (Continued)

Secondary management (Cont.)
Inform surgeons if difficulty in maintaining oxygenation persists
Check for retractors causing difficulty with ventilation
Check that patient in the prone position has not slipped off chest supports (placing pressure on the diaphragm)
Prepare to transfer the patient to the supine position emergently
Arrange for ICU transfer for postoperative care
Obtain ABGs
Ask blood gas laboratory to check for abnormal hemoglobin if clinically indicated e.g., methemoglobin, carboxyhemoglobin
Restore adequate circulating blood volume to maintain cardiac output and hemoglobin levels
Do not fixate on pulse oximeter function. Monitor the patient carefully while ruling out artifacts and transients. To verify function of the pulse oximeter:
Correlate oximeter readings with activation of electrocautery
Check the probe position
Shield the probe from ambient light
Assess adequacy of oximeter signal amplitude
Change the site of the probe (from finger to ear)

Text in BLUE CAPITAL LETTERS refers to other cognitive aids
Reproduced from Veterans Health Administration.[29] Originally from Gaba DM, Fish KJ, Howard SK. Crisis Management in Anesthesiology. New York: Churchill Livingstone; 1994. Copyright © Elsevier. Reproduced with permission. (Reference 27).

TEAMWORK

There is growing appreciation for the importance of sound communication skills between care providers in healthcare. Good teamwork and communication are essential for delivering high-quality patient care. Communication errors are a major root cause of patient harm,[8] while effective team communication skills have been shown to increase staff[35] and patient[36] satisfaction and to improve clinical outcomes.[37,38] In the OR, approximately 30% of procedurally relevant exchanges can be defined as communication failures.[9] Improving information transmission between team members can prevent adverse events associated with anesthesia administration.[7]

There are several communication tools and team skills, which when applied together, can establish a common mental model among team members and create an environment that empowers providers to speak up when they have safety concerns[35] (Table 2–3). The first is **leadership**: team leaders, whether designated or impromptu, play an important role in promoting good teamwork by organizing teams, articulating goals clearly, making decisions based on team members' input, and making members feel safe challenging their superiors when clinically necessary. Leaders also facilitate briefs (planning sessions), debriefs (process improvement discussions), and huddles (ad hoc problem-solving meetings), three important tools to ensure that all team members are "on the same page"[39] (Table 2–4). In thoracic procedures, teams can be large and diverse, including members from anesthesia,

Table 2-3. Teamwork and Communication Tools and Skills

Leadership
Team organization
Goal articulation
Decision making through collective input of team members
Briefs, debriefs, and huddles
Creation of an environment that promotes effective communication

Shared mental model
Situation awareness
Cross monitoring
Situation monitoring

Mutual support
Task assistance
Patient advocacy
Assertion

Structured communication
SBAR (Situation, Background, Assessment, Recommendation)
Check back
Handoff

Table 2-4. Important Elements of Team Briefs, Huddles, and Debriefs

Briefs
Planning
  Form the team
  Designate team roles and responsibilities
  Establish climate and goals
  Engage team in short- and long-term planning

Huddles
Problem solving
  Ad hoc, "touch-base" meetings to regain situation awareness
  Discuss critical issues and emerging events
  Anticipate outcomes and likely contingencies
  Assign resources
  Express concerns

Debriefs
Process improvement
  Brief, informal information exchange and feedback sessions
  Occur after an event, shift, or surgery
  Designed to improve teamwork skills
  Designed to improve outcomes
    An accurate reconstruction of key events
    Analysis of why the event occurred
    What should be done differently next time

Reproduced with permission from Department of Defense Patient Safety Program and Agency for Healthcare Research and Quality.[39]

surgery, intensive care, nursing, pathology, laboratory, pharmacy, blood bank, and other disciplines. Team members often have varying levels of training and experience, team composition may change frequently, and different leaders may be responsible during different phases of the perioperative period. Enabling good teamwork can be more challenging in these circumstances than when coordinating small teams with consistent team members.[40]

Another skill that characterizes high-performing teams is the establishment of a **shared mental model**.[41] Teams that share a common mental model understand the current system state, can interpret what it means for team members, and are able to deduce their future actions and expectations.[41] Individuals that have good **situation awareness**, acquired through situation monitoring (actively observing the situation and environment) and cross monitoring (monitoring other team members in order to support their work and prevent errors), facilitate the creation of a shared mental model.[39] It is critical for anesthesia providers in thoracic cases to maintain situation awareness when the patient's airway and breathing are shared with the surgical team. Understanding the surgeon's current and planned actions can help the anesthesia provider anticipate changes in patient ventilation and react appropriately. A shared mental model is also important when positioning the patient. Correct positioning to avoid patient injury is particularly difficult and time-consuming in thoracic procedures. Inefficiency can be prevented and safety achieved through preoperative discussions between surgeons, anesthesiologists, and nurses during the Sign In or preoperative briefing.[9]

Mutual support is also an essential component of good teamwork. Mutual support includes offering task assistance to colleagues and advocating for the patient. **Advocacy** is invoked when a team member's viewpoint regarding patient care does not coincide with that of the decision maker. In this situation, the team member should assert his or her position in a firm, respectful manner. If ignored, the team member should voice concern at least twice and, if the outcome is still not acceptable, speak with a person higher up in the chain of command.[39] **Assertion** is likely the most important—and most difficult—team skill to apply. Its goal is to prevent medical errors from occurring, but assertion requires a care provider to challenge another provider, usually his or her superior, in a culture that has traditionally been very hierarchical and discouraging of such practice. Therefore, it is important to first set up a supportive environment, one that "flattens" hierarchy, creates familiarity, and makes providers feel safe to speak up.[35] In contrast to surgeons, anesthesia providers and nurses are not as comfortable intervening when they have concerns about patient status.[42,43] However, anesthesia providers are perceived as "patient advocates," "diplomats," and "diffusers" by nursing, surgery and by themselves,[44] and in this capacity they can help create a supportive climate that encourages equality and openness in the OR.

The high-stakes, high-reliability domain of commercial aviation has shown that the adoption of standardized communication tools is a very effective strategy for improving teamwork and reducing risk.[35] Structured communication can be useful in many clinical situations. Here we'll mention **SBAR**, **check-back**, and **handoffs** as examples. SBAR is a framework for effectively relaying information about a patient during briefings, phone calls, or any situation that calls for a concise description of a patient's condition. SBAR stands for Situation (what is going on with the patient?), Background (what is the clinical context?), Assessment (what do I think the problem is?), and Recommendation (what would I do to correct it?).

Check-back is a communication loop in which the receiver of a message repeats it back to the sender and the sender verifies its correctness.[39] Check-backs are valuable for transmitting crucial information such as medication doses or laboratory results. Thoracic anesthesiologists will recognize this communication loop as a vital part of the OR conversation between perfusionists, surgeons, and anesthesiologists during cardiopulmonary bypass procedures (eg, Surgeon "Go on bypass," followed by Perfusionist "On bypass, now at full flow").

Finally, standardizing patient handoffs can reduce errors and omissions in information transfer while improving the efficiency of the patient transfer process.[45-47] Handoffs have been shown to be a high-risk, error-prone point of patient care[46] (with trainees being particularly prone to communication failures in this process),[46,48] and their standardization has been required by the Joint Commission.[49] One method for structuring handoffs is the use of tools such as SBAR when communicating patient information. Another method involves development of protocols and checklists for specific disciplines and situations. For example, Catchpole and colleagues created a protocol for handing off pediatric cardiac surgery patients who were being transferred from OR to ICU.[45] This protocol had specific roles for different providers at predefined times, such as "the anesthetist checks the equipment and that the patient is appropriately ventilated and monitored and is stable" during equipment transfer. A checklist—the information transfer *aide mémoire*[50]—was created for use by the surgeon, anesthetist, and receiving ICU team to ensure that important patient information was communicated during the handoff. Like pediatric heart surgery patients, postoperative thoracic surgical patients are in a compromised physical state, and it is essential that the receiving ICU team establish a shared mental model with the OR team through a comprehensive discussion of patient status and surgery, anesthesia, and other team member concerns. Standardizing this process can improve patient care by ensuring information completeness and accuracy.

MONITORING AND ALARMS

Anesthesia providers use many sources of information to track patient status. In addition to gathering data directly from the environment (eg, viewing the surgical procedure or observing the patient), the anesthesia provider operates the patient monitor, which displays as many as 30 distinct physiological variables,[51] as well as the anesthesia machine, ventilator, infusion pumps, and record-keeping systems. Additional monitors may be required for certain procedures and patients, such as a transesophageal echocardiograph (TEE). Performing anesthesia-related tasks while monitoring the patient can be cognitively demanding. Manipulation or observation of the TEE, for example, has been shown to increase workload and adversely affect vigilance in normal working conditions.[52] When patient status begins to change unexpectedly, this information-rich environment can also lead to attention overload. In these situations, the anesthetist's decision-making and problem-solving behaviors are generally concentrated at higher levels of abstraction than the information provided by standard OR monitors. For example, the anesthesiologist will focus on entire physiological systems, rather than single measured variables that only partially map the patient's state.[53] Numbers and waveforms can only indicate that a problem exists; they do not support the anesthesia provider in diagnosing it, defining its etiology, or in making treatment decisions.

Equipment designers and purchasers often fail to consider the usability of perioperative monitoring systems and the implications of systems that lack in functionality or usability on providers' performance.[3,54] One possible outcome is clumsy automation, a poor fit between humans and machines that leads to increased cognitive workloads during critical periods.[54,55] The effects of poorly designed monitors include inefficiency and frustration. Inadequate system design can also promote human error or prevent successful recovery from errors.[3,56] Human factors tools such as usability testing, simulation-based training, and human-centered design can help identify and correct problems with clinical monitoring systems before they are implemented in the OR.

The anesthesia provider's first line of defense in crisis management is the auditory alarm. Most patient monitors feature single-sensor single-indicator limit alarms, which are activated whenever a physiological variable deviates from a predefined range. There is general agreement that these threshold alarms have failed at their role of redirecting the anesthesia provider's attention to clinically important changes in patient state.[57-60] Perhaps the leading reason that alarms have proven ineffective is that the false alarm rate is substantial: in the OR, 75% of alarms are spurious, caused by patient movement, interference, or mechanical problems. Only 3% indicate actual risk to patients.[57,61] Another problem is that different alarm conditions can generate similar sounds and the same condition can generate different alarms on different devices.[60] Often, when the patient's condition is deteriorating, multiple alarms go off simultaneously, increasing the anesthesia provider's workload rather than decreasing it.[54] Alarms lack context sensitivity, that is, they are not "aware" of artifacts caused by patient positioning, intubation, and other extraneous circumstances that can cause physiologic disturbances.[58,60] They also cannot project the clinical urgency of the alarm-triggered condition.[60] As a result of these limitations, many anesthesia providers simply disable bedside monitor alarms. In the United States, 84% of 115 anesthesiologists surveyed indicated that they sometimes turned off anesthesia alarms. The percentage of respondents who regularly turned off the alarm ranged from 12% (low inspired oxygen) to 77% (low mean blood pressure).[60] In thoracic anesthesia, where the amount of monitored data is greater than in other, less complex procedures, false alarms are more common and, therefore, more disruptive. Specific stages of thoracic anesthesia, such as the transition to OLV or interruption of ventilation, are particularly prone to irrelevant alarms.

Various attempts have been made to alleviate the alarm problem in ORs, ICUs, and other care settings. Several studies evaluated the use of continuous auditory streams of physiological data, similar to the pulse oximetry tone, and of auditory icons and "earcons" to support the identification of the type and origin of changes in patient's state.[62,63] Other efforts have examined visual alarms, delivered via a head-mounted display, as a possible replacement of auditory alarms.[62] Intelligent (or integrated) alarms, which synthesize multiple physiological variables to produce a single status assessment, have also been proposed.[64-66] These alarms, based on artificial intelligence engines, are intended to reduce the number of low-level nuisance alarms. A similar approach uses redundant signals to identify deviations of a single physiological variable. The arterial blood pressure waveform, for example, was used as a secondary source of information to validate ECG arrhythmia alarms.[67] Finally, delays have also been suggested as a simple method of reducing clinically irrelevant alarms.[59] Each of these solutions is promising, but each introduces new problems to clinical monitoring which have to be addressed prior to field testing and widespread implementation.

MEDICATION ERRORS

On average, a hospital patient may be subject to at least one medication error per day, yet at least a quarter of all adverse drug events may be preventable.[68] Drug-administration errors are particularly concerning in anesthesia practice, where providers administer large numbers of drugs. Drug errors are committed in as many as 1 in 133 anesthetics,[69] and up to 21.7% of these errors result in patient harm (not including awareness).[70] The most common medication errors are syringe swaps, ampoule labeling errors, and preparation errors (eg, morphine dilution).[70]

A category of wrong-drug errors that is particularly relevant to thoracic anesthesia is tubing misconnections, the cross-connection of tubes and catheters. A broad range of medical devices, which have different functions and access the body through different routes, are often outfitted with similar connectors. These interchangeable connectors can lead providers to unintentionally connect intravenous (IV) infusions to epidural lines and, conversely, epidural solutions to IV catheters.[71] A fail-safe solution to this problem, the creation of different connectors for epidurals, IVs, enteral feeding tubes, dialysis catheters, etc, is not widely available or utilized. Less reliable approaches include labeling and color-coding tubes and catheters and training clinicians to trace tubes from origin to patient.[71]

Although similar drug names and confusing labels are commonly blamed, they are involved in relatively few perioperative medication errors. More common causes of error are performance deficits, inattention, communication failures, and failure to follow protocols.[72] An observational study of anesthesia provider activities in the OR sheds some light on these findings. Its authors found the drug preparation and administration tasks to be complex, yet inefficient and error-prone. An analysis of the preparation and administration of a single bolus of IV drug identified 41 distinct steps. Drug and fluid-related tasks comprised 50% of anesthetists' clinical activities during set-up and 20% of activities during surgery. The authors also found that searches for medications in the anesthesia cart were frequent; that the workspace was often disorganized, littered with sterile packaging, used and unused syringes, and airway equipment; that IV tubes and poles were commonly in the way; and that objects, including drug-filled syringes, were frequently dropped on the floor and retrieved (sometimes without assuring their sterility).[73] What is surprising, in an environment that is so unfit for the performance of such intricate tasks as drug preparation and administration, is not that errors occur; it's that they occur so rarely.

Several methods have been proposed for reducing the incidence of perioperative medication errors. Simple tools include increasing the legibility of drug labels, color-coding by class of drug, carrying out double checks, prefilling syringes with the most commonly used anesthetic drugs, labeling syringes, and organizing the anesthesia cart and workspace.[73-76] A more sophisticated solution could include bar-code automation that speaks the name of the scanned drug out loud, verifies its correctness, and documents its use.[73-75] Although no single method will prevent all medication errors from occurring, a combination of methods can reduce their likelihood.

RESPIRATORY EVENTS

Management of the patient's respiratory system and the anesthesia equipment attached to it is a demanding task. The ventilation system is complex, composed of a large number of biological and equipment-related variables. There is tight coupling among processes within this system and with other physiological systems. These factors and the dynamic, uncertain, risk-laden nature of the ventilation system combine to create a challenging environment for managing respiratory events.[77]

A large fraction of anesthesia-related critical incidents can be attributed to airway and respiratory problems. For example, the Australian Incident Monitoring Study (AIMS) found that 16% of all anesthesia-related incidents involved ventilation problems.[78] In a closed claims analysis of anesthesia cases resulting in death or permanent brain damage, 35.6% of events were associated with the respiratory system, most commonly due to difficult intubation or inadequate ventilation/oxygenation. Concurrent with the introduction and gradual adoption of pulse oximetry and capnography monitoring (recognized in 1990 and 1991, respectively, as standards for intraoperative monitoring by the American Society for Anesthesiologists) was a decrease in the proportion of respiratory-related events leading to death or brain damage.[79] Although association does not prove causation, it is possible that the improved ability to monitor patient oxygenation and ventilation led to this reduction.

Respiratory concerns are intensified in thoracic procedures requiring one-lung patient ventilation, although the frequency of patient injury related to the use of one-lung anesthesia is not well-known. Hypoxemia is common in these procedures.[80] Airway devices like double-lumen endotracheal tubes and bronchial blockers (BBs) are frequently misplaced or in suboptimal position for lung isolation, and can become dislodged during patient positioning and surgical manipulations.[81,82] Placing these devices may increase the risk of airway trauma, and their use can be challenging for providers who have limited experience in thoracic anesthesia.[81, 83] In thoracic surgery, respiratory failure accounts for approximately half of the 30-day postsurgery mortality.[84] Although data on respiratory events in thoracic anesthesia are not available, their incidence is likely greater than the incidence in nonthoracic cases due to the complexity of surgery and frequency of OLV.

Anesthesia providers are trained in the management of difficult airways and ventilation problems, but they receive few opportunities to practice these skills since life-threatening intraoperative airway and respiratory events are uncommon. Although periodic retraining is important to reinforce airway management skills, simulation-based training, for example, Anesthesia Crisis Resource Management, is particularly useful for augmenting airway skills with aspects of crisis management and decision making not usually taught in postgraduate and residency education.[85] In certain circumstances, checklists can be useful in resolving difficult airway issues. The evidence-based American Society of Anesthesiologists Difficult Airway Guidelines can facilitate the management of patients who are difficult to ventilate or intubate.[86] A checklist for supplies to be stocked in emergency carts can prevent the occurrence of missing equipment during critical periods.

Patient Safety Issues Raised in Case Vignette

1. Standard fire precautions (control of oxidizers [oxygen] and fuel [alcohol]) whenever an ignition source (electrosurgical unit) is used during surgery.
2. Operating room Time Out to include fire precautions and assurance that surgical preparation is dry prior to incision and use of electrosurgical unit.
3. Team roles, communication, and assertion, including need for all team members to "speak up" when they detect problems. This includes anesthesia staff that detected a circuit leak and needed to increase fresh gas oxygen flow, and nursing staff that detected something unusual during the case but failed to mention this to other staff members.

Glossary

Active failure—an unsafe act committed by care providers at the "sharp end" of the system, that is, providers whose actions can have immediate, adverse consequences.
Advocacy—arguing in favor of the patient when a team member's viewpoint does not coincide with that of the decision maker.
Assertion—requesting corrective action from a team member in a firm, clear, respectful, nonthreatening manner.
Check-back—a communication loop in which a sender initiates a message, the receiver provides feedback confirmation, and the sender verifies that the message was received.
Checklist—a list of action items or criteria arranged in a systematic manner, allowing the user to record the presence/absence of the individual items listed to ensure that all are considered or completed. Checklists lie somewhere in between an informal cognitive aid, such as a post-it note, and a protocol, which typically entails mandatory items for completion to lead the user to a predetermined outcome.

Deferred task—a task to be performed following a delay, that is, a task that requires prospective memory. Deferred tasks can be classified as event-based or time-based. Event-based tasks are to be executed when a certain external event occurs, while time-based tasks are to be executed at a certain time.

Handoff—the transfer of information (along with authority and responsibility) during transitions in care. Handoffs should include an opportunity to ask questions, clarify, and confirm information.

Human factors engineering—a field which is involved in conducting research regarding human psychological, social, physical, and biological characteristics, and in applying that information with respect to the design, operation, or use of products or systems for optimizing human performance, health, safety, and/or habitability.[87]

Latent condition—a condition that is created as a result of decisions made in management positions. Their consequences may lie dormant for a long time, only becoming evident when they combine with active failures and local triggering factors to create a medical error.

Leadership—providing guidance and direction within a team framework. An effective leader organizes teams, articulates goals clearly, makes decisions based on team members' input, empowers members to challenge their superiors when clinically necessary, and is skillful at conflict resolution.

Mistake—a failure of intention: the plan is inadequate, though its execution may be carried out as planned.

Mutual support—the support that team members render each other to protect from work overload.

Prospective memory—the ability of humans to remember intentions to perform actions after a delay, such as remembering to purchase milk on the way home.[88]

SBAR—situation, background, assessment, recommendation. A tool for effectively and concisely communicating about patients by stating what is going on with the patient, the clinical context, what the problem is, and how it can be corrected.

Shared mental model—the perception of, understanding of, or knowledge about a situation or process that is shared among team members through communication.

Situation awareness—the state of knowing the current conditions affecting a team's work, such as the status of a particular event or of the team's patients.

Slip—a failure of execution: the plan is adequate, but its execution is not as intended. A slip is caused by attention failure.

Violation—a deviation from safe operating practices, procedures, standards, or rules. Deliberate violations differ from errors in that they are associated with motivational problems.

REFERENCES

1. Gaba DM. Anesthesiology as a model for patient safety in health care. *BMJ.* 2000;320:785-788.
2. Aspden P, Corrigan JM, Wolcott J, Erickson SM. *Patient Safety: Achieving a New Standard for Care.* Washington, DC: National Academies Press; 2004.

3. Weinger MB. Anesthesia equipment and human error. *J Clin Monit Comput.* 1999;15:319-323.
4. Longnecker DE, Brown DL, Newman MF, Zapol WM. *Anesthesiology.* New York: McGraw-Hill Medical; 2007.
5. Reason J. Human error: models and management. *BMJ.* 2000;320(7237):768-770.
6. Reason J. Safety in the operating theatre—Part 2: human error and organisational failure. *Qual Saf Health Care.* 2005;14(1):56-60.
7. Cooper JB, Newbower RS, Kitz RJ. An analysis of major errors and equipment failures in anesthesia management: considerations for prevention and detection. *Anesthesiology.* 1984;60(1):34-42.
8. Joint Commission on Accreditation of Healthcare Organizations. *Sentinel Event Statistics.* Oakbrook, IL: Joint Commission on Accreditation of Healthcare Organizations; 2005.
9. Lingard L, Espin S, Whyte S, et al. Communication failures in the operating room: an observational classification of recurrent types and effects. *Qual Saf Health Care.* 2004;13:330-334.
10. Parasuraman R, Wickens C. Humans: still vital after all these years of automation. *Hum Factors.* 2008;50(3):511-520.
11. Chapanis A. To communicate the human factors message, you have to know what the message is and how to communicate it. *Human Factors and Ergonomics Society Bulletin.* 1991;34(11):1-4.
12. Malignant Hyperthermia Association of the United States. *Emergency Therapy for Malignant Hyperthermia.* Sherburne, NY: Malignant Hyperthermia Association of the United States; 1995.
13. Einstein GO, McDaniel MA. Normal aging and prospective memory. *J Exp Psychol Learn Mem Cogn* 1990;16(4):717-726.
14. Groot YCT, Wilson BA, Evans J, Watson P. Prospective memory functioning in people with and without brain injury. *J Int Neuropsychol Soc.* 2002;8:645-654.
15. Reason JT. *Human Error.* New York: Cambridge University Press; 1990.
16. Williamson JA, Webb RK, Sellen AJ, Runciman WB, Van der Walt JH. Human failure: an analysis of 2000 incident reports. *Anaesth Intensive Care.* 1993;21(5):678-683.
17. McDaniel MA, Einstein GO. *Prospective Memory: An Overview and Synthesis of an Emerging Field.* Thousand Oaks, CA: Sage Publications; 2007.
18. Morris AH. Treatment algorithms and protocolized care. *Curr Opin Crit Care.* 2003;9:236-240.
19. Hales BM, Pronovost PJ. The checklist—a tool for error management and performance improvement. *J Crit Care.* 2006;21:231-235.
20. Institute of Medicine. *To Err Is Human: Building a Safer Health System.* Washington, D.C.: National Academies Press; 1999.
21. Craig J, Wilson ME. A survey of anaesthetic misadventures. *Anaesthesia.* 1981;36(10):933-936.
22. American Society of Anesthesiologists. Guidelines for pre-anesthesia checkout procedures 2008; http://www.asahq.org/clinical/FINALCheckoutDesignguidelines02-08-2008.pdf. Accessed August 24, 2009.
23. March MG, Crowley JJ. An evaluation of anesthesiologists' present checkout methods and the validity of the FDA checklist. *Anesthesiology.* 1991;75:724-729.
24. Joint Commission. *National Patient Safety Goals: Universal Protocol.* Oakbrook Terrace, IL: Author; 2008.
25. World Health Organization. Surgical Safety Checklist 2008; http://www.who.int/entity/patientsafety/safesurgery/tools_resources/SSSL_Checklist_finalJun08.pdf. Accessed August 27, 2009.
26. Haynes AB, Weiser TG, Berry WR, et al. A surgical safety checklist to reduce morbidity and mortality in a global population. *N Engl J Med.* 2009;360(5):491-499.
27. Gaba DM, Fish KJ, Howard SK. *Crisis Management in Anesthesiology.* New York: Churchill Livingstone; 1994.
28. Runciman WB, Kluger MT, Morris RW, Paix AD, Watterson LM, Webb RK. Crisis management during anaesthesia: The development of an anaesthetic crisis management manual. *Qual Saf Health Care.* 2005;14(3):e1-e12.
29. Veterans Health Administration. *Cognitive aid for anesthesiology.* Ann Arbor, MI: VA National Center for Patient Safety; 2003.
30. Jordan S, Evans TW. Predicting the need for intensive care following lung resection. *Thorac Surg Clin.* 2008;18(1):61-69.
31. Arbous MS, Meursing AEE, van Kleef JW, et al. Impact of anesthesia management characteristics on severe morbidity and mortality. *Anesthesiology.* 2005;102:257-268.

32. Morris AH. Decision support and safety of clinical environments. *Qual Saf Health Care.* 2002;11:69-75.
33. Bosk CL, Dixon-Woods M, Goeschel CA, Pronovost PJ. Reality check for checklists. *Lancet.* 2009; 374(9688):444-445.
34. Harrison TK, Manser T, Howard SK, Gaba DM. Use of cognitive aids in a simulated anesthetic crisis. *Anesth Analg.* 2006;103(3):551-556.
35. Leonard M, Graham S, Bonacum D. The human factor: the critical importance of effective teamwork and communication in providing safe care. *Qual Saf Health Care.* 2004;13:i85-i90.
36. Uhlig PN, Haasa CK, Nason AK, Niemann PL, Camelio A, Brown J. Improving patient care by the application of theory and practice from the aviation safety community. *17th International Symposium on Aviation Psychology.* Vol Columbus, OH2001.
37. Morey JC, Simon R, Jay GD, et al. Error reduction and performance improvement in the emergency department through formal teamwork training: evaluation results of the medteams project. *Health Serv Res.* 2002;37:1553-1580.
38. Mann S, Marcus R, Sachs B. Lessons from the cockpit: how team training can reduce errors on L&D. *Contemporary OB/GYN.* 2006;51:34-45.
39. Department of Defense Patient Safety Program and Agency for Healthcare Research and Quality. TeamSTEPPS: team strategies and tools to enhance performance and patient safety. 2006; http://teamstepps.ahrq.gov/. Accessed November 20, 2009.
40. Hackman JR. Why teams don't work. Interview by Diane Coutu. *Harv Bus Rev.* 2009;87(5):98-105.
41. Rouse WB, Cannon-Bowers JA, Salas E. The role of mental models in team performance in complex systems. *IEEE Trans Syst Man Cybern.* 1992;22(6):1296-1308.
42. Mills P, Neily J, Dunn E. Teamwork and communication in surgical teams: implications for patient safety. *J Am Coll Surg.* 2008;206(1):107-112.
43. Makary MA, Sexton JB, Freischlag JA, et al. Operating room teamwork among physicians and nurses: teamwork in the eye of the beholder. *J Am Coll Surg.* 2006;202(5):746-752.
44. Lingard L, Garwood S, Poenaru D. Tensions influencing operating room team function: does institutional context make a difference? *Med Educ.* Jul 1 2004;38(7):691-699.
45. Catchpole KR, De Leval MR, McEwan A, et al. Patient handover from surgery to intensive care: using formula 1 pit-stop and aviation models to improve safety and quality. *Paediatr Anaesth.* 2007;17: 470-478.
46. Dunn W, Murphy JG. The patient handoff: medicine's formula one moment. *Chest.* 2008;134(1): 9-12.
47. Berkenstadt H, Haviv Y, Tuval A, et al. Improving handoff communications in critical care: utilizing simulation-based training toward process improvement in managing patient risk. *Chest.* 2008;134(1):158-162.
48. Nemeth C, Nunnally M, O'connor M, Brandwijk M, Kowalsky J, Cook R. Regularly irregular: how groups reconcile cross-cutting agendas and demand in healthcare. *Cogn Tech Work.* 2007;9(3): 139-148.
49. Joint Commission. The joint commission accreditation program: hospital national patient safety goals. 2009; http://www.jointcommission.org/NR/rdonlyres/31666E86-E7F4-423E-9BE8-F05BD1CB0AA8/0/HAP_NPSG.pdf. Accessed August 24, 2009.
50. Catchpole KR. Surgery to cardiac critical care handover protocol. 2007; http://emcrit.org/pdf/Handover%20Protocol%20ISSUE%20v1.0a.pdf. Accessed August 27, 2009.
51. Michels P, Gravenstein D, Westenskow DR. An integrated graphic data display improves detection and identification of critical events during anesthesia. *J Clin Monit.* 1997;13(4):249-259.
52. Weinger MB, Herndon OW, Gaba DM. The effect of electronic record keeping and transesophageal echocardiography on task distribution, workload, and vigilance during cardiac anesthesia. *Anesthesiology.* 1997;87(1):144-155; discussion 129A-130A.
53. Hajdukiewicz JR, Vicente KJ, Doyle DJ, Milgram P, Burns CM. Modeling a medical environment: an ontology for integrated medical informatics design. *Int J Med Inform.* 2001;62:79-99.
54. Cook RI, Woods DD. Adapting to new technology in the operating room. *Hum Factors.* 1996;38(4): 593-613.
55. Wiener EL. Human factors of advanced technology ("glass cockpit") transport aircraft. Springfield, VA: National Technical Information Service;1989. *NASA Tech.* Report 117528.

56. Dalley P, Robinson B, Weller J, Caldwell C. The use of high-fidelity human patient simulation and the introduction of new anesthesia delivery systems. *Anesth Analg.* 2004;99:1737-1741.
57. Watson M, Russell WJ, Sanderson P. Anesthesia monitoring, alarm proliferation, and ecological interface design. *AJIS.* 2000;7(2):109-114.
58. Seagull F, Sanderson P. Anesthesia alarms in context: an observational study. *Hum factors.* 2001;43(1):66.
59. Görges M, Markewitz BA, Westenskow DR. Improving alarm performance in the medical intensive care unit using delays and clinical context. *Anesth Analg.* 2009;108(5):1546-1552.
60. Block FE, Nuutinen L, Ballast B. Optimization of alarms: a study on alarm limits, alarm sounds, and false alarms, intended to reduce annoyance. *J Clin Monit Comput.* 1999;15(2):75-83.
61. Kestin IG, Miller BR, Lockhart CH. Auditory alarms during anesthesia monitoring. *Anesthesiology.* 1988;69(1):106-109.
62. Sanderson P, Watson MO, Russell WJ, et al. Advanced auditory displays and head-mounted displays: advantages and disadvantages for monitoring by the distracted anesthesiologist. *Anesth Analg.* 2008;106(6):1787-1797.
63. Loeb RG, Fitch WT. A laboratory evaluation of an auditory display designed to enhance intraoperative monitoring. *Anesth Analg.* 2002;94(2):362-368.
64. Becker K. A fuzzy logic approach to intelligent alarms in cardioanesthesia. 1998:1-5.
65. Oberli C, Urzua J, Saez C, et al. An expert system for monitor alarm integration. *J Clin Monit Comput.* 1999;15(1):29-35.
66. Becker K, Thull B, Käsmacher-Leidinger H, et al. Design and validation of an intelligent patient monitoring and alarm system based on a fuzzy logic process model. *Artif Intell Med.* 1997;11(1):33-53.
67. Aboukhalil A, Nielsen L, Saeed M, Mark RG. Reducing false alarm rates for critical arrhythmias using the arterial blood pressure waveform. *J Biomed Inform.* 2008;41:442-451.
68. Institute of Medicine. *Preventing Medication Errors.* Washington, DC: National Academies Press; 2007.
69. Webster CS, Merry AF, Larsson L, McGrath KA, Weller J. The frequency and nature of drug administration error during anaesthesia. *Anaesth Intensive Care.* 2001;29(5):494-500.
70. Abeysekera A, Bergman IJ, Kluger MT, Short TG. Drug error in anaesthetic practice: a review of 896 reports from the Australian Incident Monitoring Study database. *Anaesthesia.* 2005;60(3):220-227.
71. The Joint Commission. Sentinel event alert: tubing misconnections—a persistent and potentially deadly occurrence. 2006; http://www.jointcommission.org/SentinelEvents/SentinelEventAlert/sea_36.htm. Accessed August 27, 2009.
72. Wanzer LJ, Hicks RW. Medication safety within the perioperative environment. *Annu Rev Nurs Res.* 2006;24:127-155.
73. Fraind DB, Slagle JM, Tubbesing VA, Hughes SA, Weinger MB. Reengineering intravenous drug and fluid administration processes in the operating room: step one: task analysis of existing processes. *Anesthesiology.* 2002;97(1):139-147.
74. Webster CS, Mathew DJ, Merry AF. Effective labelling is difficult, but safety really does matter. *Anaesthesia.* 2002;57:201-202.
75. Webster CS, Merry AF, Gander PH, Mann NK. A prospective, randomised clinical evaluation of a new safety-orientated injectable drug administration system in comparison with conventional methods. *Anaesthesia.* 2004;59:80-87.
76. Jensen LS, Merry AF, Webster CS, Weller J. Evidence-based strategies for preventing drug administration errors during anaesthesia. *Anaesthesia.* 2004;59:493-504.
77. Sowb YA, Loeb RG. Cognitive analysis of intraoperative critical events: a problem-drien approach to aiding clinicians' performance. *Cognition, Technology & Work.* 2002;4:107-119.
78. Russell WJ, Webb RK, Van der Walt JH, Runciman WB. The Australian incident monitoring study. Problems with ventilation: an analysis of 2000 incident reports. *Anaesth Intensive Care.* 1993;21(5):617-620.
79. Cheney FW, Posner KL, Lee LA, Caplan RA, Domino KB. Trends in anesthesia-related death and brain damage: a closed claims analysis. *Anesthesiology.* 2006;105(6):1081-1086.
80. Sticher J, Junger A, Hartmann B, et al. Computerized anesthesia record keeping in thoracic surgery—suitability of electronic anesthesia records in evaluating predictors for hypoxemia during one-lung ventilation. *J Clin Monit Comput.* 2002;17(6):335-343.

81. Miller RD, Eriksson LI, Fleisher LA, Wiener-Kronish JP, Young WL. *Miller's Anesthesia.* Vol II. 7th ed. Churchill Livingstone; 2009, Philadelphia, PA.
82. Hurford WE, Alfille PH. A quality improvement study of the placement and complications of double-lumen endobronchial tubes. *J Cardiothorac Vasc Anesth.* 1993;7(5):517-520.
83. Campos JH. Which device should be considered the best for lung isolation: double-lumen endotracheal tube versus bronchial blockers. *Curr Opin Anaesthesiol.* 2007;20(1):27-31.
84. Ramsay JG, Murphy M. Postoperative respiratory failure and treatment. In: Kaplan JA, Slinger PD, eds. *Thoracic Anesthesia.* 3rd ed. Philadelphia, PA: Churchill Livingstone; 2003.
85. Gaba DM, Howard SK, Fish KJ, Smith BE, Sowb YA. Simulation-based training in anesthesia crisis resource management (ACRM): a decade of experience. *Simul Gaming.* 2001;32:175-193.
86. American Society of Anesthesiologists Task Force on Management of the Difficult Airway. Practice guidelines for management of the difficult airway: an updated report by the American Society of Anesthesiologists Task Force on management of the difficult airway. *Anesthesiology.* 2003;98(5):1269-1277.
87. Stramler JH. *The Dictionary for Human Factors/Ergonomics.* Boca Raton, LA: CRC Press; 1993.
88. Dieckmann P, Reddersen S, Wehner T, Rall M. Prospective memory failures as an unexplored threat to patient safety: results from a pilot study using patient simulators to investigate the missed execution of intentions. *Ergonomics.* 2006;49(5):526-543.

Physiology of One-Lung Ventilation

3

Raquel R. Bartz
Richard E. Moon

Optimal operating conditions for many cardiothoracic procedures require collapse of one lung, producing a challenge for the anesthesiologist who must maintain arterial PO_2, PCO_2, and hemodynamics within tolerable levels while ventilating the single remaining lung. One-lung ventilation (OLV) for thoracic surgery is usually performed while the patient is in the lateral decubitus position, with the nondependent lung collapsed. For other types of procedures, for example whole lung lavage, the patient may be in the supine position and the nonventilated lung remains inflated with saline resulting in different physiologic consequences. Therefore, a thorough understanding of pulmonary physiology will help facilitate the delivery of anesthesia for procedures requiring OLV.

PULMONARY VENTILATION

Flow of gas into the lungs is dependent upon the pressure difference between the upper airway (or endotracheal tube) and the alveoli. This pressure change can be induced either by inspiratory muscle contraction (spontaneous breathing) or positive pressure ventilation. Time-related variation in lung and chest wall mechanical properties induce variable tidal volumes and airway pressures during both spontaneous breathing and in some modes of positive pressure ventilation. To expand the lungs and overcome elastic recoil and resistive loads, a sufficient transpulmonary pressure gradient must either be generated with the use of positive pressure breathing or from negative pressure by the contraction of the diaphragm and muscles of inspiration as occurs during spontaneous breathing.

Elastic Effects

The lungs can be considered as many small, interconnected balloons inside the chest cavity, the elastic properties of which produce a recoil force. During lung expansion, recoil force of the lung is generated due to smooth muscle, elastin, and collagen as well as from other surface forces. The latter are due to surface tension generated by liquid within the alveoli. This is attenuated by surfactant produced by type II pneumocytes present at the alveolar-air interface. Changes in lung volume are accompanied by parallel changes in the volume of the chest wall, which has its own elastic properties. There is also a resistive component, mostly due to the properties of the airways, discussed below.

The lungs expand due to an increase in transpulmonary pressure (P_{tp}), equal to the difference between alveolar pressure (P_A) and pleural pressure (P_{pl}) ($P_{tp} = P_A - P_{pl}$). The pressure generated within the lungs to produce lung inflation must also be great enough to overcome forces independent of the lung including the chest wall, diaphragm, and abdomen (defined collectively as "chest wall").

The change in a given unit volume (eg, lung volume) per unit change in pressure is termed compliance. Compliance (C) is calculated by the following equation:

$$C = (V_1 - V_2)/(P_1 - P_2) \text{ or } \Delta V/\Delta P$$

Where V is intrapulmonary gas and P is transthoracic pressure. Lung compliance (C_L) in a normal awake human is typically in the range 150 to 250 mL/cm H_2O. Because elastic recoil forces increase at maximal lung volumes, compliance decreases as the lung inflates. Lung compliance is also decreased in diseases that result in scarring, fibrosis, and pulmonary edema. Although lung compliance normally increases with aging, diseases that disrupt the lung architecture of the alveolar septa, such as emphysema, will accelerate this process. Changes of lung compliance also occur with general anesthesia. Measurements before and after induction of anesthesia have typically revealed a 15% to 50% decrease in C_L.[1]

Because transpulmonary pressure is difficult to measure, the most clinically relevant ΔP is transrespiratory pressure, P_{TR}, defined as the pressure required to expand both lungs and the chest wall, which in a mechanically ventilated patient is equal to airway pressure. P_{TR} can be used to calculate total respiratory system compliance (C_{RS}), which is typically 90 to 120 mL/cm H_2O. Compliances for individual hemithoraces in normal anesthetized volunteers in the lateral decubitus position have been reported as 39 mL/cm H_2O (nondependent hemithorax) and 29 mL/cm H_2O (dependent hemithorax).[2]

Several factors affect lung compliance including lung volume, patient position, pulmonary blood volume, age, restriction of chest wall expansion, smooth muscle tone, lung diseases, and general anesthesia. After induction of general anesthesia there is a 20% to 35% reduction in C_{RS}. In common clinical usage, respiratory system compliance is defined as flow-dependent inflation (dynamic compliance) and non-flow-dependent inflation or static compliance. Dynamic and static compliance can be easily measured during positive pressure ventilation. Dynamic compliance represents the function of airway resistance on pressure changes whereas static compliance is measured when gas flow is static at the end of inspiration and thus mostly represents the compliance of the alveolar units. Changes in peak airway pressure measured by the mechanical ventilator at the end of inspiration reflect changes of dynamic compliance whereas changes of the plateau pressure (alveolar pressure) reflect changes in static compliance (Figure 3–1). Measurement of lung expansion and deflation, however, show that deflation pressures exceed inflation pressures. This difference in the volumes between inflation and deflation within the lung represents the affects of airway resistance and hysteresis, which is mostly due to the air–water surface forces at the beginning of inflation. The change in compliance during inflation and deflation can also be graphically plotted as pressure/volume loops, which many mechanical ventilators on anesthesia machines now display. The conventional clinical definition of dynamic compliance described

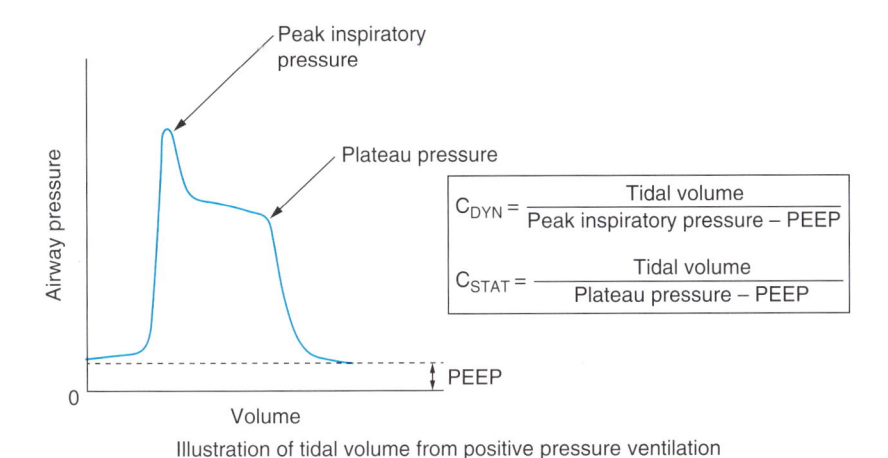

Figure 3-1. Measurement of respiratory system (thoracic compliance). The pressure-volume relationship (peak and plateau pressures, positive end-expiratory pressure (PEEP), and tidal volume, V_T) during delivery of a positive pressure tidal volume can be used to calculate clinically defined static and dynamic respiratory system compliances (CDyn, CStat).

$$C_{DYN} = \frac{\text{Tidal volume}}{\text{Peak inspiratory pressure} - \text{PEEP}}$$

$$C_{STAT} = \frac{\text{Tidal volume}}{\text{Plateau pressure} - \text{PEEP}}$$

above for mechanically ventilated patients differs from the classic definition, in which inspiratory and expiratory pressures are obtained at zero flow.

Resistive Effects

The airways of the respiratory system not only serve as the conducting vessels for gas transport but also contribute to the overall homeostasis of the lungs. In the noninstrumented patient, air is humidified in the upper airway and ciliated epithelial cells clear particles as they move down respiratory passages. Airway diameters, and thus resistance (R), change in response to sympathetic, cholinergic and nonadrenergic noncholinergic (NANC) systems, which act on bronchial smooth muscle and mucus glands. NANC mediators include substance P, neurokinins A and B (which cause bronchoconstriction) and vasoactive intestinal peptide (VIP, which causes bronchodilation). Bronchodilation also occurs as a result of local generation of nitric oxide (NO), which induces smooth muscle relaxation through soluble guanylate cyclase-dependent mechanisms. Like compliance, airway resistance changes with lung volume and differs during inspiration and expiration. During inspiration, lung expansion tends to increase airway diameter and thus decrease resistance; during expiration the decreasing lung volumes can result in compressed airways and increased airway resistance. Clinically, this may be an issue for patients with pathological narrowing of the airways, such as asthma, which may result in intrinsic positive end-expiratory pressure at the end of expiration or auto PEEP. Because inhaled anesthetics inhibit smooth muscle contraction of the airways, they produce a significant decrease in airway resistance and in the past have been used successfully to treat severe asthma exacerbations.

NORMAL LUNG VOLUMES AND EFFECTS OF ANESTHESIA, POSITIONING, AND POSITIVE PRESSURE VENTILATION

Lung volumes can be divided into different components (Figure 3–2). Normal, resting breathing occurs with a tidal volume (V_T) of approximately 5 to 7 mL/kg of ideal body weight. The volume of gas that can be exhaled beyond a resting expiration is termed the expiratory reserve volume (ERV), which is approximately 1000 mL in males and 600 mL in females. A small amount of gas is always present within the lungs at the end of maximal expiration and is termed the residual volume (RV). The summation of RV and ERV make up the functional residual capacity (FRC), which represents the point where alveolar pressure equals ambient pressure and the expansive chest wall forces are balanced by the elastic recoil of the lungs. Several factors influence FRC. Stiffening of the chest wall from aging and a decrease in the elastic forces of the lung leads to a gradual increase in RV and FRC over time. FRC is linearly related to height and decreases significantly due to obesity. In women, FRC is about 10% lower than in men. FRC is also decreased by the supine position and is affected by general anesthesia. FRC decreases during general anesthesia by 10% to 20% primarily due to a change in the shape of the ribcage.[3] In awake volunteers in the lateral decubitus position, the dependent lung has a lower FRC than the nondependent lung, which during anesthesia can lead to atelectasis and regions of poor ventilation. In studies in anesthetized volunteers after being turned from supine to lateral decubitus position, the normal reduction in FRC due to anesthesia was partially reversed, due to an increase in the nondependent lung FRC.[2] In the supine position each lung contributes approximately the same proportion of ventilation. However, in

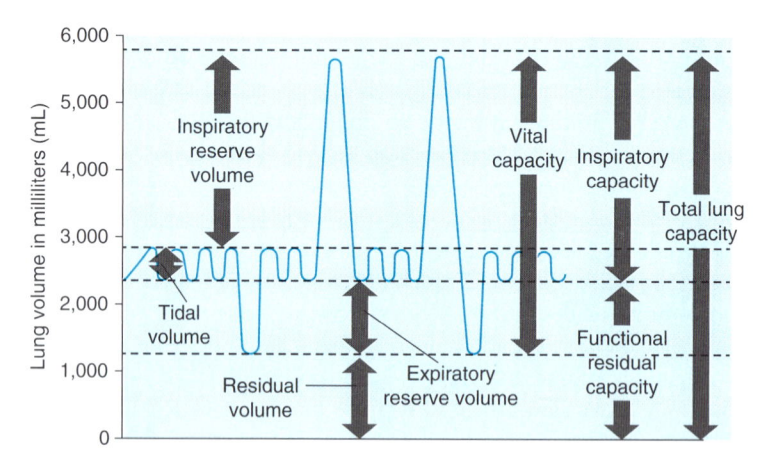

Figure 3–2. Subdivision of lung volumes. Several factors can different subdivisions of the lung volumes especially Functional Residual Capacity (FRC). FRC is linearly related to height, which increases FRC. Obesity and the supine position cause a reduction in FRC. (Adapted with permission from Shier D, Butler J, Lewis R. *Hole's Human Anatomy and Physiology*. New York: McGraw-Hill; 2004).

the lateral decubitus position during spontaneous breathing ventilation of the dependent lung is greater than the nondependent lung,[2,4] while during positive pressure ventilation the reverse is true.[2]

VENTILATION AND PULMONARY GAS EXCHANGE

Ventilation exchanges air from the environment to the lungs by producing a transpulmonary pressure gradient that facilitates transport of oxygen from the upper airway to the alveoli and movement of carbon dioxide in the opposite direction. Several factors influence both the alveolar oxygen and carbon dioxide pressure. The main determinants of alveolar PO_2 (P_AO_2) are inspired PO_2 and alveolar ventilation ($\dot{V}_A$). Arterial PO_2 (PaO_2) also depends on ventilation/perfusion matching, right-to-left (intrapulmonary and intracardiac) and alveolar-capillary diffusion, although the latter is rarely a limiting factor in clinical medicine except during exercise in patients with interstitial disease.

After leaving the right heart, deoxygenated blood enters the pulmonary capillaries and flows into the pulmonary veins. Hypoxemia results from desaturated blood (venous admixture) emanating from abnormal gas exchange units with low ventilation/perfusion ratio <1) or shunt $\dot{V}_A/\dot{Q}$ ($\dot{V}_A/\dot{Q}$ ratio = 0) units. Pulmonary arteriovenous right-to-left shunts have been described within the normal lung and are detectable when pulmonary artery flow and pressure are high, such as during exercise. Two other physiological sources of deoxygenated blood include the bronchial and thebesian veins, which drain directly into the pulmonary veins and left atrium, respectively ("left-to-left" or post-pulmonary shunt). Normally these account for <1% of the cardiac output (CO) and therefore do not significantly affect arterial oxygenation. However, in patients with severe bronchiectasis, where the bronchial circulation can increase several fold, left-to-left shunt may contribute significantly to arterial hypoxemia.

Secondary factors affecting PaO_2 include CO and second gas effect. The alveolar/arterial PO_2 difference in a young healthy adult breathing air is usually < 10 mm Hg but increases with age and lung disease. This difference results from physiological shunt or venous admixture. In diseased lungs this difference may increase significantly and is the main cause of arterial hypoxemia.

In the steady state, PCO_2 in arterial blood is determined by the amount of CO_2 produced from metabolism and the amount eliminated by ventilation. Total ventilation (minute ventilation, [$\dot{V}_E$], which is the product of respiratory rate [f] and tidal volume [V_T]), is made up of alveolar ventilation and dead space ventilation ($\dot{V}_D$). Dead space is composed of the volume of the upper airway and conducting airways ("anatomic" or "series" dead space) and unperfused or hypoperfused distal gas exchange units (physiological or parallel dead space). Alveolar PCO_2 is determined by the following equation:

$$P_ACO_2 = 0.863\ \dot{V}CO_2/\dot{V}_A \text{ where } \dot{V}CO_2 \text{ is the } CO_2 \text{ production rate.}$$

Alveolar ventilation can be written as:

$$\dot{V}_A = \dot{V}_E \times (1 - V_D/V_T)$$

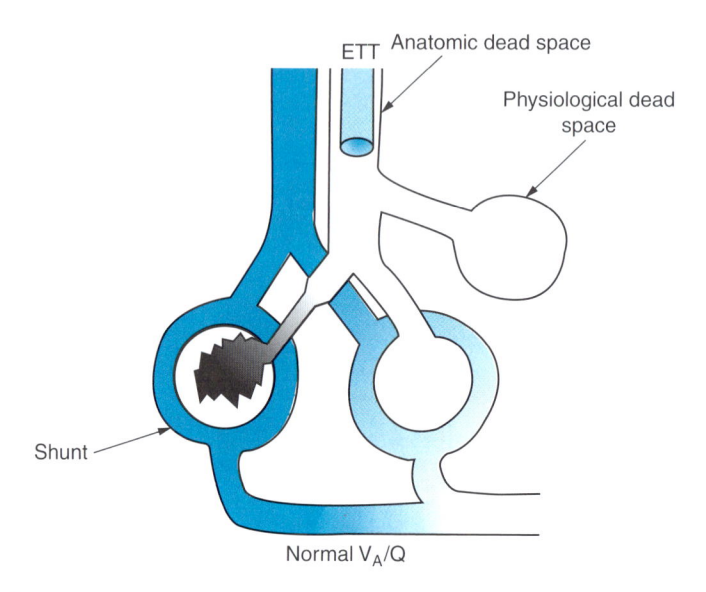

Figure 3-3. Alveolar ventilation is determined by the amount of anatomic and physiologic dead space as well as the minute ventilation, which is a function of respiratory rate and tidal volume.

Where V_D/V_T is dead space/tidal volume ratio. Therefore, since $\dot{V}_A$ is a function of both $\dot{V}_E$ and V_D/V_T, any variation in $\dot{V}CO_2$, $\dot{V}_E$, or V_D/V_T will also affect PCO_2. O_2 consumption ($\dot{V}O_2$), and hence $\dot{V}CO_2$, decreases slightly during general anesthesia, to a large extent because of the frequently associated reduction in body temperature (Figure 3-3).

During OLV, maintenance of $PaCO_2$ at preinduction levels will require $\dot{V}_E$ at or slightly higher than during two-lung ventilation. This is to account for the effect of right-to-left shunt and less efficient $\dot{V}_A/\dot{Q}$ matching. Indeed, the majority of individuals requiring OLV have lung disease, which may limit the degree to which isocapnia can be maintained. In particular, obstructive lung disease is associated with increased V_D/V_T. Airways obstruction may limit the adequacy of expiration and lead to dynamic hyperinflation also known as auto PEEP, particularly during OLV,[5] which in turn can reduce pulmonary blood flow and lead to systemic hypotension.

PULMONARY CIRCULATION

The pulmonary arteries divide several times to form arterioles that have larger diameters and thinner vessel walls than their counterparts in the systemic circulation. This interconnected network of vessels leads to small single-cell layered capillaries where alveolar-capillary exchange of O_2 and CO_2 occurs via diffusion. While the majority of pulmonary gas exchange occurs in the capillaries, a significant portion also occurs in the larger arterioles of the pulmonary vasculature. During air breathing, pulmonary blood may acquire as much as 15% of its O_2

load before reaching the capillaries; during 100% oxygen breathing the pulmonary arterial blood may be fully oxygenated before traversing the capillaries.[6]

Because the pulmonary circulation is a large and highly compliant interconnected network of vasculature under relatively low pressure and normal physiologic conditions, the right ventricle requires less contractile force to generate blood flow into the capillary network of the lungs than the force generated by left ventricle for the systemic circulation. For this reason, the right ventricle has less musculature than its counterpart on the left side. Adequate ejection of blood from the right ventricle and the distensibility or resistance of the pulmonary vasculature are the main determinants of pulmonary arterial blood flow.

Positional changes in pulmonary blood flow distribution would be expected when the patient is turned to the lateral decubitus position. While animal studies suggest in fact that very little flow redistribution occurs; human data support increased blood flow in the dependent lung.[4,7,8] This facilitates V_A/Q matching and maintenance of arterial oxygenation during OLV in the lateral decubitus position.

PULMONARY CIRCULATION PRESSURE-FLOW RELATIONSHIPS

The relatively low-pressure pulmonary arterial system contains approximately 450 mL of blood at any given time or about 9% of total circulatory blood volume. Normal pulmonary arterial pressure is typically 25/5 mm Hg, mean pressure 10 to 12 mm Hg. Pulmonary blood flow or perfusion exhibits significant heterogeneity among lung regions. This was described in the 1960s and thought to be primarily related to gravity.[9] West first proposed the idea of gravity-dependent forces being responsible for regional heterogeneity of pulmonary perfusion, with blood in the erect position flowing preferentially to the most dependent areas of the lung and the least amount to the lung apices (Figure 3–4).

West proposed the existence of three lung zones. In the uppermost zones (zone 1) at apices of the lung, pulmonary blood flow is lacking given the pressure exerted by the alveoli (P_A) is greater than pressure in the pulmonary arteries (P_a) or veins (P_V); $P_A > P_a > P_V$. This zone is therefore largely dead space. In the middle zone (zone 2) $P_a > P_A > P_V$, flow depends on the pressure difference between arterial and alveolar pressures. In the basal lung units (zone 3) $P_a > P_V > P_A$, blood flow is continuous, and ventilation and perfusion are well-matched. The practical implications of West zones are that if lung volume in zone 3 is atelectatic then better oxygenation may ensue if it can be recruited. Some authors have added a zone 4 region to reflect those areas in the lung where interstitial pressure (P_{is}) is higher than P_V, and blood flow is disproportionately reduced.

Methods that appeared to confirm the West's original gravitational hypothesis were quite crude at the time,[11] and newer evidence has led to other models. Glenny and his colleagues, using microsphere studies of the lungs during the 1990s, were able to determine that gravity dependent mechanisms, while present, play a lesser role, the major factor being branching and path length of the vessels.[12] Due to these factors, pulmonary blood flow is highest in hilar regions compared with the lung periphery. Previously, recruitment of apical pulmonary vessels was thought to

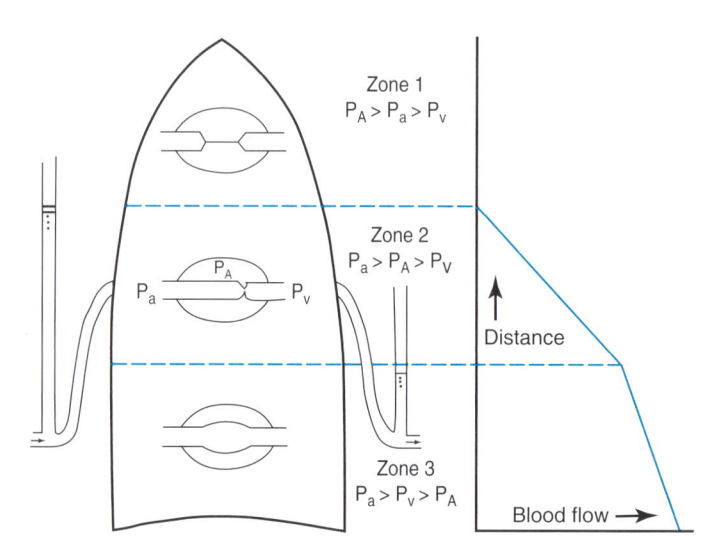

Figure 3-4. The Zones of West. In the uppermost zones (zone 1) $P_A > P_a > P_v$, thus there is no blood flow. In the middle zone (zone 2) $P_a > P_A > P_v$, thus flow depends on the pressure difference between arterial and alveolar pressures. In the basal lung units (zone 3) $P_a > P_v > P_A$, thus blood flow is continuous, and ventilation and perfusion are well matched. (Redrawn permission from West JB, Dollery CT, Naimark A.[10])

occur during increased cardiac output (CO) with exercise, however recent studies suggest that increasing CO above resting levels results in a very modest redistribution of blood flow.[13] A gravitational effect will be most evident in a well-expanded lung, with pulmonary vessels dilated and low pulmonary artery pressure, and least evident in a low volume, vasoconstricted lung with high pulmonary artery pressure. For example, no gravitational effect has been demonstrated *within* the dependent lung in the lateral decubitus position.

PULMONARY VASODILATION AND VASOCONSTRICTION

Pulmonary arteriolar vasodilation and vasoconstriction play an important role in distribution of pulmonary blood flow and maintain matching of pulmonary ventilation ($\dot{V}$) with pulmonary perfusion ($\dot{Q}$). Pulmonary arterioles constrict in response to low oxygen tension (hypoxic pulmonary vasoconstriction or HPV). This is unique to the lung vessels; blood vessels in the systemic circulation dilate in response to hypoxemia. HPV occurs in response to alveolar hypoxia at an P_AO_2 less than 50 mm Hg[14] and are also somewhat dependent on mixed venous PO_2. The precise intracellular mechanisms leading to pulmonary arteriole smooth muscle contraction in response to oxygen sensing have yet to be defined. However, multiple components for intracellular smooth muscle contraction are thought to play a role including L-type calcium channels, K_v channels, nonspecific cation channels, Rho-kinase, reactive oxygen species, and release or uptake of NO by hemoglobin.[15-17] Hypoxia has also been shown to stimulate the release of endothelin, a powerful vasoconstrictor.[18-20] In response to activation of the endothelin (ET_A and ET_B) receptors by endothelin, the pulmonary arterial smooth muscle myocytes constrict leading to increased pulmonary vascular resistance.[18,21] Proposed mechanisms are shown in Figure 3–5. There is little evidence that HPV plays a major role in matching under normal conditions. However, in the presence of lung pathology, HPV facilitates the diversion of pulmonary blood flow away from hypoxic regions to regions with better oxygenation.[22] Due to the same mechanism, whole lung hypoxia can cause an increase in pulmonary artery pressure, which if severe enough can lead to decreased right ventricular function.

Pulmonary arterial smooth muscle contraction and dilation also occur in response to systemic factors other than low or normal arterial oxygen tensions. For instance, the pulmonary vessels dilate in response to a high pH or alkalosis and contract in response to a low pH or acidosis. Several drugs, such as inhaled anesthetics, sodium nitroprusside, nitroglycerin, and calcium channel blockers, can also cause vasodilation and inhibition of HPV. In the presence of lung pathology or collapse, these agents can reduce arterial oxygenation. Some halogenated anesthetic agents can attenuate HPV by as much as 30%. However, most commonly used anesthetics such as isoflurane, sevoflurane, and desflurane appear to have modest inhibition of HPV at clinically relevant levels close to 1 MAC.[23]

APNEIC OXYGENATION

If nitrogen has been washed out of the lung and the airway is connected to a source of 100% oxygen, apneic oxygenation can occur. Adequate oxygenation occurs despite apnea due to the relatively slow rise in PCO_2 (typically 8 to 12 mm Hg during the first minute, 2 to 3 mm Hg/min thereafter[24] and ongoing convective delivery of oxygen from airway to alveoli due to the ratio of CO_2 production:O_2 consumption (R = respiratory exchange ratio) less than 1 (typically 0.8). For a normal individual approximately 250 mL/min of oxygen leave the alveoli and enter the blood. In parallel, the body produces 200 mL of carbon dioxide each minute. Some of this enters the alveoli, with the rest remaining in dissolved form in the blood. Provided the airway remains open and connected to an oxygen source, the discrepancy between oxygen uptake and carbon dioxide release will force oxygen to flow continuously from airway to alveolus despite the lack of active ventilation. When using apneic oxygenation, it has been shown that arterial hemoglobin-O_2 saturation of 100% can be maintained for nearly an hour.[25] During OLV this principle can be used to augment arterial PO_2 if the nonventilated lung remains connected to a source of oxygen.

PHYSIOLOGY OF ONE-LUNG VENTILATION (OLV)

When transitioning from two- to one-lung ventilation, ventilation of the lung on the operative side will be discontinued, either with the aid of an endobronchial blocker or double-lumen endotracheal tube that allows independent lung ventilation. The isolated lung will then gradually collapse of its own accord or due to external compression by the surgeon, facilitating exhalation of gas via the bronchial tree. Lung collapse can be accelerated by absorption of soluble gases into

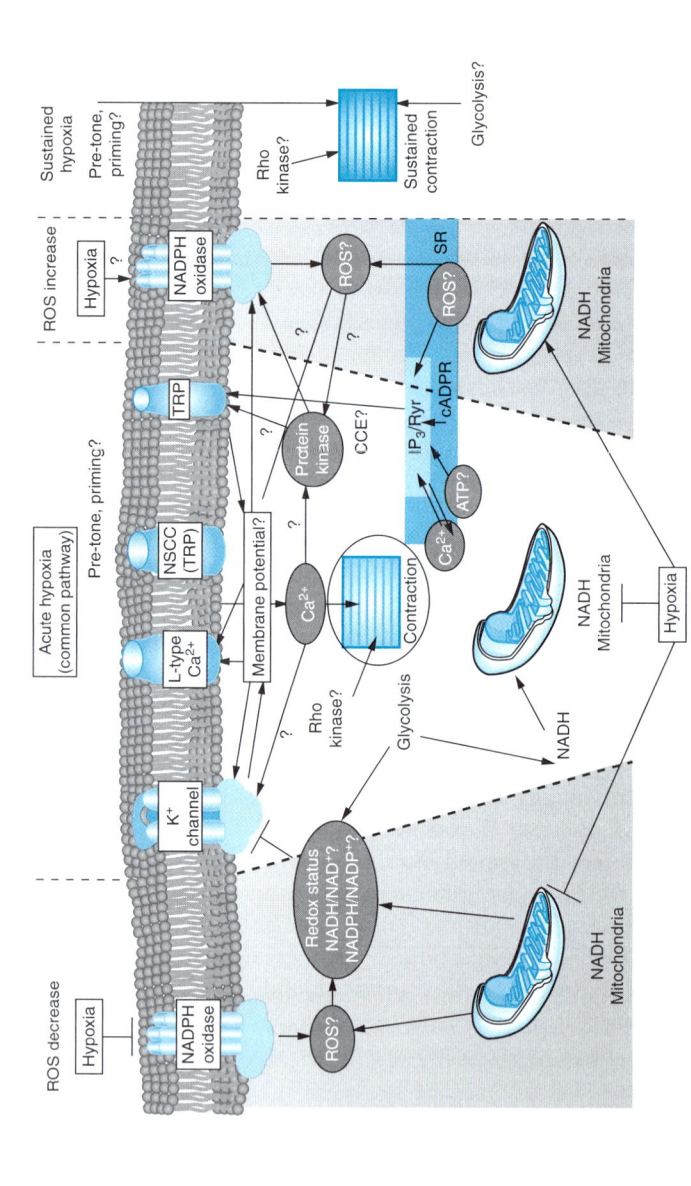

Figure 3–5. Pathways involved in hypoxic pulmonary vasoconstriction. Acute hypoxia results in an increase of intracellular calcium in pulmonary arterial smooth muscle cells and thus contraction. This increase in calcium is achieved by inflow of extracellular calcium through plasmalemmal calcium channels and release of intracellularly stored calcium. Hypoxic effects could be mediated or modulated by a decrease (left side) or increase (right side) of reactive oxygen species (ROS). NADPH: reduced nicotinamide adenine dinucleotide phosphate; NSCC: nonspecific cation channels; TRP: transient receptor potential; NADH: reduced nicotinamide adenine dinucleotide; NAD: nicotinamide adenine dinucleotide; NADP: nicotinamide adenine dinucleotide phosphate; CCE: capacitative calcium entry; ATP: adenosine triphosphate; IP$_3$: inositol triphosphate; cADPR: cyclic ADP-ribose; SR: sarcoplasmatic reticulum. (Adapted with permission of the European Respiratory Society Sommer, N., A. Dietrich, et al. (2008). Regulation of hypoxic pulmonary vasoconstriction: basic mechanisms. *Eur Respir J.* 32(6):1639-1651. doi:10.1183/09031936.00013908.)

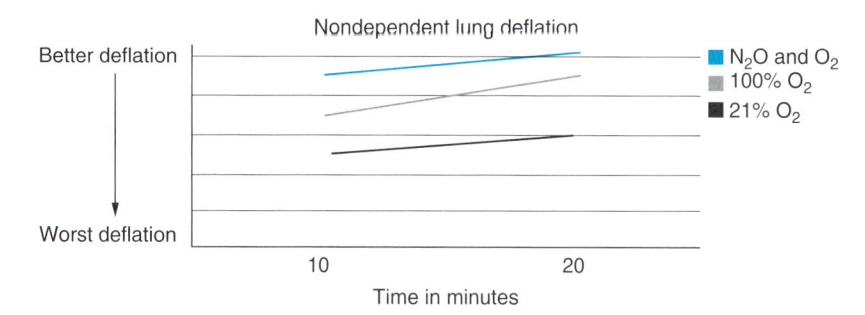

Figure 3-6. Nondependent lung deflation is best (high "lung deflation score") when a ventilating gas of high blood solubility is used, either 100% O_2 or O_2-N_2O, compared with air. (Adapted from with permission Ko R, McRae K, Darling G, et al.[26])

the bloodstream. Predictably, this occurs faster if the lung has been ventilated with N_2O-O_2 or 100% O_2 compared with N_2-O_2 mixtures (Figure 3–6).

Collapse of the nonventilated lung results in a reduction in its blood flow, due to the combination of mechanical effects and HPV. The degree of right-to-left shunt through the nonventilated lung to a large extent governs the PaO_2. A high blood flow through the nonventilated lung reduces PaO_2 and vice-versa (see below). Factors that reduce blood flow through the nonventilated lung include surgical retraction,[27] and in the case of whole lung lavage, the hydrostatic pressure of the lavage fluid (typically 50 cm H_2O at the end of each fill cycle).

HEMODYNAMIC CHANGES DURING OLV

Hemodynamic effects can be seen when the nonventilated lung collapses due to the reduction in available pulmonary vasculature. However, the reduction in pulmonary blood flow through the nonventilated lung during OLV, in most individuals, is accompanied by only a modest increase in pulmonary vascular resistance and mean pulmonary artery pressure (typically a 2-4 mm Hg increase); however, the increase may be augmented in the presence of hypoxemia or hypercapnia.

OXYGENATION DURING OLV

Because right-to-left shunt plays a dominant role in blood oxygenation during OLV, the major factors that affect PaO_2 during OLV are fractional blood flow through the nonventilated lung and mixed venous oxygen content ($C\bar{v}O_2 = S\bar{v}O_2 \times 1.34 \times$ Hb) + $0.003 \times PaO_2$).

Mixed Venous Oxygen Content

$C\bar{v}O_2$ is determined by oxygen consumption ($\dot{V}O_2$) and tissue oxygen delivery (the product of CO and arterial oxygen content). Since $\dot{V}O_2$ and hemoglobin concentration are relatively constant over short-time periods, changes in $C\bar{v}O_2$ reflect O_2 delivery. In Figure 3–7, arterial Hb-O_2 saturation is plotted as a function of shunt fraction (Qs/Qt) and, for convenience, $S\bar{v}O_2$. Due to the absence of an

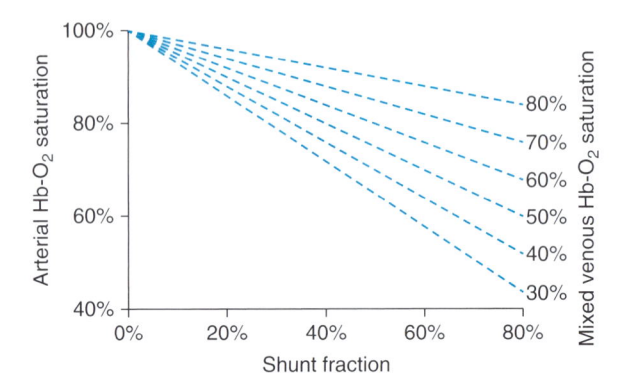

Figure 3–7. At any given shunt fraction, arterial oxygenation depends on mixed venous oxygen content (displayed here as mixed venous Hb-O_2 saturation). In the presence of right-to-left shunt (or V_A/Q mismatch) low $S\bar{v}O_2$ is associated with arterial hypoxemia. In the presence of shunt or V_A/Q mismatch a reduction in arterial oxygenation can also be caused by a drop in cardiac output (see text). Anemia would have the same effect as low $S\bar{v}O_2$.

increase in CO, anemia will cause a decrease in $S\bar{v}O_2$. In the presence of V_A/Q mismatch or right-to-left shunt, any change in O_2 delivery, caused by changes in CO or Hb, will influence $S\bar{v}O_2$ and hence PaO_2. An increase in CO or Hb, by delivering more oxygen to tissues, will cause an increase in $S\bar{v}O_2$, and hence a rise in PaO_2 and vice-versa.

Positioning

During OLV, lateral decubitus position improves oxygenation compared with the supine position due to gravitational diversion of blood from the nondependent to the dependent lung, thus decreasing shunt fraction. The effect of position on arterial PO_2 at different inspired oxygen fractions is shown in Figure 3–8. V_A/Q

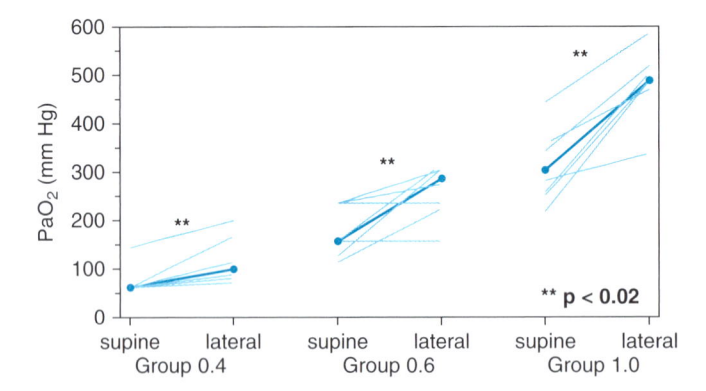

Figure 3–8. Arterial PO_2 during OLV as a function of position and inspired oxygen fraction (0.4, 0.6, and 1.0). (Reproduced with permission from Bardoczky GI, Szegedi LL, d'Hollander AA, Moures JM, de Francquen P, Yernault JC.[30])

relationships and the effect of selective PEEP are shown in Figure 3–9. Shunt may also be affected during OLV by head-up or head-down tilt. Head-down tilt during OLV has been associated with worsening of arterial oxygenation, and head-up tilt, an improvement.[28] The increase in PaO_2 during head-up tilt has been attributed to a decrease in shunt.

EFFECTS OF DRUGS AND ANESTHESIA ON BLOOD FLOW DISTRIBUTION

Vasodilators such as calcium channel blockers, nitrates, and nitroprusside tend to inhibit HPV, and thus may disproportionately increase flow to the nonventilated lung. Inhaled anesthetics can also inhibit HPV.[29] However, this is not normally seen clinically, perhaps because the concentrations of inhaled agents commonly used (≈1 MAC) are insufficient to offset the degree of HPV actually encountered. Alternatively, HPV may be relatively unimportant in determining PaO_2 during anesthesia. An additional possibility is that while the effects of inhaled anesthetics on pulmonary blood flow may tend to impair $\dot{V}_A/\dot{Q}$ matching, this could be offset by their bronchodilatory effects, which may engender a parallel improvement in intrapulmonary gas distribution. In any event, although inhaled anesthetics may attenuate the HPV response, their effect is usually reduced over time.

Intravenous anesthetics do not directly affect HPV, although high doses could reduce oxygenation due to a reduction in CO, causing a decrease in mixed venous oxygen content. Thoracic epidural anesthesia has no significant effect except at high doses (eg, 6-8 mL 0.75% ropivacaine at T_{7-8}); this tends to cause a reduction in arterial oxygenation,[31] which could similarly be due to decreased CO.

Improved oxygenation can be achieved through the use of an agent that increases HPV. One such agent is almitrine, a pulmonary vasoconstrictor, which has been shown during OLV to enhance arterial oxygenation when used in conjunction with an α_1-adrenergic receptor agonist. These agents have been suggested as useful adjuncts in conjunction with inhaled nitric oxide to treat severe hypoxemia during OLV. Nitric oxide (NO), because it is inhaled and works locally at gas exchange sites where it is distributed, is a selective vasodilator of well-ventilated gas exchange units and thus improves $\dot{V}_A/\dot{Q}$ matching. The combination of inhaled NO and intravenous almitrine may be especially effective at raising PaO_2 during OLV.

Gas Exchange Effects of pH Manipulation

Acidosis produces pulmonary vasoconstriction; alkalosis causes, pulmonary vasodilation. Hypocapnia has been shown in animals to inhibit HPV[32-34] and in dogs can be virtually abolished at a $PaCO_2$ of 20 mm Hg (pH ≈ 7.6). However, in humans more modest degrees of alkalosis (pH ≈ 7.5) induced by administration of tris buffer or sodium bicarbonate appear to have little or no effect.[35] Although acute respiratory acidosis induces pulmonary vasoconstriction, it does not appear to augment HPV.[33]

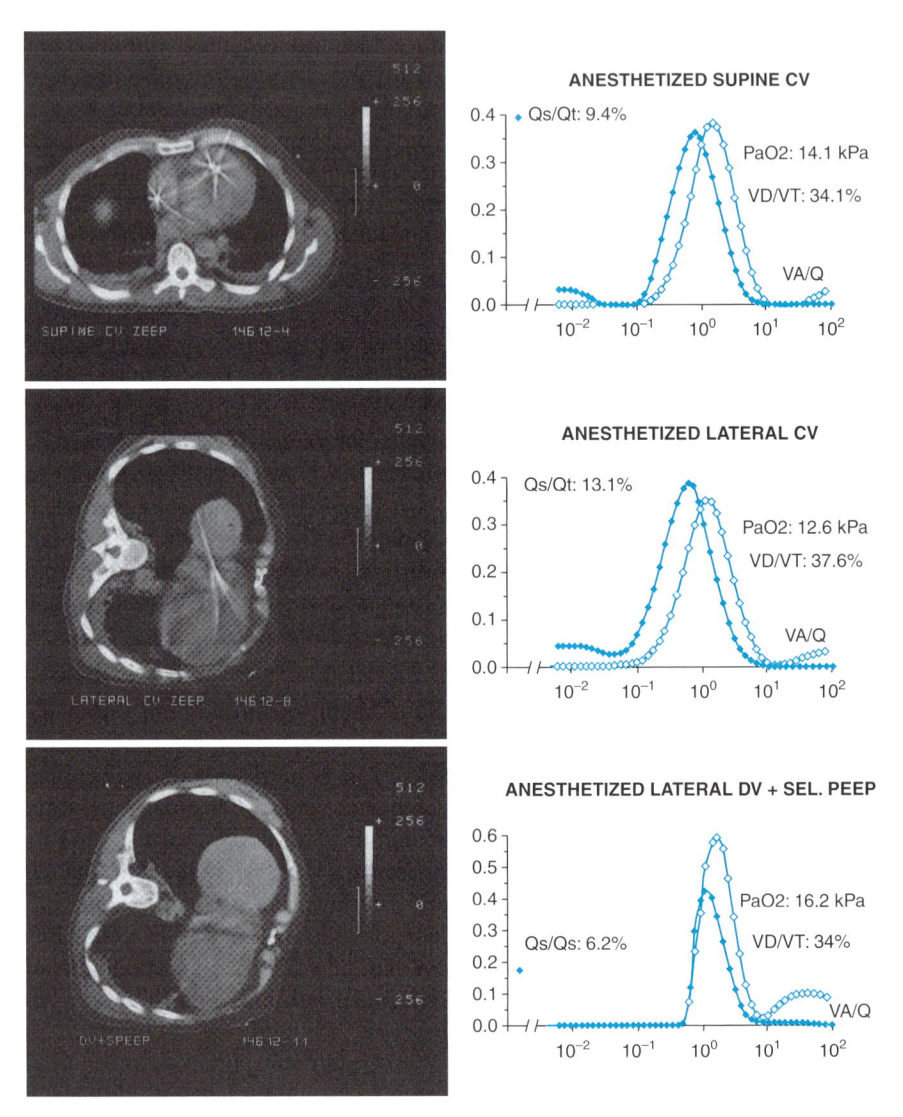

Figure 3–9. CT scans and V_A/Q distributions during anesthesia (open circles: ventilation, closed circles: blood flow, l/min) in a male (age 52, non-smoker). Upper panel: controlled ventilation (CV) with ZEEP supine; Middle panel: CV with zero end-inspiratory pressure (ZEEP), lateral; Lower panel: differential ventilation (DV) and selective PEEP, lateral. There are atelectatic areas in both lungs while supine, with a large shunt. Atelectatic areas in non-dependent lung are diminished in the lateral position, but shunt has not decreased and the number of regions with low V_A/Q ratios has increased. Atelectasis in the dependent lung and shunt flow were both reduced by DV + selective PEEP. (Reproduced from Klingstedt C, Hedenstierna G, Baehrendtz S, Lundqvist H, Strandberg A, Tokics L, Brismar B. Ventilation-perfusion relationships and atelectasis formation in the supine and lateral positions during conventional mechanical and differential ventilation. *Acta Anaesthesial Scand.* 1990;34:421-429. With permission of John Wiley & Sons, Inc.)

Mechanical Effects of Ventilation

Mechanical ventilation will increase pressure on the dependent hemithorax and thus tend to redistribute blood flow toward the nondependent lung, an effect that is augmented by hyperventilation and high levels of PEEP. If there is insufficient time to exhale fully, auto-PEEP can occur, which has the same effect (Figure 3–10).

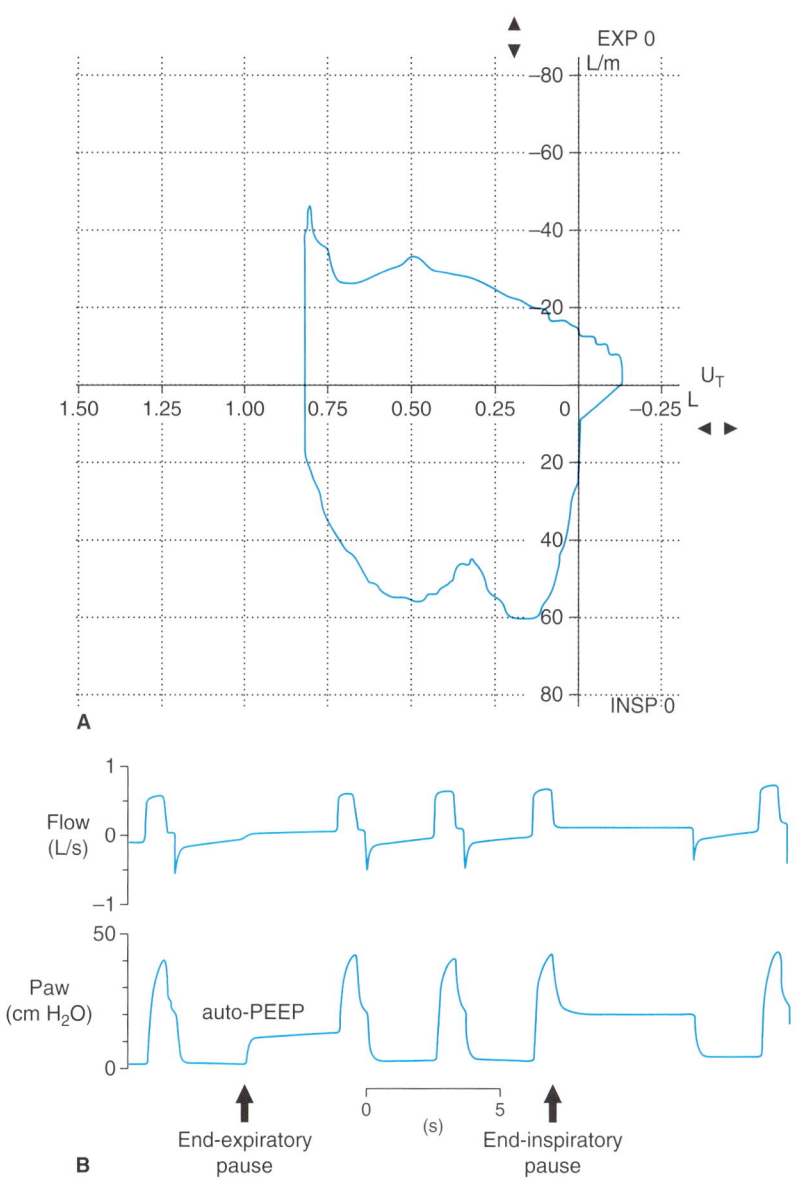

Figure 3–10. Detection of auto-PEEP. Flow and airway pressure (Paw) waveforms from a patient with chronic obstructive pulmonary disease, receiving mechanical ventilation.

Auto-PEEP is more likely to occur when airways resistance is high. Low levels of PEEP or auto-PEEP in the dependent lung may actually be helpful in reducing atelectasis, however auto-PEEP can increase dead space fraction, and hence $PaCO_2$, especially in patients with underlying emphysema. Auto-PEEP can also lead to decreased venous return and hypotension. It may also further augment redistribution of blood flow to the nonventilated lung, leading to a decrease in PaO_2. Auto-PEEP can be transiently eliminated by removal of the patient from the ventilator circuit and allowing adequate time for complete exhalation. It can be minimized by decreasing the amount of time spent in inspiration, by increasing the inspiratory:expiratory time (I:E ratio) or decreasing the minute ventilation and allowing the $PaCO_2$ to rise (permissive hypercapnia).

Positive pressure ventilation with high tidal volumes and unrecognized auto-PEEP can cause unintended pulmonary parenchymal damage. Studies on mechanically ventilated ICU patients who have underlying lung injury in the form of ARDS have consistently shown that minimizing lung volumes not only decreases inflammatory cytokines within the circulation but also decreases mortality associated with ARDS.[36-38] This may be a factor even within the relatively short time-frame of a surgical procedure, particularly if the transition from two-lung ventilation to OLV is not accompanied by a reduction in tidal volume. During OLV, maintenance of $PaCO_2$ within an acceptable range requires approximately the same ventilation as when both lungs are ventilated. However, after the transition from two-lung ventilation to OLV if tidal volume is not decreased, stretch injury is very likely to occur. This is particularly true for most surgical patients since the majority of thoracic procedures are performed on patients with significant underlying pulmonary parenchymal disease.

Pattern of Ventilation

Customary ventilatory strategy during general anesthesia incorporates constant tidal volume and rate (constant inter-breath interval). This however is very different from the normal ventilatory pattern, in which tidal volume and inter-breath interval vary from breath to breath. On cursory inspection this pattern appears random, although it is not. In fact, breathing usually exhibits fractal properties, where the inter-breath interval and tidal volume of a given breath are influenced by characteristics of breaths in the distant past.[39] Successful incorporation of a physiological breathing pattern into mechanical ventilation has been demonstrated in a porcine model of acute lung injury, using a pattern derived from a spontaneously breathing anesthetized pig.[40] The advantage of such "biologically variable ventilation (BVV)" has subsequently been shown for low tidal volume ventilation in ARDS.[41] In humans undergoing abdominal aortic aneurysm repair, BVV produced higher PaO_2, lower $PaCO_2$, lower dead space ventilation, increased compliance and lower mean peak inspiratory pressure.[42] Improved PaO_2 using BVV during OLV has been demonstrated in pigs.[43] Human studies during OLV have not yet been published, however evidence thus far available suggests that of biologically variable ventilation may provide an additional method of improving arterial oxygenation.

SUMMARY

Pulmonary gas exchange during OLV is governed by several factors, including mechanical factors that govern the distribution of pulmonary blood flow, such as ventilation of the single lung and collapse of the nondependent lung, hypoxic pulmonary vasoconstriction, CO, and mixed venous oxygen content. Vasodilators can attenuate HPV and thus may lower PaO_2, although this may be offset by increased CO. Manipulation of these factors during OLV can usually achieve acceptable $PaCO_2$ and PaO_2. Stretch injury of the ventilated lung is a serious concern when inappropriately high tidal volumes are used.

REFERENCES

1. Don H. The mechanical properties of the respiratory system during anesthesia. *Int Anesthesiol Clin.* 1977;15(2):113-136.
2. Rehder K, Hatch DJ, Sessler AD, Fowler WS. The function of each lung of anesthetized and paralyzed man during mechanical ventilation. *Anesthesiology.* 1972;37(1):16-26.
3. Warner DO, Warner MA. Human chest wall function while awake and during halothane anesthesia. II. Carbon dioxide rebreathing. *Anesthesiology.* 1995;82(1):20-31.
4. Kaneko K, Milic-Emili J, Dolovich MB, Dawson A, Bates DV. Regional distribution of ventilation and perfusion as a function of body position. *J Appl Physiol.* 1966;21(3):767-777.
5. Ducros L, Moutafis M, Castelain MH, Liu N, Fischler M. Pulmonary air trapping during two-lung and one-lung ventilation. *J Cardiothorac Vasc Anesth.* 1999;13(1):35-39.
6. Conhaim RL, Staub NC. Reflection spectrophotometric measurement of O2 uptake in pulmonary arterioles of cats. *J Appl Physiol.* 1980;48(5):848-856.
7. Mure M, Domino KB, Robertson T, Hlastala MP, Glenny RW. Pulmonary blood flow does not redistribute in dogs with reposition from supine to left lateral position. *Anesthesiology.* 89(2):483-492.
8. Chang H, Lai-Fook SJ, Domino KB, et al. Spatial distribution of ventilation and perfusion in anesthetized dogs in lateral postures. *J Appl Physiol.* 2002;92(2):745-762.
9. West JB. Effects of ventilation-perfusion inequality on over-all gas exchange studied in computer models of the lung. *J Physiol.* 1969;202(2):116P+.
10. West JB, Dollery CT, Naimark A. Distribution of blood flow in isolated lung: relation to vascular and alveolar pressures. *J Appl Physiol.* 1964;19:713-724.
11. West JB. Studies of pulmonary and cardiac function using short-lived isotopes oxygen-15, nitrogen-13 and carbon-11. *Prog At Med.* 1968;2:39-64.
12. Glenny RW. Blood flow distribution in the lung. *Chest.* 1998;114(1 Suppl):8S-16S.
13. Robertson HT, Hlastala MP. Microsphere maps of regional blood flow and regional ventilation. *J Appl Physiol.* 2007;102(3):1265-1272.
14. Sommer N, Dietrich A, Schermuly RT, et al. Regulation of hypoxic pulmonary vasoconstriction: basic mechanisms. *Eur Respir J.* 2008;32(6):1639-1651.
15. Archer SL, Weir EK, Reeve HL, Michelakis E. Molecular identification of O_2 sensors and O_2-sensitive potassium channels in the pulmonary circulation. *Adv Exp Med Biol.* 2000;475:219-240.
16. Sham JS, Crenshaw BR Jr, Deng LH, Shimoda LA, Sylvester JT. Effects of hypoxia in porcine pulmonary arterial myocytes: roles of K(V) channel and endothelin-1. *Am J Physiol Lung Cell Mol Physiol.* 2000;279(2):L262-272.
17. McMahon TJ, Moon RE, Luschinger BP, et al. Nitric oxide in the human respiratory cycle. *Nat Med.* 2002;8(7):711-717.
18. O'Brien RF, Robbins RJ, McMurtry IF. Endothelial cells in culture produce a vasoconstrictor substance. *J Cell Physiol.* 1987;132(2):263-270.
19. Hieda HS, Gomez-Sanchez CE. Hypoxia increases endothelin release in bovine endothelial cells in culture, but epinephrine, norepinephrine, serotonin, histamine and angiotensin II do not. *Life Sci.* 1990;47(3):247-251.

20. Rakugi H, Tabuchi Y, Nakamaru M, et al. Evidence for endothelin-1 release from resistance vessels of rats in response to hypoxia. *Biochem Biophys Res Commun.* 1990;169(3):973-977.
21. MacLean MR, McCulloch KM, Baird M. Endothelin ETA- and ETB-receptor-mediated vasoconstriction in rat pulmonary arteries and arterioles. *J Cardiovasc Pharmacol.* 1994;23(5):838-845.
22. Domino KB, Hlastala MP, Eisenstein BL, Cheney FW. Effect of regional alveolar hypoxia on gas exchange in dogs. *J Appl Physiol.* 1989;67(2):730-735.
23. Rogers SN, Benumof JL. Halothane and isoflurane do not decrease PaO2 during one-lung ventilation in intravenously anesthetized patients. *Anesth Analg.* 1985;64(10):946-954.
24. Eger EI, Severinghaus JW. The rate of rise of PaCO2 in the apneic anesthetized patient. *Anesthesiology.* 1961;22:419-425.
25. Frumin MJ, Epstein RM, Cohen G. Apneic oxygenation in man. *Anesthesiology.* 1959;20:789-798.
26. Ko R, McRae K, Darling G, et al. The use of air in the inspired gas mixture during two-lung ventilation delays lung collapse during one-lung ventilation. *Anesth Analg.* 2009;108(4):1092-1096.
27. Ishikawa S, Nakazawa K, Makita K. Progressive changes in arterial oxygenation during one-lung anaesthesia are related to the response to compression of the non-dependent lung. *Br J Anaesth.* 2003;90(1):21-26.
28. Park SY, Kim DH, Kim JS, Lee SS, Hong YW. Effects of head-up tilt on intrapulmonary shunt fraction and oxygenation during 1-lung ventilation in the lateral decubitus position. *J Thorac Cardiovasc Surg.* 2010;139(6):1436-1440.
29. Bjertnaes LJ, Hauge A, Nakken KF, Bredesen JE. Hypoxic pulmonary vasoconstriction: inhibition due to anesthesia. *Acta Physiol Scand.* 1976;96(2):283-285.
30. Bardoczky GI, Szegedi LL, d'Hollander AA, Moures JM, de Francquen P, Yernault JC. Two-lung and one-lung ventilation in patients with chronic obstructive pulmonary disease: the effects of position and FiO$_2$. *Anesth Analg.* 2000;90(1):35-41.
31. Xu Y, Tan Z, et al. Effect of thoracic epidural anesthesia with different concentrations of ropivacaine on arterial oxygenation during one-lung ventilation. *Anesthesiology.* 2010;112(5):1146-1154.
32. Lloyd TC, Jr. Influence of blood pH on hypoxic pulmonary vasoconstriction. *J Appl Physiol.* 1996;21(2):358-364.
33. Benumof JL, Wahrenbrock EA. Blunted hypoxic pulmonary vasoconstriction by increased lung vascular pressures. *J Appl Physiol.* 1975;38(5):846-850.
34. Benumof JL, Mathers JM, Wahrenbrock EA. Cyclic hypoxic pulmonary vasoconstriction induced by concomitant carbon dioxide changes. *J Appl Physiol.* 1976;41(4):466-469.
35. Bergofsky EH, Lehr DE, Fishman AP. The effect of changes in hydrogen ion concentration on the pulmonary circulation. *J Clin Invest.* 1962;41:1492-1502.
36. Ventilation with lower tidal volumes as compared with traditional tidal volumes for acute lung injury and the acute respiratory distress syndrome. The Acute Respiratory Distress Syndrome Network. *N Engl J Med.* 2000;342(18):1301-1308.
37. Kallet RH, Jasmer RM, Pittet JF, et al. Clinical implementation of the ARDS network protocol is associated with reduced hospital mortality compared with historical controls. *Crit Care Med.* 2005;33(5):925-929.
38. MacIntyre N. Ventilatory Management of ALI/ARDS. *Semin Respir Crit Care Med.* 2006;27(4):396-403.
39. Fadel PJ, Barman SM, Phillips SW, Gebber GL. Fractal fluctuations in human respiration. *J Appl Physiol.* 2004;97(6):2056-2064.
40. Lefevre GR, Kowalski SE, Girling LG, Thiessen DB, Mutch WA. Improved arterial oxygenation after oleic acid lung injury in the pig using a computer-controlled mechanical ventilator. *Am J Respir Crit Care Med.* 1996;154(5):1567-1572.
41. Boker A, Graham MR, Walley KR, et al. Improved arterial oxygenation with biologically variable or fractal ventilation using low tidal volumes in a porcine model of acute respiratory distress syndrome. *Am J Respir Crit Care Med.* 2002;165(4):456-462.
42. Boker A, Haberman CJ, Girling L, et al. Variable ventilation improves perioperative lung function in patients undergoing abdominal aortic aneurysmectomy. *Anesthesiology.* 2004;100(3):608-616.
43. McMullen MC, Girling LG, Graham MR, Mutch WA. Biologically variable ventilation improves oxygenation and respiratory mechanics during one-lung ventilation. *Anesthesiology.* 2006;105(1):91-97.

Perioperative Management of the Patient with Pulmonary Hypertension

4

E. Andrew Ochroch

Pulmonary hypertension is a common but underappreciated pathological condition in patients who undergo thoracic surgery, and being unaware of this condition or underestimating its severity can lead to significant perioperative complications. Management of this condition requires foresight and preparation as discussed in this chapter. Thus, this chapter will serve to: (1) review the pathogenesis of pulmonary hypertension, (2) describe the preoperative preparation and evaluation of patients with pulmonary hypertension who present for thoracic surgery, (3) explain the effects of anesthesia and surgery on the pulmonary vasculature, and (4) define the proper use of the pharmacological aids to control pulmonary hypertension.

NORMAL PULMONARY PHYSIOLOGY AND HYPOXIC PULMONARY VASOCONSTRICTION

At rest, the normal pulmonary vascular system is noted as a high-compliance, high-flow, low-pressure system. This stands in contrast to the systemic circulation, which has much higher resting level of arterial and venous tone. This difference stems partly from the anatomy because the pulmonary precapillary arterioles have a thinner media and less smooth muscle than their systemic counterparts. Furthermore, at rest, there are far more recruitable vessels in the pulmonary bed, which permits dramatic increases in flow with minimal impact on pressure.

The difference between the systemic and arterial systems is also due to the response of the pulmonary vascular endothelium to the challenges of hypoxia (hypoxic pulmonary vasoconstriction: HPV). This vasoconstriction is known as the Euler-Lijestrand reflex. Mitochondria play a key role as the primary sensor of hypoxia, with intracellular calcium increasing as a key response, but the basic mechanism is controversial.[1] Figure 4–1 displays several of the key pathways for hypoxic vasoconstriction in which voltage gated potassium (K^+) channels directly alter mitochondrial responses. L-type calcium (Ca^{2+}) channels are facilitated by the depolarization of the K^+ channels; they then directly increase intracellular Ca^{2+}. Further, classical transient receptor potential channel 6 (TRPC6) also increases intracellular Ca^{2+} as do store operated channels (SOC) and sodium (Na^+)/Ca^{2+} exchangers (NCX).[1] This rise in intracellular Ca^{2+} also triggers release from sarcoplasmic reticulum via activation of the ryanodine receptors. The end result is

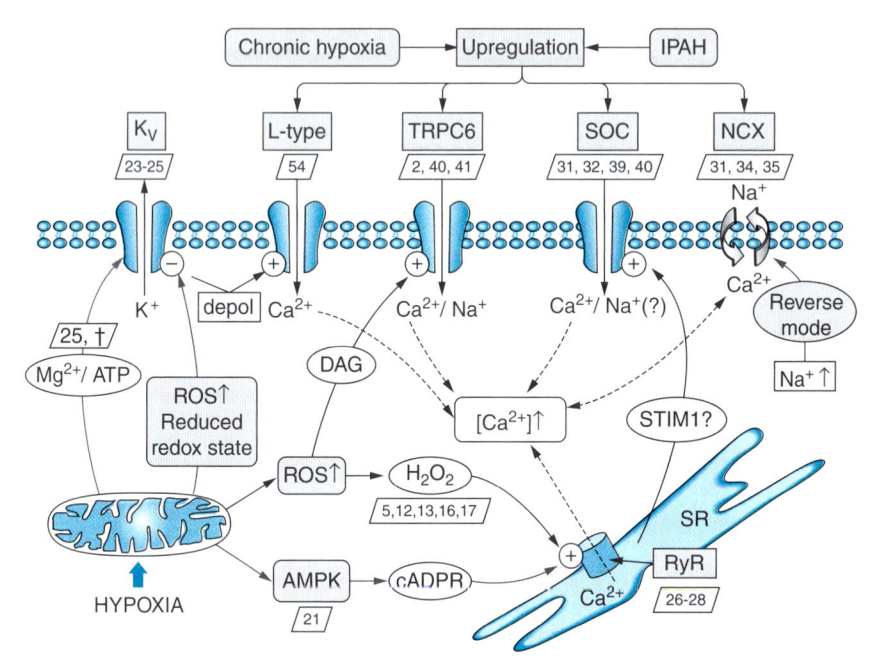

Figure 4-1. Ca^{2+} mobilization in HPV: mechanisms that have been implicated in the hypoxia-induced elevation of [Ca^{2+}], and their potential signaling pathways. Note that some mechanisms are probably only applicable to one phase of HPV (see text). Not shown for clarity: possibility of functionally different types of SOC and Ca^{2+} store. Note that Na^+ entry via NSCC would also contribute to depolarization. y: action of Mg^{2+} and ATP on K_V channels depends on membrane potential (see text). DAG, diacylglycerol; cADPR, cyclic ADP ribose; depol, depolarization; K_V, voltage-gated K^+ channels; L-type, voltage-gated Ca^{2+} channels; NCX, Na^+-Ca^{2+} exchanger; RyR, ryanodine receptors; SOC, store-operated channels. TRPC6, classical transient receptor potential channel 6. (From: Ward J, McMurtry I. Mechanisms of hypoxic pulmonary vasoconstriction and their roles in pulmonary hypertension: new findings for an old problem. *Curr Opin Pharmacol.* 2009;9(3):287-296, with permission. Copyright © Elsevier.)

constriction of the smooth muscle of the precapillary sphincters and pulmonary arterioles. This calcium-dependent vasoconstriction is the primary phase of HPV and lasts 15 to 30 minutes. The Ca^{2+} independent phase (the sustained phase) of pulmonary vascular constriction starts at 15 minutes and can last for hours. It is highly dependent on RhoA/Rho kinase (ROCK) mediated Ca^{2+} sensitization,[2] and may be a key to the development of pulmonary hypertension.[3] Interestingly, nitric oxide (NO)-induced relaxation and endothelin-1-induced vasoconstriction of pulmonary arteries have been shown to be due to regulation of ROCK-mediated Ca^{2+}-sensitization, rather than altered Ca^{2+} metabolism.[4,5] See Figure 4–1.

Anesthetics can influence pulmonary vascular function and inhibit HPV. Inhalational agents (halothane, enflurane, isoflurane, desflurane, and sevoflurane) will all inhibit HPV, but at concentrations of greater than 1 MAC,[6] However, intravenous anesthetics such as propofol have a less profound impact on HPV than the inhalational agents.[7] Opioids, benzodiazepines, and epidural analgesia/anesthesia have minimal impact. For further discussion on the effect of anesthetic drugs on HPV see Chapter 3.

PULMONARY HYPERTENSION

The pathologic changes of pulmonary hypertension (PH) stem directly from a derangement of the basic mechanisms that lead to HPV. The increased vasoconstriction of the pulmonary arteries in PH has been attributed to a reduced expression or activity of voltage-gated K⁺ channels and dysfunction of the endothelium and platelets; this leads to imbalances in the production and release of both vasodilators such as NO and prostacyclin (PGI_2) as well as vasoconstrictors such as endothelin-1 (ET-1) and serotonin (5-HT).[8] Many of these regulators of vascular tone also have roles in the control of cell proliferation and apoptosis and thus may also contribute to the characteristic remodeling of the pulmonary vasculature in PH.[3] Much of the pharmacologic management of PH is directed toward modulating these known mechanisms.

Pulmonary hypertension is diagnosed by measurements indicating that mean pulmonary arterial pressure (mPAP) exceeds 25 mm Hg at rest and 30 mm Hg during exercise. To make the diagnosis of primary PH left ventricular end diastolic pressure or pulmonary capillary wedge pressure has to be ≤15 mm Hg and the pulmonary vascular resistance (PVR) greater than 3 Wood units (mm Hg/L: 1 Wood unit = 80 dyn.cm.sec-5).[9] Secondary PH is due to the increase in pulmonary vascular impedance from intrinsic parenchymal lung disease. Increased PVR, which requires the right ventricle (RV) to raise pulmonary artery pressure (PAP) to maintain cardiac output, can cause failure of the afterload-intolerant RV, ultimately leading to death. Median survival time for untreated idiopathic PH (formerly included in primary PH) in a historical series was 2.8 years.[10]

There are a myriad of causes of PH, and the World Health Organization's list of causes is shown in Table 4–1.[11] The most common cause of PH in patients presenting for lung cancer resection is cigarette smoking. Acute exposure to tobacco smoke increases vasoconstriction through multiple routes including increased expression of endothelin-1 (ET-1).[12] Tobacco smoke also causes a widespread injury to the lung with epithelial and endothelial apoptosis and necrosis.[13,14] Further, the normal healing mechanisms for the lung are inhibited by apoptosis of alveolar macrophages and release/expression of other inflammatory mediators.[15] The "earliest" pathology in the lungs of smokers is the development of intimal thickening of pulmonary arteries, the severity of which is correlated to the pack-year history.[16] Thus, the lung and vascular changes seen in PH associated with chronic obstructive pulmonary disease (COPD) may represent alternate pathways and responses to the damage of tobacco smoke.[17]

Table 4–1. World Health Organization Classification of Pulmonary Hypertension

Group 1: PAH Idiopathic Familial Associated with Collagen vascular disease Congenital systemic-to-pulmonic shunt Portal hypertension HIV infection Drugs and toxins Other: thyroid disorders, glycogen storage disease, Gaucher's disease, hereditary hemorrhagic telangiectasia, hemoglobinopathies, myeloproliferative disorders, splenectomy associated with significant venous or capillary involvement Pulmonary veno-occlusive disease Pulmonary capillary hemangiomatosis Persistent pulmonary hypertension of the newborn
Group 2: Pulmonary hypertension with left heart disease Left-sided ventricular or atrial disease Left-sided valvular disease
Group 3: Pulmonary hypertension associated with lung disease and/or hypoxemia Chronic obstructive lung disease Interstitial lung disease Sleep-disordered breathing Alveolar hypoventilation disorders Chronic exposure to high altitude Developmental abnormalities
Group 4: Pulmonary hypertension due to chronic thrombotic and/or embolic disease Thromboembolic obstruction of proximal pulmonary arteries Thromboembolic obstruction of distal pulmonary arteries
Group 5: Miscellaneous Sarcoidosis, histiocytosis X, lymphangiomyomatosis, compression of pulmonary vessels (adenopathy, tumor, fibrosing mediastinitis)

Based on the 2003 World Symposium.[11]

EFFECTS OF PULMONARY RESECTION ON RIGHT VENTRICULAR AND PULMONARY VASCULAR DYNAMICS

Lung resection reduces the available cross section of pulmonary vasculature. This is typically very well-tolerated at rest. However, when post-thoracotomy patients are examined in detail, cardiac output and stroke volume decrease, while pulmonary and systemic resistance increase.[18] One study examined 40 "normal" subjects and 40 subjects with PH or restrictive pulmonary disease for thoracotomy utilizing transthoracic echocardiography and PA catheter data, preoperatively and postoperatively. They found that preoperatively the subjects with PH had higher right ventricular end diastolic volume (RVEDV), lower RV ejection fraction (RVEF), and higher pulmonary artery wedge pressures. After lobectomy or bi-lobectomy, all subjects demonstrated a rise in RVEDV, PVR and wedge pressure with a fall in RVEF. Subjects with preexisting PH or restrictive lung disease had a greater rise in RVEDV, PVR and wedge and a greater fall in RVEF than "normal" subjects.[19] The authors comment that the rise in RVEDV and RV end diastolic pressure in subjects with PH caused a trend toward new postoperative wall motion abnormalities in the RV, suggesting that the myocardium was at significant risk.

PREOPERATIVE MEDICAL MANAGEMENT OF PATIENTS WITH PULMONARY HYPERTENSION

Many patients with PH receive warfarin, diuretics, digoxin, and oxygen. These treatments are often referred to as background or conventional therapy. Diuretics and digoxin provide symptomatic relief but are not thought to affect the course of the disease. Warfarin might provide a survival advantage due to altered platelet and endothelial function in PH, but its contribution is difficult to estimate.[20] Calcium channel blockers, such as nifedipine, offer considerable benefit to the patients that respond to them, although these account for only around 6% of patients with PH.[21]

Patients with PH have reduced production of prostacyclin (PGI_2), a product of the arachidonic acid cascade that promotes vasodilation and inhibits vascular proliferation and platelet aggregation.[22] Activation of the prostacyclin receptor by PGI_2 produces activation of the enzyme adenylate cyclase, increased intracellular cyclic adenosine monophosphate levels, and opening of Ca^{2+}-activated K^+ channels.[23] Increased K^+ conductance produces hyperpolarization of the cell membrane, blockade of L-type Ca^{2+} channels, and decreased cytosolic Ca^{2+}. The net result of this process in the vascular smooth muscle cell is relaxation with consequent vasodilation. Epoprostenol was the first PGI_2 replacement to be studied; in addition to symptomatic improvement, it has been shown to offer a survival advantage.[22,24,25] However, its administration (intravenous, via an indwelling catheter) is complex and it causes adverse effects such as decreased platelet function, hypotension, headache, nausea, and diarrhea.

Other prostanoid analogues have since been studied, including iloprost (inhalation),[26] treprostinil (IV)[27] and beraprost (oral).[25] The duration of hemodynamic effect of nebulized iloprost averages approximately 90 minutes after inhalation; the drug requires 6 to 9 nebulizer treatments per 24 hours, with each treatment requiring up to 10 to 20 minutes. While iloprost improved 6-minute walk performance similar to epoprostenol, its use is cumbersome for outpatients. Treprostinil was developed as a longer acting intravenous epoprostenol, so that brief interruptions of the delivery would not have dramatic consequences. Beraprost is an oral drug that is under evaluation. Data from clinical trials support the short-term benefits of these drugs[22] but their cost-effectiveness has been challenged by the United Kingdom's National Institute for Health and Clinical Excellence.[28]

As previously discussed, in PH there is an imbalance between endogenous production of vasodilators and vasoconstrictors, with decreased levels of PGI_2 and increased levels of endothelin-1.[22] Endothelin-1 is a vasoconstrictor which acts via two receptors, ET_A and ET_B to both regulate vascular tone and cell proliferation.

Both receptor subtypes are found on vascular smooth muscle cells and their activation causes vasoconstriction, probably by augmenting Rho kinase Ca^{2+} sensitivity,[4] while the ET_B receptor activation on endothelial cells increases NO and prostacyclin release. There are three clinically available ET blockers: bosentan, a nonspecific blocker, and ambrisentan and sitaxsentan, which selectively block ET_A. These drugs improve 6-minute walk distance, improve functionality and delay progression of PH.[29] Hepatotoxicity limits their usefulness in some patients, and anemia is common. These drugs are eliminated through the cytochrome P450 system, and thus may alter anesthetic drug half-life.[29]

Pulmonary vascular tone can also be reduced through phosphodiesterase inhibitors. Sildenafil is a selective inhibitor of phosphodiesterase type 5 (PDE_5). Present throughout the body, PDE_5 is found in high concentrations in the lungs. Inhibition of PDE_5 enhances the vasodilatory effects of nitric oxide in PH by preventing the degradation of cyclic guanosine monophosphate (cGMP).[30,31] When added to conventional therapy, sildenafil increased exercise capacity in patients with PH due to both decreased PVR and improved ventilation-perfusion matching.[31] Sildenafil was also associated with improvements in the World Health Organization functional class and hemodynamic parameters. Sildenafil has a short half-life, and it requires dosing three times a day for clinical effectiveness.

PREOPERATIVE PREPARATION

Preoperative preparation of patients with lung cancer is typically foreshortened due to the threat of metastasis. Several reviews and meta-analyses have focused on perioperative pulmonary complications and strategies to reduce morbidity and mortality. Collectively, these reviews indicate that most risk factors are not modifiable; the surgical incision site has been identified as the single most important risk factor, with thoracic incisions placing the patient at significant risk (odds ratio [OR] of 4.24) for perioperative morbidity and mortality.[32-34] Age was the most important patient-related predictor with postoperative pulmonary complication rates being linearly related: age 50 to 59: 6.1%, age 60 to 69: 8.1% and 70 to 79: 11.9%.[35] In a multivariate model that adjusted for cardiac and pulmonary comorbidities, the OR of postoperative pulmonary complication also varied by age 50 to 59 years OR 1.5 (CI 1.31–1.74), 60 to 69 OR 2.28 (CI 1.86–2.8), and 70 to 79 OR 3.9 (CI 2.7–5.7).[33] Traditional spirometry did not stratify risk, and smoking cessation within 8 weeks of surgery did not impact risk.[32-34]

Although it is important to consider the risk of pulmonary complications in patients undergoing thoracic operations, epidemiologic studies have shown that perioperative cardiac complications remain the leading cause of death after anesthesia and surgery.[36-38] Most of the data regarding perioperative myocardial risk comes from studies of noncardiac surgical patients, of whom thoracic surgical patients were only a small proportion. For example, The Coronary Artery Surgery Study (CASS) registry reported 1600 operations over a 3-year period. However, only 89 of the 1600 were thoracic operations.[39] Consequently, the published estimates of perioperative cardiac morbidity do not address the risks incurred specifically from the perturbations of the thoracic procedure itself on the typical patient presenting for thoracic surgery. Instead, they address the average risk of a patient with coronary risk factors undergoing either high-risk or low-risk procedures. While few studies have addressed the incidence of perioperative cardiovascular complications in thoracic surgical patients selectively, it is likely that cardiovascular events are a major cause of perioperative mortality in this subgroup. Further discussion on cardiac and pulmonary complications following thoracic surgery procedures may be found in Chapter 24.

Pulmonary Rehabilitation

Pulmonary rehabilitation combines optimizing bronchodilator management, improving anti-inflammatory therapy, treating preexisting pneumonia/atelectasis, increasing exercise capacity, and optimizing oxygen therapy. Typical regimens last 4 to 9 weeks. Although lung mechanics are usually not altered, exercise capacity, severity of dyspnea and quality of life are improved.[40] One small trial of pulmonary rehabilitation in patients with Stage 1 lung cancer indicated that while exercise capacity increased, no discernable effect on perioperative morbidity was found.[41] Specifically for PH, only prolonged oxygen therapy has been shown to stop the progression of the disease, but not to reverse the condition.[42]

Determination of Presence of Pulmonary Hypertension

Pulmonary hypertension is an uncommon and underdiagnosed disease. Although the effect of PH on perioperative outcome of thoracic procedures has not been extensively studied, preoperative diagnosis should promote optimal intra- and postoperative care. Determining whom to evaluate for PH is difficult, because the typical presenting symptoms of PH, such as breathlessness, decreased exercise tolerance, and fatigue, are nonspecific and easily attributable to COPD. In patients with COPD significant enough to be evaluated for lung volume reduction surgery, pulmonary function tests did not distinguish between those with and without PH. A study by Bach et al, determined that PaO_2 while breathing room air was significantly lower in PH patients (51.5 +/− 1.4 vs 69 +/− 1.3 mm Hg, p = 0.000008), but this finding had a poor positive and negative predictive value.[43] Similarly, end tidal CO_2 did not distinguish those with and without PH. However, this study only examined the criteria for PH at rest. When patients with significant or severe COPD were examined for PH during exercise, one-third met criteria with mean PA pressures greater than 30 mm Hg.[44] Consequently, patients with COPD may have limited cardiopulmonary reserve to deal with exercise or perioperative challenges due to rises in pulmonary artery pressures.

In patients with PH, or those suspected of it, further testing may help to delineate risk. Trans-thoracic echocardiography (TTE) can provide significant data on cardiac function. Of 207 subjects with significant COPD studied prior to surgery with TTE, 98% had adequate studies of right and left ventricular wall motion. Right heart abnormalities were found in 40% of subjects and included right atrial enlargement (32%), right ventricular hypertrophy (12%), and RV systolic dysfunction (7%).[43] Unfortunately, pulmonary arterial pressure could not be consistently measured as it relies on detection and measurement of tricuspid regurgitant jet, not attainable in all patients.

Right heart catheterization has also been used in an attempt to better assess risk. Patients who had exercise induced decreases in RVEF were at significantly greater risk for developing postoperative cardiopulmonary complications than patients who had exercise induced increases in RVEF.[45] The authors claim that decreases in RVEF in response to exercise indicated a limited cardiopulmonary reserve. Further reduction of the pulmonary vascular bed after lung resection may stress this limited reserve leading to an increased risk of cardiopulmonary decompensation and complications.[45] Similarly, unilateral pulmonary artery occlusion has been used to determine if the right heart can compensate for a decrease in the vascular bed by assessing the subsequent rise in total pulmonary vascular resistance.[46] Unfortunately, both of these methods are highly invasive and risky, and neither have been prospectively evaluated in randomized, blind studies; neither methods are commonly used.

There are no studies in which pulmonary pressures have been linked to outcome after thoracic surgery. The oft-quoted cutoff of 35 mm Hg for maximal pulmonary pressure for pulmonary resection candidates is an arbitrary number that originated from guidelines for lung volume reduction surgery patients.[45] It remains unclear if there is a better test to determine likelihood of postsurgical survival than having the patient walk two flights of stairs, as it is primarily a broad test of cardiopulmonary reserve.

PERIOPERATIVE CARE

Coagulation and Epidural Analgesia

All preoperative medications for the management of PH should be continued except warfarin. Perioperative management of coagulation will depend on the patient's history of thromboembolic disease with the understanding that all patients with PH are at increased risk of embolism due to increased platelet adhesion.[47] This embolic risk needs to be balanced against the significant benefit of epidural analgesia. Similarly, if patients are receiving intravenous prostacyclin, epidural catheterization needs to be considered in the light of the significant platelet inhibition. Acute withdrawal of intravenous prostacyclin puts the patient at significant risk of rebound pulmonary hypertension. A discussion with the patient's pulmonologist needs to occur to determine if the patient can be safely transitioned to inhaled prostacyclin immediately prior to the operation. The 5-minute half-life of IV prostacyclin would allow for epidural placement 15 to 20 minutes after transition to inhaled medication. While the use of epidural analgesia is both desirable and important, the amount of sympathetic blockade of the epidural must be increased slowly to allow time for adequate right heart preload to occur, to prevent hypotension and to avoid decreased myocardial perfusion.

Central Venous Catheterization

Central venous pressure (CVP) monitoring can provide valuable information used to direct perioperative therapy and permit indirect monitoring of right heart function. Typically the CVP should be placed on the operative side due to the small risk of pneumothorax. Once the patient is positioned, the CVP waveform itself should be closely analyzed and printed out, because the waveform can indicate right ventricular and valvular abnormalities.[48] A central catheter is also preferred for delivery of concentrated cardiac and vascular medications.

Pulmonary Artery Catheterization

The usefulness of pulmonary artery catheterization (PAC) in CABG and vascular surgery is hotly debated as a PAC has never been demonstrated to improve outcome.[49-52] Further, PAC use in thoracic surgery has never been studied prospectively in humans in sufficient numbers to determine the effect on outcome. Despite the paucity of data, PAC catheters are successfully used in clinical care,[53,54] but authors note a need for caution;[55] it has been recommended that a PAC needs to be placed preoperatively with fluoroscopic guidance to ensure placement into the nonoperative lung. The alternative is the process of: (1) placing the catheter during two-lung ventilation, (2) withdrawing the catheter into the main PA or RV prior to OLV, and (3) readvancing the catheter once the operative lung is collapsed due to the continued uncertainty of the placement of the catheter in the surgical field. Although the surgeon can place a temporary clamp on the main PA on the surgical side prior to readvancement of a PAC, this procedure increases cardiac stress; PH patients are especially at risk and the temporary clamp may be enough to trigger right heart failure. Regardless of the choice of positioning techniques, the CVP and PA waveforms need to be closely analyzed and printed out, as their baseline shape holds information that is probably more important than the absolute number.[48] Waveform changes can indicate ventricular failure, regurgitant valvular lesions, and changes in volume status.

Transesophageal Echocardiography

Transesophageal echocardiography (TEE) is a profoundly powerful tool for perioperative hemodynamic measurement. TEE in thoracic surgical patients has been reviewed, with most of the data derived from lung transplant patients.[56] The TEE probe is best placed while the patient is supine, but can be placed with the patient in the lateral position; prior planning and coordination are optimal. While the presence of a double lumen tube may make passage more difficult and increase the risk of oral and/or esophageal injury, TEE probes have been successfully placed for many types of thoracic surgery using caution and skill. However, an option to be considered is the use of a single lumen tube and a bronchial blocker when intraoperative TEE monitoring is planned. TEE has the advantage of determining volume status, ventricular performance, and valvular function.

Comparison of Echocardiography and PA catheter

No prospective human data has been collected to compare the accuracy of PA catheters and echocardiography during the dynamic changes of RV and PA function with lateral positioning, OLV, and/or hypoxemia. When pigs were ventilated with hypoxemic mixtures, the PA catheter accurately tracked pulmonary pressures and RV area (loading), but could not track pulmonary vascular resistance.[57] Consequently, TEE maybe preferable for intraoperative management during thoracic surgery.

Induction and Maintenance

Typical goals of induction for thoracic surgery patients and patients with PH are nearly identical. Maintenance of hyperoxia and hypocarbia require a plan to maintain a patent airway and adequate ventilation at all times. Sympathetic stimulation of laryngoscopy and intubation needs to be thoroughly blunted without producing deleterious hypotension. Significant analgesia can be achieved from short-acting intravenous narcotics in 2 to 5 minutes;[58] this peak effect should be timed to occur during laryngoscopy. Lidocaine can also be used to reduce the response to laryngoscopy. Propofol, muscle relaxants, and mask ventilation are then used as usual. In the event of hypotension, as discussed below, phenylephrine is not the best agent for hypotension in PH patients; norepinephrine and vasopressin have theoretical advantages.

Maintenance of anesthesia during thoracic surgery requires attention to the activities of the surgeon. Given the typically long duration between induction and incision, epidural bupivacaine loaded after induction should blunt the majority of the reaction to the incision. Manipulation of the visceral pleura and bronchi stimulates vagal and phrenic afferents, which will not be blocked by epidural anesthesia (see Chapter 24) and may require supplemental inhalational agents.

The placement of the patient into the lateral decubitus position from the supine position can lead to abrupt hemodynamic changes including a decrease in preload due to venous pooling from bed flexion, particularly if the patient has a sympathectomy from the epidural anesthetic. Further, movement of the endotracheal tube with position changes can cause sympathetic stimulation. All of these positioning maneuvers may especially alter the stability of PH patients.

The initiation of OLV can also be fraught with risk in patients with PH and COPD. Hypoxemia and hypercarbia can lead to HPV with subsequent shunting of blood to the oxygenated, dependent lung. This will increase PVR, worsen PH and place the RV at risk of failure. However, without HPV, the shunt fraction could remain greater than 25% to 30%, which would also lead to hypoxemia. A typical maneuver to decrease shunt is the use of continuous positive airway pressure (CPAP) to the operative, nonventilated lung. If CPAP is unsuccessful, temporary occlusion of the operative pulmonary artery can be considered. Results of a preoperative pulmonary artery occlusion test will tell the anesthesiologist if intraoperative temporary clamping of the operative PA is an option, but this test is rarely performed. Two-lung ventilation should be maintained as long as possible and reinitiated as soon as possible.

INTRAOPERATIVE HYPOTENSION

There are four primary reasons for a thoracic surgical patient to become hypotensive:

1. Decreased SVR from the epidural analgesia/sympathectomy or inhaled anesthetics
2. Inadequate RV preload leading to inadequate left heart filling

3. RV failure from myocardial ischemia, increased PVR, embolism, LV failure, or new mitral regurgitation from myocardial ischemia
4. LV failure from myocardial ischemia

The detection of hypotension should be prompt and the treatment guided by clinical acumen and hemodynamic monitors. These issues are covered in depth in most major anesthesia and cardiovascular texts. They are briefly outlined in Table 4–2.

Table 4–2. Diagnosis of Hypotension with PAC

	CVP	PAD	PAS	PCWP	CO	SVR	Rx
↓**SVR**	↔↓	↓	↓↔	↓↔	↓↔	↓↓	volume vasopressin norepinephrine
↓**RV preload**	↓	↓	↓↔	↓↔	↓	↔	volume
RV failure LV failure	↑↔	↑	↑	↑↑	↓↓	↔↑	Optimize preload ↑systemic diastolic pressure epinephrine dobutamine IABP
RV failure ischemia	↑	↑	↑↔	↔↓	↓↓	↔	Optimize preload ↑systemic diastolic pressure epinephrine milrinone
RV failure embolism	↑↑	↑	↑	↓↓	↓↓	↑↔	Optimize preload ↑systemic diastolic pressure epinephrine milrinone
RV failure Mitral regugitation	↑↔	↑	↑↑: altered wave form	cannot obtain wedge	↓↓	↑↔	Optimize preload ↓ SVR HR ~ 100 bpm
RV failure Pulmonary	↑						
LV failure	↑↔	↑	↑↑	↑↑	↓↓	↔↑	Optimize preload ↑systemic diastolic pressure epinephrine dobutamine IABP

CVP = central venous pressure, PAD = pulmonary artery diastolic pressure, PAS = pulmonary artery systolic pressure, PCWP = pulmonary capillary wedge pressure, CO = cardiac output, SVR = systemic vascular resistance, Rx = suggested therapy, ↑= increased, ↔ = unchanged, ↓ = decreased, IABP = intra aortic balloon pump, HR = heart rate

Determination of Intraoperative Pulmonary Hypertension

Without CVP, PA, or TEE monitoring, determining PH as the cause of intraoperative hemodynamic compromise will be difficult, but it can be done as a matter of exclusion. The typical causes for hemodynamic compromise must be addressed. Hypoxemia and hypercarbia need to be corrected. Left ventricular failure is the most common cause of RV failure[59]; it should be addressed with fluid boluses and consideration for the use of inotropic support to optimize hemodynamics and ensure myocardial perfusion. Simultaneously, discussion with the surgeon needs to occur to determine if two-lung ventilation can be resumed, which will augment oxygenation, reduce pulmonary vascular tone and thus unload the right ventricle. Epinephrine is the agent of choice in a patient with hemodynamic compromise of undetermined etiology.[59]

Intraoperative echocardiography can be sought to quickly guide therapy. If the patient has significant esophageal disease, the experienced surgeon may perform an epicardial echocardiographic examination; very atypical images will be obtained, which will need to be evaluated by a person expert in echocardiography. While this application of echocardiography is a non-continuous monitor, it can provide valuable information.

INITIAL MANAGEMENT OF INTRAOPERATIVE PULMONARY HYPERTENSION

Once PH is determined, the initial management is to optimize ventilation to achieve hyperoxia, hypocarbia, and alkalosis.[60] This metabolic milieu minimizes HPV, optimizes ventilation/perfusion matching, and decreases PVR. However, careful attention to ventilatory patterns is crucial as over distension of the alveoli through high-ventilatory pressures, excessive PEEP or auto-PEEP can further increase PVR. With the diagnosis of PH, inhalational agents should be reduced to less than 1 MAC so as not to interfere with pulmonary vascular tone. After goal-oriented ventilation, RV inotropic support may be required with the recognition that the failing RV is volume dependent. End-diastolic RV volume should be optimized by intravascular volume expansion and maintenance of sinus rhythm. The heart rate should be high–normal, typically 90 to 100 beats per minute, since the failing RV is also rate sensitive.[59,61,62] (Table 4–3).

Milrinone, as an inodilator, not only augments RV systolic function but also decreases PVR, and therefore unloads the RV. Milrinone is a phosphodiesterase inhibitor and prevents breakdown of cyclic guanosine monophosphate (cGMP).[63] Higher intracellular cGMP levels explain milrinone's inodilatory effects. cGMP increases intracellular calcium levels which increase myocardial inotropy. Milrinone will often also cause systemic hypotension. Epinephrine, vasopressin or norepinephrine should be considered for the treatment of this hypotension, instead of phenylephrine.

Epinephrine directly increases intracellular myocardial cAMP through activation of β_1 adrenergic receptors; its inotropic effect is thus synergistic with milrinone, since they both increase myocardial second messengers by different mechanisms. Similar to epinephrine, dobutamine primarily activates β_1 adrenergic receptors. It has been used as a

Table 4-3. Initial Management of Pulmonary Hypertension

Intervention	Mechanism	Effect	Clinical Use
Metabolic measures	ensure hyperoxia, hypocarbia, alkalosis, normothermia and nomotension	↓ PVR unloads RV	initial strategy titrated to clinical effect and serial blood gases
Epinephrine (intravenous)	direct cAMP increase	↑ RV contractility ↑ PVR	dosage titrated to clinical effect and increase in PVR
Milrinone (intravenous)	inodilator and phosphodiesterase inhibitor indirect cAMP increase	↑ RV contractility ↓ PVR	synergistic effect with epinephrine limited by systemic hypotension
Iloprost (Inhaled)	selective pulmonary vasodilator	↓ PVR unloads RV	50 ng/min
Nitric Oxide (inhaled)	selective pulmonary vasodilator	↓ PVR unloads RV	In combination with inotropic support and/or intravenous prostaglandin

PVR = pulmonary vascular resistance, RV = right ventricle, cAMP = cyclic AMP

sole agent[64-66] or in conjunction with other inotropes and pulmonary vasodilators[59,64,67] to treat PH, left and right ventricular heart failure.

A selective pulmonary vasodilator should only be considered after all the aforementioned approaches have been implemented, particularly if RV failure or its inotropic state is in question.

SELECTIVE PULMONARY VASODILATORS

Inhaled NO (iNO) results in relaxation of pulmonary vascular smooth muscle. The intracellular mechanism involves activation of guanylate cyclase to produce cGMP. NO is then rapidly inactivated by binding to hemoglobin in the pulmonary vascular compartment, and therefore never reaches the systemic circulation.[68,69] This explains its lack of systemic effects; its pulmonary selectivity is due to its route of administration and its rapid inactivation. The clinical dosage of iNO is typically 5 to 40 parts per million.[69] The routine clinical application of iNO has been limited by a multitude of factors:

- High per day expense of administration (on the order of thousands of dollars per day of treatment).
- Reaction with oxygen in the lung to form nitrogen dioxide, a known trigger of pulmonary edema and bronchospasm. NO and nitrogen dioxide levels must be continuously monitored during iNO administration.
- Reaction with hemoglobin to form methemoglobin, which also must be monitored during iNO administration. Methemoglobin levels above 5% may cause hypoxia and thus may require management with methylene blue.[69]

- Possible pulmonary edema in isolated left ventricular dysfunction. Since NO decreases PVR, it may increase pulmonary blood flow, and hence acutely increase left ventricular end-diastolic volume. This may trigger left ventricular failure.[70]
- Rebound PH with hypoxemia and RV failure during rapid iNO weaning.[69] The iNO wean should be gradual, titrated to hemodynamics/gas exchange and should include alternative pulmonary vasodilators.

Intravenous prostacyclin (PGI_2, Epoprostenol, Flolan) has a half-life of 5 to 6 minutes due to spontaneous hydrolysis; there are no known toxic effects or metabolites. It is a pulmonary vasodilator and a potent platelet inhibitor; it may act as an anticoagulant in vivo.[26] The primary mechanism of its vasodilation is via the production of cAMP, an endovascular smooth muscle relaxant.[68,71] Inhalational delivery of PGI_2 ($iPGI_2$) has been studied and is equivalent to iNO in its effect on the pulmonary vasculature while sparing the systemic vasculature.[26] The cost of $iPGI_2$ 50 ng/kg/min is significantly less than iNO, both with respect to actual drug and to the delivery system. $iPGI_2$ has no significant systemic effects. It is effective in decreasing PVR, improving RV performance, and it can also improve systemic oxygenation by improving V/Q matching and thus reducing shunt.

The clinical administration of $iPGI_2$ is also more straightforward, less expensive, and more readily available than iNO. Its lack of toxicity means that no monitoring of the drug or its metabolites is required, in distinction to iNO. The nebulized prostacyclin is added to the inspiratory limb of the breathing circuit[72] (Table 4–4). There should be continuous nebulization with an external gas source. The dose range for clinical effect is 5 to 50 ng/kg/min, but most practitioners start with 50 ng/kg/min.[73] Further, unlike iNO, the dose of $iPGI_2$ is weight-based. When using an in-circuit nebulizer that is fed off of a separate oxygen source, volume cycled ventilation (with pressure limit) is preferred to pressure controlled ventilation; alteration in delivered volumes with pressure

Table 4–4 Iloprost/Epoprostenol Continuous Aerosol Delivery Protocol

Epoprostenol reconstituted in pharmacy
- Epoprostenol and NSS to IV pumps
- IV pump to mini-heart nebulizer in inspiratory limb
- O_2 flow @ 2 L/min for output = 8 mL/H
- Pumps adjusted for dosage = 10-50 ng/kg IDBW/min
- Titration charts used to adjust IV pump flows

Or

- Epoprostenol reconstituted in pharmacy
  Concentration based on patient weight
  Set for 50 ng/kg IDBW/min
- Fill mini-heart nebulizer in inspiratory limb
- O2 flow @ 2 L/min for output

control may occur, due to the possibility of the pressure from the nebulizer being falsely sensed.

If intravenous PGI$_2$ is to be used, the infusion is initiated at a rate of 2 ng/kg of body weight per minute and increased by increments of 2 ng/kg/min every 10 to 15 minutes.[22] Significant systemic hypotension and platelet inhibition can occur, putting the patient at risk for systemic and epidural bleeding.

SUPPORTIVE MEDICATIONS

Nesiritide is recombinant human B-type natriuretic peptide (BNP), an endogenous peptide produced by the ventricular myocardium.[74,75] BNP achieves endovascular smooth muscle cell relaxation by boosting intracellular cGMP, the second messenger for vasodilation of veins and arteries. The half-life of BNP is 18 minutes.[74,75] It is administered as a 2 mcg/kg intravenous bolus, followed by an infusion of 0.01 mcg/kg/min. BNP significantly decreases PVR, improves pH and cardiac index, promotes diuresis and natriuresis, and rarely causes more than mild systemic hypotension. Pharmacologic tolerance to BNP has not been reported in any of the clinical studies.[74,75] These properties prompted its pilot evaluation in cardiac surgical patients. In PH after coronary artery surgery, BNP significantly reduced PH and PVR, improved cardiac index, facilitated withdrawal of inotropic support, and enhanced diuresis.[76]

As described above, milrinone, dobutamine, and epidural anesthetics have the potential to cause hypotension, which should be avoided due to the increased oxygen demands of a stressed RV. Vasopressin may be advantageous for the treatment hypotension in patients with PH as it is a selective systemic vasoconstrictor. It results in the maintenance of SVR, without a concomitant increase in PVR, unlike systemic vasopressors such as phenylephrine. Vasopressin is also a pulmonary vasodilator; this effect is mediated by vasopressin 1 receptor activation, subsequent pulmonary endothelial NO release[77] and cGMP effects, with NO as an intermediary. Vasopressin's mild pulmonary vasodilatory effect has been established in animal models of hypoxemia.[78] Although vasopressin has been extensively investigated as a systemic vasoconstrictor, it has not been widely evaluated as a pulmonary vasodilator in humans. In vasodilatory shock, boluses of 1 to 4 units and infusion rates of 0.04 to 0.1 unit/min are acceptable, but for intraoperative use infusions should be less than or equal to 0.04 units/min.

Norepinephrine is also preferred over phenylephrine due to its β_1 effects, which should assist with the maintenance of myocardial performance. Typical bolus doses are 1 to 5 micrograms with infusions of 1 to 10 mcg/min.

POSTOPERATIVE RECOVERY

The postoperative period is fraught with danger for the patient with PH who has undergone lobectomy. Supplemental oxygen should be used and oxygen saturation should be kept above 93%. Aggressive pulmonary toilet needs to be enforced because hypoxemia, atelectasis, and pneumonia can increase PVR and risk RV failure. Inhaled beta agonists should be routinely used. Noninvasive ventilation should be considered as an early intervention to elevate oxygenation and promote CO_2 elimination. All measures described for intraoperative management of PH should be used postoperatively. For example, inhaled prostacyclin has been effectively used via facemask. Preoperative therapy for PH should be reinstituted as soon as appropriate.

Epidural and multimodal analgesia need to be maintained to optimize analgesia, leading to improved pulmonary function, thus promoting the prevention of atelectasis, hypoxemia, and hypercarbia. The sympathetic response to surgery can further increase the thromboembolic risk of patients with PH, so subcutaneous heparin and thromboprophylactic compression stockings or mechanical devices should be used.

REFERENCES

1. Ward J, McMurtry I. Mechanisms of hypoxic pulmonary vasoconstriction and their roles in pulmonary hypertension: new findings for an old problem. *Curr Opin Pharmacol.* 2009;9(3):287-296.
2. Aaronson PI, Robertson TP, Knock GA, et al. Hypoxic pulmonary vasoconstriction: mechanisms and controversies. *J Physiol.* 2006;570(Pt 1):53-8.
3. Rhodes CJ, Davidson A, Gibbs JS, Wharton J, Wilkins MR. Therapeutic targets in pulmonary arterial hypertension. *Pharmacol Therapeut.* 2009;121(1):69-88.
4. Weigand L, Sylvester JT, Shimoda LA. Mechanisms of endothelin-1-induced contraction in pulmonary arteries from chronically hypoxic rats. *Am J Physiol Lung Cell Mol Physiol.* 2006;290(2):L284-L290.
5. Jernigan NL, Walker BR, Resta TC. Chronic hypoxia augments protein kinase G-mediated Ca2+ desensitization in pulmonary vascular smooth muscle through inhibition of RhoA/Rho kinase signaling. *Am J Physiol Lung Cell Mol Physiol.* 2004;287(6):L1220-L1229.
6. Nagendran J, Stewart K, Hoskinson M, Archer SL. An anesthesiologist's guide to hypoxic pulmonary vasoconstriction: implications for managing single-lung anesthesia and atelectasis. *Curr Opin Anaesthesiol* 2006;19(1):34-43.
7. Abe K, Shimizu T, Takashina M, et al. The effects of propofol, isoflurane, and sevoflurane on oxygenation and shunt fraction during one-lung ventilation. *Anesth Analg.* 1998;87(5):1164-1169.
8. Humbert M, Sitbon O, Chaouat A, et al. Pulmonary arterial hypertension in France: results from a national registry. *Am J Respir Crit Care Med.* 2006;173(9):1023-1030.
9. Barst RJ, McGoon M, Torbicki A, et al. Diagnosis and differential assessment of pulmonary arterial hypertension. *J Am Coll Cardiol.* 2004;43(12 Suppl S):40S-7S.
10. D'Alonzo GE, Barst RJ, Ayres SM, et al. Survival in patients with primary pulmonary hypertension. Results from a national prospective registry. *Ann Intern Med.* 1991;115(5):343-349.
11. Simonneau G, Galie N, Rubin LJ, et al. Clinical classification of pulmonary hypertension. *J Am Coll Cardiol.* 2004;43(12 Suppl S):5S-12S.
12. Wright JL, Tai H, Dai J, Churg A. Cigarette smoke induces rapid changes in gene expression in pulmonary arteries. Laboratory Investigation. 2002;82(10):1391-1398.
13. Spira A, Beane J, Shah V, et al. Effects of cigarette smoke on the human airway epithelial cell transcriptome. *Proceedings of the National Academy of Sciences of the United States of America.* 2004;101(27):10143-10148.
14. Yokohori N, Aoshiba K, Nagai A, Respiratory Failure Research Group in Japan. Increased levels of cell death and proliferation in alveolar wall cells in patients with pulmonary emphysema. *Chest.* 2004;125(2):626-632.
15. Aoshiba K, Tamaoki J, Nagai A. Acute cigarette smoke exposure induces apoptosis of alveolar macrophages. *Am J Physiol Lung Cell Mol Physiol.* 2001;281(6):L1392-L1401.
16. Hale KA, Niewoehner DE, Cosio MG. Morphologic changes in the muscular pulmonary arteries: relationship to cigarette smoking, airway disease, and emphysema. *Am Rev Respir Dis..* 1980;122(2):273-278.

17. Higenbottam T. Pulmonary hypertension and chronic obstructive pulmonary disease: a case for treatment. *Proc Am Thorac Soc.* 2005;2(1):121-9.
18. Girard F, Couture P, Boudreault D, et al. Estimation of the pulmonary capillary wedge pressure from transesophageal pulsed Doppler echocardiography of pulmonary venous flow: influence of the respiratory cycle during mechanical ventilation. *J Cardiothorac Vasc Anesth.* 1998;12(1):16-21.
19. Jovev S, Tager S, Spirovski Z, et al. Right heart haemodynamics after lung resection; the role of the transthoracic echo-Doppler cardiography. *Makedonska Akademija na Naukite i Umetnostite Oddelenie Za Bioloshki i Meditsinski Nauki Prilozi.* 2006;27(2):201-216.
20. Johnson SR, Mehta S, Granton JT. Anticoagulation in pulmonary arterial hypertension: a qualitative systematic review. *Eur Respir J.* 2006;28(5):999-1004.
21. Rubin LJ. Calcium channel blockers in primary pulmonary hypertension. *Chest.* 1985;88(4 Suppl):257S-260S.
22. Chin KM, Rubin LJ. Pulmonary arterial hypertension. *J Am Coll Cardiol.* 2008;51(16):1527-1238.
23. Schubert R, Serebryakov VN, Engel H, Hopp HH. Iloprost activates KCa channels of vascular smooth muscle cells: role of cAMP-dependent protein kinase. *Am J Physiol.* 1996;271(4 Pt 1):C1203-C1211.
24. Lee SH, Rubin LJ. Current treatment strategies for pulmonary arterial hypertension. *J Intern Med.* 2005;258(3):199-215.
25. Gomberg-Maitland M, Olschewski H. Prostacyclin therapies for the treatment of pulmonary arterial hypertension. *Eur Respir J.* 2008;31(4):891-901.
26. Hsu HH, Rubin LJ. Iloprost inhalation solution for the treatment of pulmonary arterial hypertension. *Expet Opin Pharmacother.* 2005;6(11):1921-1930.
27. Skoro-Sajer N, Lang I, Naeije R. Treprostinil for pulmonary hypertension. *Vasc Health Risk Manag.* 2008;4(3):507-513.
28. National, Institute, for et al. Pulmonary arterial hypertension (adults) - drugs: appraisal consultation document. http://www.nice.org.uk/guidance/index.jsp?action=article&o=39688 2008.
29. Steiner MK, Preston IR. Optimizing endothelin receptor antagonist use in the management of pulmonary arterial hypertension. *Vasc Health Risk Manag.* 2008;4(5):943-952.
30. Croom KF, Curran MP, Abman SH, et al. Sildenafil: a review of its use in pulmonary arterial hypertension. *Drugs.* 2008;68(3):383-397.
31. Ghiadoni L, Versari D, Taddei S. Phosphodiesterase 5 inhibition in essential hypertension. *Cur Hypertens Rep.* 2008;10(1):52-57.
32. Lawrence VA, Cornell JE, Smetana GW, American College of P. Strategies to reduce postoperative pulmonary complications after noncardiothoracic surgery: systematic review for the American College of Physicians. *Ann Intern Med.* 2006;144(8):596-608.
33. Smetana GW, Lawrence VA, Cornell JE, American College of Physicians. Preoperative pulmonary risk stratification for noncardiothoracic surgery: systematic review for the American College of Physicians. *Ann Intern Med.* 2006;144(8):581-595.
34. Qaseem A, Snow V, Fitterman N, et al. Risk assessment for and strategies to reduce perioperative pulmonary complications for patients undergoing noncardiothoracic surgery: a guideline from the American College of Physicians. *Ann Intern Med.* 2006;144(8):575-580.
35. Turrentine FE, Wang H, Simpson VB, Jones RS. Surgical risk factors, morbidity, and mortality in elderly patients. *J Am Coll Surg.* 2006;203(6):865-877.
36. Mangano DT. Perioperative cardiac morbidity—epidemiology, costs, problems, and solutions. *West J Med.* 1994;161(1):87-89.
37. Her C, Lees DE. Preoperative predictors of perioperative cardiac morbidity. *Anesthesiology.* 1990;73(3):579.
38. Mangano DT. Perioperative cardiac morbidity. *Anesthesiology.* 1990;72(1):153-184.
39. Foster ED, Davis KB, Carpenter JA, et al. Risk of noncardiac operation in patients with defined coronary disease: The Coronary Artery Surgery Study (CASS) registry experience. *Ann Thorac Surg.* 1986;41(1):42-50.
40. Casaburi R, ZuWallack R. Pulmonary rehabilitation for management of chronic obstructive pulmonary disease. *N Engl J Med.* 2009;360(13):1329-1335.
41. Bobbio A, Chetta A, Ampollini L, et al. Preoperative pulmonary rehabilitation in patients undergoing lung resection for non-small cell lung cancer. *Eur J Cardio-Thorac Surg.* 2008;33(1):95-98.
42. Girgis RE, Mathai SC. Pulmonary hypertension associated with chronic respiratory disease. *Clin Chest Med.* 2007;28(1):219-232.

43. Bach DS, Curtis JL, Christensen PJ, et al. Preoperative echocardiographic evaluation of patients referred for lung volume reduction surgery. *Chest.* 1998;114(4):972-980.
44. Holverda S, Bogaard HJ, Groepenhoff H, et al. Cardiopulmonary exercise test characteristics in patients with chronic obstructive pulmonary disease and associated pulmonary hypertension. *Respiration.* 2008;76(2):160-167.
45. Okada M, Okada M, Ishii N, et al. Right ventricular ejection fraction in the preoperative risk evaluation of candidates for pulmonary resection. *J Thorac Cardiovasc Surg.* 1996;112(2):364-370.
46. Tanita T, Tomoyasu M, Deguchi H, et al. Review of preoperative functional evaluation for lung resection using the right ventricular hemodynamic functions. *Ann Thorac Cardiovasc Surg.* 2004;10(6):333-339.
47. Mandegar M, Fung Y-CB, Huang W, et al. Cellular and molecular mechanisms of pulmonary vascular remodeling: role in the development of pulmonary hypertension. *Microvasc Res.* 2004;68(2):75-103.
48. Malov SS, Body SC. Importance of monitoring both pressure waveforms during pulmonary artery catheterization. *J Cardiothorac Vasc Anesth.* 1999;13(4):517-518.
49. Binanay C, Califf RM, Hasselblad V, et al. Evaluation study of congestive heart failure and pulmonary artery catheterization effectiveness: the ESCAPE trial. *JAMA.* 2005;294(13):1625-1633.
50. American Society of Anesthesiologists Task Force on Pulmonary Artery C. Practice guidelines for pulmonary artery catheterization: an updated report by the American Society of Anesthesiologists Task Force on Pulmonary Artery Catheterization. *Anesthesiology.* 2003;99(4):988-1014.
51. Bernard GR, Sopko G, Cerra F, et al. Pulmonary artery catheterization and clinical outcomes: National Heart, Lung, and Blood Institute and Food and Drug Administration Workshop Report. Consensus Statement. *JAMA.* 2000;283(19):2568-2572.
52. Huter L, Schwarzkopf K, Preussler N-P, et al. Measuring cardiac output in one-lung ventilation: a comparison of pulmonary artery and transpulmonary aortic measurements in pigs. *J Cardiothorac Vasc Anesth.* 2004;18(2):190-193.
53. Zaune U, Knarr C, Kruselmann M, et al. Value and accuracy of dual oximetry during pulmonary resections. *J Cardiothorac Anesth.* 1990;4(4):441-452.
54. Nomoto Y, Kawamura M. Pulmonary gas exchange effects by nitroglycerin, dopamine and dobutamine during one-lung ventilation in man. *Can J Anaesth.* 1989;36(3 Pt 1):273-277.
55. Kaplan JA. Monitoring technology: advances and restraints. *J Cardiothorac Anesth.* 1989;3(3):257-259.
56. Myles PS, Snell GI, Westall GP. Lung transplantation. *Curr Opin Anaesthesiol.* 2007;20(1):21-26.
57. Vedrinne JM, Curtil A, Martinot S, et al. The hemodynamic effects of hypoxemia in anesthetized pigs: a comparison between right heart catheter and echocardiography. *Anesth Analgesia.* 1998;87(1):21-26.
58. Servin FS, Billard V. Remifentanil and other opioids. *Handbook Exp Pharmacol.* 2008(182):283-311.
59. Steendijk P. Right ventricular function and failure: methods, models, and mechanisms. *Crit Care Med.* 2004;32(4):1087-1089.
60. Cohen E. One lung ventilation: prospective from an interested observer. *Minerva Anestesiol.* 1999;65(5):275-283.
61. Hemnes AR, Champion HC. Right heart function and haemodynamics in pulmonary hypertension. *Int J Clin Pract.* 2008;(160):11-19.
62. Haddad F, Doyle R, Murphy DJ, Hunt SA. Right ventricular function in cardiovascular disease, part II: pathophysiology, clinical importance, and management of right ventricular failure. *Circulation.* 2008;117(13):1717-1731.
63. Bayram M, De Luca L, Massie MB, Gheorghiade M. Reassessment of dobutamine, dopamine, and milrinone in the management of acute heart failure syndromes. *Am J Cardiol.* 2005;96(6A):47G-58G.
64. Acosta F, Sansano T, Palenciano CG, et al. Effects of dobutamine on right ventricular function and pulmonary circulation in pulmonary hypertension during liver transplantation. *Transplant Proc.* 2005;37(9):3869-3870.
65. Kerbaul F, Rondelet B, Motte S, et al. Effects of norepinephrine and dobutamine on pressure load-induced right ventricular failure. *Crit Care Med.* 2004;32(4):1035-1040.
66. Pagnamenta A, Fesler P, Vandinivit A, et al. Pulmonary vascular effects of dobutamine in experimental pulmonary hypertension. *Crit Care Med.* 2003;31(4):1140-1146.
67. Bradford KK, Deb B, Pearl RG. Combination therapy with inhaled nitric oxide and intravenous dobutamine during pulmonary hypertension in the rabbit. *J Cardiovasc Pharmacol.* 2000;36(2):146-151.

68. Granton J, Moric J. Pulmonary vasodilators—treating the right ventricle. *Anesthesiol Clin.* 2008; 26(2):337-53.
69. Kavanagh BP, Pearl RG. Inhaled nitric oxide in anesthesia and critical care medicine. *Int Anesthesiol Clin.* 1995;33(1):181-210.
70. Augoustides JG, Culp K, Smith S. Rebound pulmonary hypertension and cardiogenic shock after withdrawal of inhaled prostacyclin. *Anesthesiology.* 2004;100(4):1023-1025.
71. Schroeder RA, Wood GL, Plotkin JS, Kuo PC. Intraoperative use of inhaled PGI(2) for acute pulmonary hypertension and right ventricular failure. *Anesth Analgesia.* 2000;91(2):291-295.
72. Augoustides JG, Ochroch EA. Inhaled selective pulmonary vasodilators. *Int Anesthesiol Clin.* 2005;43(2): 101-114.
73. Lowson SM. Inhaled alternatives to nitric oxide. *Crit Care Med.* 2005;33(3 Suppl):S188-S195.
74. Potter LR, Yoder AR, Flora DR, et al. Natriuretic peptides: their structures, receptors, physiologic functions and therapeutic applications. *Handbook Exp Pharmacol.* 2009;(191):341-366.
75. Alsaddique AA. Recognition of diastolic heart failure in the postoperative heart. *Eur J Cardio-Thorac Surg.* 2008;34(6):1141-1148.
76. Moazami N, Damiano RJ, Bailey MS, et al. Nesiritide (BNP) in the management of postoperative cardiac patients. *Ann Thorac Surg.* 2003;75(6):1974-1976.
77. Russ RD, Walker BR. Role of nitric oxide in vasopressinergic pulmonary vasodilatation. *Am J Physiol.* 1992;262(3 Pt 2):H743-H747.
78. Eichinger MR, Walker BR. Enhanced pulmonary arterial dilation to arginine vasopressin in chronically hypoxic rats. *Am J Physiol.* 1994;267(6 Pt 2):H2413-H2419.

Lung Separation Techniques   5

Andrew D. Shaw
Katherine Grichnik
Atilio Barbeito
Javier Campos

Lung separation allows the anesthesiologist to provide one-lung ventilation (OLV) in patients undergoing lung resection surgery. It is also utilized to facilitate access to other thoracic structures such as the heart, the esophagus, mediastinal lymph nodes, the thoracic aorta, and the thoracic vertebrae.[1,2] In addition to facilitating surgical exposure, lung separation is also indicated for prevention of contamination of the contralateral lung from bleeding, pus material, or saline lavage (in cases of hemoptysis, purulent drainage, and lung lavage, respectively), and to allow positive pressure ventilation and adequate gas exchange in the presence of a large bronchopleural fistula.

Two main techniques are used for lung separation. The first one involves a device made of disposable polyvinylchloride material, the double-lumen endotracheal tube (DLT).[3] The DLT is a bifurcated tube with both an endotracheal and an endobronchial lumen and can be used to achieve isolation of either the right or left lung. The second technique involves blockade of a mainstem bronchus to allow lung collapse distal to the occlusion.[4]

This chapter reviews the insertion techniques and complications for both types of devices and will provide some practical recommendations for their safe and effective use.

DOUBLE-LUMEN ENDOTRACHEAL TUBES

Double-lumen endotracheal tubes (DLT) have been used in thoracic anesthesia for lung separation and one-lung ventilation (OLV) for more than 50 years, since the report of Carlens and Bjork in 1950.[5] They provide excellent operating conditions when sized and placed correctly, and allow access to both ventilated and collapsed lungs for secretion clearance, independent ventilation, and bronchoscopic inspection. Today they are the commonest method of securing lung isolation and are available in sizes ranging from 26 to 41 F, with the Bronco-Cath DLT from Mallinckrodt being the most popular in North America. Other manufacturers include Argyle (Sheridan), Rusch and Portex. The Silbroncho, a newer DLT by Fuji Systems, is also available in a left-sided version only (Figure 5–1A). This device features a shorter, wire-reinforced endobronchial tip and a reduced bronchial cuff size.[6] This design should provide a greater margin of safety, although its clinical effectiveness has not been reported.

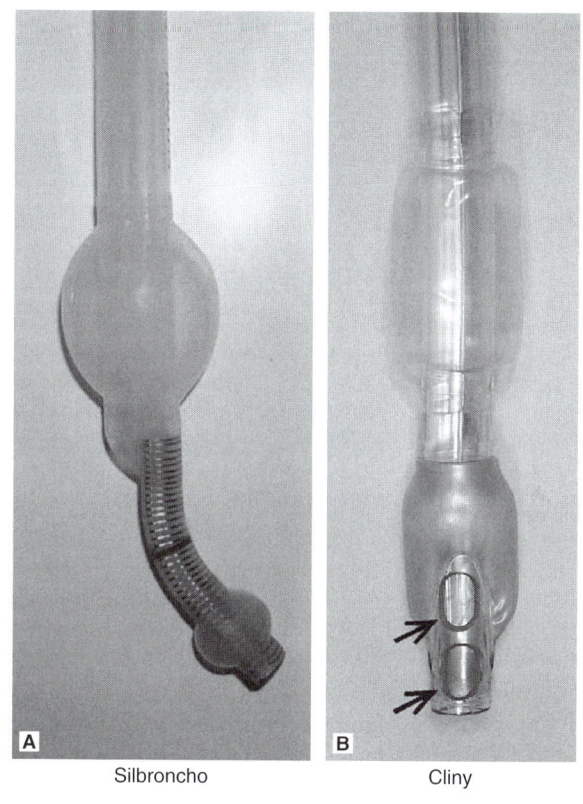

Figure 5-1. **A.** The Silbroncho left-sided DLT. **B.** The Cliny right-sided DLT. Notice the long oblique bronchial cuff and the two ventilation slots for the right upper lobe (arrows). (Reproduced with permission from Campos J. Lung isolation. In: Slinger P., ed. *Principles and Practice of Anesthesia for Thoracic Surgery.* New York: Springer, 2011, p. 235. Copyright © Springer Science + Business Media, LLC 2011.)

Choices—Left or Right?

Traditionally, thoracic anesthesiologists would place a DLT on the side contralateral to the surgical procedure. However, before the advent of routine fiberoptic bronchoscopy, incorrect placement was common and lead to a high incidence of avoidable hypoxemia secondary to right upper lobe obstruction. In light of this, it became the norm to place a left-sided tube for all procedures except a left pneumonectomy or left-sided main bronchial *sleeve* resection. This practice has become widespread and is probably the most common policy in use today. Some practitioners even advocate that a left-sided tube be used for *all* procedures, and withdrawn into the trachea when necessary. It is true that a right-sided tube is harder to insert and place correctly, but it is also true that a well-placed right-sided tube makes surgery on the proximal left lung airways far easier. Indications for right-sided tube placement are summarized in Table 5–1.

Table 5–1. Indications for a Right-Sided Double-Lumen Endotracheal Tube

- Distorted anatomy of the entrance of left mainstem bronchus by intrabronchial mass or external compression
- Compression of the entrance of the left mainstem bronchus from to a descending thoracic aortic aneurysm
- Left lung transplantation
- Left-sided *sleeve* resection
- Left-sided pneumonectomy
- Any contraindication to placement a left-sided DLT

There are important anatomic differences between the two main bronchi, and appreciation of these allows understanding of the problems one is likely to encounter when placing a DLT. The right main bronchus is shorter, arises from the carina at a more acute angle, and gives off the right upper lobe bronchus much earlier (ie, closer to the carina—usually at about 1.5-2 cm) than its left-sided equivalent. As a result, it is very easy to inadvertently occlude the right upper lobe with the bronchial portion of the tube and thus leave only the middle and lower lobes available for ventilation. There are some design features of right-sided tubes that reduce the chance of this happening, but they do not eliminate this problem entirely.

All the currently available right-sided DLT have an orifice cut through the bronchial portion of the tube, usually distal to the cuff, which may itself be offset (Figure 5–2). This is to permit ventilation of the right upper lobe (RUL), and ideally the orifice is placed directly opposite the right upper lobe bronchus. In practice this is difficult and most practitioners are happy if they can see the RUL bronchus through the orifice, as this usually permits good ventilation of the RUL during OLV. Newer designs attempt to facilitate positioning and ventilation of the RUL. An example is the right-sided DLT by Cliny (Create Medic Co. Ltd, Yokohama, Japan), which has a long bronchial cuff with two ventilation slots for the right upper lobe (Figure 5–1B). This device may prove useful in patients with a very short right mainstem bronchus.[7]

In about 1 in 250 patients a porcine bronchus will be encountered.[8] Here, the right upper lobe bronchus originates directly from the trachea, usually within 2 cm of the carina, but sometimes as much as 6 cm. In this situation, a right-sided tube necessarily occludes the RUL, and a left-sided tube is preferable.

Sizing-Practical Considerations

Much has been written about the *best* size DLT to use, and how best to make the selection. In general, most female patients will be well served with a 37-F size, and most male patients with a 39 F. This is of course an oversimplification, but is not a bad starting point. When considering whether to vary from this policy, patient height is more important than weight as it better predicts tracheal length, which is the prime determinant of whether a

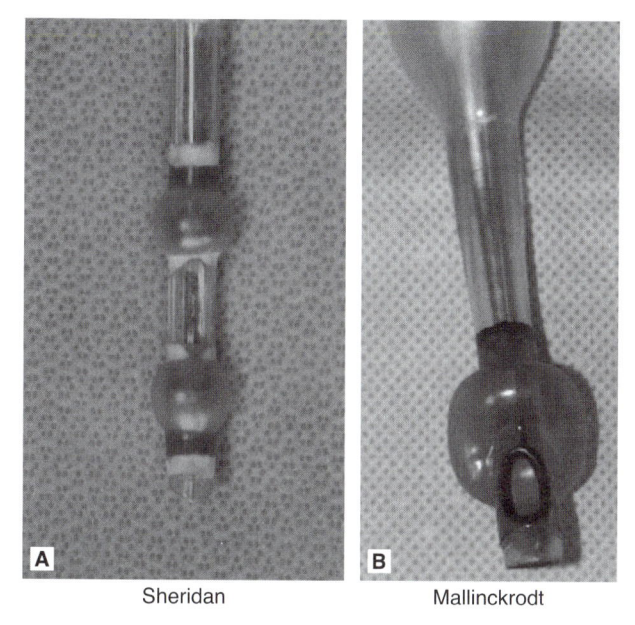

Figure 5–2. A. The Sheridan right-sided DLT. **B.** The Mallinckrodt right-sided DLT.

tube of a given size provides effective lung isolation. Tubes that are too small cause far more trouble than tubes that are too large, because the problems they cause do not declare themselves until the case is well underway and lung isolation unsatisfactory. A tube that is too large will not fit, a situation that declares itself much earlier in the case, when there is still time to correct the problem. Tubes that are too small do not sit well in the main bronchus, require higher cuff volumes (the bronchial cuffs are not designed to contain more than 3 mL of air) and become dislodged easily. This leads to repeated attempts to improve their position, disruption to the surgery, repeated need for bronchoscopy, and repeated interruptions to ventilation. A correctly sized tube passes smoothly through the glottis and comes to rest at a distance of approximately 29 cm from the incisors in both men and women. In one study performed in adult cadavers, it was shown that the cricoid ring diameter never exceeds the diameter of the glottis. Thus, if a DLT encounters resistance when passing the glottis, it is likely that the DLT would also encounter resistance while passing the cricoid ring.[9]

Sizing—Reported Studies

Most of the published literature focuses on the left-sided DLT in part because the right-sided DLT is used less commonly. There are reports of complications related to the use of an undersized DLT. A tension pneumothorax and pneumomediastinum occurred after the endobronchial tip of an undersized DLT had migrated too far into the left lower bronchus, and the whole tidal volume was delivered into a single lobe.[10] Smaller DLTs also provide more resistance to gas flow and will develop more auto-positive end-expiratory pressure when compared with larger DLTs.[11] Airway-related complications have similarly been reported with the use of undersized left-sided DLTs.[12]

Brodsky et al[13] reported that measurement of the tracheal diameter at the level of the clavicle on the preoperative posteroanterior chest radiograph can be used to determine the proper left-sided DLT size. This approach lead to the use of larger left-sided DLTs (ie, 41 F in men and 39 F in women). However, a study involving Asian patients by Chow et al[14] using the same method found this approach less reliable. In their study, Chow et al found that the overall positive predictive value for the correct size of a left-sided DLT was 77% for men and 45% for women. Therefore, this method may be less useful in patients of smaller stature such as women and people of Asian descent.

Amar et al[15] have shown that the use of a smaller DLT (35-F left-sided) was not associated with any difference in clinical intraoperative outcomes, regardless of patient size or gender. However, in their study, of the 35% of patients who received a DLT, 92 (65%) were female. In practice, many women will usually receive a 35 F DLT anyway; therefore the question of whether or not a 35 F for all patients is favorable remains unclear.

A different alternative that has been suggested in order to predict the proper size of a right-sided or left-sided DLT is a three-dimensional image reconstruction of tracheobronchial anatomy generated from spiral computed tomography (CT) scans combined with superimposed transparencies of DLTs.[16] This is unlikely to become an everyday habit however, because of the time required to generate the 3D images, and the fact that most of the time a 37- or 39-F tube will suffice.

Taken as a group, these studies suggest that chest radiographs and CT scans may be valuable tools for selection of the correct DLT size. As such these images should certainly be reviewed before placement of a DLT as they will alert the operator to the presence of abnormal anatomy. In addition, the preoperative CT scan will provide the distance to the epidural space should an epidural catheter be part of the anesthetic plan.

DLT Insertion Technique

Double-lumen tubes may be placed "blind" or using a fiberoptic bronchoscope. In the blind technique the DLT is introduced into the glottis during direct laryngoscopy. The tip is passed through the glottis with the tip pointing anteriorly and the entire tube then turned 90 degrees to the left (for a left-sided DLT) or right (for a right-sided DLT) after the endobronchial cuff has passed beyond the vocal cords. The DLT is then advanced further into the trachea until the depth of insertion at the teeth is approximately 29 cm (for patients who are at least 170 cm tall).[17] Rotating the patient's head slightly to the opposite side as the tube is advanced into its final position helps the tip of the DLT find the correct main bronchus. Correct location may then be confirmed using a fiberoptic bronchoscope—see the following pages for details.

The second technique employs fiberoptic bronchoscopy, where the tip of the endobronchial lumen is guided into position bronchoscopically after the DLT passes the vocal cords. A study by Boucek et al[18] compared the blind technique with the fiberoptic technique and showed that of the 32 patients who underwent the blind technique, primary success occurred in 30 patients. In contrast, in the 27 patients receiving the bronchoscopy-guided technique, primary success was achieved only in 21 patients and eventual success in 25 patients. This study also showed that the time spent placing a DLT was an average of 88 seconds for the blind technique and 181 seconds for the fiberoptic method. Although both methods resulted in successful placement in the majority of patients, more time was required when the fiberoptic technique was used. Figure 5–3 shows both the blind technique and the fiberoptic technique for placement of a left-sided DLT. The most important aspect of the fiberoptic technique is to confirm visualization of the trifurcation of the RUL bronchus from the right main bronchus—there is no other place in the tracheobronchial tree where this image is seen, and it therefore confirms that the position is correct. Figure 5–4A and B illustrates the optimal position of a right- and left-sided DLT, respectively, together with the bronchoscopic views that should be obtained in each case.

With either technique, the final position will be confirmed fiberoptically prior to surgery commencing. This is best performed immediately after tube placement and again once the patient is placed in the lateral position for surgery. Tubes often migrate out during patient positioning, and often a small degree of neck flexion will replace the tip of the bronchial lumen into its correct location. Ideally, the blue edge of the bronchial cuff will be visible in the main bronchus when it is inflated and in good position. The bronchial cuff is unlike the tracheal cuff and is not designed to minimize inflation pressure. It is essential therefore that the bronchial cuff is not *overinflated* as all this will do is increase the pressure applied to the bronchial mucosa and increase the risk of an ischemic lesion.

Problems and Complications

The most common problems and complications arising from the use of DLTs are incorrect placement and damage to the airways. A malpositioned DLT does not permit collapse of the operative lung, and may partially collapse the ventilated or dependent lung, producing hypoxemia. A common cause of malposition is dislodgement of the endobronchial cuff because of overinflation, surgical manipulation of the bronchus, or extension of the head and neck during or after patient positioning.[19]

Airway trauma and damage to the membranous part of the trachea or main bronchus continue to be associated with the use of DLTs.[12,20] This complication can develop at any time the DLT is in position or during extubation.[21-23] A 25-year review of the literature by Fitzmaurice and Brodsky[24] found that most airway injuries were associated with undersized DLTs, particularly in women who received a 35- or 37-F disposable DLT. It is likely that airway damage occurs when an undersized DLT migrates distally into the bronchus and the main tracheal body of the DLT comes into contact with the bronchus, producing lacerations or rupture of the airway. Airway damage during the use of DLTs can present as unexpected air leaks, subcutaneous emphysema, and

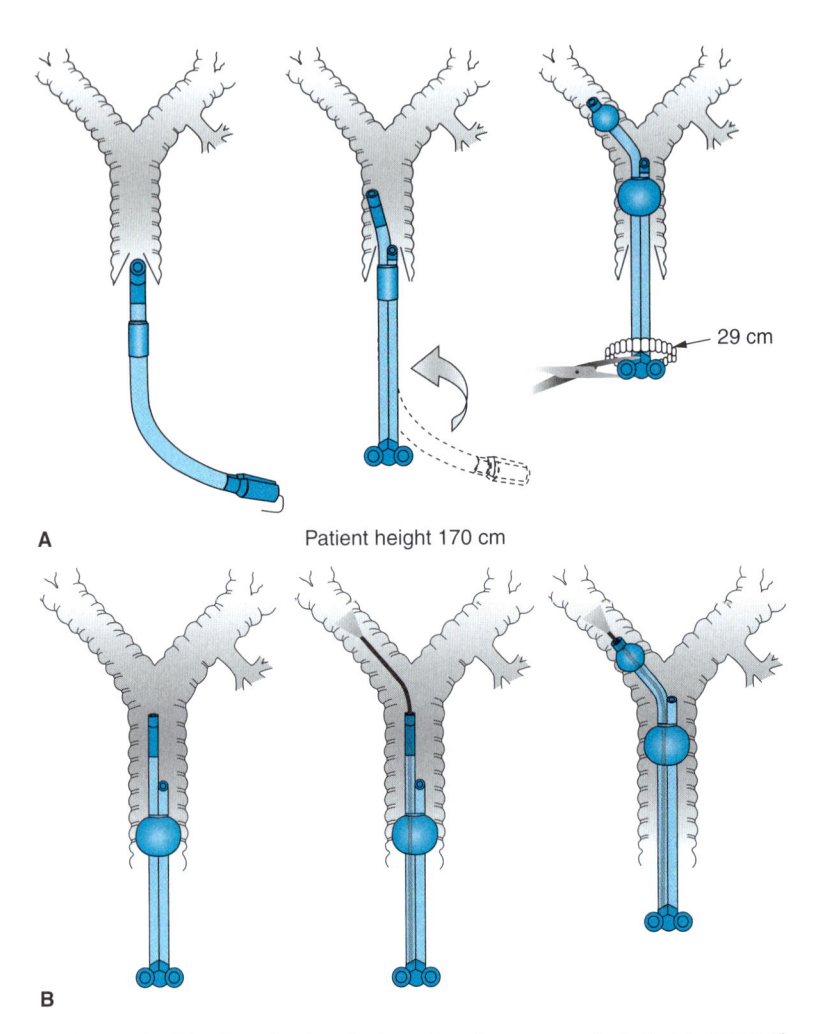

Figure 5–3. A. The blind method technique for placement of a left-sided DLT. The endobronchial lumen is in an anterior position during initial insertion (left figure); the DLT is then passed through the glottic opening using direct laryngoscopy and rotated 90 degrees to the left (center figure); the DLT is finally advanced until moderate resistance is felt, indicating the endobronchial lumen of the DLT has entered the bronchus (right figure). (Reproduced with permission from Campos JH.[68])
B. The fiberoptic bronchoscopy guidance technique for placement of a left-sided DLT. The DLT is inserted into the trachea using direct laryngoscopy (left figure). The fiberoptic bronchoscope is then inserted through the endobronchial lumen and the tracheal carina and the left main stem bronchus visualized (center figure). The DLT is rotated 90 degrees to the left and, with the aid of the fiberoptic bronchoscope; the tube is advanced to the optimal position into the left main stem bronchus (right figure). (Reproduced with permission from Campos JH.[68])

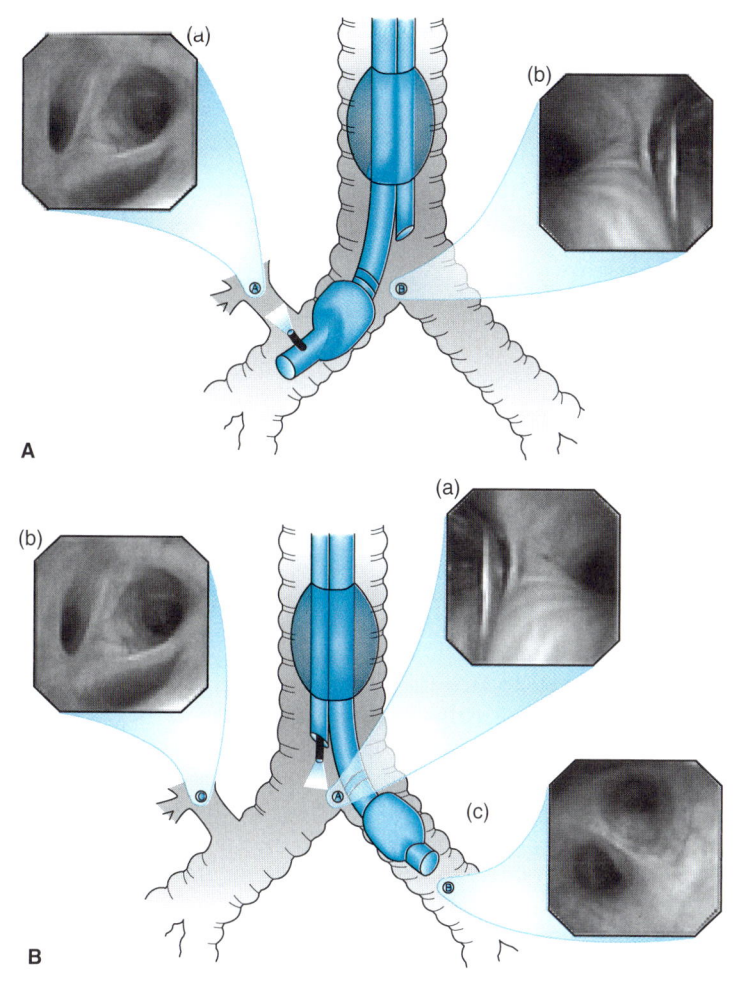

Figure 5–4. **A.** Optimal position of a right-sided DLT. Insert A shows the take-off of the right-upper lobe bronchus with its three segments (apical, anterior and posterior) as seen when the fiberoptic bronchoscope emerges from the opening slot located in the endobronchial lumen of the DLT. Insert B shows an unobstructed bronchoscopic view of the entrance of the left mainstem bronchus when the fiberscope is passed through the tracheal lumen of the DLT and the edge of the fully inflated endobronchial cuff is positioned below the tracheal carina in the right mainstem bronchus. (Reproduced with permission from Campos JH.[67]) **B.** Optimal position of a left-sided DLT. Insert (a) shows an unobstructed bronchoscopic view of the entrance of the right mainstem bronchus when the fiberscope is passed through the tracheal lumen of the DLT and the edge of the fully inflated endobronchial cuff is below the tracheal carina in the left mainstem bronchus. Insert (b) shows the take-off of the right-upper lobe bronchus with its three segments (apical, anterior and posterior); this landmark should be used to reconfirm the location of the right bronchus. Insert (c) shows an unobstructed bronchoscopic view of the left-upper and left-lower bronchi when the fiberoptic bronchoscope is advanced through the endobronchial lumen of the DLT. (Reproduced with permission from Campos JH.[67])

massive airway bleeding into the lumen of the DLT, or protrusion of the endotracheal or endobronchial cuff into the surgical field.

Another serious problem that may occur is the development of tension pneumothorax in the dependent, ventilated lung.[25,26] This complication is particularly important to detect promptly as the treatment is immediate decompression of the non-operative-side pneumothorax. This can be achieved either directly, across the mediastinum, or by turning the patient and placing a cannula through the chest wall. If the diagnosis is wrong however, the patient now has an extra pneumothorax and chest tube to deal with postoperatively. We routinely place an esophageal stethoscope (a regular stethoscope attached to an esophageal temperature probe) and confirm auscultation of breath sounds during OLV in order to either confirm or rule this diagnosis out whenever it is suspected.

Less serious complications with the use of the DLT have been reported by Knoll et al.[27] In their comparative study between the DLT and the endobronchial blocker, the development of postoperative hoarseness occurred significantly more commonly in the DLT group when compared to the endobronchial blocker group; however, the incidence of bronchial injuries was comparable between groups.

BRONCHIAL BLOCKERS

Balloon blockade of the right or left mainstem bronchus offers another strategy for achieving lung separation to facilitate thoracic surgical procedures.[4] As blockage of the endobronchial lumen results in distal lung collapse; this method can also be used to selectively achieve lobar collapse when the bronchial blocker is placed in a more distal bronchus.[28-34] There are multiple types of endobronchial blockers including independent catheters that are inserted into a normal endotracheal tube (ETT) after intubation (Arndt blocker,[35] Cohen tip-deflecting endobronchial blocker,[36] Fuji Uniblocker)[37,38] and those that are mounted within a specialized endotracheal tube (the Univent tube).[4]

Independent Bronchial Blockers

There are multiple independent bronchial blockers, which are designed to be inserted into an in situ endotracheal tube after successful intubation. The three major types commonly used in the United States are the Arndt endobronchial blocker, the Cohen endobronchial blocker, and the Fuji Uniblocker.[37,38]

The primary advantage of an independent blockers include the ability to use the blocker in a patient with a preexisting ETT,[39] after a difficult airway is secured through any variety of mechanisms,[40] for use in trauma patients who may urgently and unexpectedly require one-lung ventilation.[41,42] Additional uses are in post-pneumonectomy patients, who may require selective one-lobe ventilation[43] or to control unilateral pulmonary hemorrhage.[44]

ARNDT BLOCKER

The Arndt blocker[35] is relatively unique in that it utilizes a wire loop attached to a FOB, which allows the anesthesiologist to guide the blocker into the correct position. This blocker is available as a 5-, 7-, or 9-F catheter and in 65 cm and 78 cm lengths; within the blocker itself is an inner 1.4 mm diameter lumen that houses a flexible nylon wire ending in a small flexible loop distally. This loop is retractable and thus can be cinched to a fiberoptic bronchoscope (FOB), which can then be used to guide the blocker into the correct position within the selected bronchus. After placement, the guidewire can be removed and the inner lumen used for lung deflation or insufflation of oxygen if needed.

Proper placement and functioning of the blocker rests on choosing the proper single lumen ETT size for use with the blocker. In general (for use in adults), a 7-F blocker requires a 7.5-mm internal diameter (ID) ETT, and a 9-F blocker requires at least an 8.0-mm ID single-lumen ETT. The balloon on the Arndt blocker is a high-volume, low-pressure cuff and comes in an elliptical or spherical shape.

Placement and Positioning of the Arndt Blocker

After intubation or with a preexisting ETT and selection of the correct size bronchial blocker, the bronchial blocker should be lubricated and the balloon checked, and the FOB should be prepared. The size of blocker may be dictated by the ETT size and the choice of a spherical versus elliptical balloon rests on the goal of the surgery; the spherical blocker is more secure with less opportunity to become malpositioned in the short right mainstem bronchus or for selective lobar intubation, whereas the elliptical or the spherical blocker may both be used in the left mainstem bronchus. Appropriate lubrication of the blocker and the FOB are encouraged for ease of insertion.

There are multiple suggestions in the literature for placement of an Arndt endobronchial blocker; the following is one stepwise process that has been advocated by many: First, the multiconnector port is examined and the various attachment ports identified for the bronchial blocker, the FOB and for attachment to the ventilator. Next, the bronchial blocker is inserted through its port (the lumen with the screw top), the FOB is inserted through its port, and, after both the FOB and the bronchial blocker are beyond the entire multiconnector port lumen, the blocker guide wire loop is tightened to secure it to the FOB. Next, the combined multiconnector port/FOB/bronchial blocker are inserted into the existing endotracheal tube, the multiport connector is attached to the top of the ETT and the ventilator tubing attached to the appropriate ventilation sideport. After resumption of ventilation with assurance of end tidal CO_2, the FOB/blocker combination should be advanced distally to the desired bronchus under fiberoptic visualization. When the deflated cuff of the blocker is beyond the entrance of the bronchus, the guide loop is loosened and the FOB withdrawn to the carina. This position allows visualization of the blocker as it advances into the correct bronchial lumen. The blocker cuff is then fully inflated under direct visualization with 4 to 8 mL of air to completely fill the bronchial lumen.

A simplified approach is possible when blocking the right lung: due to the ease of insertion of the blocker into the right mainstem bronchus given its alignment with the trachea, it is possible to insert the Arndt blocker and the FOB in the lumen of the endotracheal tube without the wireguide loop attachment. The blocker can then be advanced into the right mainstem bronchus under FOB visualization. However, due to the relatively shorter right mainstem bronchus, the blocker's cuff should be deflated and the blocker advanced 1 cm before repositioning the patient into the left lateral decubitus position, to avoid blocker retraction into the trachea with the move. It is always necessary to reconfirm blocker position after the surgical positioning is completed.

After corroboration of the correct position of the blocker and its balloon, the wire loop can be withdrawn to convert the 1.4 mm channel into an open port to allow lung deflation. One version of the Arndt blocker has a cone-shaped device that can be attached to this 1.4 mm channel for connection to a low level of suction. This may both facilitate lung collapse but could also be used to suction very thin secretions.[45] Of note, the wire loop must be at least retracted into the central lumen, if not removed from the channel, to avoid inclusion in the stapling line of the bronchus with any proximal surgical resection.[46] Prior to inflation of the bronchial balloon, many practitioners choose to hold patients apneic for 1 to 2 minutes to facilitate operative lung collapse. Optimal positioning of the Arndt blocker is achieved when the blocker balloon's outer surface is visualized fiberoptically about 5 mm below the tracheal carina in the operative side bronchus and no leakage of air is noted around the blocker. Figure 5–5 illustrates the placement of an Arndt blocker.

COHEN FLEXITIP ENDOBRONCHIAL BLOCKER

The Cohen bronchial blocker was designed with a wheel-controlled device to achieve deflection of the distal blocker tip and a torque grip at 55 cm for blocker rotation, both designed to facilitate guidance of the blocker into the desired bronchus.[2,36] This blocker also features a pre-angled distal tip to improve the maneuverability of the device. Of note, when viewed through a FOB, one can see an arrow at the distal tip above the balloon to indicate which direction the tip deflects. This blocker is only available in size 9 F and 65 cm in length and has a spherically shaped high-volume, low-pressure balloon and side holes near the distal end to facilitate lung deflation. The Cohen blocker also comes with a multiport adaptor for in situ use of the blocker while maintaining ventilation.

Placement and Positioning of the Cohen Endobronchial Blocker

The Cohen blocker should be used with an 8.0-mm ID or greater single-lumen ETT; preparation includes testing the blocker balloon, deflation of the balloon and lubrication of the blocker prior to attachment and insertion into the ETT lumen. After securing the multiconnector port and placing the endobronchial blocker into the ETT, FOB is used to observe the movement of the blocker into the desired mainstem bronchus. The wheel device is used to deflect the blocker tip and the torque grip to guide and position the blocker correctly.

The blocker is relatively easy to place in the right mainstem bronchus and the inflated balloon (with 4-8 mL of air) should be visualized with the FOB 5 mm caudal to the tracheal carina on the right. Intubation of the left mainstem bronchus may be more challenging; guiding the blocker into the left mainstem bronchus can be facilitated by advancing the tip of the single-lumen ETT to the carina, just

Chapter 5 / Lung Separation Techniques   93

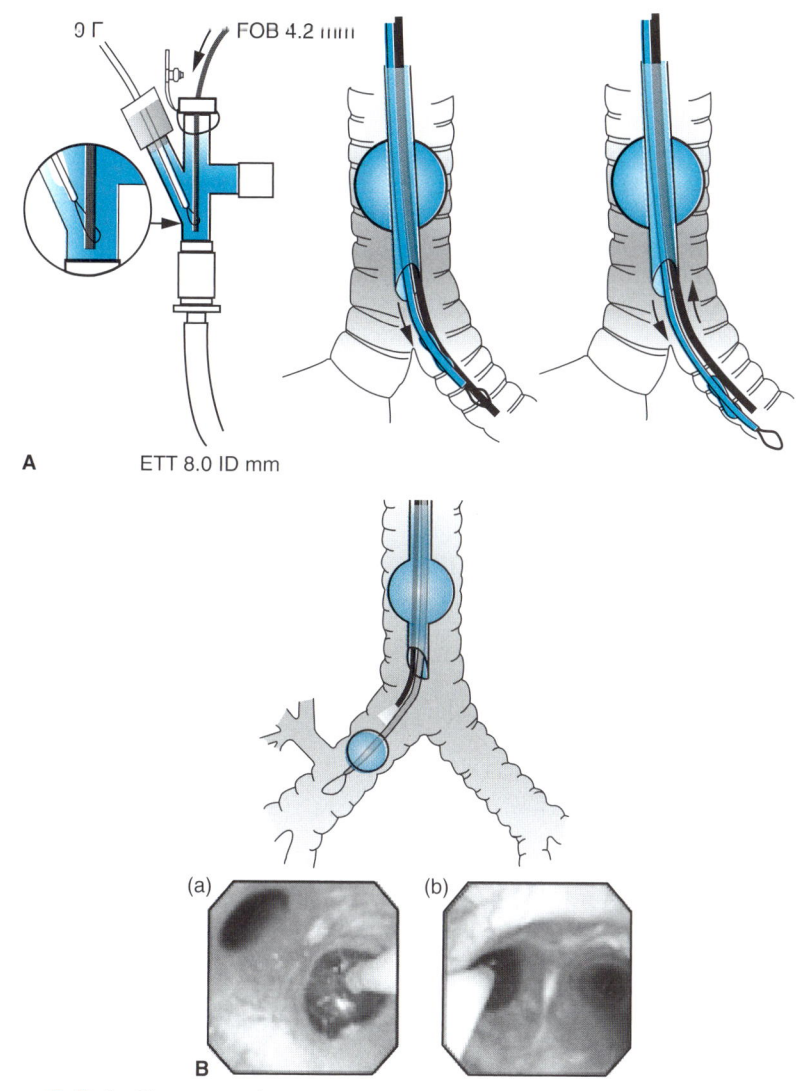

Figure 5-5. **A.** Placement of an Arndt bronchial blocker through a single-lumen endotracheal tube. Note how the fiberoptic bronchoscope is advanced through the loop of the bronchial blocker guidewire. (Reproduced with permission from Campos JH.[68]) **B.** Optimal position of a bronchial blocker in the left mainstem bronchus. The proximal edge of the fully inflated cuff is approximately 5 to 10 mm below the tracheal carina. Inserts (a) and (b) are bronchoscopic views of a bronchial blocker in the right and left mainstem bronchi respectively. (Reproduced with permission from Campos JH.[2] © Elsevier.)

cranial to the entrance of the left bronchus. Then, a leftward twist of the Cohen blocker facilitates entrance to the left mainstem bronchus. After the blocker is observed within the left bronchus, the single-lumen ETT is withdrawn a few centimeters. Similar to the right side, the blocker's balloon should be positioned approximately 5 mm distal to the trachea carina.

FUJI UNIBLOCKER

The Fuji Uniblocker bronchial blocker is available in 4.5 and 9 F sizes; it is 65 cm in length and features a high-volume balloon made of silicone. This blocker has two unique features. One is that the balloon is made of a material that impairs the diffusion of gas into or out of the cuff. Thus, with a maximal inflation of 6 mL of air, the blocker's transmitted pressure is always less than 30 mm Hg, a pressure thought to be safe for the bronchial mucosa.[47] Second, the Fuji Uniblocker features a swivel connector with torque control built into the shaft of the blocker to optimize control of the blocker's movements.

Placement and Positioning of the Fuji Uniblocker

An 8.0 ETT is required for placement of the Fuji Uniblocker most commonly used in adults—the size 9 F. Similar to the other blockers, the Fuji Uniblocker is advanced into and through an ETT using a FOB and the torque control shaft used to position the blocker within the desired bronchus. Also similar to the other endobronchial blockers, the edge of the blocker's inflated balloon should be viewed 5 mm below the tracheal carina on the right but on the left should it should be seen at least 5 to 10 mm below the trachea carina.

COMPARISON OF INDEPENDENT BRONCHIAL BLOCKERS

A study was conducted comparing the Fuji Uniblocker, the Arndt and the Cohen bronchial blockers to left-sided DLTs for thoracoscopic procedures and open thoracotomy[37]; all of the bronchial blockers took a longer time to position and required more intraoperative repositioning compared to left-sided DLTs, but resulted in similar surgical exposure. Another report[48] examined the Fuji Uniblocker for patients undergoing video-assisted thoracic surgery; the quality of lung collapse was deemed to be greater for left-sided compared to right-sided procedures. Table 5–2 displays the characteristics of the Arndt blocker, the Cohen endobronchial blocker, and the Fuji Uniblocker.

UNIVENT ENDOTRACHEAL TUBE

The Univent tube consists of an endotracheal tube combined with a bronchial blocker; it is a modified single-lumen tube with an attached, enclosed and movable bronchial blocker within the tube itself. The non-latex blocker is designed as a flexible shaft to facilitate positioning of the blocker past the tip of the endotracheal tube into the right or left mainstem bronchus.[49] Of note, the balloon inflates in a high-pressure, low-volume manner that requires 4 to 6 mL of air for selective lobar blockade or 6 to

Table 5–2. Characteristics of the Arndt Blocker, the Cohen Flexitip Endobronchial Blocker, and the Fuji Uniblocker

	Cohen Blocker	**Arndt Blocker**	**Fuji Uniblocker**
Size	9 F	5, 7, and 9 F	4.5, 9 F
Balloon shape	Spherical	Spherical or elliptical	Spherical
Guidance mechanism	Wheel device to deflect the tip	Nylon wire loop that is coupled with the FOB	None, preshaped tip
Smallest recommended ETT for coaxial use	9 F (8.0 ETT)	5 F (4.5 ETT), 7 F (7.0 ETT), 9 F (8.0 ETT)	4.5 (4.5 ETT), 9 F (8.0 ETT)
Murphy eye	Present	Present in 9 F	Not present
Center channel	1.6 mm internal diameter	1.4 mm internal diameter	2.0 mm internal diameter

ETT = single endotracheal tube.
Modified with permission from Campos JH.[38]

8 mL of air for mainstem bronchial blockade. Given that it is a high-pressure cuff, it is important to manually palpate and evaluate the bronchial pilot balloon pressure to prevent excessive pressure to the bronchial mucosa; the minimum amount of air needed to seal a bronchus should be used to inflate the blocker balloon. The Univent blocker is useful for selective lung isolation in a patient with a difficult airway, which may preclude dual lumen endotracheal tube placement.[50-55] Another attribute of the Univent blocker is an indwelling 2-mm diameter lumen that can be used for suctioning or for oxygen administration into the deflated lung. A potential disadvantage is the smaller internal diameter of the specialized endotracheal tube when compared to an equal size outer diameter regular endotracheal tube, which may result in a relatively higher airflow resistance during mechanical ventilation.

Placement of the Univent blocker/endotracheal tube should include the following steps:

Prior to standard endotracheal intubation, the enclosed bronchial blocker should be lubricated and then fully retracted into its lumen within the endotracheal tube. Intubation of the trachea is achieved through any means chosen (dependent on the difficulty of the airway) followed by FOB placement through a Portex swivel adaptor. Under direct visualization, the bronchial blocker is advanced into the bronchus on the operative side and the bronchial balloon inflated to achieve unilateral lung collapse.

COMPLICATIONS WITH THE USE OF BRONCHIAL BLOCKERS

Serious complications are rare with bronchial blockers and are usually less severe than those related to double-lumen ETT tubes. The most common complication is actually failure to achieve adequate lung isolation and/or separation. This may be due to abnormal bronchial anatomy but may also be due to operator error. Abnormal anatomy is noted when the right upper lobe bronchus branches from the trachea instead of the right mainstem bronchus, precluding the ability of a bronchial blocker to deflate the right upper, middle and lower lobe bronchi simultaneously. More commonly, the bronchial balloon is not inflated or positioned properly, leading to an inadequate seal of the bronchus.[56,57] The bronchial balloon can be mistakenly inflated in the trachea or an overinflated bronchial balloon cuff can also migrate cranially and move back into the trachea; both situations cause complete tracheal occlusion with subsequent respiratory failure.[58] Air trapping has occurred distal to the blocker leading a pulseless electrical activity arrest; prompt deflation of the bronchial blocker cuff resolved the problem.[59] The distal portion of the bronchial blocker and/or the guidewire have been included in the surgical staple line during lobectomy.[46,60] Adequate communication with the surgical team regarding the presence of a bronchial blocker is crucial. Structural complications from the blockers themselves that have been reported include shearing the balloon with retraction of the blocker through the multichannel port with an Arndt blocker and a fracture of the blocker cap connector with the Univent blocker.[61,62] It has been recommended that independent bronchial blockers be removed with the multiport connector in place rather than through the connector. There have not been any reports of tracheal or bronchial rupture.

LUNG SEPARATION IN THE TRACHEOSTOMIZED PATIENT

The anesthesiologist occasionally encounters a patient that has a tracheostomy in place and requires OLV. Although the stoma provides direct, easy access to the lower airway, it is important to note that the tracheal segment above the carina where the endotracheal tube's tracheal cuff is to be positioned is short in these cases, and hence more prone to positioning complications. Also, the stoma may be small and restrictive, which may limit the size of the tube or cannula used. Appropriate lubrication should always be used and forceful maneuvers should be avoided in order to avoid airway bleeding, which invariably complicates visualization during FOB.

There are three main alternatives for achieving successful lung separation in the tracheostomized patient: (a) orotracheal intubation using a DLT, (b) insertion of a single-lumen endotracheal tube through the stoma and into the right or left mainstem bronchus, as indicated; or (c) use of a bronchial blocker, either attached to a single-lumen endotracheal tube such as the Univent blocker,[63,64] passed independently through a tracheostomy cannula,[43] or placed through a single-lumen endotracheal tube.[65]

The first technique has all the limitations of DLT insertion, plus the difficulty in passing the larger diameter DLT through the site of the stoma, which may be narrow and friable. The second technique, insertion and "mainsteming" of a single lumen tube through the stoma, prevents full deflation and aspiration of secretions in the collapsed lung. Use of a bronchial blocker is generally the most versatile and stable technique, and therefore the preferred one in the authors' opinion.

When passing a 9-F bronchial blocker through a tracheostomy tube, the recommended flexible FOB size should be 3.5-mm ID, so the independent blocker and the fiberscope can navigate together to achieve optimal position of these devices into the designated bronchus. Alternatively, a smaller diameter bronchial blocker should be chosen for lung isolation, since the internal diameter of an 8.0 tracheostomy cannula is often smaller than a conventional 8.0 ETT.

In some instances when using a tracheostomy cannula, the multiport connector is attached to the ventilating port of the tracheostomy cannula to maintain the bronchial blocker in place. A short-breathing circuit extension may be used to facilitate access to the device and to prevent the weight of the multiport connector and anesthesia circuit from dislodging the tracheal cannula. As in other lung separation techniques, optimal position is achieved with FOB aid.

LUNG COLLAPSE FOLLOWING LUNG SEPARATION

Correct placement of a lung separation device is not necessarily followed by immediate, complete lung collapse. In fact, spontaneous lung deflation may take more than 25 minutes depending on the device used.[49] Strategies that may be used to aid lung deflation during lung isolation include de-nitrogenation using 100% inspired oxygen concentration prior to lung collapse,[66] a period of apnea prior to inflation of the bronchial blocker cuff, and gentle aspiration of the airways using the fiberoptic endoscope suction channel prior to lung separation.

It is important to note that once lung isolation is achieved, the overall clinical performance is similar for both DLTs and bronchial blockers.[37] In one study, the bronchial blockers required longer time to position and were more prone to intraoperative reposition, however. Table 5–3 displays the advantages and disadvantages of DLTs and bronchial blockers.

Table 5–3. Advantages and Disadvantages of Double-Lumen Endotracheal Tubes and Bronchial Blockers

Double-Lumen Endotracheal Tubes	Bronchial Blockers (Arndt, Cohen, Fuji)
Advantages	*Advantages*
• Large lumen facilitates suctioning • Best device for absolute lung separation • Conversion from 2- to 1-lung ventilation easy and reliable	• Easy recognition of anatomy if the tip of a single tube is above carina • Best device for patients with difficult airways • No cuff damage during intubation • No need to replace a tube if mechanical ventilation is needed
Disadvantages • Difficulties in selecting proper size • Difficult to place during laryngoscopy • Damage to tracheal cuff • Major tracheobronchial injuries	*Disadvantages* • Small channel for suctioning • Conversion from 1- to 2- then to 1-lung ventilation (problematic for the novice) • High maintenance device (dislodgement or loss seal during surgery)

Modified with permission from Campos JH.[38]

SUMMARY

Prerequisites for successful lung isolation include knowledge of the normal tracheobronchial anatomy, a thorough preoperative assessment of the patient, including review of the chest x-ray and chest CT scan when available, and familiarity with fiberoptic bronchoscopy equipment and techniques. Additionally, it is important for the anesthesia provider to be familiar with several different lung separation techniques, such as DLT placement and one or more types of bronchial blockers.

Left-sided DLTs are generally used for most thoracic surgery cases given their ease of insertion and the quality of lung separation achieved. A right-sided DLT is recommended for a left-sided pneumonectomy or left-sided bronchial *sleeve* resection. Bronchial blockers are indicated in patients with a difficult or abnormal airway or those who have a tracheotomy in place, but these devices require more time for placement and are more prone to intraoperative dislodgement. Lung collapse is facilitated by a de-nitrogenation technique using 100% inspired oxygen concentration prior to lung collapse, and a period of apnea and/or gentle aspiration of the airways using the fiberoptic endoscope suction channel prior to lung separation.

Placement of any of these lung isolation devices requires auscultation followed by fiberoptic bronchoscopy in order to obtain a high success rate during lung separation. The optimal position of these devices (DLTs and bronchial blockers) is best achieved using fiberoptic bronchoscopy in both the supine and the lateral decubitus position or whenever repositioning of the device is needed.

REFERENCES

1. Campos JH. Current techniques for perioperative lung isolation in adults. *Anesthesiology.* 2002;97(5):1295-1301.
2. Campos JH. Progress in lung separation. *Thorac Surg Clin.* 2005;15(1):71-83.
3. Lewis JW Jr, Serwin JP, Gabriel FS, Bastanfar M, Jacobsen G. The utility of a double-lumen tube for one-lung ventilation in a variety of noncardiac thoracic surgical procedures. *J Cardiothorac Vasc Anesth.* 1992;6(6):705-710.
4. Campos JH. An update on bronchial blockers during lung separation techniques in adults. *Anesth Analg.* 2003;97(5):1266-1274.
5. Bjork VO, Carlens E. The prevention of spread during pulmonary resection by the use of a double-lumen catheter. *J Thorac Surg.* 1950;20(1):151-157.
6. Lohser J, Brodsky JB. Silbronco double-lumen tube. *J Cardiothorac Vasc Anesth.* 2006;20(1):129-131.
7. Hagihira S, Takashina M, Mashimo T. Application of a newly designed right-sided, double-lumen endobronchial tube in patients with a very short right mainstem bronchus. *Anesthesiology.* 2008;109(3):565-568.
8. Stene R, Rose M, Weinger MB, Benumof JL, Harrell J. Bronchial trifurcation at the carina complicating use of a double-lumen tracheal tube. *Anesthesiology.* 1994;80(5):1162-1164.
9. Seymour AH, Prakash N. A cadaver study to measure the adult glottis and subglottis: defining a problem associated with the use of double-lumen tubes. *J Cardiothorac Vasc Anesth.* 2002;16(2):196-198.
10. Sivalingam P, Tio R. Tension pneumothorax, pneumomediastinum, pneumoperitoneum, and subcutaneous emphysema in a 15-year-old Chinese girl after a double-lumen tube intubation and one-lung ventilation. *J Cardiothorac Vasc Anesth.* 1999;13(3):312-315.
11. Bardoczky G, d'Hollander A, Yernault JC, Van Meuylem A, Moures JM, Rocmans P. On-line expiratory flow-volume curves during thoracic surgery: occurrence of auto-PEEP. *Br J Anaesth.* 1994;72(1):25-28.
12. Sakuragi T, Kumano K, Yasumoto M, Dan K. Rupture of the left main-stem bronchus by the tracheal portion of a double-lumen endobronchial tube. *Acta Anaesthesiol Scand.* 1997;41(9):1218-1220.

13. Brodsky JB, Macario A, Mark JB. Tracheal diameter predicts double-lumen tube size: a method for selecting left double-lumen tubes. *Anesth Analg.* 1996;82(4):861-864.
14. Chow MY, Liam BL, Lew TW, Chelliah RY, Ong BC. Predicting the size of a double-lumen endobronchial tube based on tracheal diameter. *Anesth Analg.* 1998;87(1):158-160.
15. Amar D, Desiderio DP, Heerdt PM, Kolker AC, Zhang H, Thaler HT. Practice patterns in choice of left double-lumen tube size for thoracic surgery. *Anesth Analg.* 2008;106(2):379-383, table of contents.
16. Eberle B, Weiler N, Vogel N, Kauczor HU, Heinrichs W. Computed tomography-based tracheobronchial image reconstruction allows selection of the individually appropriate double-lumen tube size. *J Cardiothorac Vasc Anesth.* 1999;13(5):532-537.
17. Brodsky JB, Benumof JL, Ehrenwerth J, Ozaki GT. Depth of placement of left double-lumen endobronchial tubes. *Anesth Analg.* 1991;73(5):570-572.
18. Boucek CD, Landreneau R, Freeman JA, Strollo D, Bircher NG. A comparison of techniques for placement of double-lumen endobronchial tubes. *J Clin Anesth.* 1998;10(7):557-560.
19. Saito S, Dohi S, Naito H. Alteration of double-lumen endobronchial tube position by flexion and extension of the neck. *Anesthesiology.* 1985;62(5):696-697.
20. Hannallah M, Gomes M. Bronchial rupture associated with the use of a double-lumen tube in a small adult. *Anesthesiology.* 1989;71(3):457-459.
21. Benumof JL, Wu D. Tracheal tear caused by extubation of a double-lumen tube. *Anesthesiology.* 2002;97(4):1007-1008.
22. Liu H, Jahr JS, Sullivan E, Waters PF. Tracheobronchial rupture after double-lumen endotracheal intubation. *J Cardiothorac Vasc Anesth.* 2004;18(2):228-233.
23. Yuceyar L, Kaynak K, Canturk E, Aykac B. Bronchial rupture with a left-sided polyvinylchloride double-lumen tube. *Acta Anaesthesiol Scand.* 2003;47(5):622-625.
24. Fitzmaurice BG, Brodsky JB. Airway rupture from double-lumen tubes. *J Cardiothorac Vasc Anesth.* 1999;13(3):322-329.
25. Sucato DJ, Girgis M. Bilateral pneumothoraces, pneumomediastinum, pneumoperitoneum, pneumoretroperitoneum, and subcutaneous emphysema following intubation with a double-lumen endotracheal tube for thoracoscopic anterior spinal release and fusion in a patient with idiopathic scoliosis. *J Spinal Disord Tech.* 2002;15(2):133-138.
26. Weng W, DeCrosta DJ, Zhang H. Tension pneumothorax during one-lung ventilation: a case report. *J Clin Anesth.* 2002;14(7):529-531.
27. Knoll H, Ziegeler S, Schreiber JU, et al. Airway injuries after one-lung ventilation: a comparison between double-lumen tube and endobronchial blocker: a randomized, prospective, controlled trial. *Anesthesiology.* 2006;105(3):471-477.
28. Ng JM, Hartigan PM. Selective lobar bronchial blockade following contralateral pneumonectomy. *Anesthesiology.* 2003;98(1):268-270.
29. Hagihira S, Maki N, Kawaguchi M, Slinger P. Case 5—2002. Selective bronchial blockade in patients with previous contralateral lung surgery. *J Cardiothorac Vasc Anesth.* 2002;16(5):638-642.
30. Espi C, Garcia-Guasch R, Ibanez C, Fernandez E, Astudillo J. Selective lobar blockade using an Arndt endobronchial blocker in 2 patients with respiratory compromise who underwent lung resection. *Arch Bronconeumol.* 2007;43(6):346-348.
31. Campos JH, Ledet C, Moyers JR. Improvement of arterial oxygen saturation with selective lobar bronchial block during hemorrhage in a patient with previous contralateral lobectomy. *Anesth Analg.* 1995;81(5):1095-1096.
32. Campos JH. Update on selective lobar blockade during pulmonary resections. *Curr Opin Anaesthesiol.* 2009;22(1):18-22.
33. Campos JH. Effects of oxygenation during selective lobar versus total lung collapse with or without continuous positive airway pressure. *Anesth Analg.* 1997;85(3):583-586.
34. Amar D, Desiderio DP, Bains MS, Wilson RS. A novel method of one-lung isolation using a double endobronchial blocker technique. *Anesthesiology.* 2001;95(6):1528-1530.
35. Arndt GA, Kranner PW, Rusy DA, Love R. Single-lung ventilation in a critically ill patient using a fiberoptically directed wire-guided endobronchial blocker. *Anesthesiology.* 1999;90(5):1484-1486.
36. Cohen E. The Cohen flexitip endobronchial blocker: an alternative to a double lumen tube. *Anesth Analg.* 2005;101(6):1877-1879.

37. Narayanaswamy M, McRae K, Slinger P, et al. Choosing a lung isolation device for thoracic surgery: a randomized trial of three bronchial blockers versus double-lumen tubes. *Anesth Analg.* 2009;108(4):1097-1101.
38. Campos JH. Which device should be considered the best for lung isolation: double-lumen endotracheal tube versus bronchial blockers. *Curr Opin Anaesthesiol.* 2007;20(1):27-31.
39. Arndt GA, DeLessio ST, Kranner PW, Orzepowski W, Ceranski B, Valtysson B. One-lung ventilation when intubation is difficult—presentation of a new endobronchial blocker. *Acta Anaesthesiol Scand.* 1999;43(3):356-358.
40. Arndt GA, Buchika S, Kranner PW, DeLessio ST. Wire-guided endobronchial blockade in a patient with a limited mouth opening. *Can J Anaesth.* 1999;46(1):87-89.
41. Grocott HP, Scales G, Schinderle D, King K. A new technique for lung isolation in acute thoracic trauma. *J Trauma.* 2000;49(5):940-942.
42. Byhahn C, Habler OP, Bingold TM, Vogl TJ, Thoerner M, Zwissler B. The wire-guided endobronchial blocker: applications in trauma patients beyond mere single-lung ventilation. *J Trauma.* 2006;61(3):755-759.
43. Campos JH, Kernstine KH. Use of the wire-guided endobronchial blocker for one-lung anesthesia in patients with airway abnormalities. *J Cardiothorac Vasc Anesth.* 2003;17(3):352-354.
44. Kabon B, Waltl B, Leitgeb J, Kapral S, Zimpfer M. First experience with fiberoptically directed wire-guided endobronchial blockade in severe pulmonary bleeding in an emergency setting. *Chest.* 2001;120(4):1399-1402.
45. Karzai W. Alternative method to deflate the operated lung when using wire-guided endobronchial blockade. *Anesthesiology.* 2003;99(1):239-240, author reply 241.
46. Soto RG, Oleszak SP. Resection of the Arndt bronchial blocker during stapler resection of the left lower lobe. *J Cardiothorac Vasc Anesth.* 2006;20(1):131-132.
47. Roscoe A, Kanellakos GW, McRae K, Slinger P. Pressures exerted by endobronchial devices. *Anesth Analg.* 2007;104(3):655-658.
48. Iizuka T, Tanno M, Hamada Y, Shiga T, Ohe Y. Use of the UNIBLOCKER®- bronchial blocker tube to facilitate one-lung ventilation during thoracoscopic surgery. *Anesthesiology.* 2007;107.
49. Campos JH, Kernstine KH. A comparison of a left-sided Broncho-Cath with the torque control blocker univent and the wire-guided blocker. *Anesth Analg.* 2003;96(1):283-289.
50. Takenaka I, Aoyama K, Kadoya T. Use of the univent bronchial-blocker tube for unanticipated difficult endotracheal intubation. *Anesthesiology.* 2000;93(2):590-591.
51. Ransom ES, Carter SL, Mund GD. Univent tube: a useful device in patients with difficult airways. *J Cardiothorac Vasc Anesth.* 1995;9(6):725-727.
52. Hagihira S, Takashina M, Mori T, Yoshiya I. One-lung ventilation in patients with difficult airways. *J Cardiothorac Vasc Anesth.* 1998;12(2):186-188.
53. Garcia-Aguado R, Mateo EM, Tommasi-Rosso M, et al. Thoracic surgery and difficult intubation: another application of univent tube for one-lung ventilation. *J Cardiothorac Vasc Anesth.* 1997;11(7):925-926.
54. Garcia-Aguado R, Mateo EM, Onrubia VJ, Bolinches R. Use of the Univent System tube for difficult intubation and for achieving one-lung anaesthesia. *Acta Anaesthesiol Scand.* 1996;40(6):765-767.
55. Baraka A. The univent tube can facilitate difficult intubation in a patient undergoing thoracoscopy. *J Cardiothorac Vasc Anesth.* 1996;10(5):693-694.
56. Peragallo RA, Swenson JD. Congenital tracheal bronchus: the inability to isolate the right lung with a univent bronchial blocker tube. *Anesth Analg.* 2000;91(2):300-301.
57. Asai T. Failure of the Univent bronchial blocker in sealing the bronchus. *Anaesthesia.* 1999;54(1):97.
58. Dougherty P, Hannallah M. A potentially serious complication that resulted from improper use of the Univent tube. *Anesthesiology.* 1992;77(4):835.
59. Sandberg WS. Endobronchial blocker dislodgement leading to pulseless electrical activity. *Anesth Analg.* 2005;100(6):1728-1730.
60. Thielmeier KA, Anwar M. Complication of the Univent tube. *Anesthesiology.* 1996;84(2):491.
61. Prabhu MR, Smith JH. Use of the Arndt wire-guided endobronchial blocker. *Anesthesiology.* 2002;97(5):1325.
62. Campos JH, Kernstine KH. A structural complication in the torque control blocker Univent: fracture of the blocker cap connector. *Anesth Analg.* 2003;96(2):630-631.

63. Dhamee MS. One-lung ventilation in a patient with a fresh tracheostomy using the tracheostomy tube and a Univent endobronchial blocker. *J Cardiothorac Vasc Anesth.* 1997;11(1):124-125.
64. Bellver J, Garcia-Aguado R, De Andres J, Valia JC, Bolinches R. Selective bronchial intubation with the univent system in patients with a tracheostomy. *Anesthesiology.* 1993;79(6):1453-1454.
65. Tobias JD. Variations on one-lung ventilation. *J Clin Anesth.* 2001;13(1):35-39.
66. Ko R, McRae K, Darling G, et al. The use of air in the inspired gas mixture during two-lung ventilation delays lung collapse during one-lung ventilation. *Anesth Analg.* 2009;108(4):1092-1096.
67. Campos JH. Update on tracheobronchial anatomy and flexible fiberoptic bronchoscopy in thoracic anesthesia. *Curr Opin Anaesthesiol.* 2009;22(1):4-10.
68. Campos JH. How to achieve successful lung separation. *SAJAA.* 2008; 14: 22-26

Mechanisms of Pain in Thoracic Surgery

6

Jessica A. Boyette-Davis
Patrick M. Dougherty

Key Points

- Acute pain can be produced from trauma sustained during surgery. This injury results in activation of the nociceptive system, including activation of primary afferent nerve fibers in the periphery, excitation of dorsal horn neurons in the spinal cord, and recruitment of key brain areas. It will further lead to the release of multiple inflammatory mediators, which then potentiate pain.
- Persistent activation of the nociceptive system can lead to chronic pain. If nerves are damaged during surgery, this chronic pain can present in the form of neuropathy. In both instances, the chronic pain seems to be predominately centrally, as opposed to peripherally, mediated.
- Analgesic interventions are generally effective for acute postoperative pain. However, for patients who develop chronic post-thoracotomy pain, pain relief is less easily achieved and may be best accomplished best by preemptive analgesia.

Pain is a sensation that is normally associated with the application of noxious or injurious stimuli. In the context of thoracic surgery, pain can develop in multiple ways. Acute pain occurs as a direct result of physical trauma sustained during thoracic surgery. This trauma can include tissue damage from surgical incisions or manipulation, fractures to ribs, and hematomas.[1] As will be discussed in this chapter, this acute pain may then develop into a chronic pain state in approximately half of all patients. Damage to nerves, most often the intercostal nerves, during surgery also contributes significantly to pain, as this damage manifests as a distinct form of chronic pain termed neuropathy. Thus, pain in thoracic surgery patients involves multiple components and mechanisms including those mediating acute somatic pain, hyperalgesia, and neuropathic pain. In the instance where these multiple components are all observed in a patient, the condition is referred to as *chronic post-thoracotomy pain*. To explain this condition in part or in its entirety, this chapter will review the basic physiology of pain, including pain pathways and neurochemistry, the neural mechanisms and neurochemical mediators of primary and secondary hyperalgesia, and the unique mechanisms of neuropathic pain.

OVERVIEW OF PAIN PATHWAYS AND NEUROCHEMISTRY
Peripheral Neural Mechanisms

In general, pain begins in a distinct class of primary afferent fibers that respond selectively to noxious stimuli. These *nociceptors* are located in the periphery, with the cell bodies located in dorsal root ganglia (DRG) outside the spinal cord, and terminate in the dorsal horn. Nociceptors respond to a number of different stimulus modalities including thermal, chemical, and mechanical stimuli.[2,3] However, there are different classifications of nociceptors, generally based on the conduction velocity of the axons of these nociceptive neurons. The *C fibers* are generally unmyelinated fibers that conduct at velocities of less than 2 m/s and constitute over 75% of afferent fibers present in peripheral nerves. Several lines of evidence indicate that C-fiber nociceptors are essential for the normal perception of pain. For instance, intraneural electrical stimulation of identified C-fiber nociceptors in humans elicits the sensation of pain, and blockade of C-fiber transmission prevents thermal pain perception at the normal heat pain threshold.[4] Absence of C fibers, either via capsaicin ablation[5] or as is seen in patients with congenital insensitivity to pain,[6] results in diminished or altogether absent pain sensation. Recordings from C fibers in humans suggest that C-fiber activity is associated with a prolonged burning sensation. In contrast, activation of faster conducting (5 to 20 m/s) myelinated *Aδ fibers* evokes a sharp, intense, tingling sensation. Combined, Aδ- and C-fiber nociceptors encode and transmit information to the central nervous system concerning the intensity, location, and duration of noxious stimuli.

Following transduction by peripheral afferents, nociceptive information is transmitted via nerves to the central nervous system. Within the thoracic cavity, it is the *intercostal nerves* of the peripheral nervous system that transmit pain signals to the spinal cord. These nerves, which are located with the intercostal space, are often damaged during thoracic surgery, leading to symptoms of neuropathic pain. The mechanisms of this pain are discussed below.

Central Neural Mechanisms

The axons of primary afferents terminate at the ipsilateral side of the dorsal horn of the spinal cord in a highly organized manner.[7,8] As can be seen in Figure 6–1, the cells of the dorsal horn are arranged in layers, or laminae,[9] with C fibers terminating primarily in the most superficial lamina (I and II outer) and Aδ fibers ending in lamina I, and in laminae III to V. Because both C and Aδ fibers terminate in lamina I, in addition to C fiber termination into lamina II, neurons within these laminae respond almost exclusively to noxious inputs[10] and are often termed nociceptive specific (NS) or high-threshold neurons.[11,12]

In addition to these NS neurons, two other classes of sensory spinal neurons make synapse with nociceptive neurons. These cells, the wide dynamic range (WDR) and the multi-receptive (MR) cells, respond to both noxious and nonnoxious stimuli with the difference being that WDR cells show a discharge

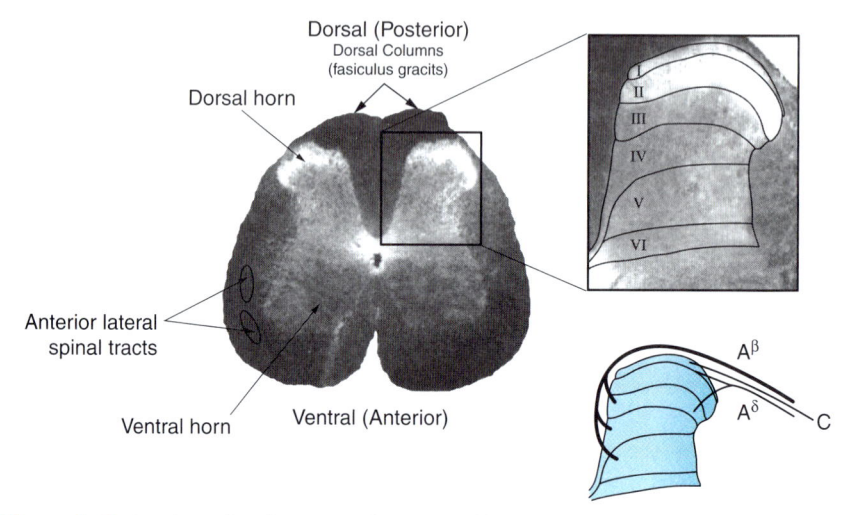

Figure 6–1. Laminae distribution and primary afferent termination within the spinal cord. The histological section on the left is labeled to show the location of the dorsal horn within the spinal cord. In the enlarged segment to the right, the layers of laminae I through VI are outlined. Primary afferent innervation to the various laminae is depicted in the schematic at the bottom. (From: Raja, SN & Dougherty, PM. Anatomy and physiology of somatosensory and pain processing. In HT Benzon, SN Raja, RE Molloy, SS Liu, & SM Fishman (eds). *Essentials of Pain Medicine and Regional Anesthesia.* 2nd ed. Figure 1-1, pg 3. Philadelphia, USA: Elsevier, Churchill, Livingstone; 2005, with permission.)

rate that is graded with stimulus intensity whereas the MR cells do not.[13,14] The WDR and MR cells in laminae III to V show responses to both cutaneous mechanical and heat stimuli, but rarely show responses from deep tissues, while cells in laminae VI and VII tend to show responses from deep tissue and visceral receptors.

Unlike for touch where information ascends ipsilaterally up the spinal cord via the dorsal column medial lemniscal system, almost all nociceptive information is transmitted to the contralateral side of the body at the level of primary afferent innervation. There the axons of WDR and NS neurons cross the midline of the spinal cord, gather into bundles and then ascend toward targets in the brainstem and diencephalon via the antereolateral system. This system is further divided into distinct tracts based primarily upon the location of projection neurons within dorsal horn laminae (Figure 6–2). For instance, the axons of WDR and NS cells that make synapse within laminae I and V-VII ascend to the medial thalamus, thus forming the spinothalamic tract.

Within the brain, several areas are especially involved in processing nociceptive information.[15] In response to pain, six brain areas are consistently recruited: the primary and secondary somatosensory cortices, the insular cortex, the anterior cingulate cortex, the prefrontal cortex (PFC), and several nuclei of the thalamus.

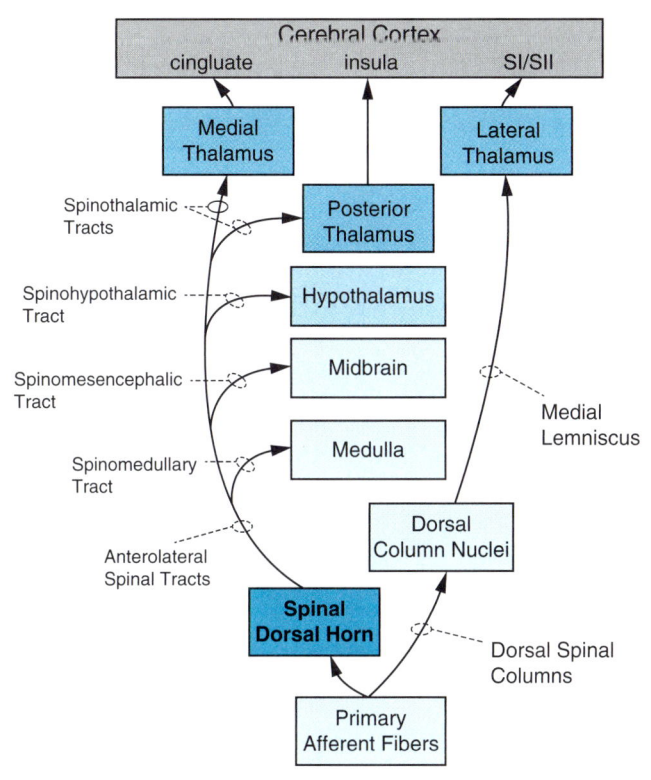

Figure 6-2. Summary of the central nociceptive pathways. Information ascends from primary afferent fibers via either the dorsal column medial lemniscal column (touch) or the anterolateral system (nociception). Projections of various nociceptive specific tracts are also depicted. (From: Raja, SN & Dougherty, PM. Anatomy and physiology of somatosensory and pain processing. In HT Benzon, SN Raja, RE Molloy, SS Liu, & SM Fishman (eds). *Essentials of Pain Medicine and Regional Anesthesia*. 2nd ed. Figure 1-4, pg 5. Philadelphia, USA: Elsevier, Churchill, Livingstone; 2005, with permission.)

The somatosensory cortices provide information regarding where in the body pain originates, and there is evidence that S2 contains a somatotopic map for nociceptive input. The insular and rostral anterior cingulate cortices are part of the limbic system, and an abundance of literature suggests these brain structures modulate the affective or emotional aspect of pain. The PFC aids not only in making a decision as to what actions should be taken to alter pain, but this part of the brain also is useful in controlling input from the limbic system. Interestingly, some research suggests that the pattern of brain activation changes during chronic pain from more limbic-related activity to significantly more activation in the PFC. Further, thalamic activation tends to be lower in chronic versus acute pain. Finally, other key areas of the brain are involved in the descending modulation of pain, primarily via serotonin-related mechanisms. These areas include the rostral ventromedial medulla, the nucleus raphe magnus, the locus ceruleus, and the periaqueductal gray matter.

Neurochemistry

Within the periphery, numerous chemicals are released following insult to tissue (Figure 6–3). These chemicals, which can directly activate nociceptors or increase the general excitability of nociceptors, are frequently referred to as an "inflammatory soup." Following injury, both bradykinin[16] and serotonin[17] directly activate nociceptors. The neuropeptides histamine, substance P, and calcitonin gene-related peptide (CGRP) are derived from activated nociceptors and produce a variety of responses, including vasodilation and edema. Further, histamine excites polymodal visceral nociceptors and potentiates the responses of nociceptors to bradykinin and heat.[18] Eicosanoids, including prostaglandins, thromboxanes, and leukotrienes, directly activate and sensitize afferents.[19, 20] Nitric oxide (NO) released by damaged

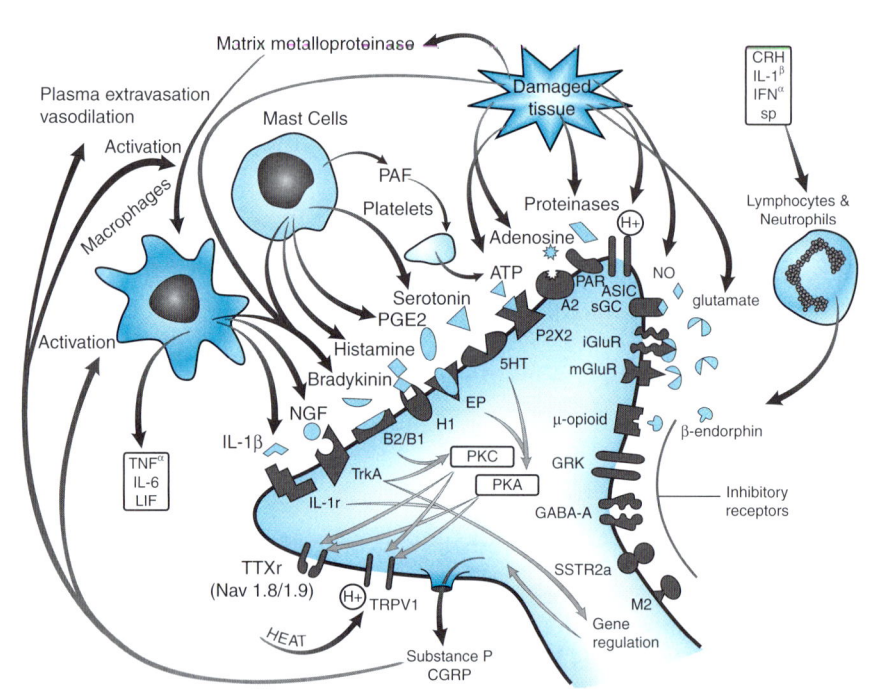

Figure 6–3. Summary of the neurochemical mediators in the periphery. Tissue injury provokes the release of numerous chemical mediators of pain. Pro-nociceptive mediators augment pain via multiple mechanisms, including directly activating nociceptors, sensitizing primary afferents, and causing the release of other known mediators. (Adapted from Dougherty, PM & Raja, SN. Neurochemistry of somatosensory and pain processing. In HT Benzon, SN Raja, RE Molloy, SS Liu, & SM Fishman (eds). *Essentials of Pain Medicine and Regional Anesthesia* 2nd ed., Figure 2-1, pg 8. Philadelphia, USA: Elsevier, Churchill, Livingstone; 2005, with permission.)

afferents can further sensitize nearby neurons, augmenting pain and inflammation.[21] Cytokines released by a variety of cells[19] can also serve to directly excite and sensitize nociceptive afferent fibers to thermal and mechanical stimuli. Cytokines also lead to increased production of nerve growth factor (NGF),[22] which in turn stimulates mast cells to release histamine and serotonin, leading to the aforementioned primary afferent fiber activation and sensitization. Proteinases such as thrombin, trypsin, and tryptase, although not traditionally considered part of the inflammatory soup, are gaining increasing attention as mediators of pain and inflammation.[23] Activation of proteinase receptors PAR1 and PAR2, which are located on primary afferent nerve fiber endings, leads to a cascade effect of histamine, substance P, CGRP, prostaglandin, bradykinin, and cytokine release.

In addition to these pro-nociceptive mediators, anti-nociceptive chemicals are also present in the periphery. For instance, opioids, which are known for their analgesic properties, are also a component in inflammatory soup.[24] The peripheral terminals of afferent fibers contain receptors for opioids, and the number of receptors is upregulated following tissue injury. Acetylcholine modulates pain primarily via its effects on muscarinic receptors. This is supported by the findings that muscarinic agonists desensitize C-fiber nociceptors to mechanical and heat stimuli.[25] Finally, somatostatin (SST) may also serve as an antinociceptive agent. The SST receptor type 2a has been identified in a small percentage of unmyelinated primary afferent fibers,[26] and administration of the SST receptor agonist octreotide attenuates bradykinin-induced nociceptor sensitization. SST also inhibits the release of cholecystokinin, which has been shown to have nociceptive properties.

Within the central nervous system, pain is modulated via a host of chemical mediators (Figure 6–4). The amino acids glutamate and aspartate constitute the main excitatory neurotransmitters within the central nervous system. Of particular interest is the glutamate receptor N-methyl-D-aspartate (NMDA). In the spinal cord, the NMDA receptor is recruited only by intense and/or prolonged stimuli, and persistent activation of NMDA receptors leads to sensitization of dorsal horn neurons that includes an increase in receptive field size, decreased activation threshold, and prolonged depolarization. The impact of spinal NMDA-mediated changes will be discussed again in regards to hyperalgesia. In the brain, NMDA receptors are also important for pain[27] and are upregulated following injury. This upregulation is associated with augmented sensitivity to inflammatory pain, excessive excitation of the brainstem, and increased expression of the transcription factor c-Fos. A multitude of research implicates c-Fos as an important facilitator of pain. Adenosine triphosphate (ATP) also serves to enhance pain. ATP receptors, especially the P2X family of receptors are present on the central terminals of primary afferent fibers innervating neurons in lamina V and II of the dorsal horn where they function to increase the release of glutamate. Like many other chemical mediators, the effects of ATP are not limited to neurons. The binding of ATP to P2 receptors on microglia activates these cells, which then begin to secrete inflammatory mediators such as cytokines, nerve growth factor, and NO. These factors then serve to sustain pain and inflammation.[28]

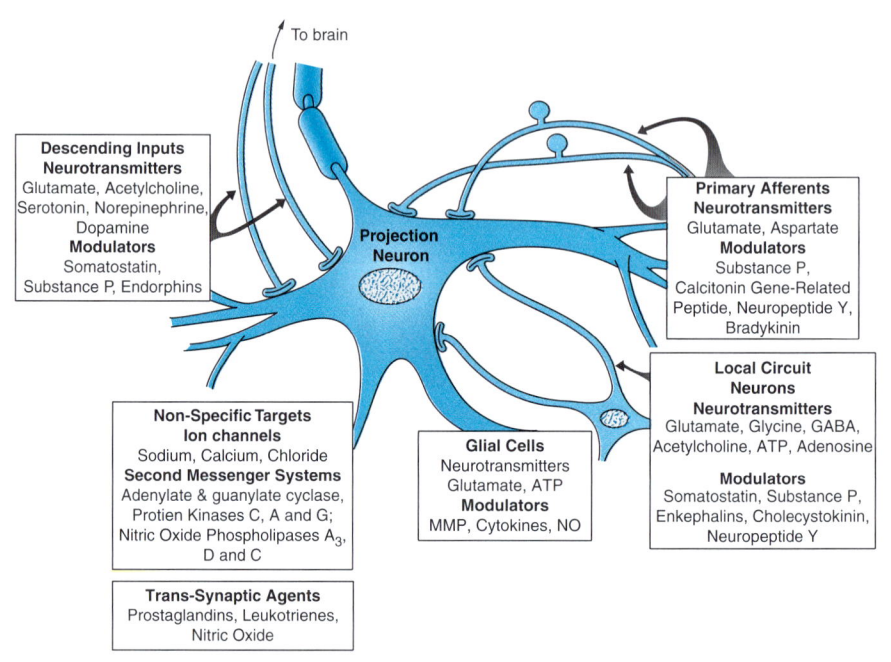

Figure 6–4. Summary of the neurochemical mediators in the spinal cord. As is seen in the periphery, many modulators are present in the spinal cord which work to increase pain transmission. In addition to these factors, nociceptive mediated changes within the spinal cord also include changes to ion channel expression and glial cell activation. These changes play a role in the transition from acute to chronic pain. (Adapted from Dougherty, PM & Raja, SN. Neurochemistry of somatosensory and pain processing. In HT Benzon, SN Raja, RE Molloy, SS Liu, & SM Fishman (eds). *Essentials of Pain Medicine and Regional Anesthesia*. 2nd ed. Figure 2-2, pg 10. Philadelphia, USA: Elsevier, Churchill, Livingstone; 2005, with permission.)

Substance P and neurokinin A serve as excitatory neuropeptides present in addition to the traditional neurotransmitters.[29,30] Activation of neurokinin receptors by either substance P or neurokinin A is an important step in the induction of sensitization and hence the expression of hyperalgesia following cutaneous injury. Spinal release of another peptide, CGRP, has an excitatory effect on WDR neurons, and administration of the CGRP antagonist CGRP8-37 reverses this activity. Interestingly, the role of CGRP released within the brain seems to be antithetic to the peripheral and spinal effects, with release of this peptide within the PAG producing antinociceptive results.

The amino acids glycine and gamma-amino-butyric acid (GABA) are the chief inhibitory neurotransmitters in the somatosensory system. Glycine is the prominent inhibitory neurotransmitter in the spinal cord, especially in local circuit neurons of spinal laminae I, II, and III. Conversely, GABA predominates at higher levels. This is evidenced by the finding that the effects of barbiturates, benzodiazepines and alcohol are mediated by GABA receptors located within the brain. Norepinephrine is another abundant inhibitory neurotransmitter, and it exerts its effects by activating inhibitory GABAergic interneurons and by also inhibiting excitatory interneurons.[31] Serotonin, like norepinephrine, is also involved in descending pathways to the spinal dorsal horn, predominately from the midbrain raphe nuclei.[32,33] The main inhibitory peptides present in the central nervous system are the opioid peptides, which bind to mu, delta and kappa receptor subtypes found at all levels of the somatosensory system. Opioids modulate pain transmission by hyperpolarizing neurons and by blocking the release of pro-nociceptive mediators, such as glutamate and substance P.

THE DEVELOPMENT OF HYPERALGESIA AND CENTRAL SENSITIZATION

Up to this point, discussion has focused on the more acute effects of tissue injury. Following surgery, patients will experience pain as a result of activation of the nociceptive system. This pain may be brief and directly related to tissue injury, but for 50% of patients, this pain will be present for months, or even years. This section, along with the following section will outline how acute pain can transition to a chronic pain state.

Injury to cutaneous and deep tissue such as that occurring with surgery will result in a state of increased sensitivity to suprathreshold stimuli at the site of injury, termed *primary hyperalgesia*, as well as in the uninjured skin surrounding the injury, termed *secondary hyperalgesia*.[34] The characteristics and mechanisms of primary and secondary hyperalgesia differ. Within the zone of primary hyperalgesia, the thresholds for both mechanical and thermal stimuli are lowered, but within the area of secondary hyperalgesia, hypersensitivity to mechanical stimuli but not to thermal stimuli is found.[35]

The driving force of primary hyperalgesia is sensitization of nociceptors.[36,37] Here, *sensitization* refers to a leftward shift of the stimulus-response function that relates magnitude of the neural response to stimulus intensity and is characterized by a decrease in threshold, an augmented response to suprathreshold stimuli, and ongoing spontaneous activity in nociceptors.[38-40] Conversely, the driving force of secondary hyperalgesia is sensitization of spinal neurons. Neurophysiological investigations have shown that the characteristics of secondary hyperalgesia are well-explained by properties of dorsal horn neurons after injury.[41-43] These neurons display increased responding and expanded receptive fields to a mechanical stimulus following an injury. As outlined above, WDR and NS cells play a key role in transmission of pain, but they appear to have differing roles in secondary hyperalgesia. Unlike NS cells, most WDR dorsal horn neurons are sensitized by a variety of peripheral injuries suggesting that this subtype of neurons are important for the detection and discrimination of tissue damaging stimuli and in the generation of secondary hyperalgesia.[44]

Finally, neurons in higher CNS areas also show enhanced responses after injury. For example, the responses of neurons in the thalamus and cortex of rats to cutaneous mechanical stimuli have been shown to increase with the induction of both experimental arthritis and experimental neuropathy.[45] Similarly, the neuronal activity in the thalamus of humans with chronic pain also show alterations.[46,47] Although these changes in responses of thalamic and cortical neurons may just reflect changes that have taken place in the primary afferents and spinal cord neurons under each of these conditions, it should be noted that anatomical and neurochemical changes also take place in the thalamus and cortex under each of these conditions.[48,49] Thus, neuronal substrates exist to support a third or even fourth component to hyperalgesia.

Unfortunately for many patients, hyperalgesia lasts long after injuries have healed. This may be due in part to the phenomenon of *central sensitization* whereby dorsal horn neurons show increased excitability as discussed above. Persistent activation of C fibers results in the release of glutamate, which then activates NMDA receptors. These receptors are an imperative part of transmission of pain signals, so much so that NMDA receptor antagonists like ketamine are often used as analgesics in surgical settings. Indeed, presurgical administration of ketamine can block the development of central sensitization and hyperalgesia.

MECHANISMS OF NEUROPATHIC PAIN

Traumatic injury to soft-tissue, bone, and/or nerve leads, in certain cases, to a chronic pain state that is characterized by ongoing pain and hyperalgesia.[50,51] Noxious stimuli during thoracic surgery may be acutely conveyed by the intercostal, vagus, and phrenic nerves.[52] For example, it is thought that the phrenic nerve is responsible for referred shoulder pain, as it is not ablated by intercostal or epidural analgesia but is treated by phrenic nerve infiltration with lidocaine.[53] Although all three nerves are at risk for mediating the development of enduring pain, in thoracic surgery, a majority of ongoing pain may be attributed to direct or indirect intercostal nerve damage.[54] The pain attributed to nerve damage is very often persistent and characterized by feelings of burning or numbness that is not responsive to typical analgesics. Intriguingly, in some patients the pain and hyperalgesia are dependent on sympathetic innervation of the affected area (sympathetically maintained pain, SMP[55]), while in others the pain is independent of the sympathetics (SIP[56]). Clinically, both SMP and SIP patients often present with similar signs and symptoms.[57]

Immediately following injury, peripheral nerves show a dramatic increase in activity, but this activity usually resolves within several minutes.[58,59] This injury barrage appears to be a very important event in provoking many of the sequelae of nerve injury, as anesthesia of a nerve prior to injury reduces both the severity and duration of the thermal hyperalgesia which later develops.[60] Along the same lines, administration an NMDA antagonist reduces the severity of partial nerve injury induced hyperalgesia.[61] Once the injury discharges subside, the activity in injured axons changes. Three to five days following nerve transection or partial nerve injury, spontaneous discharges develop in the severed nerves[62,63] which then peak at around 14 days after injury. Although this activity slowly tapers to a lower level, altered patterns of activity are sustained for many weeks.

Neurons of the CNS, like primary afferents, also show a large discharge at the time of nerve damage,[64] and the time course of the injury discharges observed in the CNS parallels that found in primary afferents. A few days following nerve injury many CNS neurons develop changes in spontaneous activity.[64-66] These neurons exhibit a pattern of continuous, regular discharges of high frequency, or they are silent except for sudden high-frequency bursts. Also, higher percentages than normal of these cells respond only to noxious stimuli.

Degenerative changes, such as the loss of inhibitory neurons in the spinal cord[67,68] and thalamus[69] following peripheral nerve injury are thought to contribute to neuropathic pain as well. Wallerian degeneration of peripheral axons and digestion of lost central neurons activates inflammatory cells, leading to increases in the levels of perineural inflammatory cytokines that can further activate nociceptive neurons and generate pain.[70-72] Following the phase of axonal/neuronal degeneration injured neurons will attempt to restore connectivity that is lost to an original innervation target and uninjured neurons will attempt to establish innervation to targets that have become deprived of neural input. As neurons grow, they discharge spontaneously thus increasing signal traffic throughout the somatosensory axis. Changes in transcription factors and other neurochemistry result in altered gene expression in neurons,[73] which then can result in widespread changes in cell phenotype, including alteration of cell surface ion channels,[74,75] neurotransmitter and neuropeptide receptors,[67] surface growth associated proteins,[76] and changes in neurotransmitter and neuropeptide content and synaptic release. Finally, the expression of nerve growth factors, which have been shown to directly produce pain when administered to experimental animals, are upregulated with neuronal proliferation.[77-79] These factors, in whole or in part, contribute to the long lasting condition of neuropathy.

ANALGESIA

Throughout this chapter, the mechanisms of pain associated with thoracic surgery have been outlined, and these principles can now be applied to pain relief. For acute pain, analgesic interventions can occur after surgery but with extremely variable success. Non-steroidal anti-inflammatory drugs (NSAIDs) are the most commonly used form of pain relief available. This class of drugs works primarily by inhibiting prostaglandin synthesis and have some success in moderating thoracic pain. However, they are most effective when combined with a form of opioid analgesia. Opioids provide almost immediate, and sometimes complete, analgesia following surgery and are the drug of choice immediately following surgery. These drugs may be administered intravenously, orally, or epidurally.

With so many patients developing chronic pain following thoracic surgery, it is important to apply the principles of chronic pain development to analgesic options. As outlined above, ongoing input to the spinal cord from nociceptors can result in a state of central sensitization. To prevent this occurrence, preemptive analgesia is now often used. While any one intervention has limited success, combining opiates, NSAIDS, and nerve blocks and administering these prior to surgery appears to decrease the incidence of chronic pain.[1]

REFERENCES

1. Hazelrigg SR, Cetindag IB, Fullerton J. Acute and chronic pain syndromes after thoracic surgery. *Surg Clin North Am.* 2002;82(4):849-865.
2. Kress M, Koltzenburg M, Reeh PW, Handwerker HO. Responsiveness and functional attributes of electrically localized terminals of cutaneous C-fibers *in vivo* and *in vitro*. *J Neurophysiol.* 1992;68(2):581-595.
3. LaMotte RH, Campbell JN. Comparison of responses of warm and nociceptive C-fiber afferents in monkey with human judgments of thermal pain. *J Neurophysiol.* 1978;41(2):509-528.10.
4. Torebjork HE, Hallin RG. Perceptual changes accompanying controlled preferential blocking of A and C fibre responses in intact human skin nerves. *Exp Brain Res.* 1973;16(3):321-332.
5. Nolano M, Simone DA, Wendelschafer-Crabb G, Johnson T, Hazen E, Kennedy WR. Topical capsaicin in humans: parallel loss of epidermal nerve fibers and pain sensation. *Pain.* 1999;81(1-2):135-145.
6. Bischoff A. Congenital insensitivity to pain with anhidrosis. A morphometric study of sural nerve and cutaneous receptors in the human prepuce. In: Bonica JJ, Liebeskind JC, Albe-Fessard DG, eds. *Advances in Pain Research and Therapy.* New York: Raven Press; 1979:53-65.
7. Ralston HJ 3rd, Ralston DD. The distribution of dorsal root axons in laminae I, II and III of the macaque spinal cord: a quantitative electron microscope study. *J Comp Neurol.* 1979;184(4):643-684.
8. Ralston HJ 3rd, Ralston DD. The distribution of dorsal root axons to laminae IV, V, and VI of the macaque spinal cord: a quantitative electron microscopic study. *J Comp Neurol.* 1982;212(4):435-448.
9. Rexed B. The cytoarchitectonic organization of the spinal cord in the cat. *J Comp Neurol.* 1952;96(3):415-466.
10. Cervero F, Bennett GJ, Headley PM. *Processing of Sensory Information in the Superficial Dorsal Horn of the Spinal Cord.* New York: Plenum Press; 1989.
11. Craig AD, Kniffki KD. Spinothalamic lumbosacral lamina I cells responsive to skin and muscle stimulation in the cat. *J Physiol.* 1985;365:197-221.
12. Han ZS, Zhang ET, Craig AD. Nociceptive and thermoreceptive lamina I neurons are anatomically distinct. *Nat Neurosci.* 1998;1(3):218-225.
13. Dougherty PM, Willis WD. Enhanced responses of spinothalamic tract neurons to excitatory amino acids accompany the generation of capsaicin-induced hyperalgesia in the monkey. *J Neurosci.* 1992;12(3):883-894.
14. Dougherty PM, Palecek J, Paleckova V, Sorkin LS, Willis WD. The role of NMDA and non-NMDA excitatory amino acid receptors in the excitation of primate spinothalamic tract neurons by mechanical, thermal, chemical, and electrical stimuli. *J Neurosci.* 1992;12(8):3025-3041.
15. Apkarian AV, Bushnell MC, Treede RD, Zubieta JK. Human brain mechanisms of pain perception and regulation in health and disease. *Eur J Pain.* 2005;9(4):463-484.
16. Beck PW, Handwerker HO. Bradykinin and serotonin effects on various types of cutaneous nerve fibres. *Pflugers Arch Physiol.* 1974;347(3):209-222.
17. Lang E, Novak A, Reeh PW, Handwerker HO. Chemosensitivity of fine afferents from rat skin in vitro. *J Neurophysiol.* 1990;63(4):887-901.
18. Mizumura K, Minagawa M, Koda H, Kumazawa T. Influence of histamine on the bradykinin response of canine testicular polymodal receptors in vitro. *Inflamm Res.* 1995;44(9):376-378.
19. Cunha FQ, Ferreira SH. Peripheral hyperalgesic cytokines. *Adv Exp Med Biol.* 2003;521:22-39.
20. Schaible HG, Ebersberger A, Von Banchet GS. Mechanisms of pain in arthritis. *Ann New York Acad Sci.* 2002;966:343-354.
21. Aley KO, McCarter G, Levine JD. Nitric oxide signaling in pain and nociceptor sensitization in the rat. *J Neurosci.* 1998;18(17):7008-7014.
22. McMahon SB. NGF as a mediator of inflammatory pain. *Philosophical Transactions of the Royal Society of London B.* 1996;351(1338):431-440.
23. Vergnolle N, Wallace JL, Bunnett NW, Hollenberg MD. Protease-activated receptors in inflammation, neuronal signaling and pain. *Trends Pharmacol Sci.* 2001;22(3):146-152.
24. Machelska H, Stein C. Pain control by immune-derived opioids. *Clin Exp Pharmacol Physiol.* 2000;27(7):533-536.
25. Bernardini N, Roza C, Sauer SK, Gomeza J, Wess J, Reeh PW. Muscarinic M2 receptors on peripheral nerve endings: a molecular target of antinociception. *J Neurosci.* 2002;22(12):1-5.
26. Carlton SM, Du J, Davidson E, Zhou S, Coggeshall RE. Somatostatin receptors on peripheral primary afferent terminals: inhibition of sensitized nociceptors. *Pain.* 2001;90(3):233-244.

27. Petrenko AB, Yamakura T, Baba A, Shimoji K. The role of N-methyl-D-aspartate (NMDA) receptors in pain: a review. *Anesth Analgesia.* 2003;97(4):1108-1116.
28. Tsuda M, Kuboyama K, Inoue T, Nagata K, Tozaki-Saitoh H, Inoue K. Behavioral phenotypes of mice lacking purinergic P2X(4) receptors in acute and chronic pain assays. *Molecular Pain.* 2009;5:28.
29. Nakanishi S. Substance P precursor and kininogen: their structures, gene organizations and regulation. *Physiol Rev.* 1987;67(4):1117-1142.
30. Carter MS, Krause JE. Structure, expression, and some regulatory mechanisms of the rat preprotachykinin gene encoding substance P, neurokinin A, neuropeptide K, and neuropeptide Y. *J Neurosci.* 1990;10(7):2203-2221.
31. Gassner M, Ruscheweyh R, Sandkuhler J. Direct excitation of spinal GABAergic interneurons by noradrenaline. *Pain.* 2009;145(1-2):204-210.
32. Basbaum AI, Fields HL. Endogenous pain control mechanisms: review and hypothesis. *Ann Neurol.* 1978;4(5):451-462.
33. Yaksh TL, Wilson PR. Spinal serotonin terminal system mediates antinociception. *J Pharmacol Exp Ther.* 1979;208(3):446-453.
34. Lewis T. *Pain.* New York: Macmillan; 1942.
35. Raja SN, Campbell JN, Meyer RA. Evidence for different mechanisms of primary and secondary hyperalgesia following heat injury to the glabrous skin. *Brain.* 1984;107(Pt 4):1179-1188.
36. LaMotte RH, Thalhammer JG, Torebjork HE, Robinson CJ. Peripheral neural mechanisms of cutaneous hyperalgesia following mild injury by heat. *J Neurosci.* 1982;2(6):765-781.
37. Meyer RA, Campbell JN. Myelinated nociceptive afferents account for the hyperalgesia that follows a burn to the hand. *Science.* 1981;213(4515):1527-1529.
38. Beck PW, Handwerker HO, Zimmermann M. Nervous outflow from the cat's foot during noxious radiant heat stimulation. *Brain Res.* 1974;67(3):373-386.
39. Beitel RE, Dubner R. Response of unmyelinated (C) polymodal nociceptors to thermal stimuli applied to monkey's face. *J Neurophysiol.* 1976;39(6):1160-1175.
40. Bessou P, Perl ER. Response of cutaneous sensory units with unmyelinated fibers to noxious stimuli. *J Neurophysiol.* 1969;32(6):1025-1043.
41. Dougherty PM, Palecek J, Willis WD Jr. Does sensitization of responses to excitatory amino acids underlie the psychophysical reports of two modalities of increased sensitivity in zones of secondary hyperalgesia? *APS J.* 1993:2(4):276-279.
42. Simone DA, Sorkin LS, Oh U, et al. Neurogenic hyperalgesia: central neural correlates in responses of spinothalamic tract neurons. *J Neurophysiol.* 1991;66(1):228-246.
43. Woolf CJ. Evidence for a central component of post-injury pain hypersensitivity. *Nature.* 1983;306(5944):686-688.
44. Willis WD. Mechanical allodynia: a role for sensitized nociceptive tract cells with convergent input from mechanoreceptors and nociceptors? *Am Pain Soc J.* 1993;2:23-33.
45. Guilbaud G, Kayser V, Attal N, Benoist JM. Evidence for a central contribution to secondary hyperalgesia. In: Willis WD, ed. *Hyperalgesia and Allodynia.* New York: Raven Press; 1992:187-201.
46. Lenz FA, Seike M, Lin YC, et al. Neurons in the area of human nucleus ventralis caudalis (Vc) respond to painful heat stimuli. *Brain Res.* 1993;623(2):235-240.
47. Lenz FA, Kwan HC, Dostrovsky JO, Tasker RR. Characteristics of the bursting pattern of action potentials that occurs in the thalamus of patients with central pain. *Brain Res.* 1989;496(1-2):357-360.
48. Casey KL. Pain and central nervous system disease: a summary and overview. In: Casey KL, ed. *Pain and Central Nervous System Disease: The Central Pain Syndromes.* New York: Raven Press, Ltd; 1991:1-11.
49. Rausell E, Cusick CG, Taub A, Jones EG. Chronic deafferentation in monkeys differentially affects nociceptive and non-nociceptive pathway distinguished by specific calcium-binding proteins and down-regulates gamma-aminobutyric acid type A receptors at thalamic levels. *Proceedings of the National Acadamey of Sciences of the USA.* 1992;89(7):2571-2575.
50. Bonica JJ. Causalgia and other reflex sympathetic dystrophies. In: Bonica JJ, ed. *Advances in Pain Research and Therapy.* New York: Raven Press; 1979;3:141-166.
51. Sunderland S. Pain mechanisms in causalgia. *J Neurol Neurosurg Psychiatry.* 1976;39(5):471-480.
52. Gottschalk AM, Cohen SP, Yang S, Ochroch, EA. Preventing and treating pain after thoracic surgery. *Anesthesiology.* 2006;V 104(3):594-600.

53. Scawn ND, Pennefather SH, Soorae A, Wang JYY, Russell GN. Ipsilateral shoulder pain after thoracotomy with epidural analgesia: the influence of phrenic nerve infiltration with lidocaine. *Anesth Analg.* 2001;93(2):260-264.
54. Rogers ML, Duffy JP. Surgical aspects of chronic post-thoracotomy pain. *Eur J Cardio-Thoracic Surg.* 2000;18(6):711-716.
55. Roberts WJ. A hypothesis on the physiological basis for causalgia and related pains. *Pain.* 1985;24(3):297-311.
56. Campbell JN, Khan AA, Meyer RA, Raja SN. Responses to heat of C-fiber nociceptors in monkey are altered by injury in the receptive field but not by adjacent injury. *Pain.* 1988;32(3):327-332.
57. Frost SA, Raja SN, Campbell JN, Meyer RA, Khan AA. Does hyperalgesia to cooling stimuli characterize patients with sympathetically maintained pain (reflex sympathetic dystrophy)? In: Dubner R, Gebhart GF, Bond MR, eds. *Proceedings of the Vth World Congress on Pain.* Amsterdam: Elsevier Science Publishers; 1988:151-156.
58. Govrin-Lippmann R, Devor M. Ongoing activity in severed nerves: source and variation with time. *Brain Res.* 1978;159(2):406-410.
59. Wall PD, Waxman S, Basbaum AI. Ongoing activity in peripheral nerve: injury discharge. *Exp Neurol.* 1974;45(3):576-589.
60. Dougherty PM, Garrison CJ, Carlton SM. Differential influence of local anesthetic upon two models of experimentally-induced peripheral mononeuropathy in the rat. *Brain Res.* 1992;570(1-2):109-115.
61. Davar G, Hama A, Deykin A, Vos B, Maciewicz R. MK-801 blocks the development of thermal hyperalgesia in a rat model of experimental painful neuropathy. *Brain Res.* 1991;553(2):327-330.
62. Kajander KC, Bennett GJ. Onset of a painful neuropathy in rat: a partial and differential deafferentation and spontaneous discharge in AB and Ad primary afferent neurons. *J Neurophysiol.* 1992;68(3):734-744.
63. Papir-Kricheli D, Devor M. Abnormal impulse discharge in primary afferent axons injured in the peripheral versus the central nervous system. *Somatosensory Motor Res.* 1988;6(1):63-77.
64. Devor M. Central changes mediating neuropathic pain. In: Dubner R, Gebhart GF, Bond MR, eds. *Proceedings of the Vth World Congress on Pain.* New York: Elsevier Science Publishers; 1988:114-128.
65. Basbaum AI, Wall PD. Chronic changes in the response of cells in adult cat dorsal horn following partial deafferentation: the appearance of responding cells in a previously non-responsive region. *Brain Res.* 1976;116(2):181-204.
66. Mendell LM, Sassoon EM, Wall PD. Properties of synaptic linkage from long ranging afferents onto dorsal horn neurones in normal and deafferented cats. *J Physiol.* 1978;285:299-310.
68. Sugimoto T, Bennett GJ, Kajander KC. Transsynaptic degeneration in the superficial dorsal horn after sciatic nerve injury: effects of a chronic constriction injury, transection, and strychnine. *Pain.* 1990;42(2):205-213.
69. Ralston DD, Dougherty PM, Lenz FA, Weng HR, Vierck CJ, Ralston HJ. Plasticity of the inhibitory circuits of the primate ventrobasal thalamus following lesions of the somatosensory pathways. In: Devor M, Rowbotham MC, Wiesenfeld-Hallin Z, eds. *Proceedings of the 9th World Congress on Pain.* Seattle, WA: IASP Press; 2000:427-434.
70. Milligan ED, Twining C, Chacur M, et al. Spinal glia and proinflammatory cytokines mediate mirror-image neuropathic pain in rats. *J Neurosci.* 2003;23(3):1026-1040.
71. DeLeo JA, Colburn RW, Rickman AJ. Cytokine and growth factor immunohistochemical spinal profiles in two animal models of mononeuropathy. *Brain Res.* 1997;759(1):50-57.
72. Sorkin LS, Doom CM. Epineurial application of TNF elicits an acute mechanical hyperalgesia in the awake rat. *J Peripher Nerv Syst.* 2000;5(2):96-100.
73. Okamoto K, Martin DP, Schmelzer JD, Mitsui Y, Low PA. Pro- and anti-inflammatory cytokine gene expression in rat sciatic nerve chronic constriction injury model of neuropathic pain. *Exp Neurol.* 2001;169(2):386-391.
74. Dib-Hajj SD, Fjell J, Cummins TR, et al. Plasticity of sodium channel expression in DRG neurons in the chronic constriction injury model of neuropathic pain. *Pain.* 1999;83(3):591-600.
75. Okuse K, Chaplan SR, McMahon SB, et al. Regulation of expression of the sensory neuron-specific sodium channel SNS in inflammatory and neuropathic pain. *Mol Cell Neurosci.* 1997;10(3-4):196-207.
76. Bennett GJ, Kajander KC, Sahara Y, Iadarola MJ, Sugimoto T. Neurochemical and anatomical changes in the dorsal horn of rats with an experimental painful peripheral neuropathy. In: Cervero F, Bennett GJ, Headley PM, eds. *Processing of Sensory Information in the Superficial Dorsal Horn of the Spinal Cord.* New York: Plenum Press; 1988:1-23.

76. Cameron AA, Cliffer KD, Dougherty PM, Garrison CJ, Willis WD, Carlton SM. Time course of degenerative and regenerative changes in the dorsal horn in a rat model of peripheral neuropathy. *J Comp Neurol.* 1997;379(3):428-442.
77. Kanaan SA, Saade NE, Karam M, Khansa H, Jabbur SJ, Jurjus AR. Hyperalgesia and upregulation of cytokines and nerve growth factor by cutaneous leishmaniasis. *Pain.* 2000;85(3):477-482.
78. Lewin GR, Ritter AM, Mendell LM. Nerve growth factor-induced hyperalgesia in the neonatal and adult rat. *J Neurosci.* 1993;13(5):2136-2148.
79. Woolf CJ, Allchorne A, Safieh-Garabedian B, Poole S. Cytokines, nerve growth factor and inflammatory hyperalgesia: the contribution of tumor necrosis factor A. *Br J Pharmacol.* 1997;121(3):417-424.

The Biology of Lung and Esophageal Cancer

Mark W. Onaitis
David H. Harpole

Over the past decades, it has become recognized that cancer is a genetic disease. Therefore, the biology of lung and esophageal cancer must be considered from the perspective of genetic changes in the epithelial cells of these organs. In this chapter, we will highlight many of these known individual genetic changes as well as groups of genetic changes.

ONCOGENES

Oncogenes are genes that lead to increased proliferative capacity of cells. Because they are activating mutations, mutation or overexpression of only one of two normal proto-oncogenes per cell is required for transformation. Oncogenes may lead to increased proliferation through a variety of mechanisms, including augmented growth rate, increased mitotic rate, and decreased rate of apoptosis.

Ras

Ras is perhaps the best-known oncogene. The Ras family of proteins consists of three members, HRas, NRas, and KRas, the last of which is implicated in 30% to 40% of human lung adenocarcinoma.[1] Wild-type Ras is a membrane-associated G protein that serves as a link between tyrosine kinase receptors at the membrane and cytoplasmic second messenger molecules. These second messenger molecules participate in a proliferative signaling cascade that activates mitogen-activated protein kinase (MAPK) resulting in increased proliferation. This proliferation is caused by mutations in KRas codons 12, 13, and 61, all of which ablate KRas' GTPase activity and constitutively activate KRas.

In both individual studies and a meta-analysis, the presence of mutated KRas in resected lung cancer portends a poor prognosis.[2-4] Although the presence of these mutations may identify aggressive tumors, a portion of the prognostic impact may be explained by poor response to adjuvant chemotherapy. In the National Cancer Institute of Canada Clinical Trials Group (NCIC-CTG) North American intergroup study, the JBR.10 trial, the subgroup of patients with Ras mutations did not experience a survival advantage.[5] Because localization of Ras to the membrane is dependent upon farnesylation, farnesyltransferase inhibitors may be more effective in patients with Ras mutation.

In addition to mutation of Ras, control of normal Ras protein levels may be important in lung cancer tumorigenesis. Recently, Ras was found to be an important target of the let-7 microRNA family. MicroRNAs are 22 nucleotide RNA molecules that negatively regulate gene expression by silencing messenger RNAs or by targeting microRNAs for destruction. Lung tumors exhibit lower levels of let-7 than normal lung,[6] and low expression levels of let-7 have been demonstrated as predictive of poor survival.[7-9]

Interestingly, oncogenic Ras mutations occur almost exclusively in adenocarcinomas of smokers.[10,11] This may relate to the effect of benzo-alpha-pyrenes on the bronchial epithelium.[12] Perhaps smoking cessation efforts will eventually lead to fewer Ras-positive tumors in the future.

In esophageal cancer, Ras mutations have also been reported in patients with high-grade dysplasia and adenocarcinoma.[9] These mutations are rarely found in Barrett metaplasia.

Epidermal Growth Factor Receptor (EGFR)

Unlike Ras, EGFR mutations most commonly occur in lung tumors of nonsmokers. They virtually never occur in the presence of Ras mutation and are most commonly present in adenocarcinomas of East Asian females.[13,14] Along with Her2, Her3, and Her4, EGFR receptors comprise one of four types of ErbB receptors. Ligands of EGFR are varied, including both epidermal growth factor and transforming growth factor alpha.[15] Ligand binding of the receptor leads to dimerization, phosphorylation, and activation of signaling pathways leading to proliferation.

Due to the availability of the EGFR-specific tyrosine kinase inhibitors, EGFR mutation has received much recent scrutiny. The majority of these mutations occur as either in-frame deletions of exon 19 or missense mutation in exon 21.[13,16-21] Epithelial cells with mutant EGFR probably become physiologically dependent on the gene's continued activity for maintenance of the transformed phenotypes.[22] As Figure 7–1 reveals, patients with tumors expressing EGFR and Her2-neu may have poorer postoperative survival than those with one or neither positive.

In esophageal carcinoma, chromosome 7 (which contains EGFR) is frequently amplified in tumors that have metastasized to lymph nodes,[23] and EGFR overexpression correlates with worse survival after induction treatment.[24]

TUMOR SUPPRESSORS

A tumor suppressor is a gene whose absence allows neoplasia to progress. Because even a small amount of wild-type protein may suppress transformation, homozygous deletion of a tumor suppressor is thought necessary for oncogenesis. When a patient is heterozygous for a gene, the term loss of heterozygosity (LOH) is used to describe deletion or inactivation of the wild-type allele.

p53

Perhaps the best-studied tumor suppressor gene is p53, which encodes a transcription factor with diverse biological functions, including the mediation of cell cycle arrest and cell death after DNA damage. The loss of wild-type (normal) p53 activity is the most common genetic abnormality in human

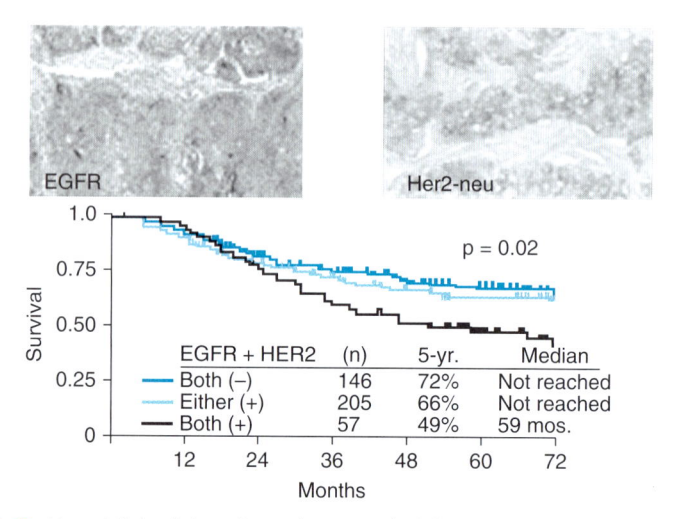

Figure 7-1. Unpublished data from the Harpole laboratory demonstrating diminished survival in Stage I patients with tumors staining positive for both EGFR and Her2-neu.

cancer and can occur through allelic deletions or point mutations, or both, that result in amino acid substitutions that alter protein function. Abnormalities in p53 are also the most frequent genetic alterations in lung cancer, occurring in 90% of SCLCs and up to 60% of NSCLCs. These alterations primarily involve inactivating point mutations, but deletions, rearrangements, and splice mutations have also been described. As with Ras mutations, p53 mutations are more common in smokers: Denissenko and co-workers reported that benzo[*a*] pyrene, a major carcinogen in tobacco smoke, preferentially forms adducts at the guanine positions in p53 that are most frequently mutated in human lung cancer.[25] In addition, Ahrendt and associates found that p53 mutations occur at a much higher frequency in lung cancers of patients with a history of significant alcohol and tobacco use.[26]

The prognostic significance of p53 abnormalities in lung cancer remains controversial. Since the half-life of mutant p53 protein is usually significantly longer than that of the wild-type protein, the detection of p53 by immunohistochemistry is considered a marker for p53 mutation, although Carbone and associates found that the concordance between positive p53 immunostaining and the presence of a p53 mutation was only 67%.[27] Numerous studies have reported that p53 mutation or overexpression is predictive of poor prognosis, whereas others have found no association between p53 mutations and survival in either NSCLC or SCLC. Two recent meta-analyses concluded that the presence of p53 mutation or overexpression correlates with a poorer prognosis in patients with NSCLC.[28,29] Data from the Harpole laboratory is in agreement with this (Figure 7–2).

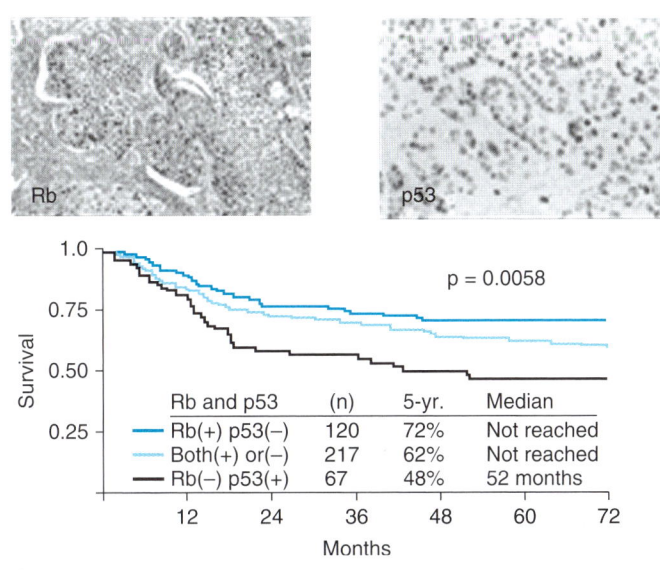

Figure 7–2. Unpublished data from the Harpole laboratory revealing diminished survival in Stage I patients with Rb deficiency and p53 overexpression.

In esophageal cancer, p53 mutation is found in up to 80% of adenocarcinomas.[30] LOH may also be important in risk stratification of patients with Barrett esophagus at risk for developing esophageal cancer.[31]

p16

Cytogenetic studies have identified chromosomal region 9p21 as one of the most commonly affected loci in human cancers, including lung cancer. The p16 (*INK4a, CDKN2A*) gene, located at 9p21, has been characterized as a tumor suppressor gene based on the high frequency of p16 mutations and deletions present in a wide variety of human tumors and the presence of germline mutations in families with hereditary melanoma. The p16 protein is one of a family of cyclin-dependent kinase (cdk) inhibitors that regulate progression through the cell cycle by inactivating cdk4 or cdk6, thereby inhibiting the phosphorylation of Retinoblastoma 1 (RB1) by cyclin D:cdk4/6 complexes. Unphosphorylated Rb1 binds E2F with resultant cell cycle arrest at the G_1/S boundary. Therefore, the loss of p16 function or the overexpression of cyclin D1 would have the same net effect as the loss of RB1 function: unregulated passage through the G_1/S checkpoint with resultant neoplastic proliferation. At least one of these three abnormalities—loss of RB1, loss of p16, or overexpression of cyclin D1—occurs in most, if not all, human cancers, suggesting that dysregulation of the RB–cyclin D–cdk4/6–p16 pathway controlling the G_1/S transition may be a necessary step during malignant transformation.

One of these cell cycle-altering pathways is active in over 90% of NSCLC tumors.[32] Although p16 inactivation is common in all NSCLCs, the mechanism of inactivation may differ between smokers and nonsmokers, with deletions and mutations primarily responsible in the former and only promoter hypermethylation being noted in the latter.[33] However, others have found hypermethylation of the gene in smokers.[34]

In esophageal cancer, alterations in p16 are common.[35,36] As with p53, p16 alterations may portend higher risk of adenocarcinoma formation in Barrett's patients.[37,38]

Inactivation of p16 may be associated with a poor outcome. Kratzke and colleagues and others have reported that the loss of p16 is associated with a poor prognosis,[39] while Kinoshita and associates found that inactivation of p16 or RB1 was associated with an increased proliferative index in tumors lacking p53 activity.

GENOMICS AND PROTEOMICS

Genomics

As technology has evolved and the human genome has been sequenced, the ability to screen samples for expression/mutation across large numbers of genes has become both possible and affordable. These techniques involve isolating either RNA (in the case of transcriptome profiling) or DNA (in the case of single nucleotide polymorphism [SNP] arrays), fluorescently labeling them, and hybridizing them to chips to which are immobilized short DNA sequences (probes) from thousands of genes of interest. After reading and analysis, an expression value for each probe is obtained. Commercially available chips now contain all known genes in the genome of humans and almost any other organism under study.

The vast amount of information obtained from these arrays has necessitated the explosion of the field of bioinformatics in that complex, computerized statistical algorithms have been developed to identify important significant differences between samples. In the case of the Affymetrix (www.affymetrix.com) human genome U133 2.0 Plus chips, expression data for over 54,000 probes is provided for each sample.

As these fields have advanced, these approaches have been applied to human lung cancer. Several groups including ours have demonstrated that squamous cell carcinoma and adenocarcinoma have markedly different transcriptome profiles.[40-43] Within these broad histologic classes, these studies have also identified subgroups that have poor prognosis. These types of studies may eventually lead to personalized treatment.

In contrast to the transcriptome array studies discussed thus far, sequencing of the human genome has led to the accumulation of single nucleotide polymorphism data. These polymorphisms represent single base pair differences between individuals and may either cause disease (if the change causes differences in protein expression) or be used as markers of disease (if a SNP is very close to a gene contributing to a disease phenotype such that recombination happens between the gene and the SNP only rarely).

Large SNP arrays are now commercially available. The protocol for their use is similar to that of transcriptome arrays except that genomic DNA is hybridized to the chips. Because this technology is relatively new, less lung cancer-specific data has been published. However, recent studies have demonstrated increased lung cancer risk with specific polymorphisms.[44-47] As the technology becomes more affordable and easier to use, more of these studies will undoubtedly be published over the next several years. Because these studies identify genetic markers in genomic DNA which can be isolated and analyzed at any time from a blood sample, a myriad of ethical considerations will inevitably arise concerning testing of healthy people for increased lung cancer susceptibility.

Proteomics

Proteomics involves study of the set of proteins in a selected group of cells and tissue. Because the protein profile represents a snapshot of the activities of a cell at any given time, proteomic study is extremely powerful. However, because of the complexity of the proteome caused by multiple amino acids comprising each protein (as opposed to just 4 bases in DNA and RNA) and extensive posttranslational modifications (glycosylation, phosphorylation, etc), methods of isolating and studying proteins lag behind those of genomics.

Despite this, proteomic analysis has proven an important tool in analysis of human cancer. The foundation of most proteomic studies is two-dimensional gel electrophoresis, in which proteins are separated on the basis of size and charge. Spots of differential expression (between differentially-labeled normal and tumor samples, for instance) are dissected from the gel and the proteins isolated. These are then analyzed by various forms of mass spectroscopy (MS) in order to sequence and identify the proteins. Such approaches have identified proteins which not only differentiate lung cancer from normal specimens[48-51] but also predict survival.[52,53]

In addition to standard 2D-gel/MS approaches, new developments in proteomic analysis have been described. Recently, proteomic microarrays have also been used in two ways. In a forward phase array, multiple protein-specific antibodies are immobilized on a glass slide and the protein sample is added to it.[54] In a reverse phase array, protein extracts are hybridized to a slide, and either antibodies or candidates for drug development are used to probe it.[55] As proteomic microarrays continue to evolve, so too does mass spectroscopy. Using surface-enhanced laser desorption/ionization mass spectroscopy (SELDI-MS), solutions of proteins are directly analyzed, allowing differentiation of cancer from normal. In addition, typical matrix-assisted laser desorption/ionization time-of-flight (MALDI-TOF), may be used to create protein profiles able to distinguish between histologic types of lung cancer and between primary and metastatic tumors.[56]

MOUSE MODELS

An exciting new area of inquiry into the molecular biology of lung cancer is mouse modeling. Modern transgenic and knockout genetic technologies have allowed manipulation of the mouse genome in order to study effects of mutation/

overexpression/deletion of specific genes. This section will briefly describe two of the present models.

This first of these models was made in Tyler Jacks' laboratory at MIT by knocking a mutant codon 12 KRas gene into the Ras locus in an inducible fashion. This mutant gene is preceded by a stop codon flanked by a certain DNA sequence termed a loxP site. These loxP sites are recognized by the Cre recombinase enzyme, which proceeds to excise the DNA between them. When Cre recombinase is delivered to specific cells of this transgenic mouse line, the stop codon is excised, and the oncogenic KRas mutant is over expressed. In order to direct recombination and oncogene expression to the bronchial epithelium in these mice, Cre recombinase was delivered via inhaled adenovirus. After the adenovirus was administered, these mice developed first atypical adenomatous hyperplasia and epithelial hyperplasia. These lesions progressed to adenomas and then to adenocarcinoma.[57] By gradually decreasing the dose of virus administered, hyperplasia was found to initiate at cells positive for both the Clara cell marker Clara Cell antigen 10 (CC10) and the alveolar Type II cell marker surfactant protein C (SPC). In a subsequent study, these "dual-positive" cells were isolated and found to exhibit stem cell properties of self-renewal and ability to differentiate into multiple lineages. These cells were termed bronchoalveolar stem cells (BASCs) and were demonstrated to proliferate after Cre-induced Ras activation in the bronchial epithelium of the above mice.[58] Thus, this inducible oncogenic Ras mouse model may have led to identification of a normal tissue stem cell in the lung. If this normal tissue stem cell is truly the cell of origin for adenocarcinoma, this would constitute proof of the cancer stem cell hypothesis, which states that tumors arise from transformed normal tissue stem cells.[59]

This mouse model also has shed light upon importance of other signaling molecules in lung cancer tumorigenesis and progression. Although the oncogenic Ras mutant produced adenocarcinomas, they did not metastasize. However, when this mouse line was crossed with an inducible knockout of p53, administration of adenoviral Cre recombinase led to adenocarcinomas which are invasive, desmoplastic, and metastatic.[60] Using the same Ras mutant in a doxycycline-inducible mouse line, the Varmus laboratory obtained the same result.[61] Another group of investigators using the same inducible Ras mutant found that inducible deletion of the Lkb1 gene, deficiency of which contributes to Peutz-Jeghers syndrome, leads to metastatic adenocarcinomas as well as a proportion of tumors which exhibit squamous histology.[62] This result indicates that, at least in a subset of lung cancers, histologic subtype may be the result of a "switch" involving Lkb1. Finally, downstream effectors of Ras may be important in tumorigenesis, as induction of oncogenic KRas in a mouse line which is null for the Ras downstream effector Rac1, leads to a markedly decreased number of tumors.[63]

Inducible mutant epidermal growth factor receptor mice also lead to adenocarcinoma. Transgenic mouse lines were made in the Varmus laboratory by injecting tetracycline-inducible oncogenic EGFR mutants driven by the Clara Cell secretory protein (CCSP) promoter. Both a point mutant at position 858

(L858R) and a deletion mutant (L747-S752) were made. When doxycycline is administered to these mice, they form tumors with histologic features similar to bronchoalveolar carcinoma (BAC). Interestingly, when doxycycline was withdrawn from these mice, the tumors regressed. The tumors also regressed upon treatment with the EGFR tyrosine kinase inhibitor erlotinib.[64] Finally, the downstream molecules in these mice were compared to those of the doxycycline-inducible mutant KRas adenocarcinoma-forming mice. In both cases, phosphorylated Erk, Akt, and Stat3 were present by immunostaining. This suggests that both models involve activation of the mitogen activated protein kinase (MAPK), phosphoinositol-3-kinase (PI3K), and signal transducer and activator of transcription-3 (STAT3) pathways.

CANCER STEM CELLS

The theory that cancers arise from small populations of cells with ability to self-renew and differentiate into multiple lineages has become very popular.[59] According to this model, stem cells may be transformed and thus become proliferative or proliferative non-stem cells may acquire the properties of stem cells. Either way, the theory holds that these cells should be targeted in order for anticancer treatments to be effective.

Across many cancer types, researchers have identified cells surface markers that differentiate cancer stem cells from the rest of the tumor.[65-69] Relevant markers include CD133, CD24, and CD44. One group has identified CD133 as identifying cancer stem cells in small cell and non-small cell lung cancer. In this study, CD133-positive cells self-renew and differentiate into all cell types in the tumor both *in vitro* (in sphere-forming assays) and *in vivo* (in immunodeficient mice) much more efficiently than CD133-negative tumor cells.[70]

However, controversy exists concerning these studies. Some have made mathematical arguments demonstrating the implausibility of these approaches[71] while others have provided direct experimental evidence that the apparent stem-like abilities of tumor subpopulations may be recapitulated by many more cells in the tumor given the correct conditions.[72,73] Thus, the cancer stem cell theory will await further confirmatory studies.

CONCLUSION

As our understanding of molecular biology increases, we will know more about both lung cancer and esophageal cancer. This may allow rapid clinical advances in the future.

REFERENCES

1. Rodenhuis S, Slebos RJ. Clinical significance of Ras oncogene activation in human lung cancer. *Cancer Res.* 1992;52(9 Suppl):2665s-2669s.
2. Slebos RJ, Kibbelaar RE, Dalesio O, et al. KRas oncogene activation as a prognostic marker in adenocarcinoma of the lung. *N Engl J Med.* 1990;323(9):561-565.

3. Sugio K, Ishida T, Yokoyama H, Inoue T, Sugimachi K, Sasazuki T. Ras gene mutations as a prognostic marker in adenocarcinoma of the human lung without lymph node metastasis. *Cancer Res.* 1992;52(10):2903-2906.
4. Mascaux C, Iannino N, Martin B, et al. The role of Ras oncogene in survival of patients with lung cancer: a systematic review of the literature with meta-analysis. *Br J Cancer.* 2005;92(1):131-139.
5. Winton T, Livingston R, Johnson D, et al. Vinorelbine plus cisplatin vs. observation in resected non-small-cell lung cancer. *N Engl J Med.* 2005;352(25):2589-2597.
6. Johnson SM, Grosshans H, Shingara J, et al. Ras is regulated by the let-7 microRNA family. *Cell.* 2005;120:635-647.
7. Yanaihara N, Caplen N, Bowman E, et al. Unique microRNA molecular profiles in lung cancer diagnosis and prognosis. *Cancer Cell.* 2006;9:189-198.
8. Yu SL, Chen HY, Chang GC, et al. MicroRNA signature predicts survival and relapse in lung cancer. *Cancer Cell.* 2008;13(1):48-57.
9. Lord RV, O'Grady R, Sheehan C, Field AF, Ward RL. K-ras codon 12 mutations in Barrett's oesophagus and adenocarcinomas of the oesophagus and oesophagogastric junction. *J Gastroenterol Hepatol.* 2000;15(7):730-736.
10. Ahrendt SA, Decker PA, Alawi EA, et al. Cigarette smoking is strongly associated with mutation of the K-ras gene in patients with primary adenocarcinoma of the lung. *Cancer.* 2001;92(6):1525-1530.
11. Slebos RJ, Hruban RH, Dalesio O, Mooi WJ, Offerhaus GJ, Rodenhuis S. Relationship between K-ras oncogene activation and smoking in adenocarcinoma of the human lung. *J Natl Cancer Inst.* 1991;83(14):1024-107.
12. Feng Z, Hu W, Chen JX, et al. Preferential DNA damage and poor repair determine ras gene mutational hotspot in human cancer. *J Natl Cancer Inst.* 2002;94(20):1527-1536.
13. Shigematsu H, Lin L, Takahashi T, et al. Clinical and biological features associated with epidermal growth factor receptor gene mutations in lung cancers. *J Natl Cancer Inst.* 2005;97(5):339-346.
14. Shigematsu H, Gazdar AF. Somatic mutations of epidermal growth factor receptor signaling pathway in lung cancers. *Int J Cancer.* 2006;118(2):257-262.
15. Harris RC, Chung E, Coffey RJ. EGF receptor ligands. *Exp Cell Res.* 2003;284(1):2-13.
16. Kosaka T, Yatabe Y, Endoh H, Kuwano H, Takahashi T, Mitsudomi T. Mutations of the epidermal growth factor receptor gene in lung cancer: biological and clinical implications. *Cancer Res.* 2004;64(24):8919-8923.
17. Pao W, Miller V, Zakowski M, et al. EGF receptor gene mutations are common in lung cancers from "never smokers" and are associated with sensitivity of tumors to gefitinib and erlotinib. *Proc Natl Acad Sci U S A.* 2004;101(36):13306-13311.
18. Huang SF, Liu HP, Li LH, et al. High frequency of epidermal growth factor receptor mutations with complex patterns in non-small cell lung cancers related to gefitinib responsiveness in Taiwan. *Clin Cancer Res.* 2004;10(24):8195-8203.
19. Tokumo M, Toyooka S, Kiura K, et al. The relationship between epidermal growth factor receptor mutations and clinicopathologic features in non-small cell lung cancers. *Clin Cancer Res.* 2005;11(3):1167-1173.
20. Paez JG, Jänne PA, Lee JC, et al. EGFR mutations in lung cancer: correlation with clinical response to gefitinib therapy. *Science.* 2004;304(5676):1497-1500.
21. Lynch TJ, Bell DW, Sordella R, et al. Activating mutations in the epidermal growth factor receptor underlying responsiveness of non-small-cell lung cancer to gefitinib. *N Engl J Med.* 2004;350(21):2129-2139.
22. Gazdar AF, Shigematsu H, Herz J, Minna JD. Mutations and addiction to EGFR: the Achilles 'heal' of lung cancers. *Trends Mol Med.* 2004;10:481-486.
23. Vissers KJ, Riegman PH, Alers JC, Tilanus HW, van Dekken H. Involvement of cancer-activating genes on chromosomes 7 and 8 in esophageal (Barrett's) and gastric cardia adenocarcinoma. *Anticancer Res.* 2001;21(6A):3813-3820.
24. Gibson MK, Abraham SC, Wu TT, et al. Epidermal growth factor receptor, p53 mutation, and pathological response predict survival in patients with locally advanced esophageal cancer treated with preoperative chemoradiotherapy. *Clin Cancer Res.* 2003;9(17):6461-6468.
25. Denissenko MF, Pao A, Tang M, Pfeifer GP. Preferential formation of benzo[a]pyrene adducts at lung cancer mutational hotspots in P53. *Science.* 1996;274(5286):430-432.

26. Ahrendt SA, Chow JT, Yang SC, et al. Alcohol consumption and cigarette smoking increase the frequency of p53 mutations in non-small cell lung cancer. *Cancer Res.* 2000; 60(12):3155-3159.
27. Carbone DP, Mitsudomi T, Chiba I, et al. p53 immunostaining positivity is associated with reduced survival and is imperfectly correlated with gene mutations in resected non-small cell lung cancer. A preliminary report of LCSG 871. *Chest.* 1994;106(6 Suppl):377S-381S.
28. Mitsudomi T, Hamajima N, Ogawa M, Takahashi T. et al. Prognostic significance of p53 alterations in patients with non-small cell lung cancer: a meta-analysis. *Clin Cancer Res.* 2000;6(10): 4055-4063.
29. Steels E, Paesmans M, Berghmans T, et al. Role of p53 as a prognostic factor for survival in lung cancer: a systematic review of the literature with a meta-analysis. *Eur Respir J.* 2001;18(4):705-719.
30. Wu TT, Watanabe T, Heitmiller R, Zahurak M, Forastiere AA, Hamilton SR. Genetic alterations in Barrett esophagus and adenocarcinomas of the esophagus and esophagogastric junction region. *Am J Pathol;* 1998;153(1):287-294.
31. Dolan K, Morris AI, Gosney JR, Field JK, Sutton R. Loss of heterozygosity on chromosome 17p predicts neoplastic progression in Barrett's esophagus. *J Gastroenterol Hepatol.* 2003;18(6):683-689.
32. Tanaka H, Fujii Y, Hirabayashi H, et al. Disruption of the RB pathway and cell-proliferative activity in non-small-cell lung cancers. *Int J Cancer.* 1998;79(2):111-115.
33. Sanchez-Cespedes M, Decker PA, Doffek KM, et al. Increased loss of chromosome 9p21 but not p16 inactivation in primary non-small cell lung cancer from smokers. *Cancer Res.* 2001;61(5):2092-2096.
34. Kim DH, Nelson HH, Wiencke JK, et al. p16(INK4a) and histology-specific methylation of CpG islands by exposure to tobacco smoke in non-small cell lung cancer. *Cancer Res.* 2001;61(8):3419-3424.
35. Barrett MT, Galipeau PC, Sanchez CA, Emond MJ, Reid BJ. Determination of the frequency of loss of heterozygosity in esophageal adenocarcinoma by cell sorting, whole genome amplification and microsatellite polymorphisms. *Oncogene.* 1996;12(9):1873-188.
36. Tarmin L, Yin J, Zhou X, et al. Frequent loss of heterozygosity on chromosome 9 in adenocarcinoma and squamous cell carcinoma of the esophagus. *Cancer Res.* 1994;54(23):6094-6096.
37. Galipeau PC, Prevo LJ, Sanchez CA, et al. Clonal expansion and loss of heterozygosity at chromosomes 9p and 17p in premalignant esophageal (Barrett's) tissue. *J Natl Cancer Inst.* 1999;91(24):2087-2095.
38. Maley CC, Galipeau PC, Li X, Sanchez CA, Paulson TG, Reid BJ. Selectively advantageous mutations and hitchhikers in neoplasms: p16 lesions are selected in Barrett's esophagus. *Cancer Res.* 2004;64(10): 3414-3427.
39. Kratzke RA, Greatens TM, Rubins JB, et al. Rb and p16INK4a expression in resected non-small cell lung tumors. *Cancer Res.* 1996;56(15):3415-3420.
40. Beer DG, Kardia SL, Huang CC, et al. Gene-expression profiles predict survival of patients with lung adenocarcinoma. *Nat Med.* 2002;8(8):816-824.
41. Bhattacharjee A, Richards WG, Staunton J, et al. Classification of human lung adenocarcinomas by mRNA expression profiling reveals distinct adenocarcinoma subclasses. *PNAS.* 2001;98(24):13790-13795.
42. Garber ME, Troyanskaya OG, Schluens K, et al. Diversity of gene expression in adenocarcinoma of the lung. *PNAS.* 2002;98(24):13784-13789.
43. Raponi M, Zhang Y, Yu J, et al. Gene expression signatures for predicting prognosis of squamous cell and adenocarcinomas of the lung. *Cancer Res.* 2006;66(15):7466-7472.
44. Cao G, Lu H, Feng J, Shu J, Zheng D, Hou Y. Lung cancer risk associated with Thr495Pro polymorphism of GHR in Chinese population. *Jpn J Clin Oncol.* 2008; Apr;38(4):308-316.
45. Kiyohara C, Yoshimasu K. Genetic polymorphisms in the nucleotide excision repair pathway and lung cancer risk: a meta-analysis. *Int J Med Sci.* 2007;4(2):59-71.
46. Nomura M, Shigematsu H, Li L, et al. Polymorphisms, mutations, and amplification of the EGFR gene in non-small cell lung cancers. *PLoS Med.* 2007;4(4):e125.
47. Oh JJ, Koegel AK, Phan DT, Razfar A, Slamon DJ. The two single nucleotide polymorphisms in the H37/RBM5 tumour suppressor gene at 3p21.3 correlated with different subtypes of non-small cell lung cancers. *Lung Cancer.* 2007;58(1):7-14.
48. Bergman AC, Benjamin T, Alaiya A, et al. Identification of gel-separated tumor marker proteins by mass spectrometry. *Electrophoresis.* 2000;21(3):679-686.
49. Chen G, Gharib TG, Huang CC, et al. Proteomic analysis of lung adenocarcinoma: identification of a highly expressed set of proteins in tumors. *Clin Cancer Res.* 2002;8(7):2298-2305.
50. Hanash S, Brichory F, Beer D. A proteomic approach to the identification of lung cancer markers. *Dis Markers.* 2001;17(4):295-300.

51. Hirano T, Franzén B, Uryu K, et al. Detection of polypeptides associated with the histopathological differentiation of primary lung carcinoma. *Br J Cancer*. 1995;72(4):840-848.
52. Chen G, Gharib TG, Wang H, et al. Protein profiles associated with survival in lung adenocarcinoma. *Proc Natl Acad Sci U S A*. 2003;100(23):13537-13542.
53. Gharib TG, Chen G, Wang H, et al. Proteomic analysis of cytokeratin isoforms uncovers association with survival in lung adenocarcinoma. *Neoplasia*. 2002;4(5):440-448.
54. Liotta LA, Espina V, Mehta AI, et al. Protein microarrays: meeting analytical challenges for clinical applications. *Cancer Cell*. 2003;3(4):317-325.
55. Huang J, Zhu H, Haggarty SJ, et al. Finding new components of the target of rapamycin (TOR) signaling network through chemical genetics and proteome chips. *Proc Natl Acad Sci U S A*. 2004;101(47):16594-16599.
56. Yanagisawa K, Shyr Y, Xu BJ, et al. Proteomic patterns of tumour subsets in non-small-cell lung cancer. *Lancet*. 2003;362(9382):433-439.
57. Jackson EL, Willis N, Mercer K, et al. Analysis of lung tumor initiation and progression using conditional expression of oncogenic K-ras. *Genes Dev*. 2001;15:3243-3248.
58. Kim CF, Jackson EL, Woolfenden AE, et al. Identification of bronchoalveolar stem cells in normal lung and lung cancer. *Cell*. 2005;121(6):823-835.
59. Reya T, Morrison SJ, Clarke MF, Weissman IL. Stem cells, cancer, and cancer stem cells. *Nature*. 2001;414:105-111.
60. Jackson EL, Olive KP, Tuveson DA et al. The differential effects of mutant p53 alleles on advanced murine lung cancer. *Cancer Res*. 2005;65(22):10280-10288.
61. Fisher GH, Wellen SL, Klimstra D, et al. Induction and apoptotic regression of lung adenocarcinomas by regulation of a K-Ras transgene in the presence and absence of tumor suppressor genes. *Genes Dev*. 2001;15(24):3249-3262.
62. Ji H, Ramsey MR, Hayes DN, et al. LKB1 modulates lung cancer differentiation and metastasis. *Nature*. 2007;448(7155):807-810.
63. Kissil JL, Walmsley MJ, Hanlon L, et al. Requirement for Rac1 in a K-ras-induced lung cancer in the mouse. *Cancer Res*. 2007;67(17):8089-894.
64. Politi K, Zakowski MF, Fan PD, Schonfeld EA, Pao W, Varmus HE. Lung adenocarcinomas induced in mice by mutant EGF receptors found in human lung cancers respond to a tyrosine kinase inhibitor or to down-regulation of the receptors. *Genes Dev*. 2006;20(11):1496-1510.
65. Al-Hajj M, Wicha MS, Benito-Hernandez A, Morrison SJ, Clarke MF. Prospective identification of tumorigenic breast cancer cells. *PNAS*. 2003;100(7):3983-3988.
66. Lawson DA, Xin L, Lukacs RU, Cheng D, Witte ON. Isolation and functional characterization of murine prostate stem cells. *PNAS*. 2007;104(1):181-186.
67. Prince ME, Sivanandan R, Kaczorowski A, et al. Identification of a subpopulation of cells with cancer stem cell properties in head and neck squamous cell carcinoma. *PNAS*. 2007;104(3):973-978.
68. Ricci-Vitiani L, Lombardi DG, Pilozzi E, et al. Identification and expansion of human colon-cancer-initiating cells. *Nature*. 2007;445(4):111-115.
69. Singh SK, Hawkins C, Clarke ID, et al. Identification of human brain tumour initiating cells. *Nature*. 2004;432:396-401.
70. Eramo A, Lotti F, Sette G, et al. Identification and expansion of the tumorigenic lung cancer stem cell population. *Cell Death Differ*. 2008;15(3):504-514.
71. Kern SE, Shibata D. The fuzzy math of solid tumor stem cells: a perspective. *Cancer Res*. 2007;67(19):8985-8988.
72. Kelly PN, Dakic A, Adams JM, Nutt SL, Strasser A. Tumor growth need not be driven by rare cancer stem cells. *Science*. 2007;317(5836):337.
73. Quintana E, Shackleton M, Sabel MS, Fullen DR, Johnson TM, Morrison SJ. Efficient tumour formation by single human melanoma cells. *Nature*. 2008;456(7222):593-598.

Anatomy, Imaging and Practical Management of Selected Thoracic Surgical Procedures

8

Betty C. Tong
Thomas A. D'Amico

ANATOMY

Chest Wall and Surface Anatomy

The thoracic viscera are protected by the chest wall and sternum. The bony framework of the chest wall is composed of 12 thoracic vertebrae, intervertebral discs, 12 pairs of ribs with corresponding cartilages, and the sternum. The thoracic vertebrae and intervertebral discs are positioned in the posterior midline; the spinous processes are relatively easy to identify as landmarks. The scapula overlies a portion of the first seven pairs of ribs posteriorly. With the arm abducted, the (vertebral) medial border of the scapula is parallel to the oblique fissure of the underlying lung.[1]

The sternum lies in the anterior midline and has three components: manubrium, body, and xiphoid process. The sternal notch, or superior border of the manubrium, is easily located between the clavicular heads. The junction of the manubrium and body of the sternum is called the sternal angle, or angle of Louis. This is an important landmark, corresponding to the level where the second costal cartilages articulate with the sternum. Since the first rib may be partially or completely obscured by the clavicle, accurate counting of ribs may commence at the sternal angle. This landmark is also important for deeper thoracic structures, marking the level of the tracheal bifurcation (carina) as well as the aortic arch.[2]

The upper seven pairs of ribs are considered to be true ribs because they form a complete circle between the sternum and vertebrae. The costal cartilages connect the ribs to the sternum anteriorly. In contrast to those of the first seven pairs of ribs, the costal cartilages of the 8th, 9th, and 10th ribs attach to the cartilage of the preceding rib. The 10th costal cartilage marks the most inferior point of the costal margin.[1] Aside from their vertebral attachments, the 11th and 12th ribs do not have other skeletal attachments and are considered to be "floating ribs."

The blood supply to the chest wall comes from the subclavian artery and aorta. The subclavian artery gives rise to the internal thoracic artery, also known as the internal mammary artery, as well as the first two intercostal arteries. Together, these vessels supply the anterior chest wall. The lateral and posterior areas of the chest wall are supplied by the remaining intercostal arteries, which arise as direct branches from the aorta posteriorly. Importantly, the intercostal bundle, consisting of the intercostal artery, vein and nerve, runs along the inferior aspect of each rib and is subject to injury during procedures such as thoracotomy or even thoracostomy tube placement.

The extrathoracic muscles of the chest wall provide both anatomic landmarks as well as substrate for surgical reconstruction of chest wall defects. The latissimus dorsi provides a large and versatile myocutaneous flap. Supplied by the thoracodorsal artery, nerve and vein, it is used most frequently for reconstruction of anterior and lateral chest wall defects. The pectoralis major is often used for anterior and midline chest wall defects, and is especially useful for coverage of sternal wounds. The rectus abdominus, external oblique and trapezius muscles may also be used for reconstruction of chest wall defects. When intrathoracic muscle flaps are needed (eg, coverage of bronchial stumps, filling a post-pneumonectomy space), the intercostal muscles and serratus anterior muscle are most frequently utilized.

AIRWAY AND LUNGS

Trachea

The trachea, palpable in the anterior neck, enters the chest just posterior to the manubrium and serves as the ventilatory conduit between the larynx and mainstem bronchi. It spans from the inferior border of the cricoid cartilage, the only complete cartilaginous ring in the airway, to the carina. There, the airway divides into the right and left mainstem bronchi. The trachea is comprised of 14 to 19 C-shaped incomplete cartilaginous rings and elastic membranous tissue.[3] During childhood, the cross-sectional area of the trachea is circular. With growth and development, it becomes elliptical in shape with its transverse length slightly longer than the anteroposterior length. However, normal anatomic variation among adults occurs frequently, and includes both circular and triangular cross-sectional shapes.[4] The average tracheal length in an adult ranges from 10 to 15 cm; in general, tracheal dimensions are slightly larger in men than women.

The posterior membranous trachea is composed of smooth muscle and respiratory epithelium, with ciliated pseudostratified columnar epithelium and mucus-producing goblet cells. The intercartilaginous tissue between the tracheal rings also contains muscle. It is this muscular tissue that is responsible for dynamic changes in tracheal size and luminal diameter.

The blood supply to the trachea is segmental, and closely related to that of the esophagus. The inferior thyroid artery arises from the thyrocervical trunk of the subclavian artery and supplies blood to both the proximal trachea and esophagus. Branches of the bronchial arteries, which arise directly from the aorta, supply the lower trachea, carina and bronchi. These arterial branches enter the tracheoesophageal groove and further divide into primary tracheal and esophageal branches. The primary tracheal branches further divide into lateral longitudinal vessels, which join together and run parallel to the longitudinal axis of the trachea, and transverse intercartilaginous arteries, which supply blood in a circumferential manner. Extensive circumferential dissection of the trachea and airways is to be avoided in order to prevent bronchial stump dehiscence or anastomotic disruption.

Bronchopulmonary Anatomy

At the carina, the trachea divides into the right and left mainstem bronchi. The lungs are divided into lobes and segments. The first branch off the right main bronchus is the right upper lobe bronchus. The ongoing airway, called bronchus intermedius, then divides into the right middle and lower lobe bronchi. The three lobes of the right lung are further divided into 10 segments (Table 8–1). The right upper lobe bronchus gives rise to the apical, anterior and posterior segments, while the right middle lobe contains the medial and lateral segments. The right lower lobe is composed of the superior segment and four basilar segments: anterior, posterior, medial and lateral.

The left lung is slightly smaller than the right lung, and has only two lobes (upper and lower) and eight segments. The lingula, the inferior portion of the left upper lobe, is anatomically analogous to the right middle lobe. From the carina, the left main bronchus gives rise to the left upper and lower lobe bronchi. The left upper lobe contains the apicoposterior and anterior segments in addition to the superior and inferior lingular segments. The left lower lobe is comprised of the superior segment, in addition to three basilar segments: anteromedial, lateral, and posterior.

Table 8–1. Lobar and Segmental Anatomy of the Lungs

Right Lung	Left Lung
Right Upper Lobe	*Left Upper Lobe*
Apical segment	Apicoposterior segment
Anterior segment	Anterior segment
Posterior segment	Superior lingular segment
Right Middle Lobe	Inferior lingular segment
Medial segment	
Lateral segment	
Right Lower Lobe	*Left Lower Lobe*
Superior segment	Superior segment
Anterior basilar segment	Anteromedial basilar segment
Medial basilar segment	Lateral basilar segment
Posterior basilar segment	Posterior basilar segment
Lateral basilar segment	

The arterial blood supply to the lungs follows the segmental bronchial anatomy. The main pulmonary artery arises from the heart and divides into the left and right pulmonary artery trunks. Branches of the right main pulmonary artery include the truncus arteriosus and posterior ascending artery, which supply the right upper lobe. The right middle lobe branch supplies its namesake, and the right lower lobe is supplied by a superior segmental artery branch as well as by branches of the basilar trunk. Similarly, the left main pulmonary artery gives rise to apical, anterior, posterior and lingular branches, which supply the left upper lobe. The superior segmental artery and common basal trunk supply the left lower lobe.

Paired pulmonary veins, superior and inferior, provide venous drainage from the lungs to the right atrium of the heart. The right superior pulmonary vein drains the right upper and middle lobes, and the right inferior pulmonary vein drains the right lower lobe. Similarly, on the left side, the superior pulmonary vein drains blood from the left upper lobe and the inferior pulmonary vein drains the left lower lobe. Rarely do the pulmonary vein branches join to form a single vessel or "common vein." However, this must be recognized during pulmonary resection in order to avoid division of the entire venous drainage from the lung, which would necessitate pneumonectomy.

ESOPHAGUS

The esophagus serves as a conduit for food and drink between the hypopharynx and stomach, and traverses three anatomic regions: the neck, thorax, and abdomen. The cervical esophagus measures approximately 5 cm in length and is located between the trachea and vertebral column. Proximally, the esophagus begins in the neck at the cricopharyngeus, or upper esophageal sphincter. Of the three areas of normal anatomic narrowing of the esophagus, the cricopharyngeus is narrowest and the most common site of iatrogenic perforation. Upon swallowing, the cricopharyngeus relaxes to accommodate the bolus traveling from the pharynx to the esophagus. The right and left recurrent laryngeal nerves reside in their respective tracheo-esophageal grooves and are at risk for injury during dissection of either the trachea or esophagus in this region.

The thoracic esophagus measures approximately 20 cm in length. From its entry at the thoracic inlet to the tracheal bifurcation, the esophagus maintains its close anatomic relationship with the posterior tracheal wall and the prevertebral fascia. Another area of normal anatomic narrowing occurs at the level of the aortic arch, where an indentation in the left lateral esophageal wall is often seen on both endoscopic examination and contrast esophagography. From this point on, the esophagus continues anterior and often slightly left of the vertebral column until it reaches the diaphragmatic hiatus, the third site of normal anatomic narrowing.

The abdominal portion of the esophagus measures 1.25 to 2 cm in length and includes part of the lower esophageal sphincter. As the esophagus traverses the diaphragmatic hiatus, it is surrounded by the phrenoesophageal membrane, a fibroelastic ligament arising from the subdiaphragmatic fascia as a continuation of the transversalis fascia of the abdomen. The lower limit of this membrane blends with the serosa of the stomach; a prominent anterior fat pad marks its end, which also marks the approximate location of the gastroesophageal junction.

The blood supply to the esophagus varies by anatomic location. Branches of the inferior thyroid artery are responsible for blood supply to the cervical esophagus. Bronchial arteries supply the thoracic esophagus. Approximately 75% of individuals have one right-sided and one- or two left-sided branches, which arise directly from the aorta. The abdominal portion of the esophagus receives arterial blood supply from branches of the inferior phrenic and left gastric arteries. One unique feature of the esophagus is the extensive collateral network of vessels in the muscular and submucosal layers. Upon entry to the esophageal wall, the arteries divide to form longitudinal anastomoses. As a result, the esophagus can undergo extensive mobilization with nominal risk of devascularization or ischemic necrosis.

Venous drainage of the esophagus occurs through a submucosal venous plexus, which then flows into a periesophageal venous plexus. The esophageal veins originate from the periesophageal venous plexus. Further drainage of the esophageal veins varies by region: in the neck, the esophageal veins drain into the inferior thyroid vein; in the thorax, esophageal veins drain into the bronchial, hemiazygos and azygos veins; and in the abdomen, drainage is into the coronary vein.

MEDIASTINUM

The mediastinum is the area of the thorax that resides between the pleural spaces, extending from the thoracic inlet to the diaphragm. It is divided into the superior and inferior mediastinum by a plane passing through the sternal angle and the fourth thoracic vertebra. There are three anatomic subdivisions of the inferior mediastinal space: anterior, middle, and posterior. The anterior mediastinum contains the internal mammary arteries and veins, lymph nodes, thymus gland, connective tissue and fat. Ectopic parathyroid or thyroid gland tissue may also be found in the anterior mediastinal compartment.

The middle mediastinum is also called the visceral compartment. It contains the pericardium, heart, great vessels, trachea and proximal mainstem bronchi, and esophagus. In addition, lymphatics, the right and left vagus and phrenic nerves, thoracic duct, connective tissue and fat are also contained within the middle mediastinum.

The posterior mediastinum includes the paravertebral sulci, or potential spaces located along each side of the vertebral column. Neurogenic structures such as the ventral ramus, thoracic spinal ganglia, and sympathetic trunk are found in the paravertebral sulci. The proximal portions of the intercostal arteries and veins, connective tissue and lymphatics are also located within the posterior mediastinum.

DIAGNOSTIC IMAGING MODALITIES

Imaging of the Lungs

Several different imaging modalities are used in the evaluation of pulmonary disorders. Plain chest radiography, done in the primary care or emergency room setting, often provides the first indication of pulmonary pathology. A standard

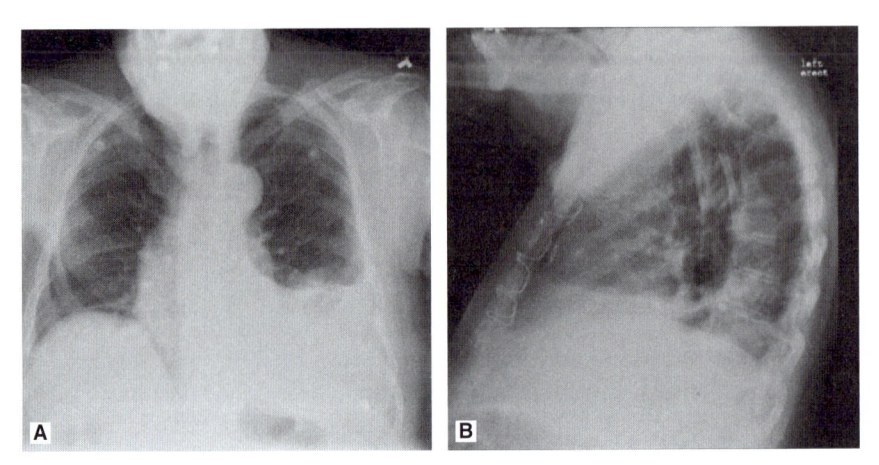

Figure 8–1. PA and lateral chest x-ray demonstrating left-sided pleural effusion. The presence of sternal wires indicates prior median sternotomy.

chest radiograph consists of two images: one taken in the posterioranterior (PA) projection and the other from the left lateral erect position (Figure 8–1). These images provide visualization of the pulmonary parenchyma, mediastinum, bony structures and diaphragm. Lateral decubitus films are often employed to evaluate the mobility of pleural effusions seen on plain films.

Computed tomography (CT) studies provide excellent anatomic detail and characterization of abnormalities or lesions detected on plain radiographs of the chest. Important features that may raise or lower the suspicion of malignancy include the following: location, appearance (cavitary vs solid, spiculated vs well-defined), involvement of adjacent structures such as chest wall or great vessels. Enlarged mediastinal lymph nodes (> 1 cm in long axis) may suggest the presence of metastatic disease and therefore warrant further evaluation. CT may also provide additional information regarding mediastinal or hilar lymphadenopathy, chest wall lesions, and diseases of the lung parenchyma such as bronchiectasis or pulmonary fibrosis (Figure 8–2). Currently, contrast-enhanced CT angiography is widely used for diagnosis of acute pulmonary embolism. With a sensitivity over 80%, it has advantages over traditional ventilation-perfusion scans, including speed, detection of venous thrombosis, and characterization of nonvascular structures.[5] However, patients with impaired renal function may not be candidates for use of intravenous contrast and in these cases, the ventilation-perfusion scan may be preferred.

In addition to CT, positron emission tomography (PET) imaging is very useful in further characterizing potentially malignant lesions. The technique uses a radio-labeled glucose (18-fluorodeoxyglucose [^{18}FDG]) to identify tissues with increased metabolic activity, such as malignant or infectious processes. In a recent meta-analysis, the sensitivity of ^{18}FDG-PET for identifying malignant lesions was 96.8% and the specificity was 77.8%.[6] However, one limitation of PET is that its resolution is limited in tumors less than 1 cm in size, and accuracy is decreased in these smaller lesions.[7]

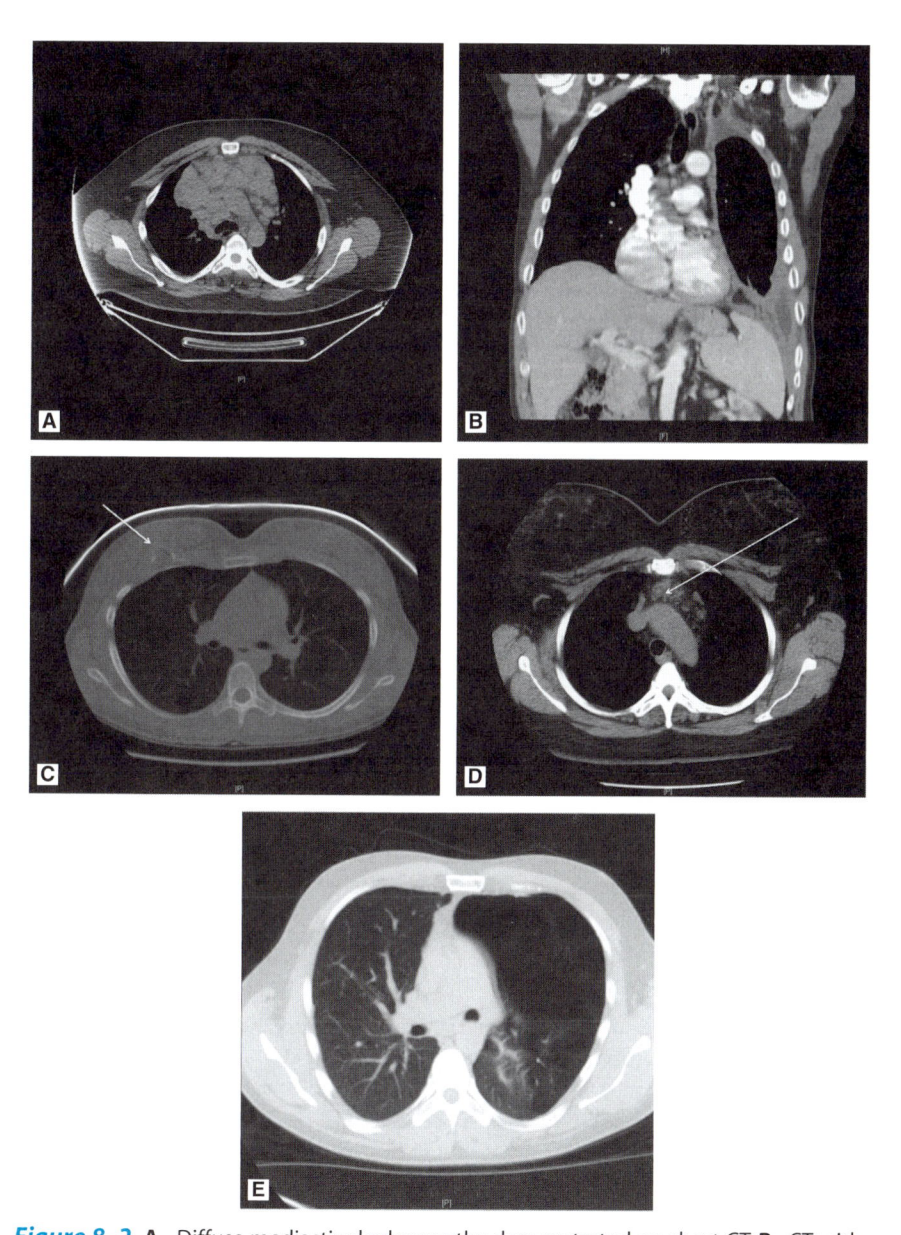

Figure 8-2. **A.** Diffuse mediastinal adenopathy demonstrated on chest CT. **B.** CT with coronal reconstruction demonstrating pleural thickening consistent with mesothelioma. **C.** Bone windows of CT scan demonstrating a lesion of the right 3rd rib (arrow). **D.** Non-contrast CT scan of the chest demonstrating thymic mass in anterior mediastinum (arrow). **E.** CT scan of the chest demonstrating the presence of left-sided giant bullous disease.

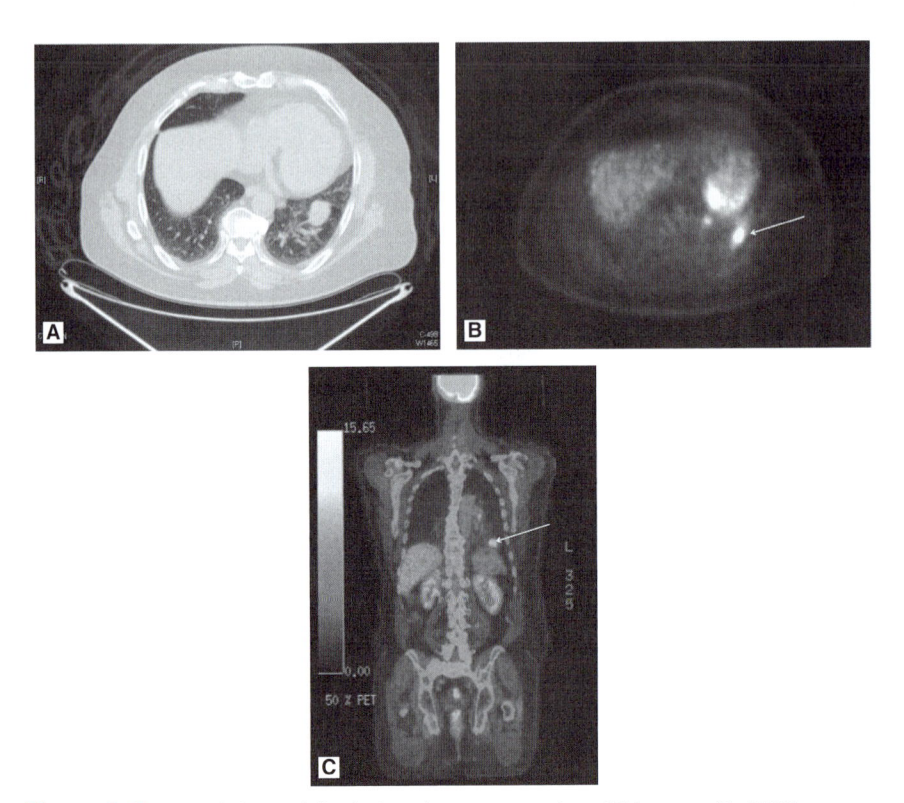

Figure 8–3. **A.** Left lower lobe lesion demonstrated on CT images. **B.** PET images of left lower lobe mass (arrow). **C.** Integrated PET/CT images of hypermetabolic left lower lobe mass.

Integrated PET/CT (Figure 8–3) and PET/CT fusion (Figure 8–4) studies combine the advantages of both modalities, providing excellent anatomic detail in addition to information regarding metabolic activity. As compared to PET alone and CT alone, integrated and fusion PET/CT studies have greater sensitivity, specificity, negative predictive value and overall accuracy for staging of mediastinal lymph nodes.[8,9] PET/CT can also be used for re-staging of the mediastinal lymph nodes following neoadjuvant therapy; however, the sensitivity of both standalone PET and integrated PET/CT are both lower after induction therapy.[10]

For evaluation of suspected superior sulcus (Pancoast) tumors, MRI is often used and preferred. It is superior to CT for evaluating tumor involvement of the brachial plexus, subclavian vessels and vertebral bodies.[11] Involvement of these structures may alter surgical management or even render the patient unresectable, thereby changing the course of recommended therapy.

The ventilation-perfusion (V/Q) scan has several uses. Historically, it was most often used in the diagnostic evaluation of suspected pulmonary embolus. More recently, however, CT angiography has supplanted the V/Q scan for patients with

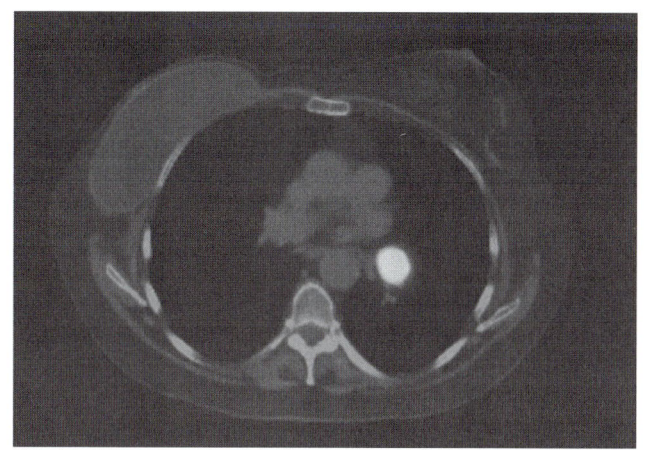

Figure 8–4. PET/CT fusion of hypermetabolic left hilar mass.

suspected pulmonary embolus. Nevertheless, the quantitative V/Q scan is often used to estimate the contribution of the upper, middle, and lower lung zones to overall lung perfusion. Patients with marginal pulmonary function may be able to tolerate resection of a lobe or segment in which there is nominal perfusion as demonstrated by the quantitative V/Q scan.

Imaging of the Mediastinum

The plain chest radiograph is often the most common initial diagnostic imaging study for mediastinal abnormalities. The posteroanterior and lateral radiograph can reveal the presence of a mediastinal mass and its location (anterior vs posterior), as well as mediastinal widening. Further evaluation is usually done with CT imaging, which provides excellent anatomic detail with regard to size and location as well as proximity to and involvement of surrounding structures and great vessels. At present, CT angiography is the test of choice for imaging the great vessels in a hemodynamically stable patient with suspected aortic dissection. In a recent study comparing helical CT and surgical findings, CT demonstrated 100% accuracy in diagnosing Type A aortic dissections and intramural hematomas.[12] For hemodynamically unstable patients, however, transesophageal echocardiography is preferred. MRI, while not used routinely, may provide improved characterization of soft tissues relative to CT and may also be used to characterize vascular structures without the need for intravenous contrast.

Esophageal Diagnostic Modalities

Barium swallow (Figure 8–5) is often one of the first tests done when esophageal pathology is suspected. Usually done under videofluoroscopy, the patient swallows a bolus of radio-opaque barium, which opacifies the esophageal lumen during its transit to the stomach. With this technique, abnormal esophageal motility as well

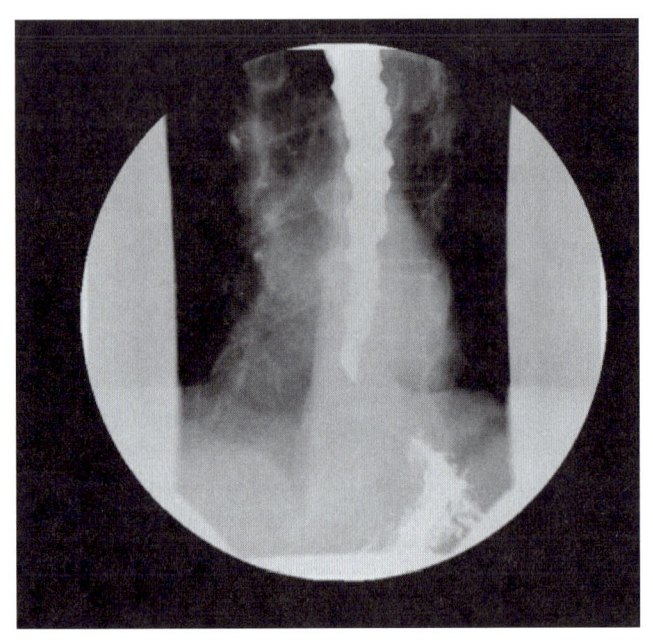

Figure 8-5. Barium swallow demonstrating tortuous esophagus with distal bird's beak deformity consistent with achalasia.

as structural changes in the esophageal lumen (eg, strictures, masses, filling defects) can be observed.

CT is also useful for evaluating the esophagus. The presence of paraesophageal fat helps to distinguish the normal esophagus from surrounding vessels, airway and other structures. Hiatal hernias, esophageal tumors, and even esophageal perforation may be diagnosed using contrast-enhanced CT.

As with other malignancies, PET and PET/CT are frequently used and recommended for the staging evaluation of esophageal cancer. While PET has a sensitivity of 91% to 95% for detecting primary esophageal tumors, accurate T staging is sometimes difficult.[13] Similarly, the sensitivity and specificity of standalone PET for detecting locoregional lymph node involvement in esophageal cancer are 51% and 84%, respectively.[14] However, PET and PET/CT are most useful for determining the presence of distant metastases.[15] The presence of distant metastatic disease may, in turn, change the clinicians' management strategy, as these patients are not candidates for surgical resection.

Endoscopic ultrasound (EUS) combines high-frequency ultrasonography with endoscopy, and is highly accurate in the locoregional staging of esophageal cancer. With the ultrasound probe, five layers of the esophagus are identified: superficial mucosa, deep mucosa, submucosa, muscularis propria and adventitia. The accuracy of predicting the depth of tumor penetration, or T stage, is approximately 85% to 90%.[16] Similarly, EUS is used for evaluation of regional lymph nodes, with a sensitivity of 73% and specificity of 77% for predicting the pathologic status of regional lymph nodes.[17] Characteristics of malignant lymph nodes include hypoechoic or homogeneous appearance, round shape, sharply demarcated borders, size > 1 cm and solitary appearance.[18-20] Fine needle aspiration of suspicious lymph nodes or liver lesions can be performed through the EUS probe to aid in staging accuracy.

PRACTICAL MANAGEMENT OF THORACIC SURGICAL PROCEDURES
General Guidelines

The complete preoperative evaluation of the thoracic surgery patient is discussed in detail in Chapter 9. For patients proceeding to surgery, several general principles are relevant for the intraoperative management of the thoracic surgical patient. First, one-lung ventilation is preferred for the vast majority of thoracic procedures, including all types of lung resection as well as esophageal surgery. Lung isolation with ventilation of the nonoperative side provides room in the thoracic cavity for the surgeon to work and facilitates performance of the operation. In addition, for cases involving massive hemoptysis or bronchopleural fistula, lung isolation can help to prevent contamination of the noninvolved side by the contralateral lung. Several methods can be used to isolate the lungs: double-lumen endotracheal tubes, bronchial blockers placed through a single-lumen endotracheal tube, and selective intubation of the right or left mainstem bronchus using a single-lumen endotracheal tube. Specific techniques for placement of these tubes and devices are discussed in Chapters 5 and 22. For the minority of patients who cannot tolerate single lung isolation, some procedures may be done with short periods of apnea and both lungs otherwise ventilated.

Patients who have had previous chemotherapy and/or radiation therapy merit special anesthetic consideration. Several chemotherapeutic agents, including those routinely used to treat lung and esophageal cancer, have been associated with pulmonary toxicity and are listed in Table 8–2. Bleomycin, most often used for patients with germ cell tumors and lymphoma, is the most studied. Oxygen administration is a recognized risk factor for bleomycin-induced pneumonitis; other risk factors include age, smoking, renal dysfunction, and history of mediastinal radiation.[21] Currently, there is no documented "safe" FiO_2 level for patients with a history of bleomycin exposure; thus, the lowest possible FiO_2 that enables the anesthesiologist to adequately oxygenate the patient is desired. Similarly, patients who have undergone mediastinal or chest radiotherapy are at risk for developing radiation pneumonitis. In lung cancer patients, the incidence of radiation pneumonitis is 5% to 15%; the proportion of breast cancer and Hodgkin's lymphoma patients who develop radiation pneumonitis is lower.[21,22] The risk of radiation pneumonitis may be increased with concomitant administration of chemotherapy, previous irradiation, total radiation dose and number of daily fractions, and recent withdrawal of steroids. Again, adequate oxygenation with the lowest possible FiO_2 is preferable for these patients.

Table 8–2. Chemotherapeutic Agents Associated with Pulmonary Toxicity

Generic Name	Other Names
Bleomycin	Blenoxane
Busulfan	Busulfex, Myleran
Carmustine	BiNCU
Chlorambucil	Leukeran
Cytosine arabinoside	Cytosar-U, Ara-C
Docetaxel	Taxotere
Etoposide*	VP-16, Toposar, VePesid, Etopophos
Fludarabine	Fludara
Gemcitabine*	Gemzar
Methotrexate	MTX, Rheumatrex, Trexall
Mitomycin	Mitomycin-C, MTC, Mutamycin
Paclitaxel*	Taxol, Onxal
Procarbizine	Matulane
Vinca alkaloids	
Vinblastine	Velban, Alkaban-AQ
Vinchristine	Oncovin, Vincasar Pfs
Vinorelbine*	Navelbine

*Often administered in lung and/or esophageal cancer
Data adapted from Carver JR, et al. American Society of Clinical Oncology clinical evidence review on the ongoing care of adult cancer survivors: cardiac and pulmonary late effects. *J Clin Oncol.* 2007;25(25):3991-4008.

Most thoracic surgical resections can be accomplished with two large bore peripheral intravenous lines and arterial line monitoring. However, central access may be desirable for cases such as standard pneumonectomy, extrapleural pneumonectomy, and resection of mediastinal tumors. If a central line is to be placed for administration of fluids and/or central venous monitoring, it should be placed on the ipsilateral side of the planned resection. In addition, for patients with complex mediastinal tumors who may require resection and reconstruction of the superior vena cava, preoperative placement of a femoral central venous line is advised.

The majority of lung resections and esophageal operations are conducted with the patient in the lateral decubitus position. Following the induction of general anesthesia and intubation, the patient is turned to the lateral decubitus position and secured to the operating table with ample padding under pressure points. Potential neurovascular injuries resulting from improper attention to the lateral decubitus position warrant discussion. The brachial plexus of the dependent arm is

Table 8–3. Common Patient Positions and Associated Thoracic Surgical Procedures

Position	Incision	Procedure(s)
Lateral decubitus	Thoracotomy or	Lung resection (wedge, lobectomy, etc)
	Thoracoscopy	Thoracoscopic pericardial window
		Decortication, pleurodesis
Supine, arms tucked at side	Cervical	Mediastinoscopy
	Median sternotomy	Cardiac surgery, mediastinal masses
	Laparotomy	Esophageal surgery, subxiphoid
		pericardial window
Supine, arms abducted	Clamshell	Lung transplant

subject to compression injury if there is inadequate padding under the dependent thorax. Careful placement of this padding is of the utmost importance, as migration into the axilla can also result in injury. The use of the bean bag has improved the ability both to stabilize the patient and to protect the axilla and the brachial plexus. The nondependent arm is also subject to brachial plexus injury; this is usually a stretch injury caused by excessive abduction of the nondependent arm, or lateral bending of the cervical spine.[23] Table 8–3 lists other patient positions and incisions for common thoracic surgical procedures.

Prevention of deep venous thrombosis (DVT) and subsequent pulmonary embolism begins in the operating room. Nearly all patients undergoing thoracic surgical procedures should be provided with measures to prevent perioperative DVT. The incidence of DVT following pulmonary resection increases with the extent of resection and ranges from 7.4% to 14% for patients undergoing pneumonectomy.[24,25] Intraoperative DVT prophylaxis usually includes intermittent calf compression with compression stockings and/or sequential compression devices (SCDs). Postoperative DVT prophylaxis includes compression stockings and SCDs in addition to the subcutaneous administration of unfractionated or low-molecular weight heparin.

Judicious fluid management is also extremely important in thoracic surgery, especially with one-lung ventilation. The incidence of acute lung injury (ALI) and adult respiratory distress syndrome (ARDS) is approximately 1% following lobectomy and 2% to 4% following pneumonectomy.[26] However, respiratory complications account for the majority of mortalities following lung resection.[27] With excessive administration of intravenous fluids, increased shunting can occur, leading to pulmonary edema of the dependent lung. Increasing perioperative fluid administration has been identified as an independent risk factor for lung injury following lung resection.[28] General guidelines also dictate that crystalloid administration does not exceed 3 L in the first 24 hours for an average adult patient; it is not necessary to ensure a urine output of > 0.5 mg/kg/h; and no fluids should be administered for "third space" losses during pulmonary resection.[23] If greater tissue perfusion is desired, invasive monitoring and administration of inotropes or vasopressors should be considered rather than additional intravenous fluid administration.

One specific intraoperative condition deserves mention here. With the patient in the lateral decubitus position, the acute onset of hypotension, hypoxia and high airway pressures can herald the onset of a spontaneous pneumothorax in the "down" or ventilated lung. This condition must be recognized and remedied quickly. Treatment includes the *immediate* return to dual-lung ventilation and placement of a thoracostomy tube into the nonoperative side to evacuate the pneumothorax. Temporary evacuation of the pneumothorax may be achieved intraoperatively by opening the contralateral pleura, either anterior to the pericardium or just anterior to the esophagus and aorta at the level of the inferior pulmonary ligament. Detection of a downside tension pneumothorax is facilitated by routine use of an esophageal stethoscope (see Chapter 13).

Maintaining normothermia can also be a challenge during thoracic surgery. However, hypothermia inhibits many of the body's normal physiologic functions, and must be avoided intraoperatively. Techniques to prevent hypothermia include use of patient warming devices, increasing the ambient room temperature, and use of fluid warmers.

Effective perioperative analgesia is mandatory for all patients undergoing lung resection, regardless of operative approach. For patients undergoing lung resection, thoracic epidural analgesia has been associated with decreased risk of postoperative pulmonary complications as well as decreased odds of postoperative death.[29,30] This is due to increased mean lung volumes resulting from improved respiratory mechanics and increased activity levels, which are effective in decreasing postoperative pulmonary complications.[31]

Selected Thoracic Surgical Procedures

MEDIASTINOSCOPY (SEE ALSO CHAPTER 10)

Mediastinoscopy is most often used for surgical staging of the mediastinal lymph nodes in patients with non-small cell lung cancer (NSCLC). It can also be used to obtain tissue diagnosis in patients with anterior mediastinal masses, such as lymphoma. Mediastinoscopy and associated procedures are discussed in detail in Chapter 10. In the procedure, a 1.5 to 2 cm low transverse cervical incision is made and the soft tissues are dissected to the trachea. The pretracheal fascial plane is dissected, and the mediastinoscope is inserted to facilitate biopsy of the mediastinal lymph nodes. While the overall complication rate from this procedure is only 1.07% in recent published series, both surgeon and anesthesiologist must be prepared for potential life-threatening complications such as major hemorrhage from injury to the great vessels (0.32% incidence).[32] Other potential complications from mediastinoscopy include vocal cord dysfunction due to injury of the recurrent laryngeal nerve, tracheal injury and pneumothorax.

For the procedure, only a single-lumen endotracheal tube is necessary. Standard monitoring includes pulse oximetry and blood pressure monitoring via a right radial arterial line. The right side is preferred because inadvertent compression of the innominate artery, which supplies the right common carotid and right subclavian arteries, can occur during the procedure. Patients with few cerebral collaterals may experience ischemia if this is not detected.

If severe hemorrhage is encountered, a number of maneuvers should be performed immediately. The surgeon should pack the wound to allow for hemodynamic stabilization as well as to potentially tamponade the bleeding source. Large-bore intravenous access should be obtained, if not done so already. In addition, blood products should be made immediately available to the anesthesiologist; blood and fluid warmers and infusers should also be brought into the operating room for use. If time permits and the surgeon believes that thoracotomy is indicated for repair of the injury, lung isolation should be obtained either using a bronchial blocker or exchange of endotracheal tubes to a double lumen tube. Once the patient has achieved hemodynamic stability, the cervical wound can potentially be re-explored; however, another approach (thoracotomy or sternotomy) to identify and repair the injury is likely more prudent.

PULMONARY RESECTION (SEE ALSO CHAPTER 13)

The most frequent indications for pulmonary resection are documented malignancy, either primary lung cancer or metastasis from an extrapulmonary site, and solitary pulmonary nodule with suspicion of primary lung cancer. Regardless of incision or approach, several oncologic principles dictate the extent of resection for lung cancer. First, the tumor should be completely resected with negative operative margins. For tumors involving the chest wall, diaphragm or other resectable surrounding structures, en bloc resection should be completed without tumor spillage. In addition to resection of the primary tumor, mediastinal lymph node sampling or dissection is done to ensure accurate pathologic staging.

Anesthetic management for patients undergoing pulmonary resection is discussed in detail in Chapter 13. In general, intraoperative management includes standard monitoring, large bore intravenous access and an arterial line. As discussed, one-lung ventilation is preferred for all pulmonary resections. For any thoracoscopic procedure, a tidal volume less than 300 cc is preferred, as higher tidal volumes can result in excessive movement of the mediastinum, which can make the surgical dissection more difficult. Patients should be kept normothermic and normotensive throughout the procedure. Ideally, all patients undergoing pulmonary resection are extubated and spontaneously breathing in the operating room prior to transfer to the postanesthesia care unit.

SUBLOBAR RESECTIONS: WEDGE RESECTION AND SEGMENTECTOMY

A wedge resection is a nonanatomic resection most often used for metastasectomy or for diagnostic purposes. It involves resection of the nodule or other focal abnormality with a margin of surrounding normal lung tissue. Segmentectomy requires anatomic dissection of one or more bronchopulmonary segments and separate division of the associated arterial and venous blood supply. This approach is most often used for management of patients who have small primary lung cancers but do not have the physiologic reserve to tolerate a lobectomy. For management of lung cancer, one advantage of segmentectomy over wedge resection is that the anatomic dissection also includes the associated lymphatics, which is desirable from an oncologic standpoint.

LOBECTOMY

The most common and standard operation for a primary lung cancer is lobectomy, an anatomic resection in which the lobar bronchus, pulmonary artery branches and pulmonary vein branch(es) are individually dissected and divided. This operation has been the mainstay of lung cancer resection since 1995, when the Lung Cancer Study Group compared limited resection (either wedge resection or segmentectomy) to lobectomy for peripheral T1 lesions.[33] Patients in the lobectomy group had significantly lower rates of local recurrence as well as a trend toward improved disease-free and overall survival.

Since the early 1990s, thoracoscopic or video-assisted thoracoscopic surgery (VATS) lobectomy has been shown to be an effective alternative to traditional thoracotomy for resection of early stage lung cancer. Relative to thoracotomy, advantages for thoracoscopic lobectomy include decreased acute postoperative pain, shorter chest tube duration, shorter hospital length of stay, and fewer overall postoperative (particularly pulmonary) complications.[34] Moreover, patients who have undergone VATS lobectomy and require adjuvant chemotherapy are able to initiate therapy sooner and have fewer reduced doses than thoracotomy patients.[35] VATS lobectomy is also cost effective.[36] While there are higher operating room costs associated with VATS lobectomy, these are counterbalanced by both shorter hospital stays and overall lower morbidity.

BILOBECTOMY, PNEUMONECTOMY, AND SLEEVE RESECTIONS

Bilobectomy or pneumonectomy may be required for complete extirpation of centrally located tumors. Bilobectomy involves the en bloc resection of the right middle and lower lobes for lesions located near or within the bronchus intermedius. For pneumonectomy, division of the mainstem bronchus, main pulmonary artery and both pulmonary vein branches is undertaken.

If pneumonectomy is considered for a centrally located lesion, then a parenchymal-sparing sleeve resection should also be contemplated. The sleeve resection involves resection of the involved lobe with removal of a segment of the adjacent bronchus. A bronchial-bronchial anastomosis is then constructed to restore bronchial continuity. While technically a more complex operation, sleeve resection offers several advantages over pneumonectomy, including preserved pulmonary function, avoidance of post-pneumonectomy complications, and improved patient quality of life.[37]

Proper fluid management is essential for patients undergoing pneumonectomy and extrapleural pneumonectomy. The sequelae of postoperative acute lung injury and pulmonary edema can be lethal, with mortality rates up to 50%.[23]

Management of hypotension should include consideration of vasopressor and/or inotropes in lieu of additional intravenous fluids, once blood losses are accounted for by the anesthesiologist. In addition, adequate pain management, usually in the form of a thoracic epidural catheter, helps to avoid respiratory compromise and postoperative pneumonia.

EXTRAPLEURAL PNEUMONECTOMY (SEE ALSO CHAPTER 14)

Extrapleural pneumonectomy is most often performed for treatment of malignant mesothelioma, a relatively uncommon but highly lethal disease associated with smoking and asbestos exposure. The operation requires extrapleural dissection of the lung with en bloc resection of the lung, pericardium and diaphragm. The pericardium and diaphragm are subsequently reconstructed, usually with gore-tex. Malignant mesothelioma, its treatment options and anesthetic implications are discussed in detail in Chapter 14.

TRACHEAL AND CARINAL RESECTIONS

Communication between the surgeon and anesthesiologist is critical for the patient undergoing tracheal and carinal resection. For patients with near-obstructing lesions, an inhalational induction technique with maintenance of spontaneous breathing is preferred, as positive pressure ventilation may result in complete obstruction.[38,39] Patients without critical stenoses may be maintained with intravenous anesthesia, which allows for prompt reversal and extubation following the procedure. Sterile anesthetic tubing and connectors should be available in the operating room for these procedures. In addition, resections involving the lower trachea and carina may require the use of an extra long, armored endotracheal tube, which can be placed into one of the mainstem bronchi using bronchoscopic guidance for ventilation during construction of the anastomosis. At the conclusion of the procedure, the orotracheal tube is replaced and the armored tube removed.

ESOPHAGEAL RESECTIONS (SEE ALSO CHAPTER 17)

Esophagogastrectomy is indicated for the treatment of esophageal cancer and for end-stage benign esophageal disease. Chapter 17 provides an in-depth review of the topic. In summary, the procedure includes resection of the esophagus, resection of periesophageal lymph nodes for accurate staging purposes, and restoration of enteric continuity. The esophageal reconstruction is usually performed using the stomach as an esophageal conduit; if the stomach is not available, other options include a pedicled segment of right or left colon, or jejunum (either pedicled or free). There are several accepted and described techniques for esophageal resection, including transhiatal, transthoracic (Ivor Lewis), 3-incision (McKeown), or minimally invasive esophagogastrectomy (MIE). The specific technique employed depends somewhat on tumor location as well as surgeon and patient preference. The specific incisions employed and some of the advantages and disadvantages to each technique are described in Table 8–4.

Anesthetic management of patients undergoing these procedures includes standard monitors, large bore or central venous access, and arterial line monitoring. For procedures involving anastomosis in the left neck, central venous access (if necessary) should

Table 8–4. Summary of Esophageal Resection Procedures

Procedure	Incisions	Comment
Transhiatal	Laparotomy	Advantage: avoids thoracotomy
	Left neck	Disadvantage: potential hemodynamic instability during intrathoracic dissection; not suitable for mid-esophageal tumors
		Does not require one-lung ventilation
		No vascular access in left neck
Ivor Lewis / Transthoracic	Right thoracotomy	Advantage: suitable for tumor in any location
	Laparotomy	Disadvantage: thoracic anastomosis
		Requires one-lung ventilation
McKeown	Right thoracotomy	Advantage: suitable for tumor in any location
	Laparotomy	Disadvantage: 3 incisions
	Left neck	Requires one-lung ventilation
		No vascular access in left neck
Minimally Invasive e	Thoracoscopy	Advantage: less perioperative pain, faster recovery
Ivor Lewis	Laparoscopy	Disadvantage: steep surgical learning curve
		Requires one-lung ventilation

be accomplished through the right internal jugular vein. The Ivor Lewis, McKeown and MIE procedures require one-lung ventilation to facilitate the dissection and mobilization of the esophagus.

The transhiatal esophagogastrectomy is accomplished through a laparotomy with anastomosis in the neck. Dissection of the intrathoracic esophagus is accomplished bluntly through the esophageal hiatus; the presence of the surgeon's hand in the mediastinum may compromise venous return, resulting in transient hemodynamic instability. Good communication between the surgeon and anesthesiologist is especially important during this portion of the operation. Normal fascial planes may be disrupted due to the presence of the tumor. As such, the transhiatal esophagogastrectomy is not suitable for mid-esophageal tumors, where the airway (adjacent to the esophagus) is at risk for injury during the blunt dissection. If an airway injury is detected during the procedure, advancing the endotracheal tube past the injury will provide a temporary means of ventilation until the defect can be repaired.

The Ivor Lewis esophagogastrectomy is a two-part operation. First, a laparotomy is performed for gastric mobilization and lymphadenectomy. Then, the patient is turned to the left lateral decubitus position and right thoracotomy is performed. There, under one-lung ventilation, the intrathoracic esophagus is mobilized and thoracic lymphadenectomy is completed. The esophagogastric anastomosis is constructed in the chest. While all anastomoses are at risk for leak, the leak rate for intrathoracic anastomoses is lower than for those constructed in the neck.[40,41] However, the morbidity and mortality associated with an intrathoracic leak is significantly higher as compared to that following cervical anastomosis.[42]

The McKeown esophagogastrectomy is a three-part operation that first utilizes a right thoracotomy or thoracoscopy with one-lung ventilation for dissection and mobilization of the esophagus. Once the chest is closed, the patient is returned to the supine position with the head turned toward the right. A laparotomy is performed for gastric mobilization and lymphadenectomy. Finally, the gastric conduit is passed through the chest and the esophagogastric anastomosis is constructed in the left neck. Again, central venous access through the left internal jugular vein should be avoided.

A minimally invasive Ivor Lewis esophagogastrectomy employs both laparoscopy for gastric mobilization and thoracoscopy or limited thoracotomy for intrathoracic esophageal mobilization. During laparoscopy, the peritoneal space is insufflated with carbon dioxide; active ventilatory management is necessary to control the patient's $PaCO_2$. One-lung ventilation is necessary to complete the intrathoracic portion of the procedure. Depending on the surgeon's experience with this procedure, operative times may be longer than that for an open operation. However, advantages to this technique include lower blood loss, less pain and shorter length of hospital stay.[43]

SUMMARY

The successful management of patients undergoing thoracic surgery requires an understanding of each patient's anatomy and physiology, the past medical and surgical history, as well as the planned operative procedure. Anticipation and management of potential intraoperative and postoperative complications will help to reduce their incidence. Clear communication between surgeon and anesthesiologist both before and during the procedure facilitates optimal patient care.

REFERENCES

1. Sayeed RA, Darling GE. Surface anatomy and surface landmarks for thoracic surgery. *Thorac Surg Clin.* 2007;17(4):449-461.
2. Miller JI, Bryant AS, Deslauriers J. Anatomy and physiology of the chest wall and sternum with surgical implications. In: Patterson GC, Cooper JD, Deslauriers J, Lerut AEMR, Luketich JD, Rice TW, eds. *Pearson's Thoracic & Esophageal Surgery.* Philadelphia, PA: Churchill Livingstone Elsevier; 2008:1197.
3. Kamel KS, Lau G, Stringer MD. In vivo and in vitro morphometry of the human trachea. *Clin Anat.* 2009;22(5):571-579.
4. Wright CD. Anatomy, physiology, and embryology of the upper airway. In: Patterson GC, Cooper JD, Deslauriers J, Lerut AEMR, Luketich JD, Rice TW, eds. *Pearson's Thoracic & Esophageal Surgery.* Philadelphia, PA: Churchill Livingstone Elsevier; 2008:189-195.
5. Tapson VF. Acute pulmonary embolism. *N Engl J Med.* 2008;358(10):1037-1052.

6. Gould MK, Maclean CC, Kuschner WG, Rydzak CE, Owens DK. Accuracy of positron emission tomography for diagnosis of pulmonary nodules and mass lesions: a meta-analysis. *JAMA*. 2001;285(7):914-924.
7. Kubota K, Matsuzawa T, Fujiwara T, et al. Differential diagnosis of lung tumor with positron emission tomography: a prospective study. *J Nucl Med*. 1990;31(12):1927-1932.
8. Magnani P, Carretta A, Rizzo G, et al. FDG/PET and spiral CT image fusion for medistinal lymph node assessment of non-small cell lung cancer patients. *J Cardiovasc Surg (Torino)*. 1999;40(5):741-748.
9. Cerfolio RJ, Ojha B, Bryant AS, Raghuveer V, Mountz JM, Bartolucci AA. The accuracy of integrated PET-CT compared with dedicated PET alone for the staging of patients with nonsmall cell lung cancer. *Ann Thorac Surg*. 2004;78(3):1017-1023; discussion 1017-1023.
10. Groth SS, Whitson BA, Maddaus MA. Radiographic staging of mediastinal lymph nodes in non-small cell lung cancer patients. *Thorac Surg Clin*. 2008;18(4):349-361.
11. Heelan RT, Demas BE, Caravelli JF, et al. Superior sulcus tumors: CT and MR imaging. *Radiology*. 1989;170(3 Pt 1):637-641.
12. Yoshida S, Akiba H, Tamakawa M, et al. Thoracic involvement of type A aortic dissection and intramural hematoma: diagnostic accuracy–comparison of emergency helical CT and surgical findings. *Radiology*. 2003;228(2):430-435.
13. Yoon HH, Lowe VJ, Cassivi SD, Romero Y. The role of FDG-PET and staging laparoscopy in the management of patients with cancer of the esophagus or gastroesophageal junction. *Gastroenterol Clin North Am*. 2009;38(1):105-120, ix.
14. van Westreenen HL, Westerterp M, Bossuyt PM, et al. Systematic review of the staging performance of 18F-fluorodeoxyglucose positron emission tomography in esophageal cancer. *J Clin Oncol*. 2004;22(18):3805-3812.
15. Erasmus JJ, Munden RF. The role of integrated computed tomography positron-emission tomography in esophageal cancer: staging and assessment of therapeutic response. *Semin Radiat Oncol*. 2006;17:29-37.
16. Patel AN, Buenaventura PO. Current staging of esophageal carcinoma. *Surg Clin North Am*. 2005;85(3):555-567.
17. Barbour AP, Rizk NP, Gerdes H, et al. Endoscopic ultrasound predicts outcomes for patients with adenocarcinoma of the gastroesophageal junction. *J Am Coll Surg*. 2007;205(4):593-601.
18. Vickers J, Alderson D. Oesophageal cancer staging using endoscopic ultrasonography. *Br J Surg*. 1998;85(7):994-998.
19. Marsman WA, van Wissen M, Bergman JJ, et al. Outcome of patients with esophageal carcinoma and suspicious celiac lymph nodes as determined by endoscopic ultrasonography. *Endoscopy*. 2004;36(11):961-965.
20. Botet JF, Lightdale CJ, Zauber AG, Gerdes H, Urmacher C, Brennan MF. Preoperative staging of esophageal cancer: comparison of endoscopic US and dynamic CT. *Radiology*. 1991;181(2):419-425.
21. Carver JR, Shapiro CL, Ng A, et al. American Society of Clinical Oncology clinical evidence review on the ongoing care of adult cancer survivors: cardiac and pulmonary late effects. *J Clin Oncol*. 2007;25(25):3991-4008.
22. McDonald S, Rubin P, Phillips TL, Marks LB. Injury to the lung from cancer therapy: clinical syndromes, measurable endpoints, and potential scoring systems. *Int J Radiat Oncol Biol Phys*. 1995;31(5):1187-1203.
23. Slinger PD, Campos JH. Anesthesia for thoracic surgery. In: Miller RD, et al, eds. *Miller's Anesthesia*. 7th ed. St. Louis, MO: Churchill Livingstone; 2009.
24. Ziomek S, Read RC, Tobler HG, et al. Thromboembolism in patients undergoing thoracotomy. *Ann Thorac Surg*. 1993;56(2):223-226; discussion 227.
25. Mason DP, Quader MA, Blackstone EH, et al. Thromboembolism after pneumonectomy for malignancy: an independent marker of poor outcome. *J Thorac Cardiovasc Surg*. 2006;131(3):711-718.
26. Grichnik KP, D'Amico TA. Acute lung injury and acute respiratory distress syndrome after pulmonary resection. *Semin Cardiothorac Vasc Anesth*. 2004;8(4):317-334.
27. Kutlu CA, Williams EA, Evans TW, Pastorino U, Goldstraw P. Acute lung injury and acute respiratory distress syndrome after pulmonary resection. *Ann Thorac Surg*. 2000;69(2):376-380.
28. Alam N, Park BJ, Wilton A, et al. Incidence and risk factors for lung injury after lung cancer resection. *Ann Thorac Surg*. 2007;84(4):1085-1091; discussion 1091.
29. Block BM, Liu SS, Rowlingson AJ, Cowan AR, Cowan JA Jr, Wu CL. Efficacy of postoperative epidural analgesia: a meta-analysis. *JAMA*. 2003;290(18):2455-2463.
30. Wu CL, Sapirstein A, Herbert R, et al. Effect of postoperative epidural analgesia on morbidity and mortality after lung resection in medicare patients. *J Clin Anesth*. 2006;18(7):515-520.

31. Warner DO. Preventing postoperative pulmonary complications: the role of the anesthesiologist. *Anesthesiology.* 2000;92(5):1467-1472.
32. Lemaire A, Nikolic I, Petersen T, et al. Nine-year single center experience with cervical mediastinoscopy: complications and false negative rate. *Ann Thorac Surg.* 2006;82(4):1185-1189; discussion 1189-1190.
33. Ginsberg RJ, Rubinstein LV. Randomized trial of lobectomy versus limited resection for T1 N0 non-small cell lung cancer. Lung Cancer Study Group. *Ann Thorac Surg.* 1995;60(3):615-622; discussion 622-623.
34. Villamizar NR, Darrabie MD, Burfeind WR, et al. Thoracoscopic lobectomy is associated with lower morbidity compared with thoracotomy. *J Thorac Cardiovasc Surg.* 2009;138(2):419-425.
35. Petersen RP, Pham D, Burfeind WR, et al. Thoracoscopic lobectomy facilitates the delivery of chemotherapy after resection for lung cancer. *Ann Thorac Surg.* 2007;83(4):1245-1249; discussion 1250.
36. Casali G, Walker WS. Video-assisted thoracic surgery lobectomy: can we afford it? *Eur J Cardiothorac Surg.* 2009;35(3):423-428.
37. Balduyck B, Hendriks J, Lauwers P, Van Schil P. Quality of life after lung cancer surgery: a prospective pilot study comparing bronchial sleeve lobectomy with pneumonectomy. *J Thorac Oncol.* 2008;3(6):604-608.
38. Lieberman M, Mathisen DJ. Surgical anatomy of the trachea and techniques of resection and reconstruction. In: Shields TW, et al, eds. *General Thoracic Surgery.* Philadelphia, PA: Lippincott Williams & Wilkins; 2009:955-966.
39. Ashiku SK, Mathisen DJ. Tracheal lesions. In: Sellke FW, del Nido PJ, Swanson SJ, eds. *Sabiston & Spencer: Surgery of the Chest.* Philadelphia, PA: Elsevier Saunders; 2005:105-117.
40. Rindani R, Martin CJ, Cox MR. Transhiatal versus Ivor-Lewis oesophagectomy: is there a difference? *Aust N Z J Surg.* 1999;69(3):187-194.
41. Crestanello JA, Deschamps C, Cassivi SD, et al. Selective management of intrathoracic anastomotic leak after esophagectomy. *J Thorac Cardiovasc Surg.* 2005;129(2):254-260.
42. Linden PA, Swanson SJ. Esophageal resection and replacement. In: Sellke FW, del Nido PJ, Swanson SJ, eds. *Sabiston & Spencer Surgery of the Chest.* Philadelphia, PA: Elsevier Saunders; 2005:627-651.
43. Luketich JD, Alvelo-Rivera M, Buenaventura PO, et al. Minimally invasive esophagectomy: outcomes in 222 patients. *Ann Surg.* 2003;238(4):486-494; discussion 494-495.

PART 2

Thoracic Anesthesia Practice

CHAPTERS

9. Preoperative Risk Stratification of the Thoracic Surgical Patient — 150
10. Bronchoscopy, Mediastinoscopy, and Chamberlain Procedure — 173
11. Therapeutic Bronchoscopy, Airway Stents, and Other Closed Thorax Procedures — 191
12. Mediastinal Masses: Implications for Anesthesiologists — 217
13. Lung Resections for Cancer and Benign Chest Tumors — 237
14. Extrapleural Pneumonectomy — 255
15. Lung Volume Reduction Surgery — 274
16. Pericardial Window Procedures — 308
17. Esophageal Cancer Operations — 322
18. Bronchopleural Fistula: Anesthetic Management — 342
19. Anesthesia for Lung Transplantation — 358
20. Thoracic Trauma Management — 378
21. Anesthesia for Pediatric Thoracic Surgery — 403

Preoperative Risk Stratification of the Thoracic Surgical Patient

9

David J. Ficke
Jerome M. Klafta

Key Points

1. All patients being considered for lung resection should have pulmonary function tests including spirometry and a DLCO (diffusing capacity of the lung for carbon monoxide) test, from which the predicted postoperative values are calculated. If the results are unfavorable, a measure of exercise capacity or peak oxygen consumption should be obtained.
2. Cardiac evaluation of the thoracic surgical patient should include surgeons, anesthesiologists, and cardiologists. Higher levels of perioperative risk may be acceptable because of the potential curative benefit of surgery for non-small-cell lung cancer.
3. A thorough history of cancer therapy that considers chemotherapy, radiation, and an evaluation of the paraneoplastic effects of the cancer identifies other potential perioperative vulnerabilities.

Case Vignette

A 69-year-old man is scheduled for a left pneumonectomy. A CT-guided biopsy 6 days ago revealed adenocarcinoma. He is obese and has hypertension, type 2 diabetes mellitus, osteoarthritis, and a 55 pack-year smoking history. When a mass was seen on his chest x-ray 2 weeks ago, he quit smoking. Pulmonary function tests show a moderately obstructive ventilatory defect with an FEV_1 of 63% of predicted. He blames limited exercise tolerance on his "bad knees" and has never been evaluated by a cardiologist. How should this case be managed? Are there any other tests that would be helpful for stratifying his perioperative risk?

Thoracic surgery can have profound effects on cardiopulmonary function in the operating room, in the immediate postoperative setting, and in the long-term. The scope of thoracic surgery ranges from a thoracoscopic sympathectomy for a healthy 20-year-old patient to an extrapleural pneumonectomy for an 80-year-old with coronary disease and emphysema. Ever since the first pneumonectomy was described in 1933,[1] physicians have been looking for a simple, effective way to evaluate patients to optimize outcomes. This chapter focuses primarily on the preoperative evaluation of patients who need pulmonary resection, but the principles apply for other thoracic surgeries as well. Esophageal surgery, for example, does not involve resection of lung tissue, but because esophageal pathology is associated with smoking, patients frequently have concurrent pulmonary disease. Several other considerations are noteworthy for esophageal surgery including the frequent presence of reflux and aspiration, poor nutritional status, and preoperative chemotherapy or radiation.

Understanding the surgical approach is critical to preparing for thoracic surgery. For example, if a patient has had coronary bypass surgery with an internal mammary artery, he is at high risk for myocardial ischemia during an ipsilateral extrapleural pneumonectomy. The unique physiology and pathophysiology of pulmonary resection necessitates several other considerations.

Pulmonary resection is generally performed on patients with lung cancer, which accounts for 160,000 deaths per year in the United States.[2] Five-year survival—only 15% for all lung cancers—is 49% for patients with surgically resectable, localized disease. It is likely that surgery is responsible for most of the long-term survivors. Lung cancers double in size within 30 to 500 days,[3] and faster growing tumors are associated with poorer prognosis.[4] Because of the aggressive nature of lung cancer, many patients (and physicians) are willing to accept higher levels of risk than they might for other types of surgery. Preoperative evaluation, ideally, should not significantly delay a surgery that is potentially curative.

We next provide a framework for the evaluation of the thoracic surgery patient with focus on the respiratory and cardiovascular systems, the potential physiologic impact of other cancer therapies such as chemotherapy and radiation, as well as other unique considerations for thoracic surgery.

Minimally invasive techniques, particularly video-assisted thoracic surgery (VATS), have become increasingly popular in the past decade. A video-assisted thoracoscopic lobectomy may have fewer and less severe complications than the same procedure performed by a conventional thoracotomy,[5,6] but preoperative evaluation of patients should be similar for both open and minimally invasive procedures. The removal of lung parenchyma and the physiologic changes this brings to the cardiorespiratory systems are not significantly different with either surgical technique–lung tissue is still removed. In addition, with VATS there is always the potential for conversion to an open procedure. Therefore, no distinction is made in this chapter between minimally invasive or open techniques with regard to preoperative risk stratification.

EVALUATION OF RESPIRATORY FUNCTION

The majority of pulmonary resections for lung cancer are performed in patients with some degree of respiratory impairment. Historically, maximum voluntary ventilation (MVV) was used to determine fitness for pulmonary resection.[7] MVV is defined as the maximal amount of air a patient can inhale and exhale in 12 seconds. In 1955, Gaensler found that patients with low MVV had a higher mortality, and subsequent studies have confirmed a correlation between MVV and perioperative mortality.[8,9] Because one of the limitations of MVV is that it depends entirely on effort, it has largely been replaced by other tests.

Spirometry

Spirometry has become the primary method by which patients are evaluated before thoracic surgery. Spirometry, which is relatively noninvasive, evaluates lung mechanics without the need for expensive equipment. The patient exhales air as fast as possible into a device that measures the pressure, flow, and volume of air exhaled. Several spirometric tests have been shown to correlate with outcome in thoracic surgery. Forced expiratory volume in 1 second (FEV_1) and forced vital capacity (FVC) are two such tests, with FEV_1 having the highest predictive value for complications.[10-12] Guidelines from the American College of Chest Physicians (ACCP)[13] and the British Thoracic Society (BTS)[14] suggest that after maximum bronchodilator therapy, an FEV_1 more than 2 L before a pneumonectomy or FEV_1 more than 1.5 L before a lobectomy is sufficient for a patient to tolerate surgery, assuming no significant dyspnea on exertion or no interstitial lung disease. The difficulty with using an absolute number for cutoffs is that FEV_1 depends on age, gender, and patient size. Because absolute values may unnecessarily exclude an elderly, small woman from surgery, FEV_1 and FVC are reported as a percentage of predicted value, which takes other factors into account. These same guidelines recommend an FEV_1 of more than 80% as sufficient to tolerate either pneumonectomy or lobectomy without further workup.

If a patient does not meet the above criterion, a more detailed approach is needed to estimate the patient's predicted postoperative FEV_1 (ppo-FEV_1). Several methods can be used to estimate ppo-FEV_1. The most basic (the anatomic method)[15] involves counting the number of segments to be removed. See Figure 9–1.

The calculation is as follows:

$$\text{ppo-FEV}_1 = \text{preop-FEV}_1\% \times (1 - \text{segments removed/total segments})$$

One advantage of this method is that postoperative lung mechanics can be calculated after a second lobectomy or completion pneumonectomy. An alternative method using radionuclide perfusion[16,17] may be better at predicting the ppo-FEV_1 after pneumonectomy than the anatomic method, which may underestimate the actual ppo-FEV_1.[18]

The risk of perioperative complications increases when the ppo-FEV_1 less than 40%.[19,20] The ACCP guidelines[13] suggest that patients with a ppo-FEV_1 less than 40% undergo exercise testing for further risk stratification (see below). A low ppo-FEV_1 is not an absolute contraindication to resection; Linden et al[21] showed that patients with a ppo-FEV_1 less than 35% could tolerate lung resections. In fact, the newly published guidelines of the European Respiratory Society and the

RUL = 3 segments

RML = 2 segments

RLL = 5 segments

LUL = 4 segments

LLL = 5 segments

For our patient with a preop FEV_1 of 63% scheduled to undergo a left pneumonectomy:

$$PPO\text{-}FEV_1 = \text{preop-}FEV_1 \times \left(1 - \frac{\text{Segments removed}}{\text{Total segments}}\right)$$

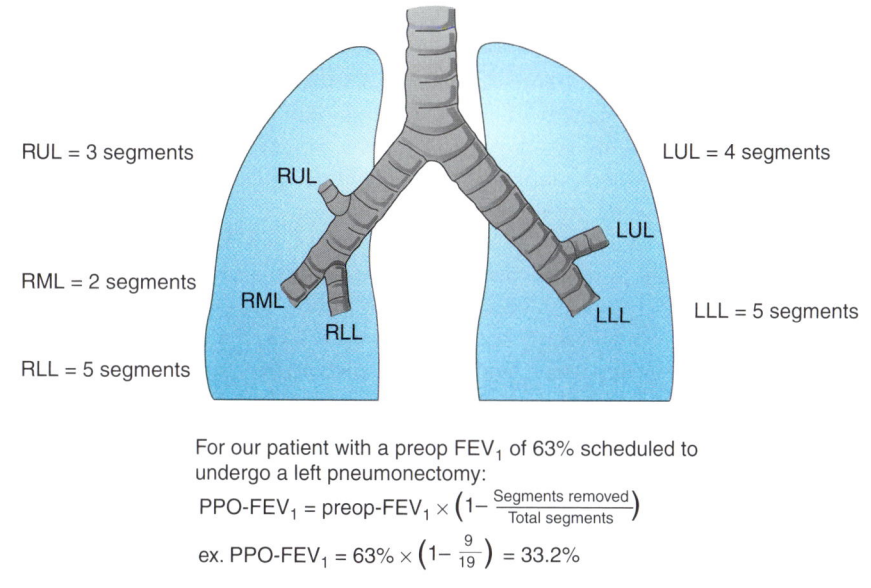

ex. $PPO\text{-}FEV_1 = 63\% \times \left(1 - \frac{9}{19}\right) = 33.2\%$

Figure 9-1. Example of anatomic method for calculating predicted postoperative FEV_1. RUL = right upper lobe, RML = right middle lobe, RLL = right lower lobe, LUL = left upper lobe, LLL = left lower lobe

European Society of Thoracic Surgery (ERS/ESTS) recommend a ppo-FEV_1 of 30% as the threshold to define high-risk patients.[22] Emerging studies also show that patients with extremely poor lung function may benefit from combined lung volume reduction surgery (LVRS) and resection of a malignant tumor.[23] It appears that the ideal candidate for combined LVRS and lung cancer resection has upper lobe emphysema with a tumor in the emphysematous upper lobe (see Chapter 15 on LVRS.). As anesthetic, surgical, and postoperative techniques improve, continuing studies are needed to determine the lowest spirometry values compatible with an acceptable surgical risk.

Gas Exchange

Unlike the measures of respiratory mechanics obtained by spirometry, other tests evaluate the capacity for gas exchange in the alveoli, including arterial oxygenation (PaO_2), arterial carbon dioxide ($PaCO_2$), and the diffusing capacity for carbon monoxide (DLCO). Historically, a PaO_2 less than 60 mm Hg breathing ambient air has been considered a contraindication for pulmonary resection. This number should be interpreted cautiously because PaO_2 may improve after lung resection when ventilation-perfusion matching has improved.[24] Similarly, a $PaCO_2$ more than 45 mm Hg has historically been the upper limit of acceptable hypercapnea before lung resection, but some studies have shown that complications do not necessarily increase with a $PaCO_2$ more than 45 mm Hg.[25]

Because of the limitations of PaO_2 and $PaCO_2$ values, DLCO is now considered the most useful test for evaluating gas exchange in the alveoli. The value is relatively easy to obtain and is often performed with other pulmonary function tests. To measure DLCO, the patient inhales a small amount of carbon monoxide and air and holds his breath for 10 seconds. When the patient exhales, the amount of exhaled carbon monoxide is measured and the diffusing capacity is calculated as the difference between the inhaled and exhaled amount.

In a retrospective analysis, Ferguson et al[26] found that DLCO correlated with surgical morbidity and mortality, perhaps even more so than FEV_1. The predicted postoperative DLCO (ppo-DLCO) can be calculated in the same manner as ppo-FEV_1 (see page 152). In another recent study, ppo-DLCO correlated with morbidity and mortality even in patients with normal spirometric values.[27]

As with ppo-FEV_1, several studies have shown that if the ppo-DLCO is less than 40%, perioperative risk is significantly increased.[19,28] The ACCP guidelines[13] suggest further risk stratification with formal exercise testing in patients with a ppo-DLCO less than 40%. Several groups have suggested that a product of % ppo-FEV_1 × % ppo-DLCO less than 1650 may be even more sensitive for revealing patients at high risk for perioperative complications.[28,29]

Split Lung Function Tests and Ventilation-Perfusion Scans

Given the strain on the cardiopulmonary system after pulmonary resection, a number of techniques have been developed to try to simulate this change and predict the body's response to the resection of a portion of lung parenchyma. Techniques involving temporary occlusion of a bronchus or pulmonary artery have been described.[30] If a pulmonary artery or lobar branch is occluded and pulmonary artery pressure does not change significantly, it is presumed that the remaining pulmonary vasculature is able to accommodate. These tests are invasive, resource intensive, and not widely used. They also may be misleading because pulmonary artery pressure may remain constant due to a failing right ventricle rather than accommodation of the pulmonary vasculature.[31]

Ventilation-perfusion scintigraphy scans (V/Q scans) have also been used in preoperative assessment to determine the relative contribution of each lung to overall ventilation.[32] A V/Q scan has two parts. The first part measures ventilation after a patient inhales a radioactive isotope that shows which parts of the lung are ventilated. The second part measures the perfusion of the lung after a separate radioactive isotope is injected to reveal which areas of the lung are perfused. V/Q scans appear to have reasonable correlation for predicting ppo-FEV_1 and ppo-FVC.[33] With this technique, an obstructed or underperfused area of lung parenchyma can be detected and the ppo-FEV_1 adjusted accordingly. If a patient has a ppo-FEV_1 less than 40% by the anatomic method, a V/Q scan may adjust the ppo-FEV_1 upwards. For example, if the patient from Figure 9–1 had a V/Q scan that showed his left lung received only 42% of the perfusion, then his revised ppo-FEV_1 would be 0.63 × (1−0.42) or 36.5%. If the revised ppo-FEV_1 still identifies the patient as high risk, exercise testing is generally recommended for further risk stratification (see page 155).

Flow-Volume Loops

Flow-volume loops are occasionally obtained before thoracic surgery to supplement other tests and are performed in the same manner as spirometry. They may be useful in the evaluation of a mediastinal mass.[34] (See also Chapter 12 on mediastinal masses.) A flow-volume loop can identify an intrathoracic airway obstruction by showing airflow limitation in the expiratory limb. Flow-volume loops were ordered frequently in the past, before more sophisticated imaging techniques of the intrathoracic airway were developed. Despite other advances in imaging, flow-volume loops have value because they measure airflow limitations throughout the entire respiratory cycle rather than at a single point in time. If a patient has few or no comorbidities and does not describe positional dyspnea or coughing, these tests are often omitted.

Exercise Testing

Patients may also undergo exercise testing before thoracic surgery. Rather than measuring isolated respiratory mechanics or gas exchange, exercise testing examines the function of the integrated cardiopulmonary system. Historically, stair climbing has been used as one functional assessment of overall cardiorespiratory status. The ability to climb three flights of stairs indicated the ability to tolerate a lobectomy; climbing five flights of stairs indicated the ability to tolerate a pneumonectomy. Surgical complications and mortality have been shown to correlate with inability to climb stairs.[35]

The lack of standardization for stair climbing makes the test somewhat problematic: the speed of ascent, duration of climbing, and number of stairs per flight may vary. Nevertheless, stair climbing still provides an easy, inexpensive estimate of the patient's exercise tolerance. In one study, patients who climbed fewer than 12 meters owing to symptoms of dyspnea had increased complications and mortality compared to those who could climb higher than 22 meters.[36] When combined with pulse oximetry, stair climbing may increase the sensitivity of predicting postoperative complications.[37]

A more objective measurement of exercise tolerance is the measure of maximal oxygen consumption (VO_2max), the gold standard for evaluation of exercise tolerance. The patient exercises—often on a treadmill—while wearing a mask that measures the volume and concentration of inhaled and exhaled gases. Many studies have shown that postoperative complications and mortality increase as preoperative VO_2max decreases.[38-41] A VO_2max less than 10 mL/kg/min is a marker for increased risk of complications and mortality. Patients with a low ppo-FEV_1 or ppo-DLCO with a VO_2max between 10 and 15 mL/kg/min also have a high rate of adverse events. Indeed the ACCP guidelines recommend that patients with a VO_2max less than 10 mL/kg/min or a VO_2max less than 15 mL/kg/min with both ppo-FEV_1 less than 40% and ppo-DLCO less than 40% be counseled about nonstandard surgery (ie, segmentectomy) or nonoperative therapies.[13]

Measuring VO_2max is time-consuming and resource intensive. Several other methods have been devised as alternatives for formal measurement of VO_2max.

The 6-minute walk test,[42] which measures how far a patient can walk in 6 minutes, correlates well with VO_2max and predicts complications after pulmonary resection.[43,44] A distance of less than 2000 feet (610 meters) correlates to a VO_2max of less than 15mL/kg/min.[45]

The shuttle walk test is another surrogate for VO_2max. In this test, the patient walks between two markers 10 meters apart, paced by an audio signal, until too tired to continue.[46] The shuttle walk test is used frequently in the nonsurgical assessment of pulmonary exercise tolerance. This test shows reasonable correlation to VO_2max.[47] Somewhat limited data suggest that a patient unable to complete 25 shuttles on two occasions is likely to have a VO_2max less than 10 mL/kg/min.[48]

Summary Recommendations for Respiratory Evaluation

Given the poor prognosis of cancer without surgery and patients' willingness to accept higher levels of risk, every effort should be made to optimize the medical condition of a patient so that surgery can be considered. All patients should have spirometry and DLCO testing. If the FEV_1 and DLCO are more than 80% predicted, no further evaluation is needed. For patients with FEV_1 less than 80% or DLCO less than 80%, a ppo-FEV_1 and ppo-DLCO should be calculated using the anatomic method. If either ppo-FEV_1 or ppo-DLCO is less than 40%, a V/Q scan can be considered to further refine predicted postoperative function. Alternatively, formal exercise testing with measurement of VO_2max should be performed. If the institution does not have the capacity to measure VO_2max, either stair climbing, the shuttle walk test, or the 6-minute walk test can be substituted. For those patients who, after exercise testing, are still at high risk for complications or death, nonstandard surgery (segmentectomy, combined LVRS/cancer resection) or nonoperative therapy should be discussed. A decision is made on a case by case basis. The algorithm in Figure 9–2 summarizes these recommendations.

CARDIAC EVALUATION

Although guidelines exist for cardiac evaluation before noncardiac surgery[49,50] (see also Figure 9–3), they are not specific to thoracic surgery. The objective of this section is to clarify some important aspects that are specific to thoracic surgical patients.

In general, the guidelines of the American College of Cardiology and the American Heart Association (ACC/AHA) classify intrathoracic surgery as a procedure of intermediate cardiac risk. That is, the risk of cardiac death or nonfatal myocardial infarction is 1% to 5%.[49] In our view, this is somewhat of an oversimplification. Even among pulmonary operations, not all resections will generate the same amount of stress on the cardiovascular system. An extrapleural pneumonectomy, for example, with its potential for blood loss and major effects on pulmonary vascular resistance, is a higher risk surgery than a wedge resection.

The revised ACC/AHA guidelines[49] recommend that if a thoracic surgical patient has an exercise tolerance of at least 4 metabolic equivalents (the ability to walk up one flight of steps), no further coronary evaluation is necessary, even in

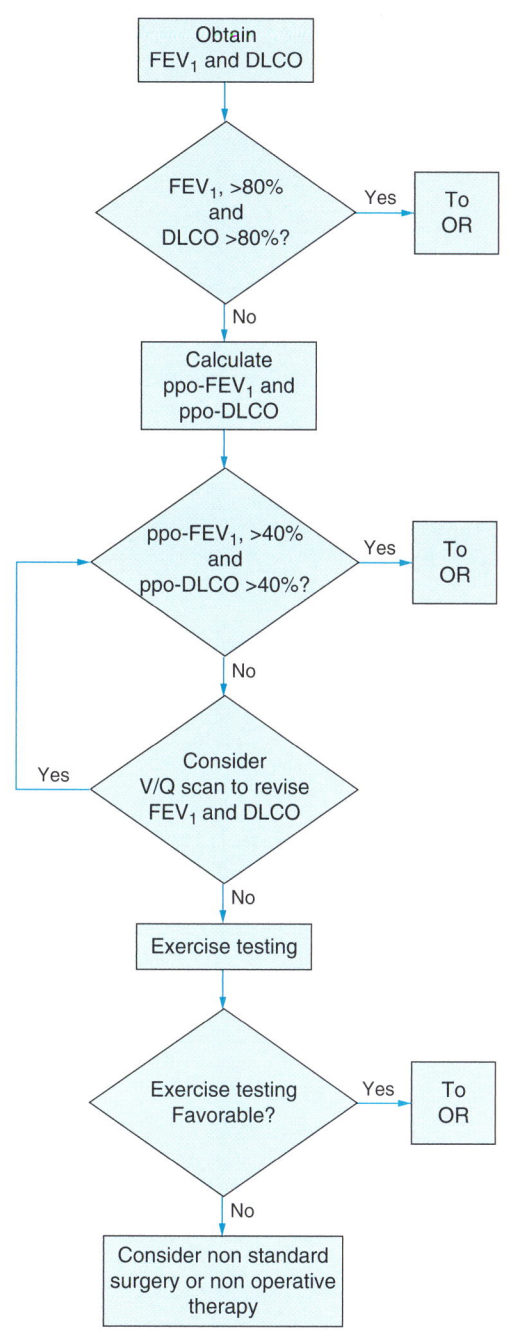

```
                    ┌─────────────────┐
                    │     Obtain      │
                    │ FEV₁ and DLCO   │
                    └────────┬────────┘
                             │
                             ▼
                    ◇─────────────────◇
                    │  FEV₁, >80%     │   Yes    ┌───────┐
                    │     and         │─────────▶│  To   │
                    │  DLCO >80%?     │          │  OR   │
                    ◇────────┬────────◇          └───────┘
                             │ No
                             ▼
                    ┌─────────────────┐
                    │    Calculate    │
                    │  ppo-FEV₁ and   │
                    │    ppo-DLCO     │
                    └────────┬────────┘
                             │
                             ▼
                    ◇─────────────────◇
                    │ ppo-FEV₁, >40%  │  Yes     ┌───────┐
                    │      and        │─────────▶│  To   │
                    │ ppo-DLCO >40%?  │          │  OR   │
                    ◇────────┬────────◇          └───────┘
                             │ No
                             ▼
         Yes        ◇─────────────────◇
        ┌───────────│    Consider     │
        │           │ V/Q scan to revise│
        │           │  FEV₁ and DLCO  │
        │           ◇────────┬────────◇
        │                    │ No
        │                    ▼
        │           ┌─────────────────┐
        │           │ Exercise testing│
        │           └────────┬────────┘
        │                    │
        │                    ▼
        │           ◇─────────────────◇
        │           │ Exercise testing│  Yes     ┌───────┐
        │           │   Favorable?    │─────────▶│  To   │
        │           ◇────────┬────────◇          │  OR   │
        │                    │ No                └───────┘
        │                    ▼
        │           ┌─────────────────────┐
        │           │ Consider non standard│
        │           │ surgery or non operative│
        │           │      therapy        │
        │           └─────────────────────┘
```

Figure 9–2. Preoperative physiologic assessment for lung resection. (Data modified from Figure 1 in Colice GL, Shafazand S, Griffin JP, et al.[13])

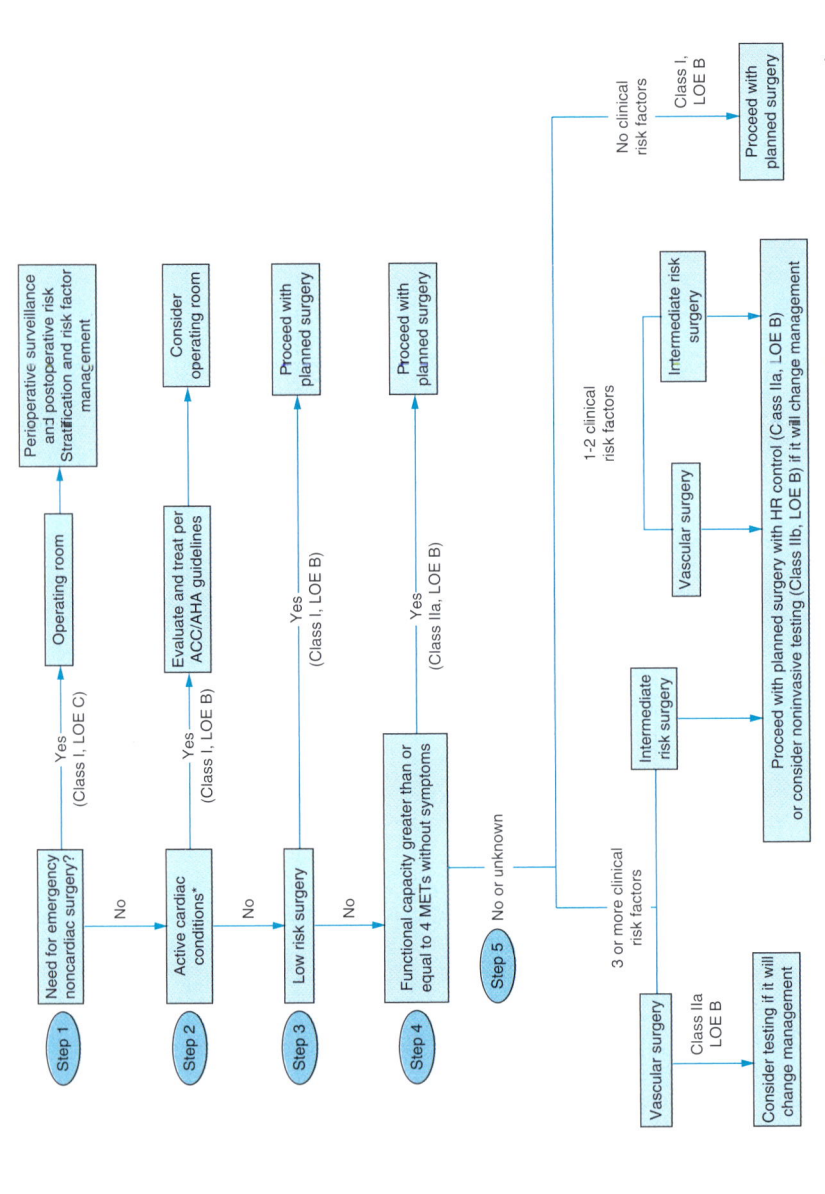

Figure 9-3. ACC/AHA guidelines for preoperative cardiac evaluation for noncardiac surgery. Thoracic surgery is categorized as an intermediate risk procedure, and preoperative cardiac evaluation is generally not indicated unless the patient exhibits an active cardiac condition, even in the presence of multiple risk factors for coronary disease. (Reprinted with permission from Circulation. 2007;116:e418-e500. ©2007 American Heart Association, Inc.)

the presence of multiple risk factors, unless such evaluation would change management. As with ordering any test, the physician should consider what is to be done with the results. A positive stress test is often followed by cardiology consultation and coronary angiography. If a flow-limiting obstruction is found during angiography, then angioplasty and stenting is considered. Stents obligate the patient to a period of anticoagulation, which may necessitate delaying surgery (see below).

Stress testing is still warranted for a patient with significant risk factors and poor exercise tolerance as an additional means of risk stratification.

We recommend involving a cardiologist in a multidisciplinary approach for patients considered at high risk for cardiovascular complications after thoracic surgery to help define the pathology, further quantify risk, and optimize preoperative management.

Coronary Stents

Patients with a flow-limiting coronary obstruction have an area of myocardium at risk for ischemia that perhaps could be relieved by stenting. Some enthusiasm for stenting in patients with stable coronary disease has been tempered by the COURAGE trial, which showed no significant reduction in death or rate of acute coronary syndrome with bare metal stents compared to medical therapy.[51] This trial, however, did not specifically focus on the perioperative setting, nor did it evaluate drug-eluting stents. As perioperative ischemia has a different pathophysiology than nonperioperative ischemia (supply-demand ratio mismatch rather than a plaque rupture and acute thrombus, in most cases), many practitioners still consider relieving the flow-limiting obstruction with stents.

When a stent is placed, the patient is obligated to a period of anticoagulation with multiple platelet-inhibiting drugs. Prematurely stopping platelet inhibitors can lead to acute thrombosis of the stent and ST elevation myocardial infarction. The practitioner must weigh the risk of stopping anticoagulation before a surgical procedure with the risk of delaying surgery. This decision is best made in consultation with a cardiologist. Compared to bare-metal stents (BMS), drug-eluting stents (DES) take a longer period of time to endothelialize,[52] which makes them prone to thrombosis for longer. Because of reports of acute thrombosis in patients 1 year after placement of DES,[53] the ACC/AHA have revised the guidelines on antiplatelet therapy after coronary stents. Dual antiplatelet therapy is recommended for at least 1 month after BMS placement, and for 1 year following a DES.[54] Again, in patients with recent stents, the risk of discontinuing antiplatelet therapy must be weighed against the risk of delaying potentially curative surgery or operating on an anticoagulated patient and necessarily foregoing postoperative epidural analgesia.

Beta Blockers

For patients at risk for perioperative myocardial ischemia, beta blockers are often recommended. Beta blockers have traditionally been withheld in patients with airway obstruction because of the concern that beta-2 blockade causes additional bronchoconstriction. However, beta-1 specific blockers are routinely used safely, eliminating this concern. Beta blockers have many potential benefits in the perioperative setting: they lower myocardial oxygen demand by lowering heart rate, decrease arrhythmias, prevent plaque rupture by decreasing sympathetic tone, and increase diastolic time thus increasing myocardial oxygen supply.

Initial trials for beta blockade before noncardiac surgery were encouraging.[55] Recent data, however, have dampened this enthusiasm. The POISE trial[56] studied 8300 patients at risk for atherosclerosis who had noncardiac surgery. Although incidence of cardiovascular death and nonfatal myocardial infarction was decreased, total mortality, stroke, and hypotension were found more often in the group treated with beta blockers. The major criticism of that study is that the patients in the beta blocker group were started on high dose beta blockers on the day of surgery. In the DECREASE IV trial[57] beta blockers were started preoperatively (median 34 days) and titrated to a heart rate of 50 to 70 bpm. Risk of death and nonfatal MI decreased without increased morbidity in patients given beta blockers. The ACC/AHA guidelines on perioperative beta blockade,[58] updated in 2009, recommend that patients who are already taking beta blockers continue them perioperatively. Patients at risk for myocardial ischemia who have not been taking beta blockers before intermediate-risk surgery may be considered for beta blockade titrated to blood pressure and heart rate, but their care should be managed in conjunction with a consulting cardiologist.

Statins

Besides beta blockade, patients at risk for myocardial ischemia are often placed on lipid-lowering therapy with statins. Statins have anti-inflammatory and plaque-stabilizing effects in addition to their effects on cholesterol (also known as pleiotropic effects). Preliminary observational trials suggest that statins may reduce perioperative risk in noncardiac surgery.[59,60] DECREASE III,[61] a randomized, controlled trial, found that fluvastatin reduced the risk of perioperative ischemia in patients undergoing vascular surgery. DECREASE IV[57] showed a trend toward improved outcome in the group treated with fluvastatin as well. Additional prospective, randomized trials are needed to further evaluate these potential benefits and the recommendation to initiate, or at least continue, statin therapy perioperatively.

Right Ventricular Impairment

In addition to the cardiovascular risks intrinsic to thoracoscopy or thoracotomy, pulmonary resection strains the cardiovascular system. Changes in preload, afterload, and contractility can cause hemodynamic instability in patients with an already compromised ventricular function. In particular, the degree of right ventricular dysfunction that occurs after lung resection is related to the change in pulmonary vascular resistance, which is proportional to the amount of lung tissue resected.[62] Right heart dysfunction may develop even without preexisting right heart abnormalities.[63] Many patients with a long history of smoking have some element of cor pulmonale or pulmonary hypertension that, with right ventricular dysfunction, may progress to overt right heart failure. Preoperative evaluation with echocardiography is not routinely recommended before thoracic surgery[64] but should be considered when left ventricular dysfunction, valvular abnormalities,[65] or pulmonary hypertension[66] is suspected.

Summary Recommendations for Cardiac Evaluation

Given the frequent coexistence of pulmonary and cardiac disease, every patient should have a thorough history and physical examination. Patients with high-risk conditions (unstable angina, decompensated heart failure, arrhythmias, valvular disease, or myocardial infarction in the past 30 days) should be evaluated by a cardiologist before thoracic surgery. If the patient has known high-risk coronary disease or a low functional capacity, stress testing is warranted to further stratify the risk. Decisions about invasive testing, beta blockers, or statins should be made in conjunction with a consulting cardiologist who can continue to follow the patient's progress beyond the immediate postoperative period. If there is a concern about pulmonary hypertension, cor pulmonale, or valvular heart disease, a preoperative echocardiogram should be performed to guide intraoperative therapy.

CHEMOTHERAPY AND RADIATION

Many thoracic surgical patients need resection of primary lung cancers, after which some are offered chemotherapy or radiation as adjuvant therapy. Other patients may have had chemotherapy or radiation before resection of a second primary lung cancer, after metastasis of another primary cancer, or for a systemic cancer. Still other patients with historically unresectable lung cancers may have undergone neoadjuvant (given before surgery) chemotherapy and radiation, in an attempt to reduce tumor size to make it resectable. Because recent studies suggest that such chemotherapy or radiation may not increase perioperative morbidity and mortality,[67,68] it is likely that the number of patients undergoing surgery after chemotherapy and radiation treatment will increase.

Preoperative chemotherapy and radiation therapy may not increase immediate perioperative morbidity and mortality, but they certainly have profound effects on perioperative and anesthetic management. A careful history with particular attention to the chemotherapeutic agents used is recommended. This section will cover many of the common chemotherapeutic agents used in lung cancer, other chemotherapy agents that influence perioperative considerations, and the serious effects of radiation therapy.

Cisplatin and Carboplatin

The most common chemotherapeutic agents for the treatment of lung cancers are the platinum-based alkylating agents cisplatin and carboplatin.[69,70] These drugs are inactive when administered into the circulation, but penetrate the cells by passive diffusion and inhibit DNA replication, RNA transcription, and protein synthesis. Because one of the serious adverse effects of platinum-based drugs is renal toxicity, a preoperative serum creatinine measurement is imperative. Impaired renal function may necessitate altered dosing of many anesthetic agents (ie, neuromuscular blockers). Some practitioners may opt to reduce the dose of NSAIDs such as ketorolac, or omit them altogether. Additionally, the platinum-based chemotherapies may be neurotoxic by affecting Schwann cells, which produce the myelin sheath that surrounds nerves. There have been reports of brachial plexus injuries possibly related to their neurotoxic effects.[71] Any preexisting neurologic deficits should be documented, and careful attention to patient positioning is warranted.

Paclitaxel, Docetaxel, and Gemcitabine

Paclitaxel, docetaxel, and gemcitabine are relatively new chemotherapy agents that are often combined with cisplatin or carboplatin for the treatment of lung cancer.[72-75] These agents can cause dose-related pulmonary toxicity in the form of pneumonitis. The pathophysiology of pneumonitis is unclear but may be related to a capillary leak.[76] Pneumonitis generally resolves after treatment with glucocorticoids but can occasionally progress to pulmonary fibrosis.[77,78] Surgery should be delayed until the acute pneumonitis resolves.

Anthracyclines

The anthracycline class of chemotherapy agents (doxorubicin, daunorubicin, epirubicin) is generally not used in the treatment of lung cancers. The anthracyclines are, however, frequently used in the treatment of breast cancers, sarcomas, and lymphomas, among others. The anthracyclines produce a cumulative dose-dependent cardiotoxicity, which is manifested by a nonischemic dilated cardiomyopathy.[79] Formal testing of left ventricular function should be considered in patients with a history of anthracycline chemotherapy, especially if there are symptoms consistent with decreased cardiac function.[80]

Bleomycin

Bleomycin is an older chemotherapeutic agent that is still used today, most commonly for germ cell tumors like testicular cancer.[81] This agent causes pulmonary fibrosis in up to 10% of patients.[82] The pathophysiology is not entirely clear but may be related to the development of free radicals.[83] It seems, however, that increased fraction of inspired oxygen concentration (F_iO_2) can exacerbate or provoke the toxicity,[84,85] perhaps even years after exposure to bleomycin.[86] The threshold of oxygen toxicity in terms of F_iO_2 or duration of exposure to high oxygen concentration is unclear, and some groups do not recommend oxygen restriction during the brief perioperative period.[87] In the authors' (and editors') opinion, it seems prudent to limit inspired oxygen to the lowest inspired concentration that adequately maintains saturation intraoperatively—a challenge during one-lung ventilation (OLV). Because the hypoxemia associated with OLV is primarily due

Table 9–1. Chemotherapeutic Agents and Their Perioperative Implications

Agent	Adverse Effects	Perioperative Implications
Carboplatin, cisplatin	Renal toxicity	Evaluate renal function and adjust medications accordingly, especially neuromuscular blockers and NSAIDs
	Neurotoxicity	Document neurological examination and position patient carefully
Paclitaxel, docetaxel, gemcitabine	Pulmonary toxicity/ pneumonitis	Delay surgery until acute pneumonitis resolves
Anthracyclines	Cardiac toxicity	Consider evaluation of left ventricular function
Bleomycin	Pulmonary toxicity/ pulmonary fibrosis	Minimize perioperative F_iO_2 to maintain adequate SpO_2
Other agents	Bone marrow suppression	Obtain complete blood count
	Nausea/vomiting	Assess for malnutrition and dehydration
	Neurotoxicity	Document neurological examination and position the patient carefully

to intrapulmonary shunt, raising the F_iO_2 may not improve systemic oxygenation profoundly anyway (see also Chapter 3 on the physiology of OLV).

Other Common Chemotherapeutic Agents

Many other chemotherapeutic agents including etoposide, pemetrexed, irinotecan and vinorelbine have been used in the treatment of lung cancers. These agents cause some degree of bone marrow suppression as well as nausea and vomiting. A complete blood count to assess the potential for anemia and thrombocytopenia, a complete metabolic panel, and a careful assessment of volume and nutritional status are indicated preoperatively. Because many agents produce neurotoxicity that may increase the risks of peripheral nerve injuries, special attention to patient positioning is warranted. A summary of chemotherapeutic agents and their perioperative implications appears in Table 9–1.

RADIATION THERAPY

Treatment of malignancy often involves therapeutic ionizing radiation. This treatment damages DNA in cells exposed to the radiation beams. Despite strategies to minimize or avoid damage to normal tissue cells, radiation therapy often damages noncancerous cells and may produce toxicities that have important perioperative implications.

Radiation causes endarteritis with vascular and capillary damage. Chronic tissue hypoxia leads to fibroblast proliferation and eventual scarring and fibrosis of the affected tissue. When natural anatomic planes are obliterated, surgical dissection is difficult, increasing the potential for blood loss. Occasionally surgical dissection is so difficult that resection may have to be abandoned.

Pulmonary toxicity is a common complication found 2 to 6 weeks after the conclusion of radiotherapy. It may be confused with other causes of pulmonary disease such as infection or chemotherapy-induced pulmonary toxicity.[88] Indeed, radiation therapy with concurrent chemotherapy may increase the risk of developing pulmonary toxicity.[89] Pulmonary toxicity generally starts as hyperemia and increased pulmonary secretions, and later progresses to pneumonitis.[90] Occasionally, pneumonitis leads to irreversible pulmonary fibrosis.[90] Patients with a history of radiation therapy should be questioned about pulmonary symptoms. Any recent dyspnea or change in symptoms requires further investigation. If a patient has acute, radiation-induced pneumonitis, surgery is ideally delayed until pneumonitis resolves. Radiation pneumonitis is often treated with a prolonged steroid taper, so patients with a history of pneumonitis may be at risk for adrenal insufficiency. Patients with extensive pulmonary fibrosis from radiation are probably not good surgical candidates. Exercise tolerance will generally be impaired and standard preoperative spirometry will likely show a restrictive defect.[91]

Besides pulmonary toxicity, radiation can cause cardiac toxicity in the form of myocardial fibrosis and diastolic dysfunction,[92] valvular abnormalities,[93] dysrhythmias,[94] and accelerated coronary artery disease if the radiation window included the heart. A careful history combined with an assessment of exercise tolerance is generally sufficient to rule out significant radiation-induced cardiotoxicity. Although the pathophysiology of the cardiotoxicity is unique, the standard method for cardiac evaluation described earlier should properly identify patients with radiation-induced cardiac injury.

PULMONARY REHABILITATION

Pulmonary rehabilitation is frequently used in the nonsurgical treatment of patients with severe chronic obstructive pulmonary disease (COPD) to reduce symptoms. Rehabilitation does not directly impact lung mechanics *per se,* but improves a patient's exercise tolerance for a higher workload without lactic acidosis.[95] Pulmonary rehabilitation often consists of supervised exercise for 3 to 4 hours a day for 6 to 12 weeks. Smaller studies suggest that preoperative pulmonary rehabilitation is beneficial, particularly before lung-volume reduction surgery.[96,97] Because pulmonary rehabilitation takes time and resources, its use preoperatively depends on the institution. It may be too time-consuming before resection of malignant lesions. The benefits of short-term pulmonary rehabilitation have not yet been thoroughly studied.

SMOKING CESSATION

Active cigarette smoking has long been known to be a risk factor for pulmonary complications after surgery.[98,99] Cigarette smoking decreases ciliary function; increases sputum production, airway reactivity, and carboxyhemoglobin levels;

and impedes wound healing, all of which affect pulmonary complications. The timing of smoking cessation before surgery, however, has been a subject of some controversy. Older studies suggest no decrease in pulmonary complications (and perhaps a paradoxical increase) if smoking cessation is within 4 to 8 weeks before surgery.[100,101] We do know that carboxyhemoglobin levels decrease (and thus shift the oxy-hemoglobin curve rightward favoring delivery of oxygen to the tissues) within 12 hours of smoking cessation.[102] Two recent studies did not show an increase in pulmonary complications with smoking cessation within 4 weeks of surgery.[103,104] In our opinion, with additional data suggesting no increase in harm, smoking cessation should be encouraged. Not doing so may neglect a powerful incentive for a patient's overall health. Further studies may help to define the optimal timing of smoking cessation with respect to pulmonary complications.

PERIOPERATIVE RESPIRATORY MEDICATIONS

Chronic lung disease such as COPD is a known risk factor for postoperative pulmonary complications.[105] Controlling the obstructive symptoms preoperatively with medications such as bronchodilators is recommended.[106,107] Long-acting bronchodilators and inhaled steroids should be continued on the morning of surgery. Acute shortness of breath or sputum production from an exacerbation of COPD should prompt postponement of an elective thoracic procedure until breathing is back to the patient's baseline.

In the intensive care setting, systemic glucocorticoids are often given to patients who are difficult to wean from mechanical ventilation or to patients with acute respiratory distress syndrome (ARDS). Some clinicians have suggested giving steroids prophylactically in the perioperative setting. As in ARDS, in which the data on steroid use are conflicting, changes in doses and dosing schedules may confound any potential benefit. The limited data available do not support prophylactic use of steroids before thoracic surgery.[108]

METASTATIC DISEASE

Patients with metastatic lung cancer generally do not undergo pulmonary resection but may need other thoracic surgeries such as pleurodesis or airway or esophageal stenting. Lung cancer may metastasize to any organ in the body, but several locations are more common and warrant special consideration including the liver, adrenals, bone, and brain. In one autopsy study, hepatic metastases were found in more than 50% of patients with lung cancer.[109] The lesions are frequently asymptomatic until late in the course of the disease. They may be detected by liver enzyme abnormalities or CT or PET scans. Metastases to the adrenal gland, often asymptomatic, do not interfere with the patient's ability to secrete glucocorticoids or mineralocorticoids. Bony metastases can cause pain and hypercalcemia. Patients with metastases to bone are likely to be taking narcotics for pain and require an evaluation of serum calcium to rule out hypercalcemia. Metastasis to a thoracic vertebra may complicate epidural placement for postoperative pain. Finally, brain metastases may cause focal neurologic deficits and seizures. Antiepileptic medicines should be continued in the perioperative period.

METABOLIC AND PARANEOPLASTIC EFFECTS OF CANCER

In addition to the possibility of metastases, any patient with cancer should be evaluated for metabolic and paraneoplastic symptoms, particularly patients with small-cell lung cancer. Many patients with cancer are malnourished, so a complete metabolic panel is indicated. As mentioned previously, bony metastases can cause hypercalcemia, which can lead to cardiac arrhythmias. If a patient is malnourished, obtaining an ionized calcium level may be useful to account for calcium's binding to albumin.

The syndrome of inappropriate anti-diuretic hormone secretion (SIADH), where the hypothalamus continues to secrete ADH despite an adequate circulating blood volume and plasma osmolarity, may be present in patients with small-cell lung cancer.[110] These patients may exhibit hyponatremia with low plasma osmolarity, urine osmolarity more than 100 mOsm/kg and high urine sodium concentration. SIADH generally resolves with treatment of the underlying lung cancer, but profound hyponatremia should be treated before a surgical procedure to avoid further fluid shifts and potential brain edema.

In Eaton-Lambert syndrome, an autoimmune syndrome associated with small-cell lung cancer, there are antibodies against the presynaptic voltage-gated calcium channels at the motor end plate.[111] The antibodies decrease the calcium influx needed to release acetylcholine. The net effect is less acetylcholine in the motor end plate and muscle weakness. Repeated stimuli typically improve the muscle weakness. Patients with Eaton-Lambert syndrome are profoundly sensitive to both non-depolarizing and depolarizing neuromuscular blockers. The symptoms of Eaton-Lambert syndrome are similar to, and often confused with, the symptoms of myasthenia gravis. Myasthenia gravis is caused by autoimmune-mediated antibodies against the nicotinic acetylcholine receptor.[112] Such patients, who may be evaluated before a thymectomy, suffer muscle weakness and fatigue with repeated muscle stimulation. They are also profoundly sensitive to non-depolarizing neuromuscular blockers but are resistant to depolarizing blockers such as succinylcholine. In summary, patients with myasthenia gravis may be resistant to succinylcholine and sensitive to non-depolarizing neuromuscular blockers; patients with Eaton-Lambert syndrome are sensitive to both types of neuromuscular blockers. Plasma cholinesterase activity may decrease in patients with myasthenia gravis after preoperative plasmapheresis or use of an anticholinesterase (eg, pyridostigmine). Thus, succinylcholine may have a prolonged effect in these patients.

Cancer is a well-known risk factor for deep vein thrombosis (DVT) and pulmonary venous thromboembolism and, combined with another risk factor, surgery, makes the perioperative period one of risk for both conditions. In one study, incidence of DVT or pulmonary embolism was 7.4% after pneumonectomy for malignancy.[113] Some form of prophylaxis is often used. Lower extremity sequential compression devices are one example. Prophylaxis with heparin or low-molecular-weight heparin may be considered as well, but timing of surgery and epidural catheter placement and removal must be carefully coordinated.

LUNG ISOLATION AND POSTOPERATIVE PAIN CONTROL

Lung isolation is covered extensively in Chapter 5 of this text but is worth consideration in the preoperative period. Lower airway difficulties may be predicted by review of the preoperative chest x-ray, CT scans, or preoperative bronchoscopy for masses that may affect airway management, such as choice of lung isolation or tube size. Similarly, pain control is also discussed in Chapter 24. However, a plan for pain management should be considered before surgery since some techniques (thoracic epidurals) are implemented before the induction of general anesthesia.

CONCLUSION AND RECOMMENDATIONS

Preoperative evaluation of the thoracic surgical patient requires a thorough, multidisciplinary approach. All patients should have spirometry and DLCO measurements. If values are less than 80% of predicted, the predicted postoperative values should be calculated. If values are less than 40% of predicted, exercise testing should be performed to further stratify the patient's risk. Cardiac evaluation requires a consultant cardiologist to help manage decisions regarding stress or invasive testing, the discontinuation of anticoagulation, and optimization of perioperative cardiac medications. Particular attention should be paid to right heart function, since lung resection adds an additional strain on the pulmonary vasculature. For patients with cancer, a thorough history pertaining to chemotherapeutic agents and radiation is needed. When applicable, the effects of metastases, masses, and metabolism should be considered as well. Finally, patients who are active smokers should be counseled about smoking cessation.

REFERENCES

1. Graham EA, Singer JJ. Successful removal of an entire lung for carcinoma of the bronchus. *JAMA.* 1933;101:137.
2. Jemal A, Siegel R, Ward E, et al. Cancer statistics 2009. *CA Cancer J Clin.* 2009;59(4):225-249.
3. Geddes DM. The natural history of lung cancer: a review based on rates of tumour growth. *Br J Diseases Chest.* 1979;73(1):1-17.
4. Arai T, Kuroishi T, Saito Y, et al. Tumor doubling time and prognosis in lung cancer patients: evaluation from chest films and clinical follow-up study. Japanese Lung Cancer Screening Research Group. *Jap J Clin Oncol.* 1994;24(4):199-204.
5. Cattaneo SM, Park BJ, Wilton AS, et al. Use of video-assisted thoracic surgery for lobectomy in the elderly results in fewer complications. *Ann Thorac Surg.* 2008;85(1):231-235.
6. Flores RM, Park BJ, Dycoco J, et al. Lobectomy by video-assisted thoracic surgery (VATS) versus thoracotomy for lung cancer. *J Thorac Cardiovasc Surg.* 2009;138(1):11-18.
7. Gaensler EA, Cugell DW, Lindgren I, et al. The role of pulmonary insufficiency in mortality and invalidism following surgery for pulmonary tuberculosis. *J Thorac Surg.* 1955;29(2):163-187.
8. Mittman C. Assessment of operative risk in thoracic surgery. *Am Rev Respir Dis.* 1961;84:197.
9. Lockwood P. Lung function test results and the risk of post-thoracotomy complications. *Respiration.* 1973;30:259.

10. Boushy SF, Billig DM, North LB, Helgason AH. Clinical course related to preoperative and postoperative pulmonary function in patients with bronchogenic carcinoma. *Chest.* 1971;59(4):383-391.
11. Colman NC, Schraufnagel DE, Rivington RN, Pardy RL. Exercise testing in evaluation of patients for lung resection. *Am Rev Respir Dis.* 1982;125(5):604-606.
12. Keagy BA, Lores ME, Starek PJ, et al. Elective pulmonary lobectomy: factors associated with morbidity and operative mortality. *Ann Thorac Surg.* 1985;40(4):349-352.
13. Colice GL, Shafazand S, Griffin JP, et al. Physiologic evaluation of the patient with lung cancer being considered for resectional surgery: ACCP evidenced-based clinical practice guidelines (2nd edition). *Chest.* 2007;132(3 Suppl):161S-177S.
14. British Thoracic Society, Society of Cardiothoracic Surgeons of Great Britain and Ireland Working Party. BTS guidelines: guidelines on the selection of patients with lung cancer for surgery. *Thorax.* 2001;56(2):89-108.
15. Juhl B, Frost N. A comparison between measured and calculated changes in the lung function after operation for pulmonary cancer. *Acta Anaesthesiol Scand Suppl.* 1975;57:39-45.
16. Olsen GN, Block AJ, Tobias JA. Prediction of postpneumonectomy pulmonary function using quantitative macroaggregate lung scanning. *Chest.* 1974;66(1):13-16.
17. Kristersson S, Lindell SE, Svanberg L. Prediction of pulmonary function loss due to pneumonectomy using 133 Xe radiospirometry. *Chest.* 1972;62(6):694-698.
18. Smulders SA, Smeenk FW, Janssen-Heijnen ML, Postmus PE. Actual and predicted postoperative changes in lung function after pneumonectomy. *Chest.* 2004;125(5):1735-1741.
19. Markos J, Mullan BP, Hillman DR, et al. Preoperative assessment as a predictor of mortality and morbidity after lung resection. *Am Rev Respir Dis.* 1989;139(4):902-910.
20. Holden DA, Rice TW, Stelmach K, Meeker DP. Exercise testing, 6-min walk, and stair climb in the evaluation of patients at high risk for pulmonary resection. *Chest.* 1992;102(6):1774-1779.
21. Linden PA, Bueno R, Colson YL, et al. Lung resection in patients with preoperative $FEV_1 < 35\%$ predicted. *Chest.* 2005;127(6):1984-1990.
22. Brunelli A, Charloux A, Bolliger CT, et al. On behalf of the European Respiratory Society and European Society of Thoracic Surgeons Joint Task Force on Fitness for Radical Therapy. ERS/ESTS clinical guidelines on fitness for radical therapy in lung cancer patients (surgery and chemo-radiotherapy). *Eur Respir J.* 2009;34:17-41.
23. McKenna RJ Jr, Fischel RJ, Brenner M, Gelb AF. Combined operations for lung volume reduction surgery and lung cancer. *Chest.* 1996;110(4):885-888.
24. Dunn WF, Scanlon PD. Preoperative pulmonary function testing for patients with lung cancer. *Mayo Clin Proc.* 1993;68(4):371-377.
25. Kearney DJ, Lee TH, Reilly JJ, DeCamp MM, Sugarbaker DJ. Assessment of operative risk in patients undergoing lung resection. Importance of predicted pulmonary function. *Chest.* 1994;105(3):753-759.
26. Ferguson MK, Little L, Rizzo L, et al. Diffusing capacity predicts morbidity and mortality after pulmonary resection. *J Thorac Cardiovasc Surg.* 1988;96(6):894-900.
27. Ferguson MK, Vigneswaran WT. Diffusing capacity predicts morbidity after lung resection in patients without obstructive lung disease. *Ann Thorac Surg.* 2008;85(4):1158-1164.
28. Pierce RJ, Copland JM, Sharpe K, Barter CE. Preoperative risk evaluation for lung cancer resection: predicted postoperative product as a predictor of surgical mortality. *Am J Respir Crit Care Med.* 1994;150(4):947-955.
29. Ribas J, Diaz O, Barbera JA, et al. Invasive exercise testing in the evaluation of patients at high-risk for lung resection. *Eur Respir J.* 1998;12(6):1429-1435.
30. Tisi GM. Preoperative evaluation of pulmonary function: validity, indications, and benefits. *Am Rev Respir Dis.* 1979;119:293.
31. Lewis JW Jr, Bastanfar M, Gabriel F, Mascha E. Right heart function and prediction of respiratory morbidity in patients undergoing pneumonectomy with moderately severe cardiopulmonary dysfunction. *J Thorac Cardiovasc Surg.* 1994;108(1):169-175.
32. Vesselle H. Functional imaging before pulmonary resection. *Semin Thorac Cardiovasc Surg.* 2001;13(2):126-136.
33. Giordano A, Calcagni ML, Meduri G, Valenti S, Galli G. Perfusion lung scintigraphy for the prediction of postlobectomy residual pulmonary function. *Chest.* 1997;111(6):1542-1547.

34. Neuman GG, Weingarten AE, Abramowitz RM, et al. The anesthetic management of the patient with an anterior mediastinal mass. *Anesthesiology.* 1984;60(2):144-147.
35. Olsen GN, Bolton JW, Weiman DS, Hornung CA. Stair climbing as an exercise test to predict the postoperative complications of lung resection. Two years' experience. *Chest.* 1991;99(3):587-590.
36. Brunelli A, Refai M, Xiume F, et al. Performance at symptom-limited stair-climbing test is associated with increased cardiopulmonary complications, mortality, and costs after major lung resection. *Ann Thorac Surg.* 2008;86(1):240-247.
37. Nikolic I, Majeric-Kogler V, Plavec D, Maloca I, Slobodnjak Z. Stairs climbing test with pulse oximetry as predictor of early postoperative complications in functionally impaired patients with lung cancer and elective lung surgery: prospective trial of consecutive series of patients. *Croat Med J.* 2008;49(1):50-57.
38. Brunelli A, Belardinelli R, Refai M, et al. Peak oxygen consumption during cardiopulmonary exercise test improves risk stratification in candidates to major lung resection. *Chest.* 2009;135(5):1260-1267.
39. Walsh GL, Morice RC, Putnam JB Jr, et al. Resection of lung cancer is justified in high-risk patients selected by exercise oxygen consumption. *Ann Thorac Surg.* 1994;58(3):704-710.
40. Smith TP, Kinasewitz GT, Tucker WY, Spillers WP, George RB. Exercise capacity as a predictor of post-thoracotomy morbidity. *Am Rev Respir Dis.* 1984;129(5):730-734.
41. Schuurmans MM, Diacon AH, Bolliger CT. Functional evaluation before lung resection. *Clin Chest Med.* 2002;23(1):159-172.
42. ATS Committee on Proficiency Standards for Clinical Pulmonary Function Laboratories. ATS statement: guidelines for the six-minute walk test. *Am J Respir Criti Care Med.* 2002;166(1):111-117.
43. Cahalin L, Pappagianopoulos P, Prevost S, Wain J, Ginns L. The relationship of the 6-min walk test to maximal oxygen consumption in transplant candidates with end-stage lung disease. *Chest.* 1995;108(2):452-459.
44. Turner SE, Eastwood PR, Cecins NM, Hillman DR, Jenkins SC. Physiologic responses to incremental and self-paced exercise in COPD: a comparison of three tests. *Chest.* 2004;126(3):766-773.
45. Solway S, Brooks D, Lacasse Y, Thomas S. A qualitative systematic overview of the measurement properties of functional walk tests used in the cardiorespiratory domain. *Chest.* 2001;119(1):256-270.
46. Singh SJ, Morgan MD, Scott S, Walters D, Hardman AE. Development of a shuttle walking test of disability in patients with chronic airways obstruction. *Thorax.* 1992;47(12):1019-1024.
47. Win T, Jackson A, Groves AM, et al. Comparison of shuttle walk with measured peak oxygen consumption in patients with operable lung cancer. *Thorax.* 2006;61(1):57-60.
48. Singh SJ, Morgan MD, Hardman AE, Rowe C, Bardsley PA. Comparison of oxygen uptake during a conventional treadmill test and the shuttle walking test in chronic airflow limitation. *Eur Respir J.* 1994;7(11):2016-2020.
49. Fleisher LA, Beckman JA, Brown, KA, et al. ACC/AHA 2007 guidelines on perioperative cardiovascular evaluation and care for noncardiac surgery: a report of the American College of Cardiology/American Heart Association Task Force on Practice Guidelines (Writing Committee to Revise the 2002 Guidelines on Perioperative Cardiovascular Evaluation for Noncardiac Surgery) developed in collaboration with the American Society of Echocardiography, American Society of Nuclear Cardiology, Heart Rhythm Society, Society of Cardiovascular Anesthesiologists, Society for Cardiovascular Angiography and Interventions, Society for Vascular Medicine and Biology, and Society for Vascular Surgery. *J Am Coll Cardiol.* 2007;50:e159-e241.
50. Guidelines for assessing and managing the perioperative risk from coronary artery disease associated with major noncardiac surgery. American College of Physicians. *Ann Intern Med.* 1997;127(4):309-312.
51. Boden WE, O'Rourke RA, Teo KK, et al. Optimal medical therapy with or without PCI for stable coronary disease. *N Engl J Med.* 2007;356(15):1503-1516.
52. Joner M, Finn AV, Farb A, et al. Pathology of drug-eluting stents in humans: delayed healing and late thrombotic risk. *J Am Coll Cardiol.* 2006;48(1):193-202.
53. McFadden EP, Stabile E, Regar E, et al. Late thrombosis in drug-eluting coronary stents after discontinuation of antiplatelet therapy. *Lancet.* 2004;364(9444):1519-1521.
54. King SB III, Smith SC Jr, Hirshfeld JW Jr, et al. 2007 Focused Update of the ACC/AHA/SCAI 2005 Guideline Update for Percutaneous Coronary Intervention: a report of the American College of Cardiology/American Heart Association Task Force on Practice Guidelines: 2007 Writing Group to Review New Evidence and Update the ACC/AHA/SCAI 2005 Guideline Update for

Percutaneous Coronary Intervention, Writing on Behalf of the 2005 Writing Committee. *Circulation.* 2008;117(2):261-295 (correction in *Circulation.* 2008;117(6):e161).
55. Wallace A, Layug B, Tateo I, et al. Prophylactic atenolol reduces postoperative myocardial ischemia. McSPI Research Group. *Anesthesiology.* 1998;88(1):7-17.
56. POISE Study Group. Devereaux PJ, Yang H, Yusuf S, et al. Effects of extended-release metoprolol succinate in patients undergoing non-cardiac surgery (POISE trial): a randomised controlled trial. *Lancet.* 2008;371(9627):1839-1847.
57. Dunkelgrun M, Boersma E, Schouten O, et al. Bisoprolol and fluvastatin for the reduction of perioperative cardiac mortality and myocardial infarction in intermediate-risk patients undergoing noncardiovascular surgery: a randomized controlled trial (DECREASE-IV). *Ann Surg.* 2009;249(6):921-926.
58. Fleisher LA, Beckman JA, Brown, KA, et al. 2009 ACCF/AHA Focused Update on Perioperative Beta Blockade Incorporated into the ACC/AHA 2007 Guidelines on Perioperative Cardiovascular Evaluation and Care for Noncardiac Surgery. A report of the American College of Cardiology Foundation/American Heart Association Task Force on Practice Guidelines. *Circulation.* 2009;120:e169-e276.
59. Lindenauer PK, Pekow P, Wang K, Gutierrez B, Benjamin EM. Lipid-lowering therapy and in-hospital mortality following major noncardiac surgery. *JAMA.* 2004;291(17):2092-2099.
60. Poldermans D, Bax JJ, Kertai MD, et al. Statins are associated with a reduced incidence of perioperative mortality in patients undergoing major noncardiac vascular surgery. *Circulation.* 2003;107(14):1848-1851.
61. Schouten O, Eric Boersma E, Hoeks SE, et al. Fluvastatin and perioperative events in patients undergoing vascular surgery. *N Engl J Med.* 2009;361(10):980-989.
62. Reed CE, Dorman BH, Spinale FG. Mechanisms of right ventricular dysfunction after pulmonary resection. *Ann Thorac Surg.* 1996;62(1):225-232.
63. Jovev S, Tager S, Spirovski Z, et al. Right heart haemodynamics after lung resection; the role of the transthoracic echo-doppler cardiography. *Pril-Maked Akad Nauk Umet Odd Biol Med Nauki.* 2006;27(2):201-216.
64. Macan JS, Karadza V, Kogler J, Majeric Kogler V. Role of transthoracic echocardiography in evaluation of cardiac risk in thoracic surgery. *Acta Med Croatica.* 2004;58(3):221-224.
65. Rohde LE, Polanczyk CA, Goldman L, et al. Usefulness of transthoracic echocardiography as a tool for risk stratification of patients undergoing major noncardiac surgery. *Am J Cardiol.* 2001;87(5):505-509.
66. Auerbach A, Goldman L. Assessing and reducing the cardiac risk of noncardiac surgery. *Circulation.* 2006;113(10):1361-1376.
67. Brouchet L, Bauvin E, Marcheix B, et al. Impact of induction treatment on postoperative complications in the treatment of non-small cell lung cancer. *J Thorac Oncol.* 2007;2(7):626-631.
68. Perrot E, Guibert B, Mulsant P, et al. Preoperative chemotherapy does not increase complications after nonsmall cell lung cancer resection. *Ann Thorac Surg.* 2005;80(2):423-427.
69. Bunn PA Jr. The expanding role of cisplatin in the treatment of non-small-cell lung cancer. *Semin Oncol.* 1989;16(4 Suppl 6):10-21.
70. Bunn PA Jr. Clinical experiences with carboplatin (paraplatin) in lung cancer. *Semin Oncol.* 1992;19(1 Suppl 2):1-11.
71. Marzetti G, Marret E, Lotz JP, Gattegno B, Bonnet F. Brachial plexus injury during anaesthesia in patients receiving cisplatin-based chemotherapy. *Eur J Anaesthesiol.* 2006;23(3):262-265.
72. Fossella F, Pereira JR, von Pawel J, et al. Randomized, multinational, phase III study of docetaxel plus platinum combinations versus vinorelbine plus cisplatin for advanced non-small-cell lung cancer: the TAX 326 study group. *J Clin Oncol.* 2003;21(16):3016-3024.
73. Bonomi P, Kim K, Fairclough D, et al. Comparison of survival and quality of life in advanced non-small-cell lung cancer patients treated with two dose levels of paclitaxel combined with cisplatin versus etoposide with cisplatin: results of an Eastern Cooperative Oncology Group trial. *J Clin Oncol.* 2000;18(3):623-631.
74. Crino L, Scagliotti GV, Ricci S, et al. Gemcitabine and cisplatin versus mitomycin, ifosfamide, and cisplatin in advanced non-small-cell lung cancer: A randomized phase III study of the Italian Lung Cancer Project. *J Clin Oncol.* 1999;17(11):3522-3530.
75. Zatloukal P, Petruzelka L. Gemcitabine plus cisplatin vs. gemcitabine plus carboplatin in stage IIIb and IV non-small cell lung cancer: a phase III randomized trial. *Lung Cancer.* 2003;41(3):321-331.

76. Briasoulis E, Froudarakis M, Milionis HI, et al. Chemotherapy-induced noncardiogenic pulmonary edema related to gemcitabine plus docetaxel combination with granulocyte colony-stimulating factor support. *Respiration.* 2000;67(6):680-683.
77. Dimopoulou I, Bamias A. Pulmonary toxicity from novel antineoplastic agents. *Ann Oncol.* 2006;17(3):372-379.
78. Vahid B, Marik PE. Pulmonary complications of novel antineoplastic agents for solid tumors. *Chest.* 2008;133(2):528-538.
79. Von Hoff DD, Rozencweig M, Piccart M. The cardiotoxicity of anticancer agents. *Semin Oncol.* 1982;9(1):23-33.
80. Jensen BV, Skovsgaard T, Nielsen SL. Functional monitoring of anthracycline cardiotoxicity: a prospective, blinded, long-term observational study of outcome in 120 patients. *Ann Oncol.* 2002;13(5): 699-709.
81. Williams SD, Birch R, Einhorn LH, et al. Treatment of disseminated germ-cell tumors with cisplatin, bleomycin, and either vinblastine or etoposide. *N Engl J Med.* 1987;316(23):1435-1440.
82. Jules-Elysee K, White DA. Bleomycin-induced pulmonary toxicity. *Clin Chest Med.* 1990;11(1):1-20.
83. Sleijfer S. Bleomycin-induced pneumonitis. *Chest.* 2001;120(2):617-624.
84. Goldiner PL, Carlon GC, Cvitkovic E, Schweizer O, Howland WS. Factors influencing postoperative morbidity and mortality in patients treated with bleomycin. *Br Med J.* 1978;1(6128):1664-1667.
85. Tryka AF, Skornik WA, Godleski JJ, Brain JD. Potentiation of bleomycin-induced lung injury by exposure to 70% oxygen. Morphologic assessment. *Am Rev Respir Dis.* 1982;126(6):1074-1079.
86. Gilson AJ, Sahn SA. Reactivation of bleomycin lung toxicity following oxygen administration. A second response to corticosteroids. *Chest.* 1985;88(2):304-306.
87. Donat SM, Levy DA. Bleomycin associated pulmonary toxicity: is perioperative oxygen restriction necessary? *J Urol.* 1998;160(4):1347-1352.
88. Kocak Z, Evans ES, Zhou SM, et al. Challenges in defining radiation pneumonitis in patients with lung cancer. *Int J Radiat Oncol Biol Phys.* 2005;62(3):635-638.
89. Rancati T, Ceresoli GL, Gagliardi G, Schipani S, Catteneo GM. Factors predicting radiation pneumonitis in lung cancer patients: a retrospective study. *Radiother Oncol.* 2003;67(3):275-283.
90. McDonald S, Rubin P. Injury to the lung from cancer therapy: clinical syndromes, measurable endpoints, and potential scoring systems. *Int J Radiat Oncol Biol Phys.* 1995;31(5):1187-1203.
91. Cudkowicz L, Cunningham M, Haldane EV. Effects of mediastinal irradiation upon respiratory function following mastectomy for carcinoma of breast. A five-year follow-up study. *Thorax.* 1969;24(3):359-367.
92. Heidenreich PA, Hancock SL, Vagelos RH, et al. Diastolic dysfunction after mediastinal irradiation. *Am Heart J.* 2005;150:977.
93. Hardenberg PH, Munley MT, Hu C, et al. Doxorubicin-based chemotherapy and radiation increase cardiac perfusion changes in patients treated for left-sided breast cancer. *Int J Radiat Oncol Biol Phys.* 2001;51:S158.
94. Orzan F, Brusca A, Gaita F, et al. Associated cardiac lesions in patients with radiation-induced complete heart block. *Int J Cardiol.* 1993;39(2):151-156.
95. Casaburi R, Patessio A, Ioli F, et al. Reductions in exercise lactic acidosis and ventilation as a result of exercise training in patients with obstructive lung disease. *Am Rev Respir Dis.* 1991;143(1):9-18.
96. Jones LW, Peddle CJ, Eves ND, et al. Effects of presurgical exercise training on cardiorespiratory fitness among patients undergoing thoracic surgery for malignant lung lesions. *Cancer.* 2007;110(3): 590-598.
97. Ries AL, Make BJ, Lee SM, et al. National Emphysema Treatment Trial Research Group. The effects of pulmonary rehabilitation in the national emphysema treatment trial. *Chest.* 2005;128(6):3799-3809.
98. Wightman JA. A prospective survey of the incidence of postoperative pulmonary complications. *Br J Surg.* 1968;55(2):85-91.
99. Morton HJV. Tobacco smoking and pulmonary complications after operation. *Lancet.* 1944;1:368-370.
100. Warner MA, Divertie MB, Tinker JH. Preoperative cessation of smoking and pulmonary complications in coronary artery bypass patients. *Anesthesiology.* 1984;60:380.
101. Bluman LG, Mosca L, Newman N, Simon DG. Preoperative smoking habits and postoperative pulmonary complications. *Chest.* 1998;113(4):883-889.

102. Akrawi W, Benumof JL. A pathophysiological basis for informed preoperative smoking cessation counseling. *J Cardiothorac Vasc Anesth.* 1997;11(5):629-640.
103. Barrera R, Shi W, Amar D, et al. Smoking and timing of cessation: impact on pulmonary complications after thoracotomy. *Chest.* 2005;127(6):1977-1983.
104. Nakagawa M, Tanaka H, Tsukuma H, Kishi Y. Relationship between the duration of the preoperative smoke-free period and the incidence of postoperative pulmonary complications after pulmonary surgery. *Chest.* 2001;120(3):705-710.
105. Smetana GW, Lawrence VA, Cornell JE. Preoperative pulmonary risk stratification for noncardiothoracic surgery: systematic review for the American College of Physicians. *Ann Intern Med.* 2006;144(8):581-595.
106. Tarhan S, Moffitt EA, Sessler AD, Douglas WW, Taylor WF. Risk of anesthesia and surgery in patients with chronic bronchitis and chronic obstructive pulmonary disease. *Surgery.* 1973;74(5):720-726.
107. Stein M, Cassara EL. Preoperative pulmonary evaluation and therapy for surgery patients. *JAMA.* 1970;211(5):787-790.
108. Bigler D, Jonsson T, Olsen J, Brenoe J, Sander-Jensen K. The effect of preoperative methylprednisolone on pulmonary function and pain after lung operations. *J Thorac Cardiovasc Surg.* 1996;112(1):142-145.
109. Stenbygaard LE, Sorensen JB, Olsen JE. Metastatic pattern at autopsy in non-resectable adenocarcinoma of the lung—a study from a cohort of 259 consecutive patients treated with chemotherapy. *Acta Oncol.*1997;36(3):301-6.
110. List AF, Hainsworth JD, Davis BW, et al. The syndrome of inappropriate secretion of antidiuretic hormone (SIADH) in small-cell lung cancer. *J Clin Oncol.* 1986;4(8):1191-1198.
111. Motomura M, Johnston I, Lang B, Vincent A, Newsom-Davis J. An improved diagnostic assay for Lambert-Eaton myasthenic syndrome. *J Neurol Neurosurg Psychiatry.* 1995;58(1):85-87.
112. Drachman DB. Myasthenia gravis. *N Engl J Med.* 1994;330(25):1797-1810.
113. Mason DP, Quader MA, Blackstone EH, et al. Thromboembolism after pneumonectomy for malignancy: an independent marker of poor outcome. *J Thorac Cardiovasc Surg.* 2006;131:711-718.

Bronchoscopy, Mediastinoscopy, and Chamberlain Procedure

10

Frederick W. Lombard
Jorn Karhausen

Key Points

- Diagnostic bronchoscopy is now usually performed using flexible equipment, whereas therapeutic bronchoscopy may be conducted with both flexible and rigid equipment. A thorough appreciation of both is essential for safe anesthetic management in the bronchoscopy suite.
- Unexpected massive bleeding is always possible during cervical mediastinoscopy, and thus anesthesiologists should be prepared to administer large volume resuscitation at a moment's notice.
- Right radial artery cannulation is preferred in order to alert the surgeon to innominate artery compression with risk of cerebral ischemia.

Case Vignette

A 75-year-old male presented with a three-month history of cough. He has been treated with two courses of antibiotic therapy after which a chest radiograph revealed a suspicious left upper lobe lesion. He is now referred for staging bronchoscopy and mediastinoscopy following a computed tomography (CT) scan, which confirmed the 3.5 × 3 cm mass, and also showed enlarged subaortic lymph nodes. He has hypertension and chronic obstructive pulmonary disease due to a 40-pack year smoking history. Medications include furosemide and aspirin.

Vital signs: BP 175/85, HR 72, room air SpO2 95%. Laboratory examination is normal except for a BUN of 25, creatinine of 1.8 and potassium of 3.2. His CXR is notable for the left upper lobe mass and mild centrilobular emphysema.

With the growing use of computed tomographic (CT) scanning, pulmonary lesions are being diagnosed with increasing frequency. In fact, incidental lesions found on chest x-ray (CXR) or CT have become the most common manifestation of lung cancer.[1] A lesion larger than 3 cm in diameter is considered a mass, and as such has a greater likelihood of being malignant.[1] A single pulmonary lesion that is less than 3 cm in diameter, completely surrounded by pulmonary parenchyma, and is not associated with atelectasis or adenopathy is defined as a solitary pulmonary nodule (SPN).[1] While as many as one-third of SPNs represent primary malignancies, and nearly one quarter may be solitary metastases, the differential diagnosis of an SPN is broad and includes vascular diseases, infections, inflammatory conditions, congenital abnormalities and benign tumors.[1]

In managing patients with suspected lung cancer, the goals are to determine an accurate histological diagnosis and stage the disease, if the lesion is malignant. This information is critical, not only to predict resectability, but also to avoid unnecessary surgery and provide the patient with prognostic information. Flexible fiberoptic bronchoscopy (FOB) and mediastinoscopy are the standard methods used for staging non-small cell lung cancer (NSCLC), the most prevalent type of lung cancer.

FLEXIBLE FIBEROPTIC BRONCHOSCOPY

Flexible fiberoptic bronchoscopy (FOB) is utilized extensively in the initial evaluation of patients suspected of having lung carcinoma. FOB enables direct visualization of the bronchial mucosa down to the level of the segmental and proximal subsegmental bronchi. At these levels direct visually guided biopsy is possible. FOB also enables endobronchial brushing and bronchoalveolar lavage (BAL) of disease beyond direct visualization.

Since its introduction into clinical practice in the early 1970s, FOB technology has undergone continuous improvement and innovation. Transbronchial needle aspiration (TBNA) was added in the early 1980s, a technique that has now been refined by the addition of image guidance, such as endobronchial ultrasound (EBUS), to enhance diagnostic precision. EBUS can be used for diagnostic aspiration of both mediastinal lymph nodes and central parenchymal lung lesions, not visible during routine bronchoscopy.[2] The more recent addition of fluorescence-reflectance bronchoscopy may also increase sensitivity in detecting early endobronchial lesions, such as moderate or severe dysplasia, carcinoma in situ and microinvasive cancer.[2]

The role of FOB in the evaluation of patients with lung cancer is twofold: (1) to confirm the diagnosis of cancer and determine the histology, and (2) to rule out the presence of endobronchial tumor in the proximal airways, ie, tumor staging.

In patients with clinical or radiographic evidence of endobronchial disease, such as hemoptysis or lobar atelectasis, FOB has a high yield, and FOB may provide a histologic diagnosis of lung cancer in up to 90% of cases. However, in patients with SPN the yield is much lower, and the level of evidence supporting bronchoscopy in this population is therefore lower. Nevertheless, almost 10% of patients with SPN may have evidence of an endobronchial lesion, and these lesions are best diagnosed using bronchoscopy.[3]

Indications for Flexible Fiberoptic Bronchoscopy

The utility of FOB extends well beyond its role in lung cancer. The diagnostic and therapeutic indications for FOB are summarized in Table 10–1.

Table 10–1. Indications for Flexible Fiberoptic Bronchoscopy

Diagnostic	Therapeutic
Lung cancer: 1. Biopsy 2. Staging	Removal of Foreign Body
Endobronchial symptoms or signs: 1. Chronic cough 2. Hemoptysis 3. Atelectasis 4. Obstructive pneumonia 5. Localized wheezing	Lung abscess: 1. Transbronchial drainage 2. Identify and remove occult lesion or foreign body
Other conditions: 1. Vocal cord paralysis 2. Elevated hemidiaphragm 3. Superior vena cava syndrome 4. Chylothorax 5. Unexplained pleural effusion	Respiratory toilet
Pneumonia or diffuse pulmonary disease: 1. Biopsy 2. Endobronchial brush biopsy 3. Bronchoalveolar lavage (BAL) 4. Transbronchial lung biopsy 5. Endobronchial ultrasound biopsy (EBUS) 6. Autofluorescence Bronchoscopy (AFB)	Dilation and stenting of tracheal stenosis
Reactive airway disease: 1. Segmental allergen challenge 2. BAL 3. Biopsy	Palliative surgery for obstructing bronchial masses: 1. Laser resection 2. Dilation 3. Stenting
Thoracic trauma or inhalational injury	Therapeutic options for carcinoma *in situ* in patients who are not surgical candidates: 1. Photodynamic therapy (PDT) 2. Electrocautery 3. Cryotherapy 4. Brachytherapy
Assessment of endotracheal tube or bronchial blocker position	Fiberoptic intubation in difficult airway

Procedural Complications

Flexible bronchoscopy, even when combined with biopsy, TBNA or BAL, is a very safe procedure. Reported mortality rates are 0.02% to 0.04%[4,5] and major complications occur in 0.12% to 0.5% of patients during simple bronchoscopies. However, when combined with TBNA complications have been reported in up to 6.8%.[4,5]

Hypoxemia

Hypoxemia is common during flexible bronchoscopy, especially when additional procedures such as BAL are performed, during which substantial decreases in arterial oxygen tension (PaO_2) may occur. Hypoventilation, the most frequent cause of hypoxemia during bronchoscopy, may result from respiratory depression due to sedation, increased airway resistance or airway circuit leaks. Oxygen supplementation is therefore required during the procedure and often following the procedure, depending on the patient's pulmonary function and degree of residual sedation.

CARDIAC ARRHYTHMIAS

Both brady- and tachy-arrhythmias have been reported during fiberoptic bronchoscopy. Arrhythmias most commonly occur as a result of autonomic stimulation due to passing the endoscope through the vocal cords, or during procedures such as TBNA or BAL. Physiological derangements such as hypoxia or hypercarbia should be ruled out as potential contributing factors.

BRONCHOSPASM

Bronchospasm seldom complicates FOB in the general population, but may be more common in patients with reactive airways disease.[6] Nevertheless, even in patients with more severe reactive airways disease (forced expiratory volume in 1 second [FEV_1] <60%) bronchoscopy, BAL and biopsy are generally well tolerated. Premedication with a bronchodilator may prevent decreases in postoperative FEV_1 and is recommended in patients with reactive airways disease.[7]

BLEEDING

While FOB is rarely complicated by significant hemorrhage, TBNA may result in substantial bleeding in 1.6% to 4.4% of cases.[8,9] Patient risk factors for bleeding include immunosuppression, uremia, pulmonary hypertension, liver disease, coagulation disorders, and thrombocytopenia. Patients with superior vena cava syndrome have a further increased risk for bleeding due to venous engorgement.

PNEUMOTHORAX

Although uncommon, pneumothorax requiring pleural drainage may complicate approximately 3.5% of cases where TBNA is performed.[10] Positive pressure ventilation increases the risk for pneumothorax during TBNA.[11] While the signs and symptoms of pneumothorax may be delayed after TBNA, it is very uncommon for a pneumothorax to develop more than 1 hour after the procedure.[12,13] It is therefore recommended to obtain a CXR at least 1 hour after TBNA to exclude this complication.

FEVER

Fever is common following FOB and may occur in up to 18.2% of patients. When combined with BAL the incidence further increases from 37% to 52.5%.[14,15] Bacteremia rates however are lower, occurring in 6.5% of patients following bronchoscopy with BAL.[16] This rate compares favorably to rates of 2.3% to 11.8% following direct laryngoscopy and intubation,[17,18] and no association with infectious sequelae has been established. Pro-inflammatory cytokines from alveolar macrophages are thought to play a role in the observed febrile reaction.[19] Therefore, unless the procedure involves incision of the respiratory tract mucosa, or drainage of an abscess or empyema, published guidelines do not recommend antibiotic prophylaxis against endocarditis.[20]

Anesthetic Management for Fiberoptic Bronchoscopy Procedures

PREOPERATIVE ASSESSMENT

Most patients with lung cancer have a history of smoking and therefore have some degree of chronic obstructive pulmonary disease. The preoperative assessment should identify reversible reactive airway disease, which warrants preoperative bronchodilator therapy.[6,7] A history of chemo or radiation therapy should alert the anesthesiologist to the possible risk of pulmonary oxygen toxicity, in which case the lowest possible inspired oxygen partial pressures (FiO_2) should be used.

MONITORING

FOB can be performed in awake patients under local anesthesia or under general anesthesia. Regardless of the anesthetic approach, standard monitoring should include ECG, pulse oximetry, and noninvasive blood pressure monitoring.

AWAKE BRONCHOSCOPY

When performed in the awake patient, adequate local anesthesia is the most important component of the anesthetic. Relying on heavy sedation to suppress laryngeal and airway reflexes could result in hypoventilation and hypoxemia, especially in patients with limited respiratory reserve. Multiple topical nasal and oral applications of any commercially available local anesthetic preparation for this use usually suffice. Blocking individual nerves or transtracheal injections of a local anesthetic solution are rarely required. A topical vasoconstrictor (such as oxymetazoline) and a systemic antisialagogue (such as glycopyrrolate) are usually administered as well. Supplemental oxygen therapy should be administered routinely.

BRONCHOSCOPY UNDER GENERAL ANESTHESIA

When FOB is scheduled in addition to surgical procedures that require general anesthesia, general endotracheal anesthesia with positive pressure ventilation is the preferred technique. Either an inhalational or intravenous anesthetic approach, combined with a short-acting muscle relaxant, would be acceptable. The endotracheal tube should be secured with the tip of the tube well above the carina to allow an unobstructed view of the carina. It is important to use an endotracheal tube with an internal diameter of at least 8.0 mm to diminish the detrimental effects of the functional reduction in internal diameter. A 5.7 mm bronchoscope will occupy only 10% to 15% of the cross-sectional area of the trachea, but 40% of a 9.0 mm tube and 66% of a 7.0 mm endotracheal tube.[7] The endotracheal tube could be trimmed in length to further reduce resistance, but this is seldom required. Additionally, PEEP should be avoided and ventilator settings should allow sufficient time for expiration. Failing to do so may result in distal air trapping.

Spontaneous ventilation should be avoided due to the increase in effective airway resistance and work of breathing. An endotracheal tube connector with a perforated diaphragm, designed to minimize circuit leaks, allows the use of positive pressure ventilation during bronchoscopy. Nevertheless, circuit leaks often render tidal volume monitoring unreliable, and ventilation should be monitored by paying attention to chest wall movement and capnography. Ventilation could be adjusted by adjusting the inspiratory pressure and respiratory rate. However, because the FOB procedure is of short duration, hypercapnia could be tolerated, and attention should rather be focused on maintaining arterial oxygen saturation and avoiding lung injury due to air trapping. Should arterial desaturation occur despite a high FiO_2, the bronchoscope should be removed and the lungs manually ventilated until oxygenation has been restored. Even though pneumothorax is rare, this complication should be ruled out if arterial desaturation does not resolve readily, or is associated with hypotension.

Some centers employ laryngeal mask airways for FOB, with either controlled ventilation (if the peak airway pressure can be maintained <25 cm H_2O) or spontaneous ventilation. Injection of local anesthetic down the suction channel of the bronchoscope facilitates passage of the instrument, and this approach permits examination of the glottis and immediate subglottic trachea. It also reduces the number of direct laryngoscopies if the case immediately precedes a lung resection.

RIGID BRONCHOSCOPY

While routine rigid bronchoscopy has been supplanted by FOB for most cases, it is still widely used and has even experienced a resurgence with the introduction of laser airway surgery and the advent of airway stents over the past 2 decades.[21] The rigid bronchoscope is a straight hollow metal tube through which direct access to the central airways can be obtained (Figure 10–1). It has a blunted distal opening, which is beveled to facilitate lifting of the epiglottis and atraumatic intubation of the airway. The distal end of the bronchoscope has side vents, which enables ventilation of the opposite lung when the distal opening is advanced into a main stem bronchus. These side vents may result in an air-leak into the pharynx during positive pressure ventilation when not advanced beyond the vocal cords. The proximal opening is adapted to accommodate attachments, provide side port ventilation, and permit insertion of surgical instruments.

Indications for Rigid Bronchoscopy

The advantages of rigid bronchoscopy over FOB are that it permits continuous assisted ventilation while simultaneously permitting access for a variety of surgical and diagnostic instruments (including FOB to inspect airways distal to the central airways). The specific indications are listed in Table 10–2.

Procedural Complications

Rigid bronchoscopy could lead to the same potential complications seen following FOB, but is associated with more trauma than with FOB.[22] Insertion of the rigid bronchoscope can result in dental damage or laceration of the mucosa of the oropharynx, larynx, or bronchial tree. In patients with cervical spine disease, hyperextension could lead to spinal injuries or even cerebral ischemia due to vertebral artery occlusion.

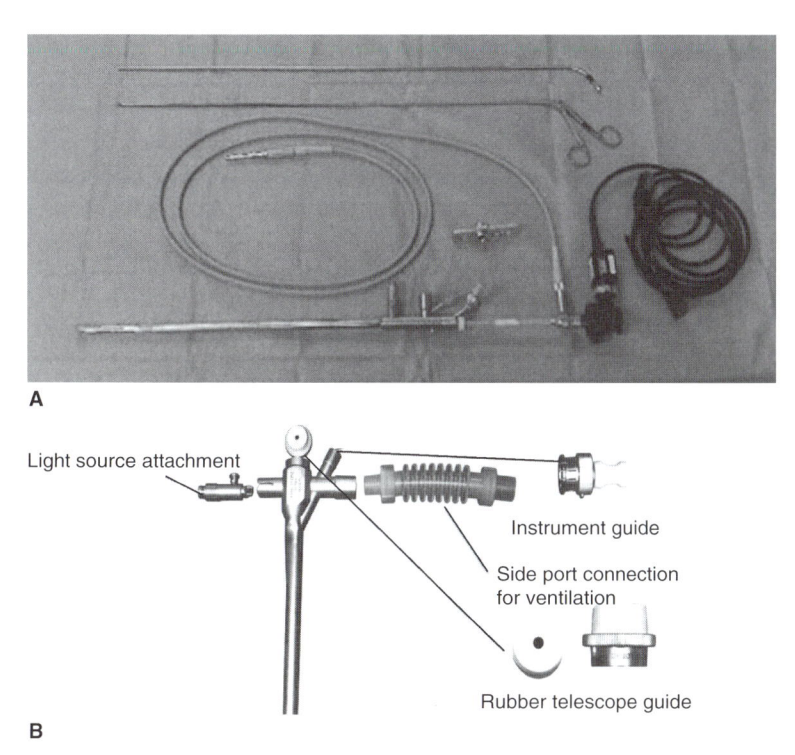

Chapter 10 / Bronchoscopy, Mediastinoscopy, and Chamberlain Procedure 179

Figure 10–1. A and B. Standard rigid bronchoscopy equipment.

Anesthetic Management for Rigid Bronchoscopy Procedurres

MONITORING

Invasive arterial pressure monitoring should be considered in addition to routine monitoring. Rigid bronchoscopy is an extremely stimulating procedure, and invasive arterial pressure monitoring enables swift detection of hemodynamic changes and

Table 10–2. Indications for Rigid Bronchoscopy

Evaluation and treatment of intrapulmonary hemorrhage
Foreign body extraction
Biopsy when fiberoptic specimen is inadequate
Dilation of tracheal or bronchial strictures
Insertion of stents
Evaluation and debulking of bronchial tumors (mechanical or laser ablation)
Pediatric bronchoscopy

the response to pharmacological intervention. It also enables monitoring of arterial carbon dioxide partial pressure ($PaCO_2$) during jet or apneic ventilation. Continuous quantitative neuromuscular monitoring should be performed to ensure adequate relaxation during the procedure and the return of normal neuromuscular function prior to emergence by assessing train-of-four (TOF) ratio. The use of bispectral index (BIS) or entropy monitoring is strongly recommended, because rigid bronchoscopy is a high-risk procedure for intraoperative awareness.

INDUCTION AND MAINTENANCE

Rigid bronchoscopy is now always performed under general anesthesia. Neuromuscular blockade facilitates atraumatic intubation and prevents sudden movement or coughing, which could result in serious airway injury. The anesthetic plan should allow for rapid emergence and extubation following completion of the surgical procedure. A routine intravenous induction can be used and mask ventilation with 100% oxygen should be established until the patient is fully paralyzed, at which time the airway is handed over to the surgeon. The choice of drugs depends on patient factors and the expected duration of the procedure. When jet ventilation is used during bronchoscopy, a total intravenous anesthetic approach, such as a propofol infusion, is required. Since surgical stimulation can be profound but postoperative pain generally minimal, remifentanil is commonly used during rigid bronchoscopy. The choice of muscle relaxant depends on the expected duration of the procedure.

VENTILATION

Ventilation can be managed by connecting the standard anesthesia circuit to the bronchoscope (ventilating bronchoscope) or by using a jet ventilator. When using a ventilating bronchoscope, positive pressure ventilation can only be applied as long as the eyepiece is closed over the bronchoscope. Ventilation must therefore be interrupted when suction catheters and surgical instruments are passed through the scope. In the absence of ventilation, adequate oxygenation can be maintained for several minutes (apneic oxygenation), especially when preceded by a period of hyperventilation with 100% oxygen to achieve hypocapnia and denitrogenation. Provided hypercapnia and respiratory acidosis can be tolerated, oxygen insufflation through a small catheter in the trachea can maintain oxygenation. Arterial PCO_2 can be expected to rise by 6 to 10 mm Hg during the first minute of apnea, and at a rate of 3 to 5 mm Hg/min thereafter. Ventilation should therefore be resumed after about 8 to 10 minutes, unless required earlier due to hypoxemia.

For prolonged rigid bronchoscopy jet ventilation is recommended (see Figure 10–1). The intermittent high-velocity oxygen jet entrains air into the bronchoscope, resulting in expansion of the lungs. Jet systems can be divided into manually triggered systems (Sanders' type) or those with automatic timing. Jet ventilation is initiated at a low frequency, using a lower driving pressure (20 psi), which is then gradually increased until adequate chest rise and breath sounds are observed. High-frequency jet ventilation (HFJV), using ventilatory rates of 150 to 300 breaths/min, will result in lower mean airway pressure and less movement in the bronchial tree, which might be desirable during laser treatment. However, low frequency jet ventilation might result in less air trapping in patients with bronchial stenoses, or improved ventilation in the opposite lung through the bronchoscope side vents during endobronchial intubation.[23]

EMERGENCE

Once the bronchoscope is removed, the patient should be intubated with an endotracheal tube prior to reversal of neuromuscular blockade and emergence. A laryngeal mask airway or face mask with or without an oral airway may also be considered, provided airway resistance and pulmonary compliance permits adequate ventilation with airway pressures less than 15 to 20 cm H_2O.[24] Full return of neuromuscular function (TOF ratio > 90%) should be confirmed prior to emergence, to enable a strong cough for clearing secretions or blood.

MEDIASTINOSCOPY

Indications

Mediastinoscopy is an invasive diagnostic procedure used to biopsy lymph nodes and masses in the mediastinum. In NSCLC, the most common indication for mediastinoscopy, the level of nodal involvement has significant prognostic importance. In general, positive mediastinal findings on CT or PET need to be confirmed histologically. Compared to less invasive diagnostic modalities, such as transbronchial fine needle aspiration and tracheal endoscopic ultrasound needle aspiration, mediastinoscopy remains the gold standard due to its superior sensitivity (>80%) and specificity (100%).[25] Mediastinoscopy also plays an important role in the diagnostic workup of other diseases presenting with mediastinal lymphadenopathy, such as sarcoidosis or lymphoma. Cervical mediastinoscopy, the most conventional form of mediastinoscopy, is used to evaluate the superior and middle mediastinal compartments. Other approaches have been devised to gain access to lymph nodes and masses that are not accessible through the cervical approach and will be described later.

Absolute contraindications to cervical mediastinoscopy are rare. Where technically not feasible, due to extreme kyphosis or previous radical laryngectomy, this procedure should not be attempted. Conditions such as superior vena cava syndrome, enlarged goiter, or previous mediastinoscopy, sternotomy, or radiation therapy do not necessarily preclude cervical mediastinoscopy. However, due to adhesions and fibrosis the procedure may be challenging under these conditions.

Anatomy

The mediastinum is anatomically one of the most complex regions of the human body. It lies between the two pleural cavities, is bounded by the sternum anteriorly

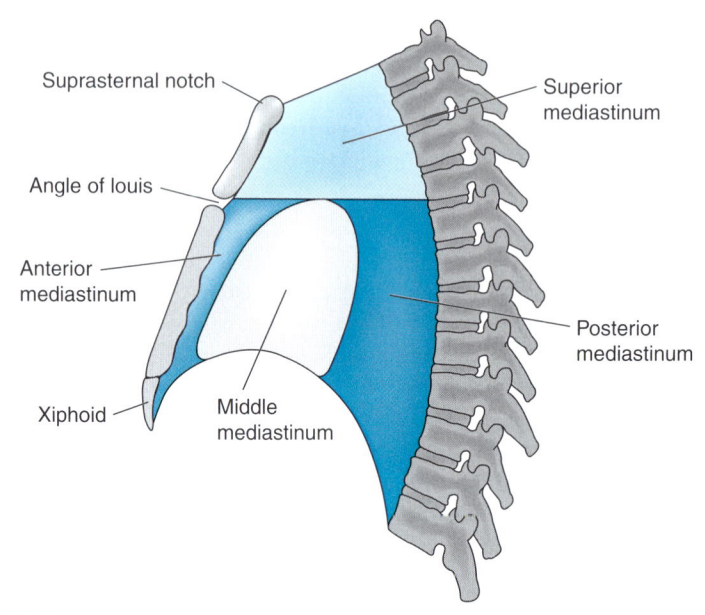

Figure 10–2. Anatomical compartments of the mediastinum.

and the vertebral column posteriorly, and extends from the thoracic inlet down to the diaphragm. For purposes of description, the mediastinum is divided into two parts by the transverse thoracic plane (Figure 10–2). This slightly oblique plane extends posteriorly from the sternomanubrial angle to the junction of the 4th and 5th thoracic vertebra. The inferior mediastinum is further divided into the posterior (behind the pericardium), middle (containing the pericardium and its contents) and anterior (in front of the pericardium) compartments. Apart from the lungs, all the thoracic viscera are contained within the mediastinum, surrounded by loose connective tissue.

The mediastinum is rich in lymph nodes, which run in parallel with the major vessels that transgress this space. Inflammatory disease, primary lymphatic tumors and metastatic disease may affect mediastinal lymph nodes. The prognostic importance of the level and extent of nodal involvement in NSCLC has led to the development of the Mountain–Dressler lymph node map (Figure 10–3).

Surgical Approaches and Considerations

A range of techniques have been developed to provide surgical access to the different regions of the mediastinum for staging mediastinoscopy. Standard cervical mediastinoscopy remains the gold standard for staging the superior mediastinal lymph nodes, but it cannot reach the subaortic (station 5) and para-aortic (station 6) nodal stations. Bronchogenic carcinoma of the left lung may metastasize to these lymph nodes, especially those tumors located in the upper

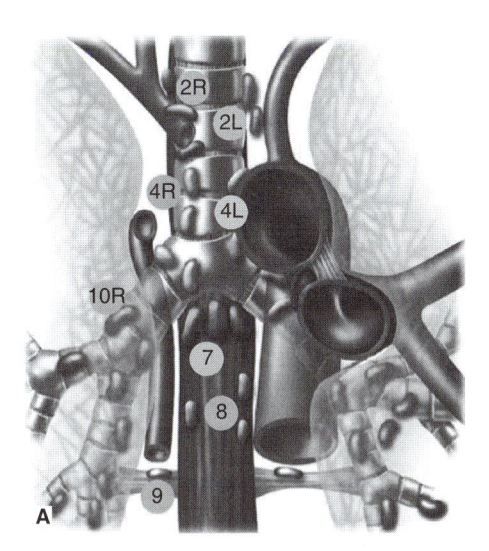

Figure 10-3A. The Mountain–Dressler lymph node map showing nodal sections used in the staging of non-small cell lung cancer. Station 1 nodes are located above the sternal notch and not routinely accessible through cervical mediastinoscopy. Station 3 nodes are not seen in this view (see Figure 10-3B). (From De Leyn P, Lerut T. Conventional mediastinoscopy. *Multimedia Man Cardiothorac Surg 2005*. doi:10.1510/mmcts.2004.000158. Schematic 2. Copyright © 2005 European Association for Cardio-thoracic Surgery, with permission.)

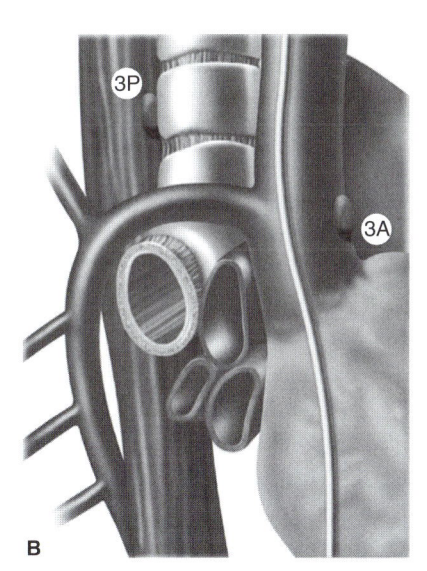

Figure 10-3B. Station 3 nodes are also not accessible by conventional cervical mediastinoscopy. Station 3A lymph nodes are anterior to the vena cava; 3P lymph nodes are reside above the tracheal bifurcation, in the upper paraesophageal region. (From De Leyn P, Lerut T. Conventional mediastinoscopy. *Multimedia Man Cardiothorac Surg 2005*. doi:10.1510/mmcts.2004.000158. Schematic 5. Copyright © 2005 European Association for Cardio-thoracic Surgery, with permission.)

lobe and hilum. Therefore, surgical staging of bronchogenic carcinoma of the left lung may require the combination of standard cervical mediastinoscopy with other surgical techniques, such as left parasternal mediastinotomy (Chamberlain's procedure), left thoracoscopy, or extended cervical mediastinoscopy to explore the subaortic and para-aortic nodal stations.

Modifications to the conventional mediastinoscope have been introduced since the 1990s. Newer devices include integrated optics that connect to a video system, and have greatly aided in the standardization and training of this procedure. A self-supported, two-bladed spreadable video-mediastinoscope developed by Linder and Dahan in 1992 allows increased exposure of mediastinal structures and bimanual dissection. This device has facilitated the development of new minimally invasive surgical techniques for the mediastinum. The best documented method is video-assisted mediastinoscopic lymphadenectomy (VAMLA), which may improve accuracy for lung cancer staging and allow definitive mediastinal surgery in selected cases.[26-28]

Cervical Mediastinoscopy

The great majority of mediastinoscopies are performed through a small cervical incision just above the suprasternal notch, as first reported by Carlens in 1959. This technique allows evaluation and sampling of upper paratracheal (station 2L and 2R), lower paratracheal (station 4L and 4R), and subcarinal (station 7) lymph nodes. The 2003 American College of Chest Physicians guidelines on lung cancer staging recommend that these five nodal stations be routinely examined and that at least one node be sampled from each location unless none is present.[29] The surgical procedure involves sharp dissection to expose the pretracheal muscles, which are then separated in the midline to reach the pretracheal fascia. Following incision of the pretracheal fascia, blunt dissection is then performed along the anterior surface of the trachea to develop the tissue plane down to the level of the carina (Figure 10–4). The rigid mediastinoscope is then passed along this tissue plane, posterior to the innominate artery and aorta. Through the mediastinoscope, lymph nodes are first mobilized using a blunt suction device, and then biopsied using a biopsy forceps.

Anterior Mediastinotomy (Chamberlain Procedure)

Anterior parasternal mediastinotomy was introduced by McNeill and Chamberlain in 1966 to access the subaortic and para-aortic stations. The traditional anterior approach is through a mediastinotomy, requiring a parasternal incision and resection of costal cartilage. However, adequate node sampling can usually be obtained through a smaller mediastinoscopy incision in the second intercostal space, through which the mediastinoscope is inserted following blunt digital dissection. The side of the incision depends on the side of the pathology. Anterior mediastinotomy and bidigital palpation of the aortopulmonary region may be performed in conjunction with cervical mediastinoscopy to locate diseased lymph nodes (see Figure 10–3). In the event of negative biopsy results, or when the nodes or the mass cannot be safely reached, the incision can be extended and the target tissue

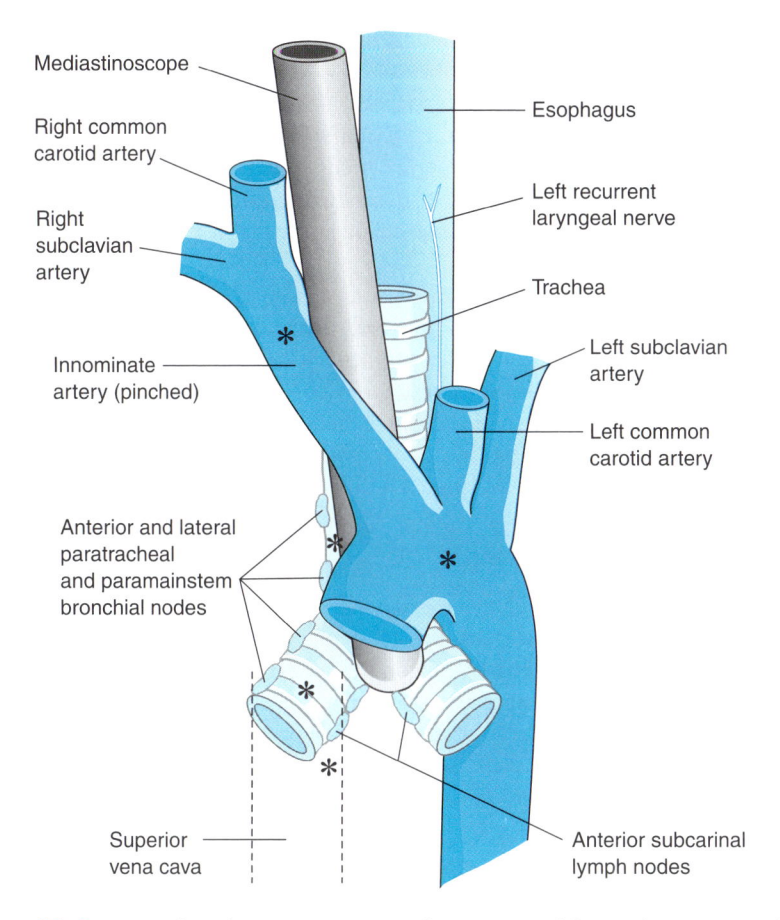

Figure 10–4. Cervical mediastinoscopy. Note the position of the mediastinoscope in relation to the anatomic structures of the mediastinum. The innominate artery is being partially occluded ("pinched") by the instrument in this example. (From: Longnecker DE, Brown DL, Newman MF, Zapol WM. *Longnecker's Anesthesiology*. Chapter 53, Thoracic Anesthesia, Figure 53-30. McGraw-Hill, Inc.: 2008, with permission.)

may be biopsied from inside the pleural space by creating an anterior thoracotomy. However, anterior thoracotomy, and to some extent anterior mediastinotomy, have largely been supplanted by video-assisted thoracoscopic (VATS) exploration of the mediastinum. The advantage of anterior mediastinotomy over VATS is that the pleural space is seldom entered, obviating the need for a pleural drain, and allowing patients to be discharged on the day of surgery.

Extended Cervical Mediastinoscopy

Extended cervical mediastinoscopy provides yet another approach for staging of subaortic and para-aortic stations. This procedure is more technically challenging, but does not require an additional skin incision following the completion of standard cervical medimediastinoscopy. It is best reserved for patients with enlarged subaortic or para-aortic nodes on CT scan. Similar to anterior mediastinotomy, it is only performed when standard cervical mediastinoscopy fails to reveal involvement of superior mediastinal lymph nodes that would make the patient inoperable. The procedure should not be performed in patients with a dilated aortic arch, excessive calcification in the aortic arch or previous median sternotomy.

For extended cervical mediastinoscopy a passage is first created using digital dissection. The mediastinoscope is then advanced over the aortic arch between the innominate artery and the left carotid artery, under the left innominate vein. (see Figure 10–4). Complications related to this technique are infrequent and some authors suggest that extended cervical mediastinoscopy has less postoperative morbidity than anterior mediastinotomy or VATS. In contrast to VATS, patients can be discharged on the day of surgery.

Video-Assisted Thoracoscopy (VATS)

Thoracoscopic exploration of the mediastinum has developed into an additional minimally invasive diagnostic staging modality. In addition to allowing access to the subaortic or para-aortic lymph node stations, it also permits access to the para-esophageal (level 8) and pulmonary ligament (level 9) stations, while also providing complete visualization of the pleural space. VATS may also provide an alternative approach when there are concerns with the alternatives, such as the presence of anatomic abnormalities, previous extensive neck surgery, sternotomy or radiotherapy.

Surgical Complications

Mediastinoscopy is well-tolerated by almost all patients with a reported complication rate of 0.6% to 3% and a mortality rate of 0% to 0.05%.[25,30-34] At least part of the reason for this is likely related to the fact that mediastinoscopy does not impair respiratory capacity. Only 0.1% to 0.5% of the reported complications are considered major, but the potential for catastrophic events is clear, given the close proximity to important anatomical structures. One of the most important considerations in avoiding complications is surgical experience. Video mediastinoscopy has enhanced surgeons' ability to teach this procedure safely. The potential complications are listed in Table 10–3.

Bleeding

The most feared complication, major bleeding, occurs at a rate of 0.1% to 0.4%. The vessels at risk for injury are the innominate artery, aorta, azygos vein, superior vena cava, and the pulmonary artery. Minor bleeding is common, and can safely be managed by electrocoagulation and packing. Temporary packing, endoscopic clipping, or repair via thoracotomy or sternotomy may be required occasionally. Most cases of major bleeding will require sternotomy, although right thoracotomy

Table 10-3. Potential Complications Following Mediastinoscopy

Vascular injury with hemorrhage
Pneumothorax
Recurrent laryngeal nerve injury with vocal cord paralysis
Infection
Tumor implantation in the wound
Phrenic nerve palsy
Esophageal perforation
Thoracic duct injury
Air embolism
Tracheobronchial laceration
Reflex bradycardia including asystole
Transient hemiparesis or stroke

may be indicated when bleeding is from the first branch of the right pulmonary artery or from the azygos vein.

Pneumothorax

Pneumothorax is also rare, but reportedly 0.08% to 0.23% of patients may require chest tube placement at the end of the procedure due to a pleural tear and trauma to the lung tissue. A small pneumothorax, detected on routine postoperative chest x-ray, can be managed conservatively in asymptomatic patients.

Tracheal laceration can lead to mediastinal emphysema and decreased ventilation. In the presence of mediastinal emphysema, FOB should be performed to rule out tracheal laceration, which may warrant operative repair.

Stroke

Compression of the innominate artery during mediastinoscopy is common, and may result in transient cerebral hypoperfusion and ischemia, in particular in patients with cerebrovascular disease and inadequate collateral blood flow. Innominate artery compression can be detected in the right arm by pulse oximetry or digital palpation of an arterial pulse, but is most reliably detected by invasive arterial pressure monitoring. Hyperextension of the cervical spine could also result in vertebral artery compression, and care should be taken to avoid or limit hyperextension in patients with a history of vertebrobasilar insufficiency. The risk of stroke appears to be highest with extended cervical mediastinoscopy, and as such appears to be related to manipulation of the innominate artery and the aorta.[35] Stroke or transient postoperative hemiparesis are most likely caused by either atherosclerotic embolization or cerebral hypoperfusion due to prolonged compression of the innominate artery.

Bradycardia, hypotension or even asystole may result from stretching of the vagus, trachea, or great vessels, and should be managed by repositioning the mediastinoscope. Persistent bradycardia may require the administration of anticholinergic drugs such as atropine.

Anesthetic Management for Mediastinoscopy Procedures

Preoperative Assessment

The preoperative assessment should identify the presence of ischemic heart disease, cardiac arrhythmias, and cerebrovascular disease. Factors that might make the surgical procedure challenging, such as limited neck extension or superior vena cava obstruction, should also be identified. When mediastinoscopy is performed in a patient with a mediastinal mass, the preoperative assessment should also include identifying associated airway, vascular or cardiac compression.

Monitoring

Apart from standard anesthetic monitoring, right radial arterial pressure monitoring will enable accurate and immediate detection of innominate artery compression. The pulse oximeter should be placed on the right side when not using invasive arterial pressure monitoring. In both instances noninvasive blood pressure monitoring should be performed on the left. Quantitative neuromuscular monitoring should be used to ensure adequate depth of neuromuscular blockade during the procedure and complete reversal prior to emergence from anesthesia.

Intraoperative Management

General anesthesia with intermittent positive pressure ventilation is the anesthetic of choice for staging mediastinoscopy. The anesthetic plan should permit rapid emergence and extubation at the end of the procedure. Because mediastinoscopy is usually combined with staging bronchoscopy, an endotracheal tube with an internal diameter of 8.0 mm or greater should be used. The endotracheal tube should be directed away from the surgical field and secured on the side toward the anesthetic machine. Connections should be secure to avoid inadvertent disconnection. Neuromuscular blockade should be maintained to prevent any sudden movement or coughing during the procedure, which may result in injury or increase the risk for bleeding due to venous engorgement. Because of the risk of intraoperative bleeding, large-bore intravenous access should be secured preoperatively and blood should be immediately available.

The patient should be positioned with the head maximally extended, with a shoulder role in place to facilitate insertion of the mediastinoscope. The anterior chest should be prepped into the field to enable immediate access for emergency median sternotomy in case of massive bleeding.

During the procedure, the primary role of the anesthesiologist should be to closely observe the patient for signs of potential surgical complications. Mediastinoscopy causes significant surgical stimulation, but this is generally of short duration and results in minimal postoperative discomfort.

Postoperative Care

Patients should be closely observed for airway or respiratory compromise in the immediate postoperative period. They should be recovered with the head in an elevated position to improve venous drainage and reduce the risk for airway edema. Pneumothorax should be excluded in all patients by chest x-ray. In patients with suspected recurrent laryngeal nerve injury, the vocal cords should be assessed by fiberoptic laryngoscopy.

REFERENCES

1. Gould MK, Fletcher J, Iannettoni MD, et al. Evaluation of patients with pulmonary nodules: when is it lung cancer?: ACCP evidence-based clinical practice guidelines (2nd edition). *Chest.* 2007; 132(3 Suppl):108S-130S.
2. Feller-Kopman D, Lunn W, Ernst A. Autofluorescence bronchoscopy and endobronchial ultrasound: a practical review. *Ann Thorac Surg.* 2005;80(6):2395-2401.
3. Chhajed PN, Bernasconi M, Gambazzi F, et al. Combining bronchoscopy and positron emission tomography for the diagnosis of the small pulmonary nodule < or = 3 cm. *Chest.* 2005;128(5):3558-3564.
4. Pue C, Pacht E. Complications of fiberoptic bronchoscopy at a university hospital. *Chest.* 1995;107:430-432.
5. Facciolongo N, Patelli M, Gasparini S, et al. Incidence of complications in bronchoscopy. Multicentre prostpective study of 20986 bronchoscopies. *Monaldi Arch Chest Dis.* 2009;71:8-14.
6. Djukanovic R, Wilson JW, Lai CK, Holgate ST, Howarth PH. The safety aspects of fiberoptic bronchoscopy, bronchoalveolar lavage, and endobronchial biopsy in asthma. *Am Rev Respir Dis.* 1991;143(4 Pt 1):772-777.
7. British Thoracic Society bronchoscopy guidelines committee asotsoccotbts. British Throacic Society guidelines on diagnostic flexible bronchoscopy. *Thorax.* 2001;56:i1-i21.
8. Hue S. Complications in transbronchial lung biopsy. *Korean J Int Med.* 1987;2:209-213.
9. Mitchell D, Emerson C, Collins J, et al. Transbronchial lung biopsy with the fibreoptic bronchoscope: analysis of results in 433 patients. *Br J Dis Chest.* 1981;75:258-262.
10. Milman N, Munch E, Faurschou P, et al. Fiberoptic bronchoscopy in local anaesthesia. Indications, results and complications in 1323 examinations. *Acta Endosc.* 1993;23:151-162.
11. O'Brien JD, Ettinger NA, Shevlin D, et al. Safety and yield of transbornchial biopsy in mechanically ventilated patients. *Crit Care Med.* 1997;25:440-446.
12. deFenoyl O, Capron F, Lebeau B, Rochemaure J. Transbronchial biopsy without fluoroscopy: a five year experience in outpatients. *Thorax.* 1989;44:956-959.
13. Hernandez-Blasco L, Sanchez-Hernandez IM, Villena-Garrido V, deMiguel-Poch E, Nunez-Delgado M, Alfaro-Abreu J. Safety of the transbronchial biopsy in outpatients. *Chest.* 1991;99:562-565.
14. Fonseca MT, Camargos PA, Abou Taam R, LeBourgeois M, Scheinmann P, DeBlic J. Incidence rate and factors related to post-bronchoalveolar lavage fever in children. *Respiration.* 2007;74:653-658.
15. Picard E, Schwartz S, Goldberg S, Glick T, Villa Y, Kerem E. A prospective study of fever and bateremia after flexible fiberoptic bronchoscopy in children. *Chest.* 2000;117:573-577.
16. Yigla M, Oren I, Bentur L, et al. Incidence of bacteraemia following fiberoptic bronchoscopy. *Eur Respir J.* 1999;14:789-791.
17. Valdes C, Tomas I, Alvarez M, Limieres J, Medina J, Diz P. The incidence of bacteraemia associated with tracheal intubation. *Anaesthesia.* 2008;63:588-592.
18. Goldstein S, Wolf GL, Kim SJ, Sierra MF, Whitmire C, Tolentino EM. Bacteraemia during direct laryngoscopy and endotracheal intubation: a study using a multiple culture, large volume technique. *Anaesth Intensive Care.* 1997;25:239-244.
19. Krause A, Hohberg B, Heine F, et al. Cytokines derived from alveolar macrophages induce fever after bronchoscopy and bronchoalveolar lavage. *Am J Respir Crit Care Med.* 1997;155:1793-1797.
20. Wilson W, Taubert KA, Gewitz M, et al. Prevention of infective endocarditis: guidelines from the American Heart Association: a guideline from the American Heart Association Rheumatic Fever, Endocarditis, and Kawasaki Disease Committee, Council on Cardiovascular Disease in the Young,

and the Council on Clinical Cardiology, Council on Cardiovascular Surgery and Anesthesia, and the Quality of Care and Outcomes Research Interdisciplinary Working Group. *Circulation.* 2007;116(15):1736-1754.
21. Wahidi MM, Ernst A. Role of the interventional pulmonologist in the intensive care unit. *J Intensive Care Med.* 2005;20(3):141-146.
22. Lukomsky GI, Ovchinnikov AA, Bilal A. Complications of bronchoscopy: comparison of rigid bronchoscopy under general anesthesia and flexible fiberoptic bronchoscopy under topical anesthesia. *Chest.* 1981;79(3):316-321.
23. Vourc'h G, Fischler M, Michon F, Melchior JC, Seigneur F. Manual jet ventilation v. high frequency jet ventilation during laser resection of tracheo-bronchial stenosis. *Br J Anaesth.* 1983;55(10):973-975.
24. Devitt JH, Wenstone R, Noel AG, O'Donnell MP. The laryngeal mask airway and positive-pressure ventilation. *Anesthesiology.* 1994;80(3):550-555.
25. Hammound ZT, Anderson RC, Meyers BF, et al. The current role of mediastinoscopy in the evaluation of thoracic disease. *J Thoracic Cardiovasc Surg.* 1999;118:894-899.
26. Leschber G, Holinka G, Linder A. Video-assisted mediastinoscopic lymphadenectomy (VAMLA)—a method for systematic mediastinal lymphnode dissection. *Eur J Cardiothorac Surg.* 2003;24(2):192-195.
27. Leschber G, Sperling D, Klemm W, Merk J. Does video-mediastinoscopy improve the results of conventional mediastinoscopy? *Eur J Cardiothorac Surg.* 2008;33(2):289-293.
28. Hurtgen M, Friedel G, Toomes H, Fritz P. Radical video-assisted mediastinoscopic lymphadenectomy (VAMLA)—technique and first results. *Eur J Cardiothorac Surg.* 2002;21(2):348-351.
29. Detterbeck FC, DeCamp MM, Jr., Kohman LJ, Silvestri GA. Lung cancer. Invasive staging: the guidelines. *Chest.* 2003,123(1 Suppl):167S-175S.
30. Cybulshky IJ, Bennett WF. Mediastinoscopy as a routine outpatient procedure. *Ann Thorac Surg.* 1994;58:176-178.
31. Kliems G, Savic B. Complications of mediastinoscopy. *Endoscopy.* 1979;11(1):9-12.
32. Kirschner PA. Cervical mediastinoscopy. *Chest Surg Clin N Am.* 1996;6:1-20.
33. Puhakka HJ. Complications of mediastinoscopy. *J Laryngol Otol.* 1989;103:312-315.
34. Lemaire A, Nikolic I, Petersen T, et al. Nine-zear single center experience with cervial mediastinoscopy: complications and false negative rate. *Ann Thorac Surg.* 2006;82:1185-1189.
35. D'Amico TA. *Complications of Mediastinal Surgery.* 1st ed. New York: Blackwell Futura; 2007.

Therapeutic Bronchoscopy, Airway Stents, and Other Closed Thorax Procedures

11

Scott Shofer
Momen M. Wahidi
Ian J. Welsby

Key Points

1. Therapeutic bronchoscopy is most commonly employed to treat patients with central airways obstruction due to malignant disease.
2. Rigid bronchoscopy provides definitive control of the airway permitting the use of general anesthesia to maximize patient comfort.
3. Patients can undergo bronchoscopy with transbronchial biopsy without stopping aspirin therapy, but clopidogrel should be stopped 5 days prior to the procedure.
4. As with any shared airway case, close communication between operator and anesthesiologist is vital for maximum patient safety.

Case Vignette

The patient is a 47-year-old female with stage 4 adenocarcinoma involving the left lung. A prior stent was placed in the left mainstem bronchus due to tumor invasion of the proximal airway. Now, the tumor has invaded the stent to the point where complete airway obstruction is imminent. She is referred for stent exchange and tumor debulking.

She has a history of 100 pack-years of smoking but no other medical problems. She is oxygen dependent at home on 2L/min nasal cannula.

Medications are alprazolam and albuterol. Vital signs: BP 110/80, HR 82, room air SpO2 85%. Laboratory examination is notable only for a WBC of 11.5.

Therapeutic bronchoscopy, previously practiced primarily by thoracic surgeons, is becoming more commonly performed by pulmonologists who receive specialized training in the performance of airway surgical techniques for the treatment of central airways obstruction. Performing these procedures involves

Table 11-1. Indications for Rigid Bronchoscopy

Massive hemoptysis
Foreign body removal
Dilation of airway stenosis
Airway stent placement
Resection of central airway tumor

the use of the rigid bronchoscope, which requires careful coordination of care between the anesthesia team and the proceduralist. Several issues around the use of rigid bronchoscopy can often lead the anesthesiologist into unfamiliar territory, including release of the airway into the hands of the proceduralist, turning the head of the patient away from the anesthesiologist during the procedure, and often ceding control of ventilation to the procedural team. Good communication regarding procedural planning, ventilatory strategy, and anesthesia management are critical to optimize patient safety and provide for a successful procedure.

Therapeutic bronchoscopy is most commonly employed to treat patients with central airways obstruction (CAO) due to benign or malignant etiology. While the incidence of CAO is unknown, it is a commonly encountered clinical problem present in 20% to 30% of patients with primary lung cancer[1] and 7% to 18% of patients post-lung transplantation.[2] Additional common causes of CAO include tracheal stenosis, either post-tracheostomy or idiopathic, tracheomalacia, and foreign body aspiration.[1] While many of the techniques that will be described in this section are amenable to use with the flexible bronchoscope, rigid bronchoscopy provides definitive control of the airway permitting the use of general anesthesia to maximize patient comfort (Table 11–1).[3] In addition, the rigid bronchoscope becomes a conduit for use of a variety of tools and suction devices to perform minimally invasive airway surgery. The bronchoscope itself can become a therapeutic tool useful for dilation of airway stenoses, and "coring out" of airway tumor providing rapid relief of central airway obstruction.[3]

RIGID BRONCHOSCOPY

The rigid bronchoscope was the only method of bronchoscopy available from the advent of the bronchoscope in 1897 by Gustav Killian, until the introduction of the flexible fiberoptic scope in 1967 by Ikeda. After the introduction of flexible bronchoscopy, use of the rigid bronchoscope declined by pulmonologists in North America. Its distinct advantages in controlling the airway while facilitating the passage of a wide variety of tools for minimally invasive airway surgery in conjunction with the development of reliable stents to promote airway patency has led to a renewal in interest in the use of rigid bronchoscopy by the pulmonary community over the past 15 years.[4]

Indications

Rigid bronchoscopy can be used for any bronchoscopic indication, however, the additional requirements of general anesthesia generally result in most centers limiting its use to therapeutic indications such as relief of central airway obstruction, foreign body removal, and for investigation of massive hemoptysis.

Patient Selection

Rigid bronchoscopy is generally well-tolerated among most patients, even those with significant respiratory disabilities due to their underlying pulmonary disease. However, several medical conditions may occur which raise the risk for complications. Major conditions to consider include ischemic or arrhythmic heart disease, bleeding diathesis (coagulopathy, thrombocytopenia, uremia), neurologic disease or head trauma, and respiratory insufficiency. Although bronchoscopy can be performed in patients who fall short of the ideal, the risk of the procedure increases accordingly, and options for more invasive manipulations (biopsies, lengthy procedures, etc) can be limited.

Preoperative laboratory studies, including platelet count, coagulation studies, blood urea nitrogen, and creatinine level, are often obtained to assess for bleeding tendencies. However, multiple studies examining the utility of preoperative laboratory examinations have determined that this is not universally necessary, but should be tailored to patients with medical histories suggesting an abnormality. In a retrospective study of 305 bronchoscopies with biopsy, Kozak and Brath identified five clinical risk factors which should prompt further pre-operative evaluation including prior anticoagulant therapy, liver disease, family or personal history of bleeding tendencies, active bleeding or recent transfusion requirements, and presence of an unreliable historian.[5]

Absolute contraindications to bronchoscopy are few and include inability to provide informed consent, status asthmaticus, severe hypoxemia, and unstable cardiovascular conditions. Detailed below are some of the main factors to consider when selecting a patient for bronchoscopy.

Asthma/Bronchospasm

Although bronchoscopy can be safely performed in asthmatic patients, it is associated with a significant drop in FEV_1 and PaO_2 post-procedure. This drop correlates inversely with the concentration of methacholine required to produce a 20% fall in FEV_1 at baseline but not with the usual measures of asthma severity such as albuterol use, symptom scoring, and peak flow variation.[6] Therefore, bronchoscopy should be approached cautiously in the patient with asthma, and avoided entirely in the setting of status asthmaticus. Elective procedures should be deferred until bronchospasm is effectively controlled.

Head Trauma/Elevated Intracranial Pressure

Increased intracranial pressure (ICP) has been anecdotally cited as a relative contraindication to bronchoscopy because of concerns that the rise in intrathoracic pressure induced by bronchoscopy-associated cough could abruptly raise ICP and precipitate herniation. A retrospective study found no increase in neurologic complications in patients with space-occupying central nervous system lesions undergoing bronchoscopy, although pretreatment with steroids was recommended to decrease cerebral edema.[7] More recently, a prospective study of 23 patients with intracranial drains in place revealed substantial, though transient, increases in ICP in patients undergoing bronchoscopy, despite adequate levels of sedation, analgesia, and paralysis.[8] No acute deterioration in the patient's clinical status was observed, but unfortunately, long-term complications or sequelae from these changes remain unknown.[8] Therefore, although fiber-optic bronchoscopy is often necessary in the care of patients after neurologic events, it should be used with caution in this patient population.

Hypoxemia/High Oxygen Requirement

Bronchoscopy carries a higher risk in patients who are hypoxemic at baseline, although determining the cause of hypoxemia is a common indication for bronchoscopy. Unfortunately, hypoxemia is also a complication of bronchoscopy, resulting from sedation related hypoventilation and ventilation-perfusion mismatch secondary to partial airway occlusion (from bronchoscope), atelectasis from frequent suctioning, airway bleeding, lavage fluid, and jet ventilation.[9] While there is no absolute amount of supplemental oxygen that is a contraindication for bronchoscopy, caution should be used in patients with high oxygen requirements. Severe hypoxemia with PaO_2 greater than 65 to 70 mm Hg despite supplemental oxygen therapy is generally considered a contraindication.[10]

Anticoagulant/Antiplatelet Therapy

Use of anticoagulant and antiplatelet agents is common among patients referred for bronchoscopy. Therefore, it is important to carefully review all medications with the patient prior to bronchoscopy and make appropriate recommendations for continuing or holding medications prior to the procedure date.

Aspirin   Aspirin was previously considered a contraindication to bronchoscopy due to its anti-platelet effects and prolongation of bleeding time. However, a large multicenter randomized trial found no difference in bleeding from transbronchial biopsies in the aspirin compared with the no aspirin group.[11] Therefore, it is generally accepted that patients can undergo bronchoscopy with transbronchial biopsy without holding aspirin therapy.

Clopidogrel   In contrast to aspirin, clopidogrel significantly increases bleeding risks following transbronchial biopsy. When the effect of clopidogrel on the incidence of bleeding was studied during transbronchial biopsy, significant bleeding rates increased to 89% compared with 3.4% in the control group.[12] In a small number of patients receiving both aspirin and clopidogrel, the incidence of significant bleeding was 100% following transbronchial biopsy.[12] Given the relatively long half-life of clopidogrel, most practices require patients to discontinue clopidogrel a minimum of 5 days prior to undergoing bronchoscopy with transbronchial biopsy.

Thrombocytopenia There is little data regarding what threshold for platelets constitutes safe levels for bronchoscopy. Transfusion guidelines and expert statements have recommended minimum platelet counts of 20,000 to 50,000/mm^3 for fiberoptic bronchoscopy and greater than 50,000/mm^3 for transbronchial biopsy.[13]

Procedure Risks and Complications

The risks of bronchoscopy and anesthesia should be specifically reviewed with the patient. The risk of major complications from bronchoscopy, including pneumothorax, pulmonary hemorrhage, infection, and respiratory failure, is 0.6%. When transbronchial biopsy is performed, the risk of serious complications reaches 1% to 6%.[14] Complications specifically related to rigid bronchoscopy include airway perforation, pneumomediastinum, and fatal hemorrhage due to injury of the great vessels, which are rare. Minor complications from bronchoscopy include fever, cough, bronchospasm, transient hypoxia, and hemoptysis. Additionally, cardiovascular complications can occur from the stress of the procedure itself, particularly in high risk patients. Cardiac events can include vasovagal reactions, arrhythmias, myocardial ischemia, angina, and cardiac arrest.[15] The mortality rate from bronchoscopy is approximately 0.01%, and has decreased in recent years as monitoring capabilities and technology have improved.[14]

Equipment

The rigid bronchoscope is essentially a stainless steel tube with a beveled tip at the distal end, while the proximal end usually contains a series of ports for ventilation, passage of suction catheters, grasping tools, a telescope, or a flexible bronchoscope (Figure 11–1). Fenestrated caps may be placed over the ports to permit closed ventilation during the procedure. Adult bronchoscopes are generally 9 to 13 mm in diameter and 40 cm long, while tracheoscopes are of similar diameter but are only 25 cm in length. Fenestrations are present in the side-wall at the distal end of the bronchoscope to allow for continued ventilation of the opposite lung if the scope is passed down one of the mainstem bronchi during the procedure.

Insertion

Prior to bronchoscope insertion, the patient must be adequately anesthetized. Many centers choose to administer a muscle relaxant as well, although this is not absolutely required. The patient's neck is hyperextended, and with the fingers of the left hand, the upper lip and teeth are covered with the operators thumb, the index finger is inserted into the patient's mouth to displace the tongue towards the left side of the mouth, and the middle finger is used to cover the lower lip and teeth to prevent injury of these structures. The bronchoscope is held in the

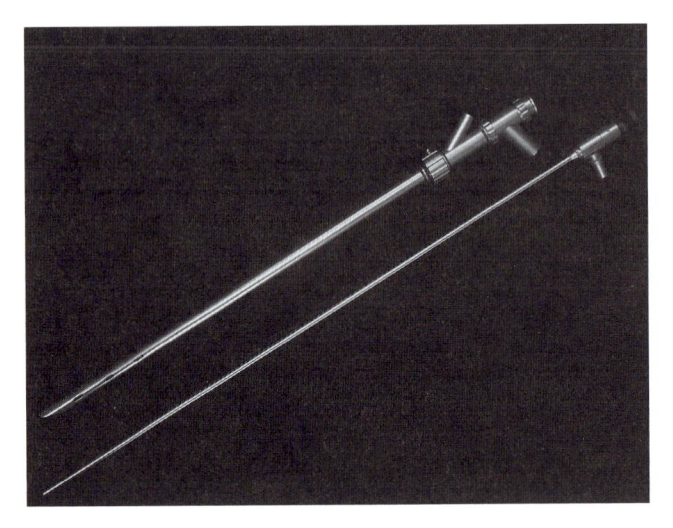

Figure 11-1. Rigid bronchoscope and telescope. Note head portion of bronchoscope with ports for passage of tools and attachment to the anesthesia circuit or jet ventilator adaptor.

right hand with the barrel of the scope resting between the thumb and first finger with the bevel of the distal end of the scope facing down. The tip of the scope is inserted into the patient's mouth against the base of the tongue. The tongue is visualized via the telescope inserted through the bronchoscope, and the scope is advanced along the base of the tongue until the epiglottis is visualized. The bevel of the scope is advanced under the epiglottis, and the tip is rotated upward, using the thumb located over the patient's upper mandible as a fulcrum to lift the epiglottis and bring the vocal cords into view. The scope is then rotated 90 degrees clockwise to allow the beveled tip to slide between the cords. Rotation is continued an additional 90 degrees as the bronchoscope enters the trachea to run the bevel against the posterior wall of the trachea to prevent injury to the membranous tracheal wall.[3]

ANESTHETIC MANAGEMENT FOR RIGID BRONCHOSCOPY

Due to the irritating nature of the rigid intubation, virtually all centers perform rigid bronchoscopy under general anesthesia. Standard American Society of Anesthesiologists' recommended monitoring should be used for these cases. Additionally, a radial arterial line is generally useful for real-time hemodynamic monitoring and for providing access for arterial blood gas analysis as indicated.

The anesthesia plan can be based on a balanced technique with positive pressure ventilation or a spontaneously breathing technique. For spontaneous assisted ventilation,[16] anesthesia is closely titrated to permit spontaneous ventilation. The rigid bronchoscope is capped and the mouth is packed with gauze to provide a seal around the barrel of the bronchoscope. Ventilation is provided by attaching the anesthesia circuit to the side port of the bronchoscope, resulting in a closed system that is suitable for delivery of oxygen and gas anesthetics to the patient if desired. Instruments are introduced into the airway through fenestrated caps on the rigid scope. The patient is lightly anesthetized for the majority of the procedure to permit continued spontaneous ventilation except during particularly noxious portions of the procedure when anesthetics are titrated up to prevent patient motion. At these times, ventilation may need to be supported with positive pressure ventilation, as the patient is likely to become apneic. While an effective technique, some operators find the need for capping the rigid bronchoscope cumbersome, because this limits the number of instruments that may be introduced into the bronchoscope. Also, in order to reduce entrainment of ambient air with subsequent dilution of inspired oxygen and anesthetic gas concentrations, high gas flows are required, which increases the consumption of inhaled anesthetics and pollutes the operating room environment.

Two basic approaches are currently practiced to provide positive pressure ventilation during rigid bronchoscopy. The most basic form uses intermittent apnea while the proceduralist performs the necessary procedures followed by capping of the rigid scope to allow intermittent positive pressure ventilation. This approach becomes quite cumbersome for longer or complex procedures and is not favored by most centers. Therefore, the majority of North American interventional pulmonologists use some form of jet ventilation during rigid bronchoscopy, either a Sander's jet ventilator or an automated jet ventilator, which allows the anesthesiologist to be freed from managing the Sander's jet during the procedure.[17,18]

Limited data exist comparing outcomes between ventilation strategies, however there is some evidence to suggest that spontaneous assisted ventilation may reduce rates of reintubation following rigid bronchoscopy.[16] This result may be partially explained by the need for muscle relaxants with jet ventilation, underscoring the importance of monitoring and avoidance of residual curarization while using this technique. Positive pressure techniques in a paralyzed patient are better suited to the more complex procedures such as airway tumor debulking and customized stent deployment. Therefore, details of the anesthetic technique discussed below focus on this.

Induction of anesthesia is typically intravenous, as this patient population is susceptible to paroxysms of coughing. Standard considerations for rapid sequence induction apply and the choice of induction agent is at the anesthesiologist's discretion, although propofol or ketamine are better suited to patients with preexisting bronchospasm. Procedures generally have a duration of 20 to 60 minutes, and choice of neuromuscular blocker should reflect this. Residual curarization or recurarization in this population will be poorly tolerated,[16] so pancuronium is rarely indicated. A balanced technique is not mandatory but avoids the cardiovascular effects of deep anesthesia that would otherwise be necessary, as bucking or coughing against the rigid bronchoscope can lead to serious tracheal injury. Depending on the circumstance, the trachea can be intubated prior to the bronchoscopic procedure, or more usually induction will occur once the pulmonologist is poised to pass the rigid bronchoscope. The rigid bronchoscope is not cuffed and may not protect against aspiration, but the airway is continuously visualized and endobronchial toilet can be immediately performed should soiling occur.

The passage of the rigid bronchoscope is very stimulating and blunting of the pressor response to intubation can be achieved with short acting opiates such as remifentanil or alfentanil, as postoperative pain is minimal and opiate induced respiratory depression will be dangerous. If the bronchoscope is capped appropriately necessitating intermittent use of the lumen for the procedure, interrupted inhalational anesthesia may be used for maintenance of anesthesia, however, a total intravenous anesthetic (TIVA) technique may better suited to rigid bronchoscopy to ensure continuous anesthesia delivery and avoid interruptions to the procedure. The TIVA should be started at the time of induction through a dedicated intravenous cannula that can easily be inspected to confirm intravenous delivery, especially if hemodynamic parameters or anesthesia depth monitors suggest inadequate anesthesia.

Assuming TIVA is used for maintenance of anesthesia, jet ventilation is used as described below, with either a jet ventilator or manually delivered using a Sanders injector. Adequate tidal volume is estimated by visually appreciating chest rise and is greatly facilitated by reverse Trendelenburg positioning. Arterial blood gas analysis or use of a percutaneous carbon dioxide monitor is advisable to avoid over or under ventilation. Prior to emergence, the patient is intubated with a cuffed endotracheal tube, reexpansion of previously collapsed lung segments is achieved with positive end expiratory pressure, and a final toilet bronchoscopy is performed with a flexible bronchoscope. Full reversal of neuromuscular blockade is confirmed prior to extubation.

This patient population is at high risk for respiratory distress after extubation and consideration should be given to nebulized bronchodilators or lidocaine for bronchospasm or excessive coughing respectively. The team should have a low threshold for awake bronchoscopy to diagnose and treat excessive secretions mobilized from newly expanded lung segments, de novo airway bleeding or stent migration.

Jet Ventilation

Jet ventilation employs a short burst of high-pressure gas delivered through a narrow (often 1-3 mm in diameter) catheter to provide ventilation through an open, uncuffed airway. Tidal volumes are usually low, often significantly less than dead space, with respiratory rates ranging from 60 to 150 breaths per minute. Given the low tidal volumes produced by the jet ventilator, mechanisms other than conventional bulk flow become important for effective gas exchange during jet ventilation.

Five mechanisms have been described to explain gas transport with jet ventilation: (1) Bulk flow or convective gas transport is responsible for gas delivery during conventional mechanical ventilation and likely plays a role in the large airways during jet ventilation as well. (2) Coaxial flow describes movement of gas in one direction down the center of an airway while movement in the opposite direction occurs along the airway periphery. This mechanism is very dependent on airway geometry and occurs more frequently at the site of bifurcations. (3) Taylor dispersion is a complex phenomenon that describes gas dispersion along the front of bulk gas flow. This probably plays the greatest role within the larger airways. (4) Molecular diffusion occurs at the alveolar level and plays a significant role in gas mixing within the alveoli in both jet and conventional ventilation. (5) Pendelluft describes the intra-alveolar mixing of gas due to impedance differences. This phenomenon may also involve airway gas as well and so result in alveolar ventilation.[19]

Other important considerations when using jet ventilation include the site of the injection catheter placement. We generally place the injection catheter at the proximal end of the bronchoscope (Figure 11–2). Others move it deeper into the airway to reduce dead space ventilation. This technique requires continuous airway pressure monitoring to prevent barotrauma, as airway obstruction related to the introduction of instrumentation through the bronchoscope may result in elevations in airway pressure.[20] In addition, caution must be used when central airways obstruction is present as placement of the catheter distal to an airway lesion may result in a ball valve mechanism leading to elevated alveolar pressures and pneumothorax.

There was some concern that ball valve induced barotrauma could also occur with ventilation proximal to sites of central airway obstruction. This question was addressed by Biro et al who used a balloon inflated to different diameters in the large airways during jet ventilation proximal to the site of obstruction and measured airway pressures proximal and distal to the site of obstruction.

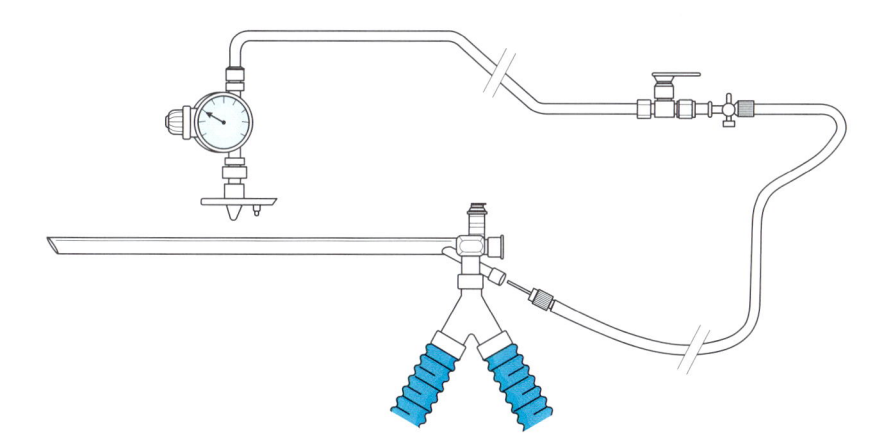

Figure 11–2. Components needed for jet ventilation through the bronchoscope (Sanders injector). Wall connector for oxygen supply, reducing valve and pressure gauge, high-pressure tubing, toggle switch, and needle injector jet. (From: Eisenkraft JB, Neustein SM. *Problems in Anesthesia.* Vol 4. Philadelphia: JB Lippincott, 1990:223, with permission.)

They found that while peak airway pressures rose at the proximal position, distally there was no change in peak pressures, but expiratory pressures rose closer to peak pressures. Since peak pressures were thought to be at a safe level, concerns of elevating airway pressures distal to a central airways stenosis were not substantiated.[21]

Determination of ventilation parameters during jet ventilation can be challenging. The variables that may be changed are frequency, inspiratory time, and inspiratory pressure. Tidal volumes are generally unknown during jet ventilation, but are titrated to the lowest pressure capable of producing a slight chest rise. Increasing respiratory rates may be used to elevate mean airway pressures and enhance oxygenation. Caution should be used when setting I:E ratios greater than 1:2 to permit adequate time for exhalation and to prevent gas trapping.[22] Our practice is to check an arterial blood gas early in the procedure to ensure adequate ventilation, while monitoring oxygenation continuously via a pulse oximeter. When available, use of transcutaneous CO_2 monitoring may be useful in assessing ventilation.

Patients with significant tracheal stenosis can prove difficult to ventilate by jet ventilation with an automated system. This situation may be addressed by performing initial attempts to open the airway using an endotracheal tube and a flexible bronchoscope. Alternatively, manual jet ventilation may provide breath-to-breath adjustment in jet duration to produce chest rise as the obstruction is addressed with conversion to automated ventilation once the initial obstruction has been relieved. Finally, determination of absolute inspired FiO_2 is difficult as gas entrainment of room air is an unpredictable but significant portion of the delivered breath. Consequently, the set FiO_2 and the actual FiO_2 may be very different. Use of additional O_2 delivered via a catheter into the rigid bronchoscope may prove useful in elevating delivered O_2 in patients who prove difficult to oxygenate.

COMPLICATIONS OF JET VENTILATION

Few studies are available detailing complications associated with jet ventilation, specifically with rigid bronchoscopy. Fernandez-Bustamante et al described their experience with 316 patients undergoing rigid bronchoscopy for interventional procedures. Complications were present in 40% of patients. The most common complications were hypercapnea, hypoxemia, and hemodynamic instability. These complications were transient and did not result in an increase in hospital stay. Serious complications included post-anesthesia laryngospasm in 2 patients, pneumothorax in 1 patient and 3 peri-operative deaths related to inability to open an obstructed airway.[23]

In a national survey of the United Kingdom otolaryngologists using high-pressure source ventilation (automated high-frequency jet ventilation and manual jet ventilation), use of manual jet ventilation was associated with greater number of complications including 3 critical care admissions and 3 deaths. Use of high-frequency jet ventilation was associated with 2 critical care admissions and no deaths. However, only 17% of study sites used high-frequency jet ventilation.[24]

THERAPEUTIC PROCEDURES

Central airway obstruction may result from benign or malignant conditions. Benign conditions include tracheal stenosis secondary to endotracheal intubation or following tracheostomy, due to tracheomalacia from disorders such as relapsing polychondritis, Wegener granulomatosis, stenosis at anastomic sites following lung transplantation, and secondary to human papilloma virus infections of the airway.[1] Virtually any type of malignancy can involve the airways, but the most common types are lung cancer, breast cancer, and renal cell carcinoma. Airway obstruction may take one of three forms; extrinsic compression, endobronchial obstruction, and mixed types composed of elements of both endoluminal obstruction and extrinsic compression.[25] Identification of the type of obstruction is important because it helps the physician determine the best course of treatment for relief of central airway obstruction, or if a procedure is likely to be effective.

A variety of therapeutic procedures are available to relieve airway obstruction due to malignancy or benign airway stenosis (Table 11–2). Rapid relief of airway obstruction may be obtained using heat therapy such as endobronchial laser, electrocautery, or argon plasma coagulation (APC).

Laser

Light amplification of stimulated emission of radiation (Laser) was first described for use in the airway in 1976,[26] and is used in many centers as the primary tool for rapid resection of central airway tumors. Several types of laser are available for use in the airway, with each type having advantages and disadvantages regarding ability to produce coagulation, vaporization, and with differing depth of tissue penetration depending on wavelength of light emitted and absorption and scattering of light energy by the tissues of the airway. The most commonly used laser is the neodymium-yttrium aluminum garnet (Nd-YAG) device, with a wavelength of 1064 nm that results in excellent coagulation and vaporization of tissues. The treatment may be applied via a flexible catheter placed through the rigid bronchoscope or via the working channel of a flexible bronchoscope. This allows for devitalization of tumor tissue followed by removal with forceps to open the airway.[25]

Other commonly used lasers include the CO_2 laser favored by ENT surgeons for work on the upper airway. This laser is a cutting laser, and has limited coagulation ability. In addition depth of tissue penetration is more superficial compared with the Nd-YAG laser due to the high degree of absorption of light energy by water in tissues at 1060 nm, which is the CO_2 laser light's wavelength. Until recently, CO_2 lasers were cumbersome to use in the lower airway because the laser light could not be conducted in flexible catheters. However, the recent release of a flexible light guide may increase the use of this device among interventional pulmonologists. The potassium–titanyl-phosphate (5-KTP) laser emits a wavelength of 532 nm with good absorption by vascular structures, and thus is good for treating vascular lesions such as angiomas.[27] The yttrium aluminium pevroskite:neodymium YAP-Nd laser wavelength of 1340 nm produces a moderately good coagulation

Table 11-2. Currently Available Bronchoscopic Ablative Therapies

Modality	Mechanism	Effect	Advantages	Disadvantages
Nd-YAG	Thermal energy produced by laser light	Coagulation and vaporization of tissue	Excellent debulking	Expensive; cumbersome setup
Electrocautery	Thermal energy produced by an electrical current	Coagulation of tissue but more superficial than laser	Excellent safety profile; multiple instrument designs; inexpensive	Contact mode requiring frequent cleaning of probe
Argon plasma coagulation	Thermal energy produced by the interaction between argon gas and an electrical current	Superficial coagulation of tissue	No undesired deep tissue effects	Ineffective for in-depth tissue coagulation or debulking
Photodynamic therapy	Injection of a photosensitizer followed by the destruction of presensitized tumor cells through illumination with nonthermal laser	Delayed destruction of tissue (24-48 h)	Relatively long-lasting effects	Expensive; need for multiple bronchoscopies; skin photosensitivity lasting up to 6 wks
Brachytherapy	Direct delivery of radiation therapy into the airway	Delayed and in-depth destruction of tissue	Long-lasting effect; synergistic with external beam radiation	Higher incidence of complications, particularly hemorrhage
Cryotherapy	Destruction of tissue by alternating cycles of freezing to extreme cold temperatures and thawing	Delayed destruction of tissue (1-2 wks)	Useful for retrieval of foreign objects and removal of large mucous plugs or clots	Not suitable for debulking in acute airway obstruction; need for multiple bronchoscopies

Adapted from Wahidi M, Herth F, Ernst A.[4] With permission from the American College of Chest Physicians.

effect but has questionable vaporization ability. This laser has otherwise similar operating characteristics as the Nd-YAG system.[27]

The principles of safe use of lasers for tumor debulking from the airway were described by Dumon et al in 1984. They emphasized application of laser light along the long axis of the airway to minimize chance of perforation through the airway wall. The laser itself is applied for brief time periods, less than 1 second intervals at modest power settings, with the primary goal of producing tissue coagulation followed by manual removal of desiccated tissue. Control of depth of penetration may be achieved by moving the laser delivery fiber between 0.3 and 1 cm from the tumor tissue. The catheter is moved closer to achieve tissue vaporization or more distant for a coagulative effect.[28] Using this technique, 70% of central airway obstructions are relieved.[25]

In the case of significant hemorrhage, the laser is applied circumferentially around the center of the bleeding to achieve hemostasis, terminating the coagulation at the center of the bleeding site. Oxygenation must remain a priority during any airway procedure, although care must be taken when using any form of heat therapy in the airway. The inspired FiO_2 should be reduced to 40% or less to avoid ignition of flammable components within the airway. Should a patient begin to desaturate, use of the laser must be stopped, FiO_2 must be increased and the airways inspected for possible collections of blood or mucous in the lower airways. The rigid bronchoscope may need to be advanced into the airway to bypass the obstructing tumor while the airway debris is removed. Once adequate oxygenation is restored, tumor debridement may be continued.[28]

The most concerning complications during use of laser therapy are perforation of a major vessel and perforation of the airway and pneumomediastinum. With cautious application of the laser along the axis of the airway, and particular care when treating tumors along the membranous posterior portion of the trachea, significant complication rates are less than 1% in most large series that have been reported.[25]

Although the use of lasers for airway debridement remains popular, the technique has significant drawbacks. Primarily, expensive equipment is required. The equipment may be cumbersome to move due to large size, although many of the newer devices are more portable. Adequate eye protection must be worn by all personnel in the operating theatre to prevent ocular injury, which may be uncomfortable to some providers. Finally, use of reflective devices in the airway must be avoided when possible to prevent inadvertent scattering of the laser beams and injury to the patient or proceduralist.

Electrocautery

Although airway laser remains the most popular technique for management of CAO due to tumor, a similar effect can be obtained using pulsed electrical field and an electrocautery probe extended through the rigid or flexible bronchoscope. In this case the tissue is devitalized using direct contact, permitting excellent control of tissue destruction. The electrocautery is fired in short bursts with frequent observation of the underlying tissue injury to avoid unwanted extension of the

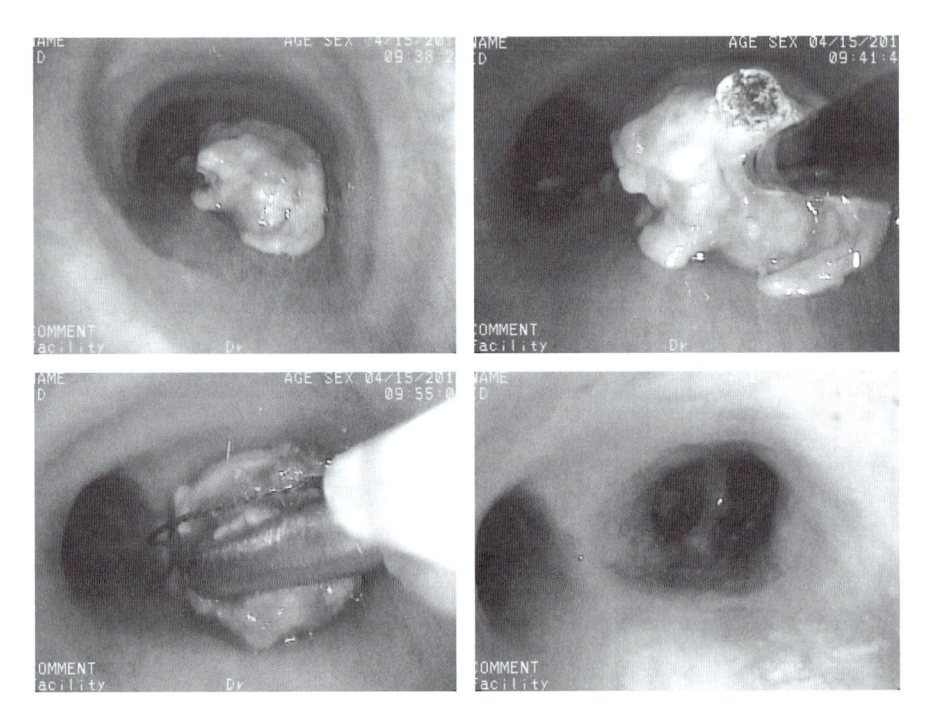

Figure 11-3. Debridement of an anaplastic large cell carcinoma. Upper left: A large polypoid mass is extending from the right upper lobe into the trachea. The lumen of the left mainstem bronchus can be seen distal to the mass. Upper right: Application of electrocautery to coagulate the proximal portion of the mass allowing safe debridement. Lower left: Application of a cautery snare to remove large portions of the tumor. The forceps are used to stabilize the piece of tissue once it has been freed from the main mass and prevent it from migrating to the left mainstem bronchus producing an obstruction of the uninvolved lung. Lower right: View from the trachea showing the right mainstem bronchus after debridement of the mass. The right upper lobe is entirely occluded with tumor, but the remaining airways of the right lung are patent.

coagulation effect. Similar to laser therapy, devitalized tissue may then be removed with the use of grasping forceps with a minimum of bleeding[1,4] (Figure 11–3). There have been no direct comparisons of laser therapy and electrocautery for the relief of central airways obstruction, however reported efficacy has been similar with both techniques. Similar precautions to those used during laser debridement must be observed, particularly when treating tumors adherent to or arising from the airway wall. Electrocautery has an advantage in that it requires less investment in equipment and does not require the use of special eye protection or the avoidance of reflective surfaces during its use. The primary disadvantage with use of electrocautery is that the probe tip may become fouled with tissue debris during repeated use requiring intermittent cleaning during the procedure.

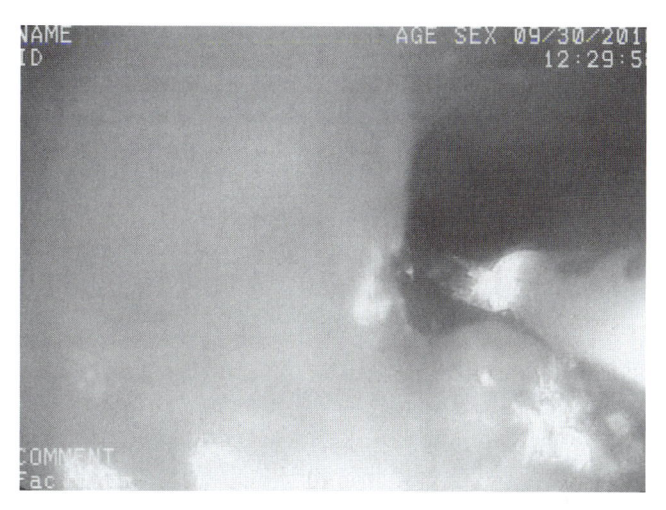

Figure 11–4. Argon plasma coagulation used to treat the base of a resected carcinoid tumor to prevent additional bleeding.

Argon Plasma Coagulation

An additional technique that uses heat therapy is argon plasma coagulation (APC). This technique employs argon gas which, when exposed to high voltage becomes ionized (plasma) and conducts electricity to underlying tissue, resulting in a superficial coagulation effect. APC is a noncontact technique, in that the electrical energy is carried by the gas to the underlying tissue, and so this technique may be used to deliver energy around corners and is difficult to reach locations in the airway. The effect of APC is more superficial than either laser or electrocautery, causing coagulation to a depth of 2 to 3 mm within the airway.[29] This limited penetration provides the ability to "spray" the coagulation effect within the airway making APC a useful tool for control of airway bleeding and devitalization of granulation tissue (Figure 11–4). The superficial coagulation effect also makes APC extremely safe resulting in lower rates of complications such as airway perforation and massive hemorrhage,[30] although there are theoretical concerns for the development of gas embolism with higher flow rates and longer pulse duration with the use of APC.[31]

Airway Fire

Special comment should be made on the concern for airway fire during the use of heat-based therapy. Airway fire has been well-recognized as a potential complication during the use of laser treatment of the airways. Risks for the development of airway fire include inspired oxygen levels greater than 40%, longer duration of treatment, increased power application, and application of heat near a combustible element such as a flexible bronchoscope or plastic endotracheal tube.[32] To reduce the risk of airway fire the FiO_2 must be reduced to 0.40 or less prior to the application of a heat based therapy. It is our practice to use the minimal amount of O_2 tolerated during these procedures. Only rarely will we use heat-based treatments with the FiO_2 greater than 0.30. Furthermore, power settings should be reduced to the minimum levels necessary to achieve effect in order to avoid excessive heating within the airway. Should an airway fire ensue, it is critical to remove the burning elements including the endotracheal tube immediately to avoid thermal injury to the airway, as well as injury from smoke inhalation.

Balloon Bronchoplasty

Treatment of airway stenosis following tracheostomy or lung transplantation may be performed using inflatable balloons or rigid dilators to disrupt the fibrous connective tissue that forms at the site of the prior airway injury.[33] Often, a combination of techniques such as use of an electrocautery knife to cut the membranous region of a stenosis followed by dilation with an inflatable balloon and removal of granulation tissue with forceps is required to achieve the desired result. Finally, the rigid bronchoscope itself can be used as a therapeutic instrument to "core out" central airway tumors after adequate desiccation and coagulation have been performed using laser therapy or electrocautery.[25]

THERAPIES WITH DELAYED EFFECT

In addition to the rapidly acting procedures above, there are several therapies that provide delayed effect in debulking airway malignancies. Cryotherapy is a safe and effective method that uses nitrous oxide gas to cool the tip of a metal probe placed through the working channel of the flexible bronchoscope. Once the gas flow is activated, the tip of the catheter rapidly cools to induce freezing of tissues at the point of contact and a small margin of surrounding tissue. The tissue thaws and the cycle may be repeated. The freeze-thawing of tissues results in delayed necrosis and sloughing of the treated area over the next several days.[34] This technique has been shown to be effective in tumor debulking and improving central airways obstruction. Cryotherapy is also useful for removal of foreign bodies.[35] The tip of the probe is placed on the foreign body, and the gas flow is activated resulting in the foreign body being frozen to the catheter tip. The foreign body is then removed from the patient by removing the flexible bronchoscope with the catheter still in the working channel without turning off the gas flow.

Additional delayed efficacy treatments include photodynamic therapy, which employs a systemically administered photosensitizing agent prior to the procedure that is preferentially concentrated by tumor cells. Photphrin is currently the only sensitizing agent licensed for use in the United States. When stimulated by light of 630 nm via an argon/dye or diode laser applied through a light guide, oxygen radicals are produced in tissues, which have concentrated the previously administered medication, resulting in tissue necrosis.[36] Often necrosis is so exuberant that a repeat procedure is needed in 24 to 48 hours after light administration to debride necrotic tumor that can cause airway obstruction. Efficacy is good in patients with central airways tumors where up to 70% report improvement in symptoms of dyspnea.[33] Primary complications include severe sunburn due to the photosensitizing effect of the medication which may last as long as 6 weeks, and bleeding due to the destruction of vascular tumor.[37]

Finally, brachytherapy is a palliative technique that employs locally delivered radionuclide for treatment of endobronchial tumor resulting in central airway obstruction. The advantages of this approach are: delivery of high-dose radiation directly to the tumor tissue with limited penetration to surrounding tissue due to the rapid drop off of radiation dose with distance from the source, ability to modify the area of treatment to conform to the shape of the tumor, and ability to precisely target the tissue of interest.[37] The radionuclide most commonly used is iridium-192 delivered in an encapsulated form via a polyethylene catheter inserted via the working channel of the flexible bronchoscope. The catheter is placed adjacent to the area to be treated and the bronchoscope removed. The catheter is then secured at the nose or mouth, and the position is confirmed using fluoroscopy. The iridium source is then afterloaded into the catheter and dwells for a period of time until the desired dose is delivered, generally 7 Gy for high-dose applications, and the catheter and source removed from the patient. Efficacy for symptom palliation ranges from 65% to 95%.[38-40] A recent Cochrane review examined efficacy between external beam radiation therapy and high-dose endobronchial therapy and showed no difference between the two treatments.[41] Complications are rare, although fatal hemoptysis is reported in 2% to 11% of treated patients.[40]

AIRWAY STENTING

Types of stents

Modern airway stenting began as a modification of the Montgomery T-tube, with silicone stents popularized by Dumon in the late 1980s.[42] Shortly afterwards, the self-expandable metal stent was developed and became widely used due to its ease of deployment without the need for rigid bronchoscopy as is required for silicone stent placement.[43] More recently, hybrid metal-silicone stents have been developed which share some of the advantages and disadvantages of each type of stent.

SILICONE STENTS

Silicone stents are composed of silicone sleeves fitted with external studs to retard stent migration in the airway (Figure 11–5). The stent wall is relatively thick at 2 mm and so significant portions of the airway lumen may be occupied in smaller (<10 mm outer diameter) stents. Stents are sized from 10 to 20 mm in outer diameter and in lengths ranging from 2 to 8 cm. In addition, Y-shaped stents are available for placement at the main carina with limbs of the Y extending proximally into the trachea and distally into each of the mainstem bronchi. The limbs of the Y are not symmetrically angled, but instead are more acute for the left mainstem bronchus take-off to accommodate the positioning of the two mainstem bronchi.

Rigid bronchoscopy is required for silicone stent placement. During deployment, the stent is rolled along the long axis and placed into a steel delivery tube sized the same length as the rigid bronchoscope (Figure 11–6). The bronchoscope is advanced to the

208 Part 2 / Thoracic Anesthesia Practice

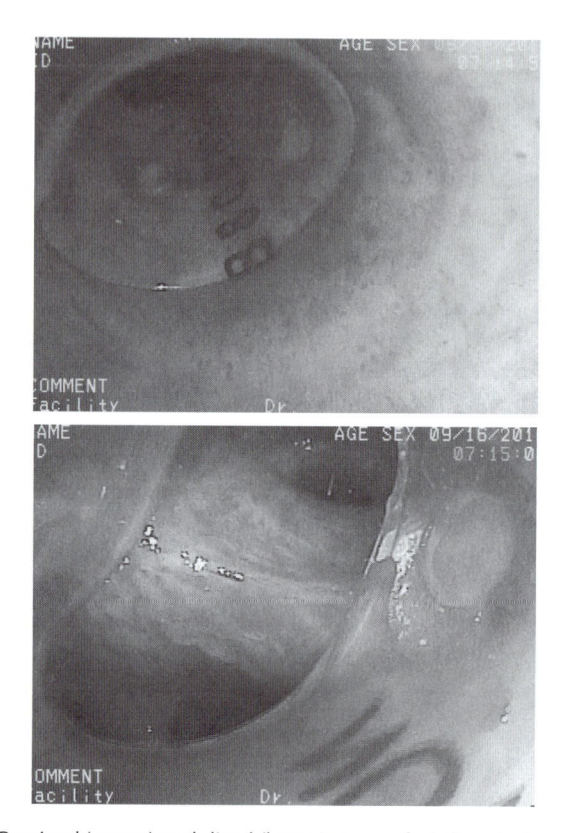

Figure 11–5. Proximal (upper) and distal (lower) views of a left mainstem silicone stent.

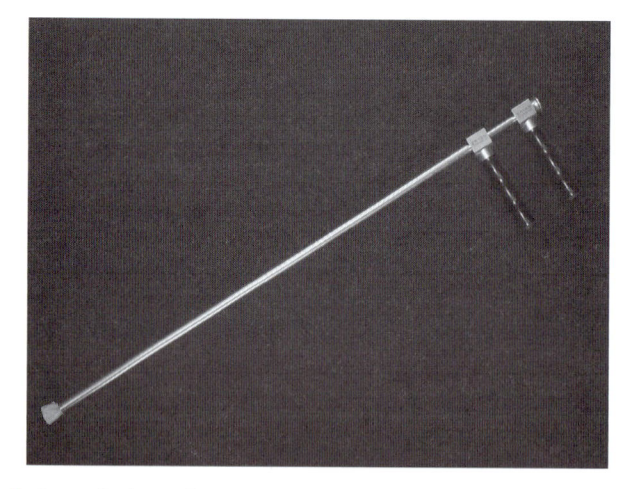

Figure 11–6. Stent deployer for Dumon style silicone stents. The deployer consists of a tube that has the stent inserted into it and a pushrod. A silicone stent can be seen partially deployed at the end of the insertion rod.

mid-point of the desired airway obstruction and the deployment tube is inserted into the bronchoscope. The stent is then pushed forward using a pushrod placed down the deployment tube, followed by removal of both the pushrod and deployment tube. The rigid scope is then withdrawn while holding the incompletely expanded stent in place until the proximal end is free from the bronchoscope. Generally, the stent will fully expand, but occasionally it may need to be opened using a dilation balloon. If the stent has been positioned distal to the area of narrowing, it may be dragged proximally using large forceps, however, stents that have been placed too proximally cannot be advanced, and must be removed and reinserted.

SELF-EXPANDING METAL STENTS

Self-expanding metallic stents were introduced in the mid-1990s as an alternative to silicone stents. The majority of these stents are constructed of nitinol, an alloy composed of nickel and titanium. This metal has the properties of being flexible while retaining excellent shape memory and so can be compressed onto a factory packaged deployment rod that will expand to its initial diameter after it is deployed. These stents are less likely to migrate than silicone stents[44] as they rapidly embed into the surrounding mucosa. They are also less likely to become occluded with secretions, because the open meshwork of the stent allows normal ciliary function of the underlying mucosa to move secretions into the upper airway. However, lumen occlusion with granulation tissue or recurrent tumor can be a significant problem with these stents. In addition, once metallic stents are placed they are rapidly incorporated into the airway wall making removal very difficult.[45] Over time, stress fractures often develop in the stents resulting in loose wires, which may migrate through the airway wall causing injury to the surrounding lung and mediastinal structures. Because of these complications, the American College of Chest Physicians and the FDA have recently issued warnings against the use of metallic airway stents for benign airway diseases.[46]

An advantage of metal stents over silicone stents is the ability to be placed without the need for rigid bronchoscopy, but rather using a flexible bronchoscope and fluoroscopic guidance. To achieve this, the patient is examined with a flexible bronchoscope under moderate sedation. The obstructed airway of interest is identified, the lesion is measured using the bronchoscope, and a guidewire is passed through the working channel of the bronchoscope across the area of stenosis. Next, the bronchoscope is positioned at the distal and proximal ends of the stenosis, and surface markers are placed on the patient's chest under fluoroscopy. The bronchoscope is removed with the guidewire left in place. The self-expandable metal stent is then passed over the guidewire, positioned in the airway between the previously placed surface markers and deployed under fluoroscopy to ensure accurate positioning.

HYBRID STENTS

Hybrid silicone and nitinol stents have recently been developed which share some of the characteristics of silicone and metallic stents. These stents are constructed of a polyurethane or silicone sleeve with supporting nitinol struts. They share many of the advantages of metal stents in that they are self-expanding and so may be deployed across a tight stenosis and act to open the lesion via the radial force exerted by the wire mesh (Figure 11–7). The silicone sleeve prevents tumor

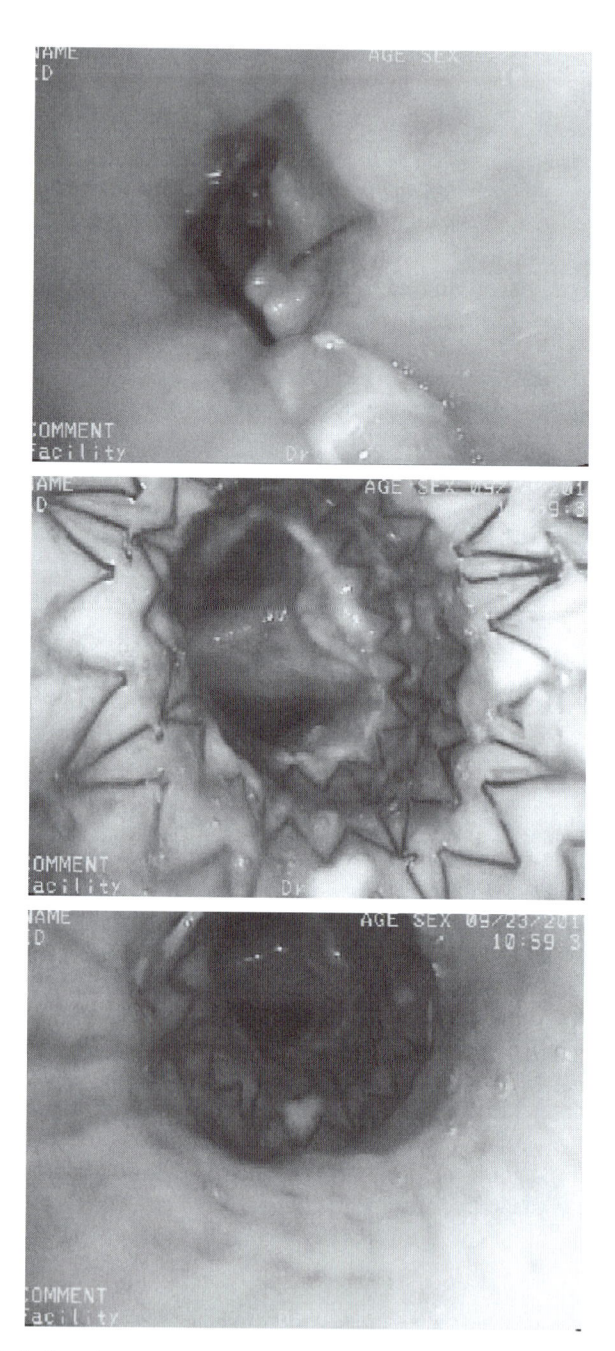

Figure 11-7. Left mainstem anastomosis stenosis in a patient after bilateral orthotopic lung transplantation. (Upper) View of the left anastomosis from the proximal left mainstem bronchus showing a 75% occlusion of the airway. (Middle) Distal view through the hybrid metal-silicone stent showing the upper and lower lobe orifices. (Lower) Proximal view of the left mainstem stent from the main carina.

in-growth through the stent, and also prevents the stent from granulating into the airway wall. This enhances patency as well as allows for removal of the stent at a later time if needed.

One disadvantage of these stents has recently been recognized related to the open nature of the nitinol struts. These struts may fold inward on themselves during vigorous coughing or breathing. Generally they will re-expand to their original dimensions, but occasionally they remain collapsed. Case reports exist describing severe shortness of breath associated with collapsed tracheal stents requiring urgent removal.[47] Due to this complication, we avoid placing these stents in the trachea when an alternative type of stent is available.

Efficacy and Complications of Stent Placement

Stents are generally effective in improving airway patency,[48] and are associated with increases in FEV_1.[49] There are no randomized trials evaluating stent efficacy, survival benefit, or head-to-head comparisons of efficacy between types of stent. In addition, optimal placement of airway stents may be more complicated than previously perceived. Miyazawa et al examined flow-limiting segments of malignant airway stenosis in 64 patients using ultrathin bronchoscopy, flow volume loops, and 3-dimensional computed tomography reconstruction before and after central airways stenting. They found that the flow limiting segment migrated distally in 15% of patients after stent placement requiring additional airway stent deployment to optimize respiratory function.[50] Significant complications are common and are as high as 50% in some series. Common complications include stent migration and occlusion by secretions, occasionally with significant airway obstruction requiring emergent procedures to clear the impacted secretions.

Choice of therapeutic approach is based on a variety of variables including the patient's degree of dyspnea, location of tumor, whether the tumor is primarily endobronchial, or if the airway obstruction is secondary to extrinsic compression, equipment availability, and the level of local experience with the various techniques.

Our approach is initially to attempt to restore airway patency using a heat-based treatment in combination with manual debridement. Stent placement is usually reserved for the treatment of some component of extrinsic compression, although it is common to encounter CAO due to mixed intrinsic and extrinsic airway disease. The optimal use of airway stents in the setting of successfully resected intrinsic tumor is still controversial and requires further study. Generally speaking, the rapid effect of heat based therapies may have a less durable effect in the absence of additional treatment such as airway stenting, palliative radiation, or chemotherapy. Treatments such as photodynamic therapy or brachytherapy may delay the recurrence of tumor, and so may result in a longer lasting tumor reduction. Currently, there is no data available comparing efficacy between techniques. There is no demonstrated increase in life expectancy with the use of any of the above treatments, but substantial data exist suggesting efficacy in providing symptomatic relief.[51-55]

CASE REPORTS

The objective of this section is to provide examples of our approach to a variety of situations and to highlight the need for a multimodality approach to central airways disorders.

Case 1

The patient is a 36-year-old female diagnosed with refractory asthma with progressive shortness of breath for over 2 years. A CT scan of the chest shows significant obstruction of the mid-trachea extending to both mainstem bronchi. Minimal diameter of the trachea is 7 mm. Due to the difficulties in providing adequate oxygenation using jet ventilation in patients with high-grade tracheal stenoses, the initial ventilation strategy employed a large laryngeal mask airway to provide ventilation. A flexible bronchoscope was placed through the LMA and electrocautery was used to perform initial desiccation of the airway tumor. Close attention was paid to aspirating any blood or mucous released into the airway during this process to prevent obstruction of the narrowed airway.

Once the tracheal lumen was enlarged enough to allow for adequate ventilation via the jet ventilator, the rigid bronchoscope was inserted. Additional electrocautery was performed at the trachea and bilateral mainstem bronchi followed by "coring out" of the tumor using the barrel of the rigid bronchoscope to further enlarge the distal trachea and mainstem bronchi to near normal diameter. Additional tumor was removed with manual debridement using large forceps through the barrel of the rigid bronchoscope. At this point the airways were adequately debulked. There was a component of extrinsic compression that warranted further treatment via deployment of self-expandable metal stents. In this case covered stents were deployed at the left and right mainstem to prevent reocclusion of the airway by tumor. Finally, to maintain patency of the trachea, a silicone stent was deployed at the distal trachea just above the takeoff of the mainstem bronchi. While the stent was in place at the termination of the procedure, it ultimately migrated proximally within the airway due to the cone shaped distal trachea secondary to distortion of the anatomy by tumor. We elected not to place a self-expanding metal stent in this area because the terminal 0.5 cm of these stents is uncovered to allow anchoring in the airway. This would allow for tumor infiltration of the stent and may cause recurrent airway obstruction in the future. A hybrid stent was not placed due to concerns for buckling of the stent resulting in airway obstruction.

The patient was diagnosed with adenoid cystic carcinoma of the central airways and initiated chemotherapy and radiotherapy with stabilization of her airway disease and has had normal respiratory function for 2 years following her diagnosis.

Case 2

The patient is a 68-year-old female who underwent a bilateral orthotopic lung transplant for treatment of endstage idiopathic pulmonary fibrosis. Her initial postoperative course was uncomplicated with the exception of mild rejection in the first postoperative month that was successfully treated with corticosteroids. Four months following transplantation her FEV_1 had declined to 0.83 liters from a posttransplantation peak of 1.51 liters. On bronchoscopy she was noted to have stenosis of her right mainstem anastomosis that was occluding 75% of the lumen diameter. This was treated with balloon dilation bronchoplasty using a 3 cm by 12 mm in diameter balloon. This resulted in improvement of her FEV_1 to 1.04 liters. Two months later, her FEV_1 had declined again to 0.93 liters and she was noted to have recurrent right mainstem stenosis on flexible bronchoscopy. She underwent rigid bronchoscopy with repeat bronchoplasty. The lesion was complex, composed of a relatively large right mainstem bronchus that substantially narrowed to a relatively small bronchus intermedius.

Post-transplant bronchial stenosis is present in up to 15% of patients. The etiology of these lesions is not entirely understood, but ischemia of the bronchial wall is thought to play an important role in the development of airway stenosis. These lesions often require airway stenting to stabilize the stenotic site. The ideal stent for treatment of stenoses at the anastomosis site should be covered to prevent in-growth and occlusion of the stent by granulation tissue, and should be removable as it is thought that the stenotic lesions will remodel over time permitting removal of the stent and avoiding complications of a foreign body in the airway. We prefer to place silicone stents in these situations for the reasons stated above.

The rapid tapering of the airway from the mainstem bronchus to the bronchus intermedius prevented the use of a conventional silicone stent, because use of a stent large enough to fit snugly in the mainstem bronchus would be too large to anchor in the bronchus intermedius. Placement of a stent in the mainstem bronchus alone would be too short distal to the stenosis and would likely migrate into the proximal airway. To overcome these obstacles we selected a tapering silicone stent with a 10 mm outer diameter distal portion and a 12 mm outer diameter proximal portion. In addition, because this stent was going to cover the orifice of the right upper lobe, we cut a window in the stent corresponding to the location of the right upper lobe to permit ventilation of that airway. Following stent placement the patient's FEV_1 increased to 1.48 liters. The patient had no complications related to the stent and it was successfully removed 5 months following placement. The underlying stenosis appeared to have remodeled, and her FEV_1 post-stent removal was 1.99 liters.

Case 3—Clinical Vignette

Considering the patient presented at the beginning of the chapter, two management decisions are required at the time of the procedure. The first relates to re-establishing airway patency. In the setting of prior endobronchial tumor, we can assume that some type of covered stent was initially deployed. This will limit our ability to provide heat-based therapy due to increased risk of airway fire or damage to a metal stent. Both lasers and electrocautery have been shown to increase risk of damage to metal stents resulting in wire breakage and loss of stent integrity. Argon plasma coagulation may be used safely in the presence of metallic stents, although stents covered with silicone or plastic coatings are still at risk for ignition. If the stent currently placed is covered metal, it has likely been infiltrated by the tumor at the uncovered ends and may prove extremely difficult to remove. In this case we would use judicious APC in combination with manual debridement to remove the obstructing mass. If a silicone or hybrid stent had been placed it may be possible to remove it, treat the underlying tumor bed, and replace the stent once adequate debridement had taken place.

The second decision would revolve around which consolidative therapy to employ in order to provide a more durable suppression of the airway tumor and maximize the palliative benefit of the procedure. In this case, consultation with the patient's oncologist and radiation oncologist will be important. If different chemotherapies are still available, a systemic therapy would be a good first choice to suppress further tumor growth. If the patient has not received maximal radiotherapy, application of external beam radiation or brachytherapy for local treatment may be viable options. If no additional chemotherapy or radiotherapy is available, we would advocate the use of photodynamic treatment for devitalization of the local tumor bed to provide a longer symptom free interval for the patient.

CONCLUSION

Therapeutic bronchoscopy may be employed for treatment of a variety of benign and malignant airway conditions. These procedures require good communication between the anesthesia and procedural teams to ensure patient safety and a satisfactory outcome for these often critically ill patients. Rigid bronchoscopic procedures often pose unusual ventilatory challenges, and a good working knowledge of different ventilator strategies, in combination with flexibility in anesthetic management is necessary for all parties involved with these procedures.

REFERENCES

1. Ernst A, Feller-Kopman D, Becker H, Mehta A. Central airway obstruction. *Am J Respir Crit Care*. 2004;169:1278-1297.
2. Santacruz J, Mehta A. Airway complications and management after lung transplantation. *Proc Am Thorac Soc*. 2009;6:79-93.
3. Beamis J. Modern use of rigid bronchoscopy. In: Bollinger C, Mathur PN, eds. *Interventional Bronchoscopy*. Basel, Switzerland: S Karger; 2000.
4. Wahidi M, Herth F, Ernst A. State of the art: interventional pulmonology. *Chest*. 2007;131:261-274.
5. Kozak E, Brath L. Do "screening" coagulation tests predict bleeding in patients undergoing fiberoptic bronchoscopy with biopsy? *Chest*. 1994;106(3):703-705.
6. Djukanovic R, Wilson J, Lai C, Holgate S, Howarth P. The safety aspects of fiberoptic bronchoscopy, bronchoalveolar lavage, and endobronchial biopsy in asthma. *Am Rev Respir Dis*. 1991;143(4 Pt 1):772-777.
7. Bajwa M, Henein S, Kamholz S. Fiberoptic bronchoscopy in the presence of space-occupying intracranial lesions. *Chest*. 1993;104(1):101-103.
8. Kerwin A, Croce M, Timmons S, Maxwell R, Malhotra A, Fabian T. Effects of fiberoptic bronchoscopy on intracranial pressure in patients with brain injury: a prospective clinical study. *J Trauma*. 2000;48(5):878-882.
9. Wahidi MM, Rocha AT, Hollingsworth JW, Govert JA, Feller-Kopman D, Ernst A. Contraindications and safety of transbronchial lung biopsy via flexible bronchoscopy. A survey of pulmonologists and review of the literature. *Respiration*. 2005;72(3):285-295.
10. Zavala D. Pulmonary hemorrhage in fiberoptic transbronchial biopsy. *Chest*. 1976;70(5):585-588.

11. Herth F, Becker H, Ernst A. Aspirin does not increase bleeding complications after transbronchial biopsy. *Chest.* 2002;122(4):1461-1464.
12. Ernst A, Eberhardt R, Wahidi M, Becker H, Herth F. Effect of routine clopidogrel use on bleeding complications after transbronchial biopsy in humans. *Chest.* 2006;129(3):734-737.
13. Rebulla P. Platelet transfusion trigger in difficult patients. *Transfus Clin Biol.* 2001;8(3):249-254.
14. Pue C, Pacht E. Complications of fiberoptic bronchoscopy at a university hospital. *Chest.* 1995;107(2):430-432.
15. Matot I, Kramer M, Glantz L, Drenger B, Cotev S. Myocardial ischemia in sedated patients undergoing fiberoptic bronchoscopy. *Chest.* 1997;112(6):1454-1458.
16. Perrin G, Colt H, Martin C, Mak M, Dumon J, Gouin F. Safety of interventional rigid bronchoscopy using intravenous anesthesia and spontaneous assisted ventilation. A prospective study. *Chest.* 1992;102(5):1526-1530.
17. Conacher I. Anaesthesia and tracheobronchial stenting for central airway obstruction in adults. *Brit J Anaesthesia.* 2003;90(3):367-374.
18. Godden D, Willey R, Fergusson R, Wright D, Compton G, Grant I. Rigid bronchoscopy under intravenous general anesthesia with oxygen venturi ventilation. *Thorax.* 1987;37(7):532-534.
19. Chang H. Mechanisms of gas transport during ventilation by high frequency oscillation. *J Appl Physiol Respir Environ Exercise Physiol.* 1984;56(3):553-563.
20. Unzueta M, Casas I, Merten A, Landeira J. Endobronchial high-frequency jet ventilation for endobronchial laser surgery: an alternative approach. *Anesth Analg.* 2003;96(1):298-300.
21. Biro P, Layer M, Becker H, et al. Influence of airway-occluding instruments on airway pressure during jet ventilation for rigid bronchoscopy. *Br J Anaesth.* 2000;85(3):462-465.
22. MacIntyre NR. High-frequency ventilation. In: MacIntyre NR, Branson RD, eds. *Mechanical Ventilation.* Philadelphia, PA: WB Saunders Co; 2001.
23. Fernandez-Bustamante A, Ibanez V, Alfara J, et al. High-frequency jet ventilation in interventional bronchoscopy: factors with predictive value on high-frequency jet ventilation complications. *J Clin Anesth.* 2006;18(5):349-356.
24. Cook T, Alexander R. Major complications during anaesthesia for elective laryngeal surgery in the UK: a national survey of the use of high-pressure source ventilation. *Br J Anaesth.* 2008;101(2):266-272.
25. Bollinger C, Sutedja T, Strausz J, Freitag L. Therapeutic bronchoscopy with immediate effect: laser, electrocautery, argon plasma coagulation and stents. *Eur Respir J.* 2006;27(6):1258-1271.
26. Laforet E, Berger R, Vaughan C. Carcinoma obstructing the trachea. Treatment by laser resection. *N Engl J Med.* 1976;294(17):941.
27. Diaz-Jimenez J, Rodriquez A, eds. *Laser Bronchoscopy for Malignant Disease*: CRC Press; 2004. Beamis J, Mathur P, Mehta A, eds. *Interventional Pulmonary Medicine: Lung Biology in Health and Disease*; No. 189.
28. Dumon J, Shapshay S, Bourcereau J, et al. Principles for safety in application of neodymium-YAG laser in bronchology. *Chest.* 1984;86(2):163-168.
29. Keller C, Hinerman R, Singh A, Alvarez F. The use of endoscopic argon plasma coagulation in airway complications after solid organ transplantation. *Chest.* 2001;119(6):1968-1975.
30. Morice R, Ece T, Ece F, Keus L. Endobronchial argon plasma coagulation for treatment of hemoptysis and neoplastic airway obstruction. *Chest.* 2001;119(3):781-787.
31. Feller-Kopman D, Lukanich J, Shapira G, et al. Gas flow during bronchoscopic ablation therapy causes gas emboli to the heart: a comparative animal study. *Chest.* 2008;133(4):892-896.
32. Casey K, Fairfax W, Smith S, Dixon J. Intratracheal fire ignited by the Nd-YAG laser during treatment of tracheal stenosis. *Chest.* 1983;84(3):295-296.
33. Vergnon J, Huber R, Moghissi K. Place of cryotherapy, brachytherapy and photodynamic therapy in therapeutic bronchoscopy of lung cancers. *Eur Respir J.* 2006;28(1):200-218.
34. Ferretti G, Jouvan F, Thony F, Pison C, Coulomb M. Benign noninflammatory bronchial stenosis: treatment with balloon dilation. *Radiology.* 1995;196(3):831-834.
35. Reddy A, Govert J, Sporn T, Wahidi M. Broncholith removal using cryotherapy during flexible bronchoscopy. *Chest.* 2007;132(5):1661-1663.
36. Mang TS. Lasers and light sources for PDT: past, present, and future. *Photodiagnosis Photodyn Ther.* 2004;1:43-48.

37. Lee P, Kupeli E, Mehta A. Therapeutic bronchoscopy in lung cancer. *Clin Chest Med.* 2002;23(1): 241-256.
38. Spratling L, Speiser B. Endoscopic brachytherapy. *Chest Surg Clin N Am.* 1996;6(2):293-304.
39. Huber R, Fischer R, Hautmann H, et al. Palliative endobronchial brachytherapy for central lung tumors: a prospective randomized comparison of two fractionation schedules. *Chest.* 1995;107(2):463-470.
40. Ozkok S, Karakoyun-Celik O, Goksel T, et al. High dose rate endobronchial brachytherapy in the management of lung cancer: response and toxicity evaluation in 158 patients. *Lung Cancer.* 2008;62(3):326-333.
41. Zorrilla AC, Reveiz L, Ospina E, Yepes A. Palliative endobronchial brachytherapy for non-small cell lung cancer. *Cochrane Database Syst Rev.* 2008;2:CD004284.
42. Dumon J. A dedicated tracheobronchial stent. *Chest.* 1990;97(2):328-332.
43. Freitag L. Tracheobronchial stents. In: Bollinger C, Mathur P, eds. *Interventional Bronchoscopy.* Vol 30. Basel: Karger; 2000:171-186.
44. Chan A, Juarez M, Allen R, Albertson T. Do airway metallic stents for benign lesions confer too costly a benefit? *BMC Pulm Med.* 2008;8:7-15.
45. Lunn W, Feller-Kopman D, Wahidi M, Ashiku S, Thurer R, Ernst A. Endoscopic removal of metallic airway stents. *Chest.* 2005;127(6):2106-2112.
46. Lund W, Force S. Airway stenting for patients with benign airway disease and the Food and Drug Administration advisory: a call for restraint. *Chest.* 2007;132(4):1107-1108.
47. Trisolini R, Paioli D, Fornario V, Agli L, Grosso D, Patelli M. Collapse of a new type of self-expanding metallic tracheal stent. *Monaldi Arch Chest Dis.* 2006;65(1):56-58.
48. Dumon J, Cavaliere S, Diaz-Jimenez J, et al. Seven-year experience with the Dumon prosthesis. *J Bronchol.* 1996;3:6-10.
49. Vergnon J, Costes F, Bayon M, Emonot A. Efficacy of tracheal and bronchial stent placement on respiratory functional tests. *Chest.* 1995;107(3):741-746.
50. Miyazawa T, Miyazu Y, Iwamoto Y, et al. Stenting at the flow-limiting segment in tracheobronchial stenosis due to lung cancer. *Am J Respir Crit Care.* 2004;169(10):1096-1102.
51. Wood D, Liu Y, Vallieres E, Karmy-Jones R, Mulligan M. Airway stenting for malignant and benign tracheobronchial stenosis. *Ann Thorac Surg.* 2003;76(1):167-172.
52. Saad C, Murthy S, Krizmanich G, Mehta A. Self-expandable metallic airway stents and flexible bronchoscopy: long-term outcomes analysis. *Chest.* 2003;124(5):1993-1999.
53. Dasgupta A, Dolmatch B, Abi-Saleh W, Mathur P, Mehta A. Self-expandable metallic airway stent insertion employing flexible bronchoscopy: preliminary results. *Chest.* 1998;114(1):106-109.
54. Bollinger C, Probst R, Tschopp K, Soler M, Perruchoud A. Silicone stents in the management of inoperable tracheobronchial stenosis: indications and limitations. *Chest.* 1993;104(6):1653-1659.
55. Lemaire A, Burfeind W, Toloza E, et al. Outcomes of tracheobronchial stents in patients with malignant airway disease. *Ann Thorac Surg.* 2005;80(2):434-438.

Mediastinal Masses: Implications for Anesthesiologists

12

Shahar Bar-Yosef

Key Points

1. The patient with an anterior mediastinal mass who undergoes general anesthesia is at risk of developing severe perioperative complications, including complete airway obstruction, severe hypoxemia, profound hypotension, and cardiac arrest.
2. Predictors of perioperative complications in these patients include significant respiratory symptomatology at baseline, greater than 50% tracheal narrowing on CT scan, pericardial effusion, and SVC syndrome.
3. The basic tenets of anesthesia for these patients include preservation of spontaneous breathing, securing the airway beyond the point of obstruction, the ability to rapidly change the patient's position, and preparation of options for managing emergencies, including rigid bronchoscopy, helium-oxygen gas mixture and CPB.

Case Vignette

A 15-year-old male patient complains of several weeks onset of cough and dyspnea, especially on lying flat. A chest x-ray taken to rule out pneumonia shows an anterior mediastinal mass. He has no other medical problems and takes no medications other than vitamins. Vital signs: BP 105/70, HR 95, room air SpO_2 96% (sitting up). Laboratory studies are unremarkable except for leukocytosis and mild anemia. He is referred for a surgical biopsy of the mass.

For the anesthesia practitioner, mediastinal masses have been described as a catastrophe waiting to happen. Complete airway occlusion and cardiovascular collapse are well-recognized complications of general anesthesia in these patients, related to pressure on and compression of nearby major airways, blood vessels, the lung and the heart. Mildly symptomatic or even asymptomatic patients might develop severe airway and vascular obstruction during induction of general anesthesia, endangering the patient's life.[1] It is important, therefore, to understand the anatomy and pathophysiology of mediastinal masses, to perform an adequate preoperative evaluation of the patient, and to formulate a clear anesthetic plan to ensure safe delivery of anesthesia.

CLINICAL ASPECTS OF MEDIASTINAL MASSES

Anatomy of the Mediastinum

The mediastinum extends from the thoracic inlet superiorly to the diaphragm inferiorly, and is bound between the left and right pleural sacs and lungs laterally, the sternum anteriorly and the vertebral column posteriorly (Figure 12–1). It is divided into the superior and inferior mediastinum by a plane passing through the sternal angle and the fourth thoracic vertebra. The inferior mediastinum is further divided into the anterior mediastinum which lays between the sternum and the heart, the middle mediastinum which includes the heart, the major airways and blood vessels and the esophagus, and the posterior mediastinum between the posterior pericardial sac and the vertebral column.[2] For clinical purposes, it is useful to consider any tumor that is anterior to a line drawn between the trachea and the posterior border of the heart as an anterior mediastinal tumor, as these are the tumors that tend to cause respiratory and vascular compression. In one series of 48 children with mediastinal masses undergoing surgery under general anesthesia, 48% (23 of 48) of patients had an anterior mediastinal mass, while of the 7 patients who developed complications during anesthesia, 6 (86%) had an anterior mediastinal mass.[3]

Pathology of Mediastinal Masses

Most mediastinal masses are neoplasms, either benign or malignant, the latter being either of primary growth or metastatic origin. In addition, abscesses, cysts, or

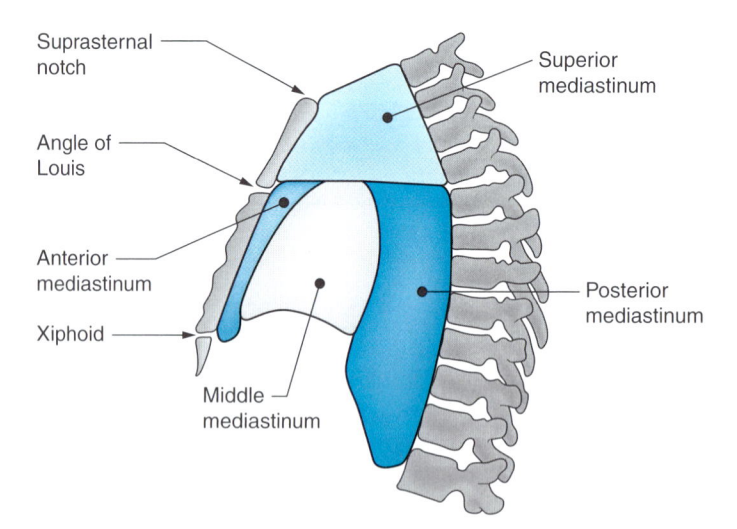

Figure 12–1. Subdivisions of the mediastinum. (Modified with permission from Benumof JL. *Anesthesia for Thoracic Surgery.* 2nd ed. Philadelphia: WB Saunders;1995:39. Copyright © Elsevier.)

Table 12-1. Types of Mediastinal Masses in Children

Location	Pathology
Anterior mediastinum (~50%)	Lymphoma (non-Hodgkin or Hodgkin)
	Teratoma
	Thymoma
	Mesenchymal tumor
Middle mediastinum (~15%)	Lymph node tumor (primary or metastatic)
	Vascular malformation
	Pericardial cyst
Posterior mediastinum (~35%)	Neurogenic tumor

vascular malformations can present as a mediastinal mass.[4] Table 12–1 summarizes the most common types of mediastinal masses in children. In adults, lymphomas (both the non-Hodgkin and the Hodgkin types), thymomas, carcinomas (either primary or metastatic), and intrathoracic thyroid goiters comprise the vast majority of mediastinal masses, while developmental abnormalities, teratomas and neurogenic tumors are much rarer.[5] While most tumor types have a predilection to specific parts of the mediastinum, a tissue biopsy is mandatory to determine the tumor type as well as its malignancy.

Signs and Symptoms

Although mediastinal masses can present with systemic symptomatology specific to their biological behavior (eg, autoimmune phenomena, neurohormonal effects), for the anesthesiologist the main concern is the effect of the mass on the respiratory and cardiovascular systems. About half of all mediastinal masses are incidental findings on chest radiograph, and tumors that do present with symptoms tend to be malignant, probably because the rapid growth tends to cause more symptoms.[4] In addition, signs and symptoms depend to a large extent on the size of the mass and its location. For example, neuroblastoma, a posterior mediastinal tumor, tends to cause systemic manifestations or neurological symptoms and only rarely respiratory distress. Children are more susceptible to severe compression because of the smaller size of their mediastinum, a larger thymus gland occupying a greater volume of the mediastinal cavity, increased collapsibility of the airways, and the smaller diameter of their airways and blood vessels. The smaller diameter also means that a relatively small reduction in the diameter will result in a relatively larger reduction of the cross-sectional area, and a greater increase in resistance to flow.

Common signs and symptoms associated with mediastinal masses are summarized in Table 12–2. The respiratory symptoms relate to pressure of the tumor on the trachea, leading to weakening of its wall (tracheomalacia), compression and narrowing of the lumen and bending of the airways. Most characteristically,

Table 12–2. Signs and Symptoms Related to a Mediastinal Mass

	Symptoms	Signs
Respiratory	Dyspnea–orthopnea	Decreased breath sounds
	Cough	Wheezing or stridor
	Hoarseness	Cyanosis
	Chest pain	Atelectasis/pneumonia
	Recurrent pulmonary infections	
Cardiovascular	Fatigue	Facial edema/jugular venous distension
	Headache	Cyanosis
	Presyncope/syncope	Pulsus paradoxus
	Dyspnea on exertion	Postural changes in blood pressure
		Hepatomegaly

symptoms are dynamic in nature, appearing mainly in the supine position or when intrathoracic pressure increases, as in expiration or while crying.

Cardiovascular symptoms can be caused by compression of the superior vena cava (SVC), pulmonary artery or the right ventricular outflow tract. Also, pericardial infiltration can result in either pericardial effusion and tamponade or in constrictive pericarditis. Rarely, intramyocardial tumor spread will lead to arrhythmias and decreased contractility. As with respiratory symptoms, changes in position or intrathoracic pressure (eg, a Valsalva maneuver), might induce cardiovascular symptoms such as syncope.

Some unique signs are associated with nerve involvement by the mediastinal tumor: hoarseness indicates recurrent laryngeal nerve involvement, Horner's syndrome indicates sympathetic ganglion involvement, and elevated hemidiaphragm on chest x-ray is associated with phrenic nerve involvement.

Several mediastinal tumors can also cause systemic syndromes. Examples include myasthenia gravis (thymoma), myasthenia-like muscle weakness (Eaton-Lambert syndrome in bronchogenic carcinoma), hyperparathyroidism (parathyroid adenomas or bronchogenic carcinoma), thyrotoxicosis (goiter), paroxysmal tachycardia and hypertension (neuroblastoma or pheochromocytoma), and von Recklinghausen disease (neurofibromatosis).[6]

Surgery for Mediastinal Masses

Most patients who present for surgery with a mediastinal mass will require either a diagnostic or therapeutic procedure related to the mass. The rare patient might present for an unrelated surgery.[7] The most common diagnostic procedures are a mediastinoscopy or mediastinotomy, though sometimes an extrathoracic lymph node biopsy can be performed. Therapeutic resection usually requires either a thoracotomy or median sternotomy.[5]

ANTERIOR MEDIASTINAL MASSES—ANESTHETIC ASPECTS
Pathophysiology of Perioperative Complications

Perioperative tracheobronchial compression with complete inability to ventilate is the most feared complication of anesthesia in a patient with a mediastinal mass. This has been described during induction of anesthesia as well as during emergence or even postoperatively.[1] While direct compression by the tumor is the more common mechanism for airway obstruction, in some patients bronchial compression has been linked to a mediastinal shift resulting from either severe atelectasis or lobar emphysema from a ball-valve type of obstruction.[8] Several physiological changes that occur during anesthesia can exacerbate the compressive effects of an existing mediastinal mass, as summarized in Table 12–3. These changes are related to supine positioning, the effect of anesthetic agents on muscle tone, effects of positive pressure ventilation and the effects of the surgical trauma. Several effects of anesthesia lead to reduced lung volume and thoracic cavity size.[9] These not only increase the relative size of the tumor mass, but also reduce the normal tethering effect that expanded lungs exert on the airways. Inhalational agents have been described to reduce activity of the intercostal

Table 12–3. Physiological Changes During Anesthesia and Surgery

Change	Consequences
Gravitational effect of tumor in a supine position	Compression of airways and blood vessels
Increased central blood volume in the supine position	Engorged tumor—increased size
Decreased rib cage excursion	Decreased thoracic cavity size
Cephalad displacement of the diaphragm	Decreased thoracic cavity size
Decreased muscle tone with inhalational agents and, even more so, with muscle relaxants	Reduced tracheal expansion leading to collapse, especially with tracheomalacia
Relaxation of bronchial smooth muscle	Increased collapsibility of the airways
Bypass of the glottis by the endotracheal tube	Prevents normal glottis narrowing that might reduce dynamic tracheal collapse
Positive pressure ventilation	Abolition of negative intrapleural pressure which dilates the airways; increase in airflow velocity leading to turbulence
Reduced venous return with positive pressure ventilation	Reduced cardiac filling (can be critical in patients with SVC* syndrome or pulmonary artery compression)
Surgical trauma	Tumor edema and bleeding, hematoma formation.

*SVC = superior vena cava

muscles, leading to mechanical instability and inward movement of the rib cage during inspiration.[10] These effects of inhalational agents can linger after extubation in the early postoperative period. While most general anesthetic agents decrease tone of the intercostal muscles and diaphragm, muscle relaxants will obviously exacerbate this. Additionally, muscle paralysis and positive pressure ventilation abolish the negative intrapleural pressure that dilates and opens the airways during inspiration.

Positive pressure ventilation also increases the velocity of gas flow, which in the presence of critical airway stenosis, will result in disruption of laminar flow and creation of turbulence, significantly increasing the resistance to airflow.[11] Induction of general anesthesia is not the only dangerous period, however. Severe respiratory compromise has been described during emergence and extubation as well.[1,12]

Changes in position and reduced negative intrathoracic pressure might also exacerbate the effects of SVC syndrome, cardiac tamponade or pulmonary artery compression, leading to sudden hypotension, hypoxemia or even cardiac arrest during induction of general anesthesia or positional changes. Both spontaneous breathing and positive pressure ventilation in the setting of partial airway obstruction can lead to dynamic hyperinflation and auto-PEEP, resulting in a decrease in venous return to the heart and exacerbation of preexisting vascular compression.

Only a few case reports of pulmonary artery obstruction from a mediastinal mass exist, probably because the main pulmonary artery and its bifurcation are relatively shielded by the bigger and high-pressure ascending aorta. However, the right ventricular outflow tract might be more susceptible because of its superficial location in the heart and low-pressure status. Indeed, an experimental study of mediastinal masses in dogs has shown significant right ventricular outflow obstruction resulting in right ventricular dilatation, leftward shift of the interventricular septum and a decrease in left ventricular size and stroke volume, leading to decreased cardiac output.[13] At baseline, the right heart can usually compensate for increased afterload caused by either pulmonary artery or outflow tract compression. However, any further decrease in preload (hypovolemia, increased intrathoracic pressure, anesthetic agents) or in contractility (anesthetic agents) might override the compensatory mechanisms, leading to hypotension, cyanosis and cardiovascular collapse.

Preoperative Evaluation

Signs and Symptoms

While asymptomatic patients are certainly not immune from developing severe cardiorespiratory compromise during anesthesia, patients with symptoms at baseline usually have the most significant reduction in airway and/or blood vessel diameter. In a large pediatric case series, 60% of the patients presented with respiratory findings, and 43% of these (13 out of 30) had significant tracheobronchial compression on computerized tomography (CT) scan, while none of 20 asymptomatic children had tracheobronchial compromise.[8] In another series of 48 children, all 7 patients who developed complications during anesthesia had at least three respiratory signs and symptoms (cough, shortness of breath, orthopnea, pleural effusion, use of accessory muscles, stridor or a history of respiratory arrest), while only 17% of patients without complications had three or more symptoms.[3]

SPIROMETRY

The importance of upright and supine spirometry to evaluate the severity of airway obstruction before surgery was initially suggested by Neuman et al in 1984.[12] Classically, reduced airflow in the inspiratory limb of the flow-volume curve is considered a sign of extra-thoracic obstruction, while reduced flow in the expiratory limb, specifically mid-expiratory flow plateau, signifies an intrathoracic obstruction. In a fixed obstruction, where the airway wall is immobile, flow is reduced in both inspiration and expiration regardless of the location of the obstruction (Figure 12–2).[14] In normal healthy adults, a change from sitting to a supine position is accompanied by only a mild decline in spirometric values.[16] Decreases of more than 10% in airflow indices when changing from sitting to supine, or around 20% upon change from standing to supine, are usually considered indicative of pathology.[17] A disproportional reduction of maximal expiratory flow can be a sign of tracheomalacia, which entails a risk of dynamic airway collapse especially after tracheal extubation. It should be stressed that simple

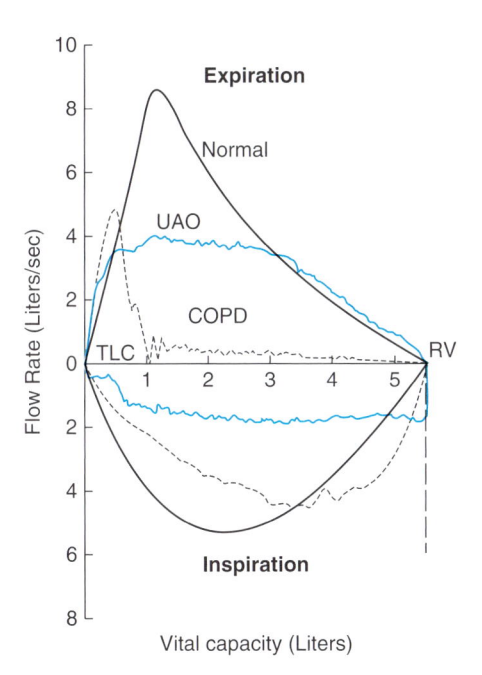

Figure 12–2. Flow-volume loops from a spirometry study of a normal subject, a patient with a fixed upper airway obstruction (UAO) and a patient with COPD. Note the reduction in both inspiratory and expiratory flows and the mid-expiratory flow plateau in the patient with upper airway obstruction. (Reproduced with permission from the American College of Chest Physicians. Diagnosis of upper airway obstruction by pulmonary function testing. *Chest*.1975;68(6):796-799.)

spirometric indices such as forced expiratory volume in 1 second (FEV_1) do not change until airway obstruction is very advanced, and therefore flow-volume loops are recommended in these cases.[15]

Recent data, however, call into question the utility of spirometry for predicting complications in patients with mediastinal masses. Hnatiuk et al have studied 37 adults with various types of mediastinal masses, all of who had undergone preoperative spirometry, and 10 of which had both supine and either upright or sitting studies. Four patients had abnormal spirometry and all had undergone surgery under general anesthesia without complications. Of the five patients with tracheobronchial compression on CT, only one had a positive spirometry test.[17]

In another study, flow-volume loops were constructed for 25 patients with intrathoracic Hodgkin lymphoma, 9 of them with radiologic evidence of moderate to severe tracheal compression. Despite this, none of the patients demonstrated variable expiratory flow pattern, and 7 of them had an inspiratory plateau typical of extrathoracic obstruction.[15] Of patients with both inspiratory and expiratory flow limitation, the same number of patients had only mild tracheal compression on CT as the number who had severe compression. The authors speculated that the classical descriptions of the effects of airway obstruction on flow-volume loops might be applicable to intraluminal obstruction, but less so for extrinsic compression of the airways typical of mediastinal masses.

Simpler to measure than flow-volume loops, peak expiratory flow rate (PEFR) has been used to evaluate patients with suspected airway obstruction. In one study on adults, PEFR less than 40% of the predicted value was associated with a 10-fold increase in the risk for postoperative respiratory complications, though no intraoperative respiratory events occurred in this group.[5] PEFR measurement requires the subject's cooperation, and therefore may not be useful in young children. More studies are required to define its place in evaluating older children and adults with a mediastinal mass.

RADIOGRAPHIC EVALUATION

A plain chest x-ray will usually show the mediastinal tumor, and may provide the clinician with a rough estimation of its size. In a study of 97 patients with Hodgkin disease, a postero–anterior chest x-ray was used to calculate the ratio between the widest diameter of the mediastinal mass and the width of the thorax at T5-6 (termed mediastinal thoracic ratio, MTR). An MTR greater than 0.5 was associated with a higher incidence of postoperative respiratory complications.[18]

However, a plain chest radiograph is not sufficient to assess the involvement of the tracheobronchial tree accurately; therefore a CT scan is always necessary (Figure 12–3).[8] The value of CT in the prediction of intraoperative complications has been demonstrated repeatedly. In one pediatric series, all 37 patients without tracheobronchial or cardiac compromise on CT scan underwent general anesthesia with no complications, while severe airway obstruction developed in 5 of 8 patients with tracheobronchial compression who underwent general anesthesia. In this series, tracheal narrowing greater than 50% in cross-sectional area was associated with an increased risk of airway obstruction during anesthesia.[8] In another

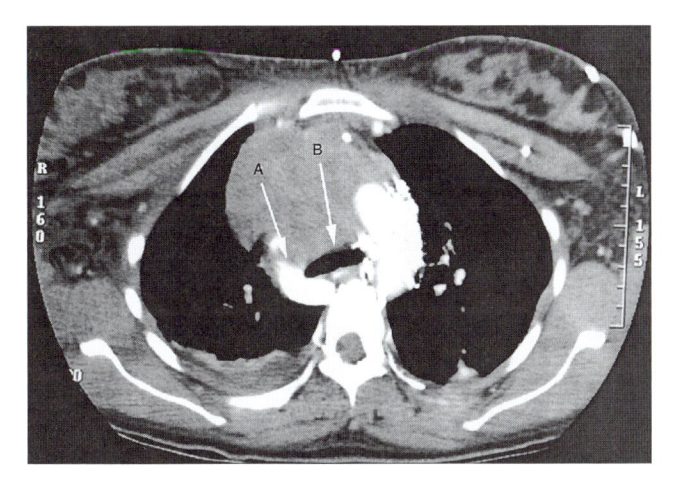

Figure 12–3. Thoracic CT scan of a 29-year-old woman with non-Hodgkin lymphoma. Arrow A points to a dilated azygos vein from SVC syndrome while arrow B points to a greater than 50% compression of the trachea just above the carina. (Reproduced with permission from Szokol JW, Alspach D, Mehta MK, Parilla BV, Liptay MJ. Intermittent airway obstruction and superior vena cava syndrome in a patient with an undiagnosed mediastinal mass after cesarean delivery. *Anesth Analg.* 2003;97(3):883-884.)

series of 48 children undergoing general anesthesia, radiologic evidence of tracheal or bronchial compression was found in all 7 patients with intraoperative complications but in only 7 of 41 patients without complications.[3] However, a more recent study described a series of 46 children with mediastinal mass, 18 with radiological evidence of tracheal compression or deviation and 24 with evidence of cardiac compromise. All of them underwent general anesthesia, about half using spontaneous ventilation. Only three patients developed respiratory complications, all benign and probably unrelated to the mediastinal mass.[19]

In a case series of 105 adults with mediastinal mass, 8 patients had tracheal compression of more than 50% cross-sectional area and 4 patients had compression of the main stem bronchus. There were no intraoperative airway problems in this series. However, tracheal compression was a risk factor for postoperative respiratory complications such as pneumonia and atelectasis. In addition, pericardial effusion on CT was a risk factor for intraoperative cardiovascular complications.[5]

MRI studies are at least as useful as CT imaging, and may offer some advantages in several specific tumor types. Both studies are done in a supine position, similar to anesthesia and surgery, and can therefore demonstrate positional compression effects of the tumor mass. It is important that the imaging studies be performed as near as possible to the time of surgery, as the tumor may grow rapidly.[6]

FLEXIBLE FIBEROPTIC BRONCHOSCOPY

While usually impractical in small children, this study can be very useful in older children and adults. Not only can it be used to explore airway anatomy and show

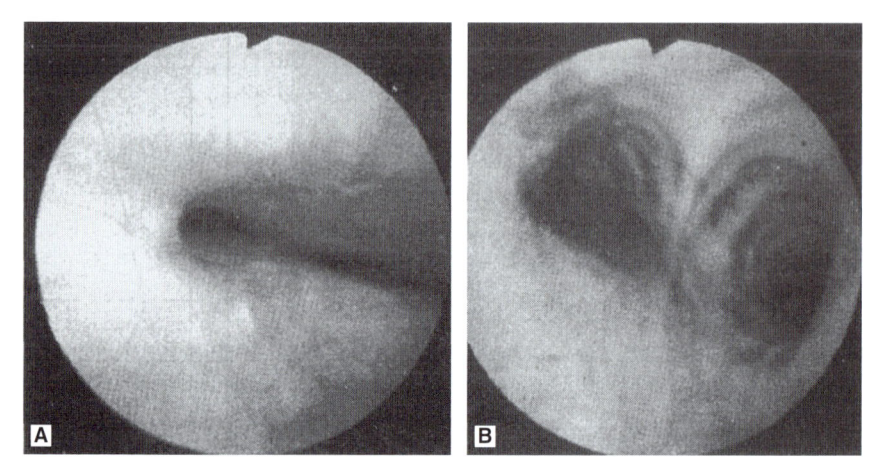

Figure 12–4. Flexible bronchoscopy views in a 24-year-old patient with Hodgkin lymphoma in supine position (A) and sitting (B). (Reproduced with permission from Prakash UB, Abel MD, Hubmayr RD. Mediastinal mass and tracheal obstruction during general anesthesia. *Mayo Clin Proc.* 1988;63(10):1004-1011.)

areas and degree of obstruction, but it can help assess the effect of change in position on the degree of obstruction (Figure 12–4).[20] It can also be used for awake intubation during spontaneous breathing or in the patient with suspected difficult visualization of the airway, or who does not tolerate the supine position without respiratory compromise.[2] Fiberoptic bronchoscopy can also be used to guide the endotracheal tube beyond the point of obstruction.

ECHOCARDIOGRAPHY

Echocardiography can delineate tumor involvement of the heart and great vessels. It can accurately assess the degree of pulmonary artery or right ventricular outflow tract encroachment, the existence of pericardial effusion and the presence of cardiac tamponade, and the degree of ventricular dysfunction related to myocardial infiltration. Some preoperative signs and symptoms that would be an indication for a preoperative echocardiography study include orthopnea, cyanosis, jugular venous distension, pulsus paradoxus and syncope.[5] Rarely, transesophageal echocardiography may show the tumor itself when it surrounds the heart.[21]

Incidence and Prediction of Perioperative Complications

Many anecdotal case reports have been published describing perioperative complications in patients with mediastinal masses.[12,20-26] While these are instructive, they do not give much information about the prevalence of these complications. However, several case series have been published and are summarized in Table 12–4. Most of the existing data is on children. Importantly, it seems that the incidence of intraoperative respiratory complications, especially airway obstruction, is much

Table 12–4. Incidence of Intraoperative Complications in Patients with Mediastinal Masses

Article	Population	# Patients with Complications / # Patients Undergoing GA* (%)	Respiratory Complications	Cardiovascular Complications	Comments
Azizkhan, 1985[8]	Children	5/45 (11%)	airway obstruction, (5)		
Ng, 2007[3]	Children	7/48 (15%)	airway obstruction, (5) respiratory arrest, (1)	hypotension, (1) cardiac arrests and death, (2)	
Stricker, 2006[19]	Children	3/46 (7%)	bronchospasm, (1) airway obstruction, (1) pneumothorax, (1)		
Bechard, 2004[5]	Adults	4/105 (4%)	hypoxemia	hypotension, (1) atrial fibrillation, (2)	(10%) postoperative respiratory complications, (11)
Hnatiuk, 2001[17]	Adults	1/35 (3%)	none	bleeding(1)	

*GA = General anesthesia

Table 12–5. Predictors of Complications during General Anesthesia in Children with a Mediastinal Mass

Risk Factor	Positive Predictive Value	Negative Predictive Value
Anterior mediastinal location	26%	96%
> 3 respiratory signs/symptoms*	50%	100%
Radiologic tracheobronchial compression	100%	98%
Radiologic vascular compression	46%	97%
Infection anywhere	45%	95%

*see text for details of signs and symptoms
Adapted from Ng A, Bennett J, Bromley P, Davies P, Morland B.[3]

smaller in adults, as might be predicted by the anatomical differences.[5,27] A search of various closed claims databases performed in 2001 found eight cases related to anterior mediastinal masses, five of them occurring in children less than 8-years old and only one case in an adult above 18 years of age.[6]

While intraoperative complications are the major source of concern for the anesthesiologist, postoperative respiratory complications have been described too and, in adults, might be more significant. These include airway edema, atelectasis and pneumonia, and usually occur within the first 48 hours.[5]

Our ability to predict which patient with a mediastinal mass will develop complications with general anesthesia is still limited. Various authors have suggested different predictors; however, most of these studies have been performed in children and their relevance for the adult population is questionable. Also, the number of subjects, and especially the number of those who developed complications, is relatively small, limiting the power of statistical multivariate analysis. The most rigorous analysis was performed by Ng et al and is summarized in Table 12–5. Important risk factors that were consistently found in various studies include an anterior (vs middle or posterior) mediastinal mass, preoperative presence of significant respiratory signs and symptoms, radiologic evidence of significant (above 35%-50%) narrowing of the tracheal cross-sectional area and the presence of SVC syndrome. In one large series in adults, only pericardial effusion was found to be a risk factor for intraoperative complications (which were mostly cardiovascular), while the presence of severe orthopnea, stridor, cyanosis or jugular vein distension, tracheal narrowing of more than 50%, PEFR less than 40% predicted, and a mixed restrictive-obstructive picture on spirometry were all predictors of postoperative respiratory complications.[5]

ANESTHETIC MANAGEMENT

The governing principle when anesthetizing a patient with a mediastinal mass is "Noli Pontes Ignii Consumere" (don't burn your bridges). Basically, the anesthesiologist should plan his interventions striving to keep available as many viable alternatives as possible should a catastrophic cardiorespiratory complication occur.

Procedures such as CT-guided needle biopsy, cervical lymph node biopsy, or diagnostic thoracentesis to obtain a tissue diagnosis should be done under local anesthesia, if at all possible. The use of EMLA cream and ketamine sedation can facilitate these procedures in young children.

If general anesthesia is essential, consideration should be given to preoperative irradiation and/or chemotherapy in an attempt to reduce the size of a large obstructing tumor, for example Hodgkin lymphoma or neuroblastoma, thereby decreasing preoperative symptoms and respiratory compromise.[8,18] In a large series of patients with Hodgkin disease who presented for surgery with a mediastinal mass, all five respiratory complications occurred in the 74 patients who did not receive preoperative radiation therapy, while none of 24 patients who did receive radiation therapy had any respiratory complication.[1] It should be taken into account, however, that such preoperative therapy might distort the histopathological appearance of the tumor and hinder accurate diagnosis. For patients with large, symptomatic pericardial effusions, preoperative drainage under local anesthesia can decrease the risk of intraoperative hypotension.

Once the decision is made to proceed with general anesthesia, a detailed plan should be formulated and discussed ahead of time with the other members of the surgical team. (Table 12–6).

Induction of Anesthesia

An important concept when inducing anesthesia is the preservation of spontaneous breathing whenever possible. This usually requires either a deeper level of anesthesia for airway manipulation (more so for endotracheal

Table 12–6. Principles of Anesthesia for the Patient with a Mediastinal Mass

Preservation of spontaneous breathing	Avoid heavy preoperative sedation
	Consider inhalational induction
	Assess hemodynamics and airway patency with positive pressure breathing
	Utilize short-acting muscle relaxants
Intubation beyond point of obstruction	Armored endotracheal tube
	Long endotracheal tube
	Double lumen endotracheal tube
	Rigid bronchoscope
Backup plan	Position change
	Helium-oxygen mixture
	CPB
	Emergency sternotomy

intubation than for a laryngeal mask airway)[28] or an awake fiberoptic intubation if difficult intubation is expected or if it is thought that the patient will not be able to tolerate the hemodynamic consequences of deep anesthesia. Topical airway anesthesia or the use of airway nerve blocks will also allow maintaining a lighter plane of anesthesia, reducing muscular hypotonicity and facilitating rapid awakening if deemed necessary. Typically, inhalational induction is chosen to preserve spontaneous breathing. If propofol is chosen for induction, slow infusion rather than a bolus dose should be used. Another choice for an IV induction agent is ketamine, which usually preserves spontaneous breathing and minimizes hemodynamic depression due to its sympathomimetic properties.[29] Some have suggested the use of PEEP of 10 to 15 cm H_2O in addition to spontaneous ventilation, to "stent" the airways open.[8]

Avoiding sedation in the premedication is advocated due to the risk of airway obstruction. In one closed claim case, an adult with a mediastinal mass developed cardiac arrest after sedation and before induction of anesthesia.[6] Antisialagogues can be helpful if awake fiberoptic intubation is contemplated.

If muscle paralysis is deemed necessary for the surgical procedure, the patient should be induced and the airway controlled while still spontaneously breathing. Then assisted breaths can be gradually added using a bag and mask, so the effect of positive pressure breaths on airway patency and hemodynamics can be evaluated before committing to a muscle relaxant, preferably a short-acting one.

Once the chest is opened, muscle paralysis can be safely employed and the patient placed on mechanical ventilation. The surgeon might be asked to mechanically lift the tumor mass to relieve airway compression.[30]

Optimal body positioning should be determined for symptomatic patients. Many will be more symptomatic in a supine position, and sitting them up by elevating the back of the operating table might alleviate the obstruction. For some tumors, positioning the patient in the lateral position might relieve pressure on the carina, especially with off-center masses. In the rare patient, severe intraoperative airway obstruction or cardiovascular collapse might only be relieved by sitting, leaning forward, or even prone positioning. Some have recommended the routine use of a semi-recumbent position for induction of general anesthesia in these patients. The danger of a massive venous air embolism in the sitting position for a thoracic or neck operation, however, is real.

Airway Management

Several options exist for instrumentation of the airway. As mentioned before, a laryngeal mask can be inserted under a relatively lighter level of anesthesia, and is an ideal solution for a spontaneously breathing patient. However, it does not allow rapid bypass of a developing complete obstruction. Also, spontaneous breathing is usually not advocated during thoracotomy, although it is not impossible.[11]

In addition to a regular endotracheal tube, several other options exist that allow passing a breathing tube beyond the point of obstruction, either preemptively or once an obstruction does develop and is not rapidly relieved by a change in patient position. This can be achieved in children by using an armored endotracheal tube passed intra-bronchially if needed[30] and in adults by either an armored endotracheal tube or by a double lumen tube. Another option is to advance two small diameter long tubes (called microlaryngeal tubes) one into each main bronchus under direct fiber-optic visualization.[23]

Management of Complications

Typically, initial signs of airway obstruction such as wheezing and reduced breath sounds are mistaken to be evidence of bronchospasm or tension pneumothorax, and precious time is lost. In a patient with suggestive anatomy, the possibility of major airway obstruction should be entertained early and adequate treatment delivered promptly.[6]

If airway obstruction develops, a change in patient position may relieve it. Passing a tube beyond the point of obstruction, as described above, is another option. A rigid bronchoscope, and a surgeon experienced in its use, should always be available in high-risk patients, as the obstruction may hinder passage of a soft tube. The use of a helium-oxygen mixture has been suggested to decrease turbulence and resistance to airflow in an obstructed airway.[31]

If hypotension develops, the experimental studies described earlier suggest that right ventricular (RV) outflow obstruction leading to RV failure is the most commonly responsible mechanism.[13] Vasopressor therapy aimed at improving coronary perfusion is the treatment of choice. However, an element of reduced preload, especially in patients with known SVC compression, might coexist, and a judicious fluid bolus should be given as well. Over-hydration, however, is counterproductive in patients with RV failure, as it will only lead to increased RV distension, more leftward displacement of the interventricular septum, and decreased left ventricular loading. It has been described that cyanosis due to pulmonary artery compression can be reversed by either resumption of spontaneous breathing[32,33] or by a change to the sitting position.[22]

If all else fails, and respiratory or hemodynamic deterioration continues, two options still exist—either rapidly awakening the patient, if possible, or emergency surgical intervention—median sternotomy with mechanical elevation of the tumor off the airways and blood vessels,[21,33] or emergency cardiopulmonary bypass (CPB).

Cardiopulmonary Bypass—Elective or on Standby?

Several reports exist in the literature where standby CPB was available in patients with a mediastinal mass; however in only a few was CPB eventually required and used.[26] It is questionable whether cannulation for CPB could be performed fast enough in a patient who develops severe cardiorespiratory compromise on the verge of arrest, and especially when the patient is not supine, eg, in a lateral position for thoracic surgery.[34] Therefore, some authors have chosen to electively cannulate the femoral vessels under local anesthesia before induction of general anesthesia, or even to commence CPB with induction of general anesthesia, instead of having CPB on stand-by status only.[32,35,36] It is highly unlikely that a study could ever be conducted to decide which approach is better. The decision should therefore be individualized, based on both the patient's risk (eg, a patient with a large mass that compresses the pulmonary artery and trachea, or with severe SVC syndrome is at a higher risk for complications around induction of anesthesia) and the preference of the surgical team (highly experienced surgeon and perfusionist could accomplish emergency cannulation and CPB faster). If the standby CPB approach is chosen, the CPB machine should be primed, the cannulation lines ready, the groins prepared and sterilely draped, and both perfusionist and cardiac surgeon available in the operating room before induction of anesthesia.

Suggested Perioperative Approach

Several algorithms have been suggested to guide the surgeon and anesthesiologist in managing patients with mediastinal masses; one is presented in Figure 12–5. Generally,

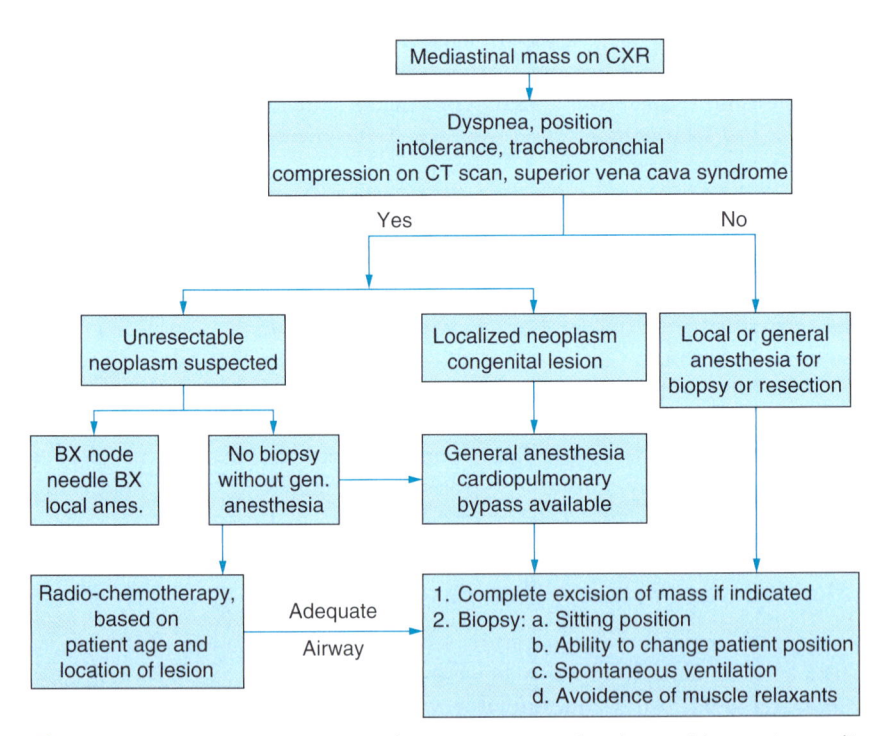

Figure 12–5. Suggested algorithm for management of patients with anterior mediastinal mass. (Reproduced with permission from Azizkhan RG, Dudgeon DL, Buck JR, et al. Life-threatening airway obstruction as a complication to the management of mediastinal masses in children. *J Ped Surg*.1985;20(6):816-822. Copyright © Elsevier.)

in the presence of clinical or radiological evidence of severe tracheobronchial obstruction, general anesthesia should be reserved for selected patients who have the prospect of a curative procedure. In this case, all the above precautions should be taken and the use of CPB should be considered. Otherwise, an attempt to achieve tissue diagnosis by biopsy under local anesthesia, or preoperative tumor shrinkage with chemotherapy or radiotherapy, is recommended. In the patient with no radiological evidence of tracheobronchial obstruction, proceeding to surgery under general anesthesia can be done relatively safely. The utility of a similar algorithm was tested in a series of 31 children with anterior mediastinal mass. Surgery under local anesthesia was chosen if either tracheal cross-sectional area or PEFR were less than 50% of predicted values, otherwise general anesthesia was used. No complications have occurred with this management policy,[37] though patient number was too small to provide a definitive proof of safety.

SUPERIOR VENA CAVA SYNDROME

The SVC syndrome results from compression of the SVC, leading to obstructed venous return from the upper half of the body. It is most commonly caused by an extrinsic compression from a mediastinal tumor, mainly bronchogenic carcinoma or lymphoma, though it has been reported to occur due to intravascular caval thrombosis.[38] The clinical manifestations depend to a large extent on the rapidity of development of the obstruction, as slow development will allow collateral veins to develop and decompress the engorged venous system. The severity of the signs and symptoms also depends on the location of the obstruction to blood flow relative to the entry point of the azygos vein into the SVC—obstruction above the insertion of the azygos vein will allow drainage of blood from the upper body through short collaterals to the azygos vein, resulting in milder symptoms. A rapidly developing SVC syndrome will result in edema and either plethora or cyanosis of the face, neck, and upper extremities, conjunctival edema, hemoptysis, dyspnea (especially on exertion), and sometimes symptoms and signs of increased intracranial pressure like headache, blurred vision, and papilledema. The distended veins in the upper torso will typically not collapse when the patient assumes the sitting position. In addition to visible edema, some patients might develop tracheobronchial and upper airway mucosal edema causing respiratory symptoms (dyspnea, cough, nasal stuffiness) or difficult airway visualization during intubation. The signs and symptoms of SVC syndrome will typically worsen while supine or leaning forward.

Evaluation of the patient with suspected SVC syndrome requires CT or a magnetic resonance imaging study to define any existing tumor, as well as an echocardiographic study to evaluate the extent of caval obstruction and any coexisting cardiac pathology (eg, pericardial effusion).[39]

Treatment of SVC syndrome is frequently palliative only, as the underlying malignant disease is usually widespread. Supportive measures include elevation of the head, oxygen, and diuretics. Steroids, chemotherapy, or radiotherapy may be used to reduce tumor size and symptoms as well as to decrease the risk of induction

Table 12–7. Anesthetic Considerations for the Patient with Superior Vena Cava Syndrome

Treat preoperative hypovolemia
Utilize anesthetics that maintain vascular tone and cardiac contractility
Consider awake fiber-optic intubation
Maintain spontaneous ventilation, if possible
Secure venous access in lower extremities
Large bore intravenous access and cross-matched blood available
Maintain cerebral perfusion pressure
Evaluate and plan for respiratory compromise

of general anesthesia (see below). Operative options include intravascular stenting, tumor debulking, thrombectomy, and vena cava bypass.[6]

Anesthetic Management

While patients might be only mildly symptomatic at baseline, induction of general anesthesia can lead to cardiovascular collapse. This is caused by a further reduction in cardiac preload, related to the vasodilatory effects of anesthetic agents, increased compression by the tumor mass, and the effect of positive pressure ventilation. Preoperative radiation or chemotherapy might be especially beneficial in alleviating SVC obstruction, if possible. Otherwise, it is very important to treat any preexisting hypovolemia before induction of anesthesia. The use of anesthetic agents with less vasodilatory and negative inotropic effects, (such as etomidate and ketamine), is preferable. Because venous return from the upper half of the body might be limited or even interrupted, it is important to secure intravenous access in the lower extremities. Bleeding might be excessive due to increased central venous pressure, so adequate venous access and cross-matched blood should be available. Central venous and pulmonary artery catheters, if planned, should also be placed through a femoral vein. All patients should be carefully evaluated for the existence of airway edema. In selected cases, awake fiberoptic intubation might be preferable over regular laryngoscopy.[40] Last, it is very important to maintain systemic blood pressure around baseline values in order to avoid a reduction in cerebral perfusion pressure, as resistance to venous outflow from the head and brain is elevated. Special neuromonitoring modalities, (cerebral oximetry, transcranial Doppler), might help to provide early clues of cerebral hypoperfusion.[41] Table 12–7 summarizes recommendations for anesthetizing patients with SVC syndrome.

REFERENCES

1. Piro AJ, Weiss DR, Hellman S. Mediastinal Hodgkin's disease: a possible danger for intubation anesthesia. Intubation danger in Hodgkin's disease. *Int J Rad Oncol Biol Phys.* 1976;1(5-6):415-419.
2. Pullerits J, Holzman R. Anaesthesia for patients with mediastinal masses. *Can J Anesth.* 1989;36(6):681-688.

3. Ng A, Bennett J, Bromley P, Davies P, Morland B. Anaesthetic outcome and predictive risk factors in children with mediastinal tumours. *Pediatr Blood Cancer.* 2007;48(2):160-164.
4. Lerman J. Anterior mediastinal masses in children. *Sem Anesth Periop Med Pain.* 2007;26:133-140.
5. Béchard P, Létourneau L, Lacasse Y, Côté D, Bussières JS. Perioperative cardiorespiratory complications in adults with mediastinal mass. *Anesthesiology.* 2004;100(4):826-834.
6. Narang S, Harte BH, Body SC. Anesthesia for patients with a mediastinal mass. *Anesthesiol Clin North Am.* 2001;19(3):559-579.
7. Crosby E. Clinical case discussion: anesthesia for Cesarean section in a parturient with a large intrathoracic tumour. *Can J Anaesth.* 2001;48(6):575-583.
8. Azizkhan RG, Dudgeon DL, Buck JR, et al. Life-threatening airway obstruction as a complication to the management of mediastinal masses in children. *J Pediatr Surg.* 1985;20(6):816-822.
9. Bergman NA. Reduction in resting end-expiratory position of the respiratory system with induction of anesthesia and neuromuscular paralysis. *Anesthesiology.* 1982;57(1):14-17.
10. Jones JG, Faithfull D, Jordan C, Minty B. Rib cage movement during halothane anaesthesia in man. *Br J Anaesth.* 1979;51(5):399-407.
11. Sibert KS, Biondi JW, Hirsch NP. Spontaneous respiration during thoracotomy in a patient with a mediastinal mass. *Anesth Analg.* 1987;66(9):904-907.
12. Neuman GG, Weingarten AE, Abramowitz RM, Kushins LG, Abramson AL, Ladner W. The anesthetic management of the patient with an anterior mediastinal mass. *Anesthesiology.* 1984;60(2):144-147.
13. Johnson D, Hurst T, Cujec B, Mayers I. Cardiopulmonary effects of an anterior mediastinal mass in dogs anesthetized with halothane. *Anesthesiology.* 1991;74(4):725-736.
14. Brookes GB, Fairfax AJ. Chronic upper airway obstruction: value of the flow volume loop examination in assessment and management. *J R Soc Med.* 1982;75(6):425.
15. Vander Els NJ, Sorhage F, Bach AM, Straus DJ, White DA. Abnormal flow volume loops in patients with intrathoracic Hodgkin's disease. *Chest.* 2000;117(5):1256-1261.
16. Vilke GM, Chan TC, Neuman T, Clausen JL. Spirometry in normal subjects in sitting, prone, and supine positions. *Respir Care.* 2000;45(4):407-410.
17. Hnatiuk OW. Spirometry in surgery for anterior mediastinal masses. *Chest.* 2001;120(4):1152-1156.
18. Turoff RD, Gomez GA, Berjian R, et al. Postoperative respiratory complications in patients with Hodgkin's disease: relationship to the size of the mediastinal tumor. *Eur J Cancer Clin Oncol.* 1985;21(9):1043-1046.
19. Stricker P, Gurnaney H, Litman R. Anesthetic management of children with an anterior mediastinal mass. *Anesthesiology.* 2006;105:A970.
20. Prakash UB, Abel MD, Hubmayr RD. Mediastinal mass and tracheal obstruction during general anesthesia. *Mayo Clin Proc.* 1988;63(10):1004-1011.
21. Lin C-M, Hsu J-C. Anterior mediastinal tumour identified by intraoperative transesophageal echocardiography. *Can J Anesth.* 2001;48(1):78-80.
22. Alkhafaji S, Mazhar R, Carr CS, Alkhulaifi AM. Extreme cardiac and pulmonary artery compression causing positional oxygen desaturation. *Emerg Med J.* 2008;25(8):541.
23. John RE, Narang VP. A boy with an anterior mediastinal mass. *Anaesthesia.* 1988;43(10):864-866.
24. Keon TP. Death on induction of anesthesia for cervical node biopsy. *Anesthesiology.* 1981;55(4):471-472.
25. Szokol JW, Alspach D, Mehta MK, Parilla BV, Liptay MJ. Intermittent airway obstruction and superior vena cava syndrome in a patient with an undiagnosed mediastinal mass after cesarean delivery. *Anesth Analg.* 2003;97(3):883-884.
26. Takeda S-i, Miyoshi S, Omori K-i, Okumura M, Matsuda H. Surgical rescue for life-threatening hypoxemia caused by a mediastinal tumor. *Ann Thorac Surg.* 1999;68(6):2324-2326.
27. Azarow KS, Pearl RH, Zurcher R, Edwards FH, Cohen AJ. Primary mediastinal masses. A comparison of adult and pediatric populations. *J Thorac Cardiovasc Surg.* 1993;106(1):67-72.
28. Hattamer SJ, Dodds TM. Use of the laryngeal mask airway in managing a patient with a large anterior mediastinal mass: a case report. *AANA J.* 1996;64(5):497-500.
29. Frawley G, Low J, Brown TC. Anaesthesia for an anterior mediastinal mass with ketamine and midazolam infusion. *Anaesth Intensive Care.* 1995;23(5):610-612.
30. Vas L, Falguni N, Veena N. Anaesthetic management of an infant with anterior mediastinal mass. *Paediatr Anaesth.* 1999;9(5):439-443.

31. Polaner DM. The use of heliox and the laryngeal mask airway in a child with an anterior mediastinal mass. *Anesth Analg.* 1996;82(1):208-210.
32. Hall KD, Friedman M. Extracorporeal oxygenation for induction of anesthesia in a patient with an intrathoracic tumor. *Anesthesiology.* 1975;42(4):493-495.
33. Levin H, Bursztein S, Heifetz M. Cardiac arrest in a child with an anterior mediastinal mass. *Anesth Analg.* 1985;64(11):1129-1130.
34. Slinger P, Karsli C. Management of the patient with a large anterior mediastinal mass: recurring myths. *Curr Opin Anaesth.* 2007;20(1):1-3.
35. Inoue M, Minami M, Shiono H, et al. Efficient clinical application of percutaneous cardiopulmonary support for perioperative management of a huge anterior mediastinal tumor. *J Thorac Cardiovasc Surg.* 2006;131(3):755-756.
36. Tempe DK, Arya R, Dubey S, et al. Mediastinal mass resection: femorofemoral cardiopulmonary bypass before induction of anesthesia in the management of airway obstruction. *J Cardiothorac Vasc Anesth.* 2001;15(2):233-236.
37. Shamberger RC, Holzman RS, Griscom NT, Tarbell NJ, Weinstein HJ, Wohl ME. Prospective evaluation by computed tomography and pulmonary function tests of children with mediastinal masses. *Surgery.* 1995;118(3):468-471.
38. Barbeito A, Bar-Yosef S, Lowe JE, Atkins BZ, Mark JB. Unusual cause of superior vena cava syndrome diagnosed with transesophageal echocardiography. *Can J Anaesth.* 2008;55(11):774-778.
39. Ayala K, Chandrasekaran K, Karalis D, Parris T, Ross J. Diagnosis of superior vena caval obstruction by transesophageal echocardiography. *Chest.* 1992;101(3):874-876.
40. Shapiro HM, Sanford TJ, Schaldach AL. Fiberoptic stylet laryngoscope and sitting position for tracheal intubation in acute superior vena caval syndrome. *Anesth Analg.* 1984;63(2):161-162.
41. Reece IJ, al Tareif H. Surgical interruption of the superior vena cava. *J Thorac Cardiovasc Surg.* 1995;109(5):1020.

Lung Resections for Cancer and Benign Chest Tumors

13

Mark Stafford-Smith

Key Points

1. Although many of the challenges to the anesthesiologist posed by lung resection surgery are similar to those with other surgeries, acute major hemorrhage is one that is particularly lethal and requires serious preparation for every case.
2. Lung resection surgeries are a highly morbid group of procedures, with mortality rates that are equivalent to or exceed elective coronary artery bypass surgery. Notably, a significant number of the serious complications of lung resection occur beyond the immediate surgical period and are related to postoperative respiratory insufficiency.
3. The anesthesiologist makes many decisions perioperatively that influence respiratory function and can conceivably contribute to postoperative insufficiency. It is imperative in caring for lung resection patients that the anesthesiologist be conscious of these issues and avoid any unwitting contribution to the burden of risk for respiratory impairment and failed tracheal extubation after lung resection surgery.

Clinical Vignette

The patient is a 59-year-old man with a 150 pack-year history of cigarette smoking. After being treated with antibiotics for a persistent productive cough, his sputum has become blood tinged over the past 2 weeks, and a chest x-ray revealed a right upper lobe coin lesion.

Health background includes longstanding hypertension, an anxiety disorder, and peripheral vascular disease, for which he underwent a left femoral-popliteal artery bypass 1 year ago. Current medications include lisinopril, atenolol, aspirin, and alprazolam.

Vital signs: BP 189/88 mm Hg, HR 55, room air SaO_2 92%.

Laboratory investigations are notable for white blood cell count 12.1 and prothrombin time 14.0 seconds (normal 12.5-13.8). Pulmonary function tests are notable for a FEV_1 of 50% predicted, FEV_1/FVC 60%, and DLCO of 45% predicted.

In the past two decades, significant research and innovation has improved both therapy and prognosis for lung cancers and benign tumors. Medical gains in imaging, better timing, prescription, and selectivity of radiation and chemotherapy have complemented surgical advances, including routine tumor staging, port access video-assistance, titanium staplers with scalpel blades, and more targeted operations designed to preserve unaffected lung tissue. Anesthesia advances have kept pace, with better lung isolation methods and a broadened pharmacologic armamentarium providing an enhanced flexibility that combines safe surgery with multiple options for postoperative analgesia and prompt wake-up and extubation, even for patients with limited respiratory reserve or when a procedure is terminated prematurely. Notably, many of these improvements have expanded the candidate pool for lung resection to include patients who would previously have been ineligible due to their marginal lung function.

Despite advances, perioperative morbidity and mortality rates for lung resection still exceed those for many major procedures (eg, aortocoronary bypass surgery), and few dispute the important role of the anesthesiologist's actions in influencing patient outcome.[1-3] The aim of this chapter is to address and integrate numerous elements of thoracic anesthesia, some outlined in more detail in other chapters, which combine to optimize anesthesia provision for lung resection surgery for cancer and benign chest tumors.

TYPES OF LUNG TUMORS

Over 170,000 primary lung tumors are diagnosed each year in the United States, with the majority being malignant (>95%). Malignant lung tumors are the largest source of cancer-related deaths in the United States. Cigarettes increase lung cancer risk for the average smoker by approximately tenfold, twentyfold for heavy smokers. Other inhalation exposures act alone or can compound smoking risk, including radiation (eg, radon, uranium), asbestos, nickel, chromate, mustard gas, arsenic, beryllium, iron, and vinyl chloride. Lung cancer is about twice as common in men as women (74 vs 31 per 100,000 per year), presenting most often during the sixth and seventh decades of life. While inhalation exposures are the major risk for lung cancer occurrence, in victims less than 40 years old (<2% patients) genetic vulnerability is also likely important.[4]

First symptoms of a primary lung cancer may include productive cough, hemoptysis, weight loss, pain or dyspnea, and less commonly clubbing, superior vena cava syndrome, Horner syndrome, muscle weakness, peripheral neuropathy, or ataxia. The most common tumors related to smoking are squamous and small cell and less frequently adenocarcinoma (Table 13–1). At diagnosis, over 80% of small cell tumors are metastatic, whereas less than half of squamous and adeno-carcinomas have spread. While most benign tumors are resectable, only 30% of malignant primary tumors are still sufficiently localized to potentially benefit from surgery.

Surgical resection of lung metastases improves survival in some situations. In the absence of other spread, one or several lung metastases can be removed on one or

Table 13-1. Classification of Lung Tumors Commonly Presenting for Lung Resection

Benign
Pleomorphic adenoma
Clear cell
Hamartoma
Plasma cell granuloma
Malignant
Primary
Small cell (20%, rarely amenable to surgery)
Non-small cell (80%)
Adenocarcinoma
Squamous cell carcinoma
Metastatic
Melanoma
Soft tissue/osteo-sarcomas
Germ cell tumors
Colorectal carcinoma
Renal cell carcinoma
Uterine carcinoma
Breast cancer
Squamous cell cancers of the head and neck

repeated occasions, often involving a simple wedge resection achieved using VATS surgery. Disease states include melanoma, soft tissue and osteo-sarcomas, germ cell tumors, colorectal, renal cell, uterine and breast cancer, and squamous cell cancers of the head and neck.[5]

LUNG RESECTION—PROCEDURE PLANNING

Minimizing loss of healthy tissue is a logical part of surgical planning for any lung resection. Limited procedures such as localized wedge or segmental lung resection are often all that is necessary for benign tumors. For cancerous lesions, evidence of tumor spread from noninvasive (eg, chest x-ray, CT, and PET scan) or invasive procedures such as bronchoscopy and mediastinoscopy provides the most important guide in avoiding unhelpful lung resection surgery. When mediastinoscopy reveals ipsilateral mediastinal lymph-node spread, subsequent response to induction chemotherapy (eg, cis-platinum, paclitaxel), evidenced by a negative re-mediastinoscopy, still indicates eligibility for curative surgery, and long-term outcomes are improved.[6]

When tumor spread is unlikely, bronchoscopy and mediastinoscopy may be scheduled at the same time as lung resection, but the anesthetic plan must always be able to adapt to early termination if staging samples return positive for cancer. Of practical clinical significance with early termination is not to have used agents with prolonged effects that delay wakeup (eg, muscle relaxants) or require prolonged observation (eg, neuraxial opioids). Delayed discharge home is particularly distressing for the patient coping with the news of their cancer spread.

Early stage cancerous tumors are treated by complete resection of the involved lung lobe. However, some early stage tumors, by reason of more extensive local spread or their relationship to major airways, are ineligible for lobectomy and have traditionally been candidates for pneumonectomy. Examples of lung-sparing alternatives to pneumonectomy for selected individuals include bi-lobectomy and upper lobe/sleeve bronchus resection with reattachment of the lower lung lobes. In high-risk patients with limited pulmonary reserve, localized wedge or segmental lung resection may be all that is possible even for malignant disease.

Video-assisted thoracic surgery (VATS) is taking an ever expanding role in the approach to lung tumor surgery. The introduction of VATS surgery for lung resection has been associated with good results and a reduction in complication rates (Table 13–2),[7,8] although some institutions have not seen improvements in outcome.[9] VATS procedures are particularly reliant on perfect lung isolation and place added responsibility on the anesthesiologist in this regard. Lung resection more extensive than lobectomy is generally not eligible for VATS, in part due to the disproportionately small size of the port incision relative to the resected tissue that must be extracted through it. However, even small tumors are sometimes so placed as to be ineligible for resection by a VATS approach (eg, hilar). Studies indicate that appropriate use of VATS procedures capably achieve surgical goals with lower dehiscence, bleeding and infection rates, reduced pain, and faster recovery. Compared to open thoracotomy, VATS also often reduces the need for rib spreading and the possibility of rib fractures. Other differences between VATS and open thoracotomy for equivalent procedures is the tendency for less pain and blood loss and quicker recovery from VATS surgery. Sources of morbidity and mortality following lung resection surgery vary by procedure and surgical approach, increasing with more extensive lung resection and open (vs VATS) surgical approaches (see Table 13–2).

PREOPERATIVE ASSESSMENT (SEE ALSO CHAPTER 9)

Beyond standard preoperative assessment, patients scheduled for lung tumor procedures commonly have considerations specific to their presenting condition and planned surgery. Perioperative risk may be increased by issues related to the origin of their cancer (eg, smoking), but tumor-derived concerns can also contribute to risk (eg, paraneoplastic syndromes). For lung tumor surgeries, a detailed assessment of airway, bleeding risk, and eligibility for neuraxial procedures is particularly relevant.

Smoking increases the risk of lung cancer, and also chronic bronchitis, reactive airway disease, and obstructive lung disease. Some patients present for surgery so affected by these accompanying conditions as to require supplemental home oxygen therapy. For these patients, preparation should include pulmonary function data to quantify their respiratory impairment and a plan for preoperative

Table 13–2. Complication Rates (%) in a Population of 1079 Patients Undergoing Lobectomy Lung Resection by Conventional Thoracotomy (*n* = 382) and video-assisted thoracoscopic surgery (VATS), *n* = 697 Approaches

Complication	Thoracotomy	VATS	*P* value
Atrial fibrillation	22	16	0.01
Atelectasis	12	5	0.0001
Prolonged air leak	19	11	0.0004
Bleeding	1.3	1	0.53
Transfusion	12	4	0.0001
Wound infection	0.8	0.1	0.13
Pneumonia	9	4	0.001
Empyema	1.6	0.6	0.18
Bronchopleural fistula	1	0.1	0.06
Sepsis	3	0.6	0.008
Renal failure	5	2	0.003
Cerebrovascular accident	0.8	0.4	0.67
Myocardial infarction	0.5	0.7	1
Ventricular arrhythmia	0.5	0.7	1
Deep venous thrombosis	0.5	0.1	0.29
Pulmonary embolus	0.8	0.4	0.67
Chest tube duration, median days (25th-75th quartile)	4 (3-6)	3 (2-4)	0.0001
Length of hospital stay, median days (25th-75th quartile)	5 (4-7)	4 (3-5)	0.0001
Death	6	2	0.003
Patients with no complication	50	70	0.0001

Adapted with permission from Villamizar NR, Darrabie MD, Burfeind WR, et al.[7] Copyright © Elsevier.

optimization. In patients with poor respiratory function, preoperative arterial blood gas assessment can also inform postoperative management (Figure 13–1). Risk for atherosclerotic heart and vascular disease is also increased in smokers, as is cor pulmonale, supraventricular tachyarrhythmias, and atrial fibrillation. Assessment of cardiac risk follows standardized protocols as for any nonscardiac surgery patient.[10]

Paraneoplastic syndromes sometimes are a presenting symptom of lung cancer. Tumor-mediated autoantibodies to calcium channels and Purkinje cells can cause Lambert-Eaton myesthenic syndrome and subacute cerebellar degeneration,

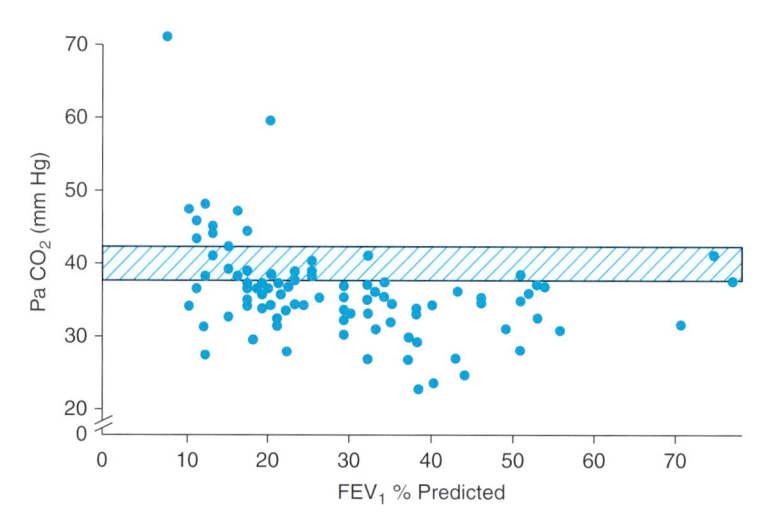

Figure 13–1. Evidence of an elevated arterial partial pressure of carbon dioxide (PaCO$_2$) while breathing spontaneously is strongly suggestive that a patient has very impaired pulmonary function, as represented in this data by severely impaired forced expiratory volume in 1 second with maximal effort (FEV$_1$). The shaded area represents normal PCO$_2$ values.

respectively.[11] The former involves muscle weakness that may be symptomatic, but whose diagnosis is sometimes missed until an exaggerated muscle relaxant response requires postoperative ventilator management; the latter is a degenerative neurologic disorder characterized by broad ataxic gait and nystagmus without other gross neurologic deficits. Lambert-Eaton syndrome contrasts with myesthenia gravis by its involvement of proximal more than distal limb muscles and improved strength with repetitive movements but not in response to acetylcholinesterase inhibitor therapy (eg, neostigmine). Other lung tumor-related hormone effects include hyponatremia due to inappropriate anti-diuretic hormone secretion, Cushing syndrome from excess adrenocorticotrophic hormone, and hypercalcemia from parathyroid hormone release. Among patients with benign lesions, those with neurofibromatosis-1 are notable for the frequent coexistence of neuroendocrine tumors including pheochromocytoma (up to 6% patients, and 20%-50% of those with associated hypertension) and carcinoids (up to 10% patients).[12-14] Although neurofibromatosis-1 is associated with an increased lung cancer risk, VATS in these patients is usually performed for neurofibroma resection with the offending tumor most often protruding from an intervertebral foramen. Presumably due to tumor friability and location, epidural hematoma with paraplegia can complicate neurofibroma resection and must be considered in the risk/benefit analysis for neuraxial analgesia.

Identification of patients with increased bleeding risk and those who may be ineligible for spinal/epidural analgesia (see Chapters 6, 9, 24) requires careful assessment of bleeding history (eg, with tooth extraction), chronic drug therapies (eg, clopidogrel), and review of coagulation tests. Neuraxial procedure guidelines are available regarding acceptable coagulation parameters and timing of anticoagulation cessation.[15] The plan for coordinated epidural catheter removal and postoperative thromboprophylaxis must also be formulated preoperatively to minimize spinal hematoma risk. In some patients presenting with conditions requiring chronic warfarin anticoagulation (eg, atrial fibrillation), heparin "bridging" therapy may be required until just prior to surgery. Concurrent infection and anatomic spinal abnormalities are also factors in determining suitability for spinal/epidural procedures.

Management of chronic drug therapies must involve attention to respiratory depressant effects, particularly in patients with marginal pulmonary reserve. Delayed tracheal extubation is a strong predictor of poor outcome, and agents such as extended release opioids can sometimes take partial blame for this complication after lung resection. Even depressant effects from well-intentioned but ill-considered "modest" preanesthetic intravenous sedative (eg, midazolam for anxiety) can complicate lung resection in high-risk patients; by compounding the respiratory depression due to agents that are arguably of more importance at the end of surgery, such as opioids for analgesia. In these circumstances, patient reassurance for anxiolysis, including an explanation of the need to limit preoperative sedation, is often sufficient, but if pharmacologic intervention is deemed essential (eg, during complicated epidural placement), then in the author's experience, for an average-sized adult, small doses of a short acting intravenous sedative (eg, 10-20 mg propofol) alone or potentiated by a *very* small dose of longer acting agent (eg, 0.25-0.5 mg midazolam) are generally very effective.

ANESTHETIC PLAN

Preinduction

Preparation for even the most "straightforward" lung surgery demands sufficient monitoring and vascular access to appropriately respond to complications that can occur, most notably including significant hemorrhage, an uncommon but ever-present risk for any intrathoracic procedure. Beyond standard monitoring requirements and two large bore peripheral intravenous catheters, invasive lines generally include a peripheral intra-arterial catheter for continuous blood pressure recording and repeated blood gas assessment. A right-sided radial arterial line is convenient if staging procedures are also planned since this location also facilitates recognition of innominate artery compression during mediastinoscopy (see Chapter 10).

Neuraxial injection or catheter placement prior to anesthesia induction (eg, epidural catheter insertion) most conveniently occurs following placement of peripheral intravenous and intra-arterial catheters but prior to central venous access. Such a sequence provides intra-arterial monitoring for recognition of intravascular or intrathecal injection of an epidural catheter test-dose and avoids the cumbersome movement required to have a patient transfer into the sitting or lateral position with a central venous line *in situ*.

While central venous access is not essential for lung resection surgery, patient and procedural factors such as comorbidities (eg, cardiac history), bleeding risk (eg, redo thoracotomy), and the likelihood of postoperative pulmonary edema (eg, pneumonectomy) may warrant such monitoring. If placement of a central venous catheter is deemed necessary, selection of the side *ipsilateral* to the operative lung is highly preferable for subclavian or internal jugular central venous puncture, due to possibilites such as unrecognized bullous lung disease and the potential for tension pneumothorax in the nonoperative lung. "Down-side" tension pneumothorax can be lethal when it manifests intraoperatively and is difficult to detect. One way is to attach a stethoscope earpiece to a suitable esophageal temperature probe and use it as an esophageal stethoscope. In the case of a "down-side" tension pneumothorax, the chest is completely silent on manual inflation of the reservoir bag.

Bladder catheter placement is not essential for all lung resection procedures and can occur after anesthesia induction. Urinary output monitoring provides some information regarding intravascular volume status in the absence of central venous pressure data and should always be used to avoid the possibility of urinary retention in patients with postoperative epidural analgesia.

Standard preinduction considerations include administration of intravenous antibiotic prophylaxis within 1 hour prior to surgical incision and planning for postoperative disposition (PACU vs stepdown vs ICU observation). Postoperative analgesia strategy often influences disposition when continuous epidural infusions are used, since the care team must be equipped and trained to recognize and treat potentially serious complications associated with their use such as hypotension from local anesthetic-mediated reductions in sympathetic tone and delayed respiratory depression due to cephalad spread of neuraxial opioids (see Chapter 6).

The potential for major hemorrhage with lung surgery is partially explained by the thin walled and high flow characteristics of the pulmonary arterial tree, making these vessels both vulnerable to injury and difficult to repair, with the same capacity for rapid blood loss as major systemic arteries. The uncommon but serious bleeding complication with lung resection mandates preparatory steps in addition to good intravenous access and monitoring. Confirmation that blood products are available and/or in the operating room is essential immediately prior to surgery. Routine availability of colloid volume expanders, use of fluid and patient warming technology, and a rapid transfusion device immediately available or nearby should also be considered.

Nonetheless, the liberal availability of blood products required in preparation for lung resection surgery must be accompanied by thoughtful application of transfusion "triggers" and strict avoidance of unjustifiable blood product administration. Poorer outcomes with "unnecessary" transfusion including pulmonary complications are particularly relevant to lung surgery. Also, a note of caution is warranted regarding the potential for resuscitation "overshoot" that can occur in any response to acute hemorrhage. An effort to keep scale in the resuscitation of hemorrhage, assisted by good communication with the surgeon, will help avoid the lung edema that can occur from fluid overload.

Intraoperative Management

Anesthesia Induction

Anesthesia induction should be immediately preceded by meticulous preoxygenation; note that compared to the standard instruction to "take a deep breath in," prolonged exhalation to expel room air *prior* to each inhalation of enriched oxygen is actually more efficient, particularly in patients with obstructive lung disease. Immediately prior to anesthesia, induction is also a convenient moment to test and/or supplement any local anesthetic block that may be developing. Standard anesthesia induction agent selection to achieve hypnosis, paralysis, and blunting of the hemodynamic intubation response should be matched to the characteristics of the lung resection procedure and patient, as highlighted above. Becoming experienced with drug selections to minimize lingering respiratory depressant effects, even for patients at low risk for delayed tracheal extubation, pays dividends when a patient is unexpectedly sick or at high risk. For example, midazolam is not essential for anesthesia induction and, while not routinely recommended, even intravenous opioids to blunt the intubation response (eg, fentanyl) can be replaced by a bolus of intravenous lidocaine (1.0-1.5 mg/kg) for the most impaired patient, particularly if postoperative continuous epidural analgesia is planned.

Choice and dose of muscle relaxant must be made to optimize conditions for tracheal intubation but also to respect any potential for a shortened procedure. When bronchoscopy and mediastinoscopy precede lung resection, a single-lumen endotracheal tube with minimum internal diameter of 7.5 to 8.0 mm is used to allow passage of an adult bronchoscope. Otherwise, tracheal intubation requires lung separation to allow for operative lung deflation and nonoperative lung ventilation.

Double-lumen endotracheal tubes provide excellent lung collapse and versatile lung isolation in most circumstances, with bronchoscopic confirmation of positioning. The course of the left mainstem bronchus under the aortic arch provides the most predictable and uninterrupted airway "landing zone" for endobronchial cuff placement. A left-sided tube is the preferred method unless tube proximity to the surgical field obliges an alternate strategy (eg, left pneumonectomy). Adult left- and right-sided double lumen tubes are identified by their endobronchial tube caliber; 32, 35, and 37 are common female adult sizes, while 37, 39, and 41 French are available for men. Both undersized and oversized double lumen tubes may complicate lung isolation and even cause difficulties with tracheal intubation.[16] Correct endotracheal tube size selection is therefore critical (see Chapter 5).

Bronchial blocker options for lung isolation are sometimes preferable. However, particular effort must be directed to assuring good lung deflation for surgery with this technique, including, (1) the earliest possible blocker inflation time to maximize absorption, and (2) prior to balloon inflation, an extended period of apneic exhalation (>60 s) following ventilation with 100% oxygen, to minimize residual lung volume and hasten gas absorption, respectively. Proximal balloon migration in the airway sufficient to lose lung isolation is common with bronchial blockers. One approach to reduce the frequency of this problem is to trap the inflated balloon at the junction of the upper lobe and mainstem bronchus. While effective, this approach should not be used for upper lobectomy surgery due to the risk of including a piece of the balloon in the resected specimen.

Secure positioning of the patient in the lateral decubitus position after anesthesia induction with the operative side up is typical for most lung resection procedures. Additional reverse-Trendelenberg and reflex positioning of the operating table is common to spread the rib spaces and level the operative chest wall. Safe positioning must include inspection of pressure points, particularly of the down-side arm, including the brachial plexus in the axilla, radial nerve at the humerus, and ulnar nerve at the elbow. In addition, reconfirmation of lung isolation in the lateral position and support of the weight of the ventilator circuit to prevent drag on the endotracheal tube is prudent.

Mild hypotension with anesthesia induction is ubiquitous but can be more common and marked in lung resection patients, often due to an evolving sympathetic epidural block, but more of concern if caused by the interaction of positive pressure ventilation with severe obstructive lung disease. Recognition of so called "dynamic hyperinflation" from inefficient exhalation (also known as breath "stacking" or "auto-PEEP") is critical both for its hemodynamic implications, but also its potential for serious complications during a procedure (eg, barotrauma, "down-side" tension pneumothorax, cardiac arrest).[17] While low levels of hyperinflation are common in patients with severe obstructive lung disease or asthma, hemodynamically significant dynamic hyperinflation is uncommon. In the author's experience, this type of dynamic hyperinflation is best diagnosed during a period of complete cessation of manual or mechanical positive pressure ventilation—a gradual rise of 10 to 20 mm Hg systolic blood pressure over a 1 to 2 minute apneic period in the absence of other stimuli is characteristic. In patients with dynamic hyperinflation, ventilator settings should be titrated to minimize breath stacking; suggested changes include eliminating positive end expiratory pressure (PEEP), adjusting ventilator settings to extend expiratory and reduce inspiratory breath times (eg, 1:4 or 1:5 ratio), and even modestly reduce breath depth and frequency (mild "permissive hypercapnia" is generally well-tolerated). If bronchoconstriction is contributing to dynamic hyperinflation, interventions such as bronchodilator therapy and inhaled volatile agent may also be helpful. Rarely, vasoactive infusions and/or fluid bolus interventions are required to support blood pressure. Periodic arterial blood gas assessment and episodic reinflation of the operative lung for ventilation, coordinated with the surgical team, may also be required for safe management of these patients. Intraoperative transesophageal echocardiography may even occasionally be considered to assess ventricular filling.

ANESTHESIA MAINTENANCE

Anesthesia for lung resection requires provision of optimal surgical conditions including the need for prolonged one-lung ventilation, while maintaining an extended period of hypnosis, muscle relaxation, and analgesia (in continuum with the postoperative period). Monitoring to minimize any chance of recall is also important (eg, bispectral index or end-tidal volatile agent monitoring), particularly with drug selection being biased away from amnestic agents. Ventilator settings must account for transitions from two to one-lung ventilation, including a goal to minimize barotrauma (eg, peak inspiratory pressures below 30 cm H_2O). Finally, strategies that keep infused perioperative fluids and inspired oxygen levels to a minimum are embraced by many thoracic surgery teams.

Major decisions in selecting agents for anesthesia maintenance include the relative roles of regional, intravenous, and inhalational anesthesia. So-called "balanced anesthesia" refers to either inhalational or infused intravenous agents to achieve "light" general anesthesia, combined with local anesthetic epidural block for surgical chest wall anesthesia. Potential advantages of balanced anesthesia include reduced need for hypnotic agents and pre-emergence establishment of analgesia. For patients with severely limited respiratory reserve who are considered at extremely high risk for failure to achieve tracheal extubation, a balanced anesthesia strategy combining intraoperative and postoperative local anesthetic epidural infusion and intraoperative light general anesthesia without the use of benzodiazepines and opioids may be useful methods to consider.

Inhalational and total intravenous anesthetic (TIVA)-based maintenance strategies without local anesthetic blockade comfortably achieve general anesthesia for most thoracic surgery patients but compared to a balanced anesthesia approach require more specific planning for transition to postoperative analgesia. Agents selected for a primarily inhalational anesthetic, such as desflurane and sevoflurane, have a low blood/gas partition coefficient that facilitates rapid emergence. Notably, the recurring requirement for 100% oxygen and the potential for air emboli surgery are clear reasons for the rare use of nitrous oxide during lung resection, although associated immune suppression also runs counter to the goals of cancer surgery. Intravenous infusion agents for TIVA are also those with "effervescent" properties that facilitate prompt emergence, such as propofol and remifentanil. Both inhalational and TIVA techniques can be combined with postoperative analgesia approaches involving longer acting opioids by intravenous bolus or epidural infusion, and/or direct local anesthetic infiltration of intercostal nerves, port wounds, and chest tube exit sites.

Purported advantages of TIVA over inhalational strategies include avoidance of volatile agent-mediated inhibition of hypoxic pulmonary vasoconstriction, thereby reducing V/Q mismatch and oxygen desaturation episodes during one-lung ventilation (OLV).[18] However, more recent clinical studies have questioned these observations.[19] One recent study comparing oxygenation and desaturation episodes with equipotent TIVA or volatile anesthesia (as judged by a bispectral monitoring target 40-60) in combination with epidural local/opioid analgesia found no difference between these approaches (Figure 13–2). In contrast, purported advantages of inhalational over TIVA include fewer episodes of hypotension and/or vasopressor use and a smoother transition to postoperative analgesia, particularly when TIVA is combined with epidural local anesthesia. In clinical terms, the impression of this author is that the anesthesiologist is the most important ingredient regardless of their selected technique.

Arterial oxygen desaturation (<90%) is common during one-lung ventilation, occuring in up to 10% of patients[20] but is rarely due to shunting alone, which

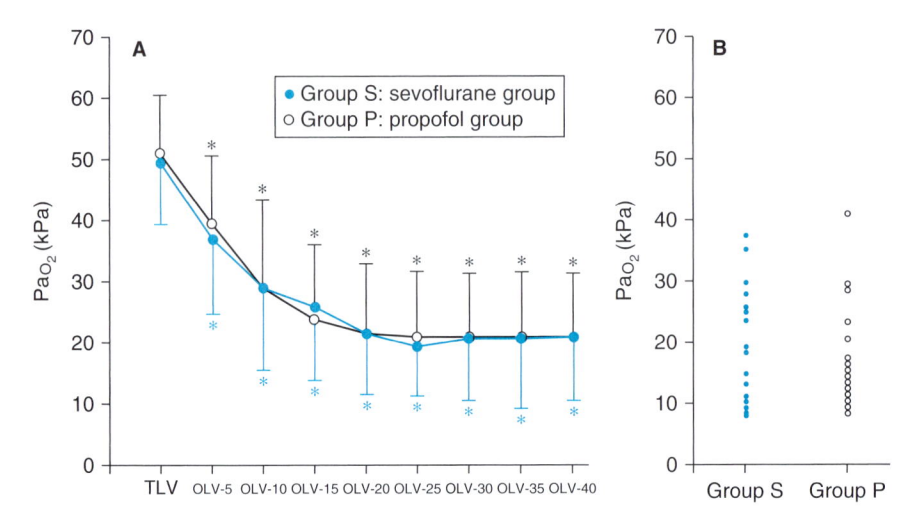

Figure 13-2. Changes in arterial oxygen levels over time (mins) with the transition from two-lung (TLV) to one-lung ventilation (OLV) during 65 thoracic surgery procedures randomized to equipotent levels of inhalational sevoflurane or intravenous propofol anesthesia (A). The lowest arterial oxygenation value observed for each patient is also depicted (B). (Used with permission from Pruszkowski O, Dalibon N, Moutafis M, et al.[31] Copyright Oxford University Press.)

amounts to only about 30% after normal adaptation to one-lung physiology. Other sources of hypoxemia with OLV are numerous, including insufficient inspired oxygen concentration, endotracheal tube obstruction or malposition, inadequate tidal volume, and low oxygen delivery from hemodilution or depressed cardiac output due to deep anesthesia, hypovolemia, or right ventricular dysfunction related to hypervolemia or myocardial dysfunction.

A logical approach to the management of arterial desaturation during OLV is an essential skill for the thoracic anesthesiologist (Figure 13–3; see also Chapter 5). The first response is to acutely rectify the clinical situation by returning inspired oxygen concentration to 100% and asking the surgeon to temporarily discontinue surgery while reinflating the operative lung by manual re-expansion. A brief period of two-lung ventilation generally returns the oxygen saturation to acceptable levels, providing a period for troubleshooting to identify addressable factors to prevent or delay its recurrence. The two main causes of hypoxemia, sources of inadequate ventilation and/or perfusion, must be promptly identified and optimized. Simple steps include suctioning of tube secretions and auscultatory and fiberoptic visual confirmation of correct tube positioning (including lung isolation and identifying any occult upper lobe obstruction from endobronchial tube malposition) and adjusting ventilator settings to 3 to 4 mL/kg tidal volume (ideal body weight) or using pressure limited ventilation (maximum peak inspiratory pressure <30 cm H_2O). The physiology of OLV increases normal demands on the right ventricle, requiring

```
┌─────────────────────────────────────┐
│   Hypoxemia during OLV: SpO₂ <90%   │
└─────────────────────────────────────┘
                  │
                  ▼
        Increase FiO₂ to 100%
```

Life threatening (SpO₂ <90%) and/or occurrence of arrhythmia and/or ST changes

Non-life threatening (SpO₂ >90%)
- Continue OLV

Improve oxygenation

Stop surgery
- Resume bipulmonary ventilation

Treatable cause
Fiberoptic bronchoscopy
- DLT position
- Secretions/blood

Hemodynamic
- Low blood pressure
- Too deep level of anesthesia
- Blood loss
- Right ventricular dysfunction

Optimize ventilation
Nonventilated lung
- Manual re-expansion (O₂ 100%)
- CPAP (O₂ 100%)

Ventilated lung
- PEEP
- Recruitment maneuver
- PEEP evaluation

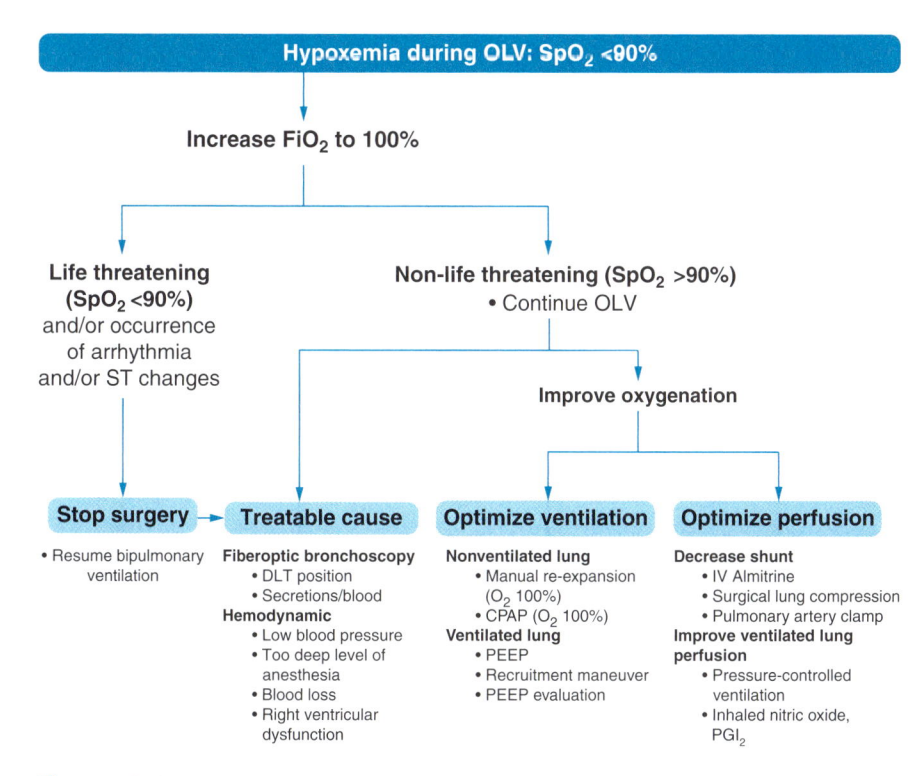

Optimize perfusion
Decrease shunt
- IV Almitrine
- Surgical lung compression
- Pulmonary artery clamp

Improve ventilated lung perfusion
- Pressure-controlled ventilation
- Inhaled nitric oxide, PGI₂

Figure 13–3. Suggested algorithm for response to hypoxemia during one-lung ventilation (OLV). CPAP - continuous positive airway pressure; DLT - double lumen tube; FiO₂ - inspired fraction of oxygen; PEEP - positive end-expiratory pressure; PGI₂ - prostacyclin; ST-ST segment. (Used with permission from Roze H, Lafargue M, Ouattara A.[20] Copyright Wolters Kluwer Health.)

higher filling pressures to maintain cardiac output—a modest colloid or crystalloid bolus (eg, 250 mL) may expose a state of volume-responsive hypovolemia. Excessively deep anesthesia should also be easily recognized and corrected.

If hypoxemia recurs during one-lung anesthesia despite the simple steps outlined above, then a sequential approach to improving oxygenation with ventilatory maneuvers may help the problem. The first simple step is to introduce continuous oxygen insufflation to the operative lung (nondependent, upside). This can be easily achieved by placing an endotracheal suction catheter into the open airway lumen attached to standard tubing with oxygen flows at 2 to 3 L/min (remember to occlude the thumb port). A more elaborate setup can be added to further recruit perfused upside lung alveoli with continuous positive airway pressure (CPAP) 5 to 10 cm H_2O; this rarely causes sufficient lung inflation to distract the surgical team.

If hypoxemia persists despite adding oxygen and CPAP to the upside lung as outlined above, then changes to improve ventilation of the nonoperative (dependent, downside) lung may be helpful. First, recruitment maneuvers for a few seconds with a peak airway pressure of 40 cm H_2O will assure that atelectasis in the dependent lung is not contributing to hypoxemia. Second, an experiment with the addition of PEEP is warranted. For some patients, the addition of 10 cm H_2O PEEP will recruit alveoli and improve oxygenation; whereas, for others, it will paradoxically shunt blood towards the upside lung, while in some individuals added PEEP will aggravate "auto PEEP" and precipitate hypotension without improving oxygenation (see also *One-lung ventilation in patients with severe chronic obstructive pulmonary disease,* in Chapter 15). Converting from volume-controlled to pressure-limited ventilation may also help for some patients.

Clearly, clamping of the arterial supply to lung being resected should reduce shunt and improve oxygen saturation, but active steps to otherwise improve hypoxemia through redistribution of blood flow during one-lung anesthesia are otherwise rarely employed. Simple retraction of the upside lung has been noted to reduce hypoxemia. As mentioned above, the importance of anesthetic agent selection is controversial, with evidence for the inhibition of hypoxic pulmonary vasoconstriction by volatile anesthetics relative to TIVA being restricted to comparisons with isoflurane; whereas, more recently, sevoflurane has even been suggested to reduce inflammatory response and improve outcomes compared to TIVA.[21] Infusions of the hypoxic pulmonary vasoconstriction potentiator almitrine have shown benefit in some studies, alone and in combination with nitric oxide. Notably, almitrine has an important toxicity profile and is not currently available in the United States.

Attentiveness to inspired air:oxygen ratios and tidal volume management during lung resection may affect outcomes, with the bulk of evidence supporting a strategy that keeps O_2 concentrations and tidal volumes at lowest tolerable levels.[22,23] For patients receiving induction therapy prior to their surgery, this has particular importance since adjuvant chemotherapy (eg, cisplatin, paclitaxel) can inflict subclinical acute lung injury making parenchyma more vulnerable to effects such as barotrauma, oxygen toxicity, and the formation of reactive oxygen species. Unacceptable oxygen desaturation clearly warrants steps to prevent hypoxemia, including recruitment maneuvers (peak airway pressure <40 cm H_2O) and inspired oxygen concentration up to 100%, but, when other options exist, avoiding high airway pressures (eg, keep peak airway pressure <30 cm H_2O) and oxygen concentrations (eg, <50%) may be beneficial. A common mistake with volume-controlled ventilation is to overlook the risk of barotrauma at the onset of one-lung anesthesia; to avoid inadvertent large breaths, minute ventilation during one-lung anesthesia can be safely achieved by more frequent smaller breaths or by changing to pressure limited ventilation and modest permissive hypercapnia.

Acute lung injury and adult respiratory distress syndrome (ALI/ARDS) is a very serious complication that arises within the first 3 to 4 days following lung resection surgery and is associated with a 40% mortality rate.[1] ALI/ARDS prevalence after pneumonectomy, lobectomy/bi-lobectomy, and sublobar resections are 8, 3, and 0.9%, respectively. Numerous patient and procedural characteristics have been associated with increased risk of ALI/ARDS, notably including high tidal volume and airway pressure during OLV.[24] Other reported factors include advanced age, male gender, chronic suppurative disease, concurrent cardiac disease, low diffusion capacity for carbon monoxide, and resection of more than 45% of lung vasculature.[2] Additional perioperative ALI/ARDS risk factors include hypervolemia, greater extent of tissue resection, extended surgery time, increased blood loss, and reoperation. While no singular cause of ALI/ARDS after lung resection has been identified, evidence supports multiple contributing mechanisms, causes and aggravating factors, including hyperoxia, reactive oxygen species and barotrauma, lymphatic disruption, microembolization, elevated pulmonary vascular pressures, and ischemia-reperfusion and inflammatory lung injury.

Concern over perioperative fluid therapy for lung resection comes from reports of ALI/ARDS associated with large volumes of intravenous fluid and hypervolemia.[2] While "excessive" fluid administration is avoidable and may be contributory, it does not always precede the onset of ALI/ARDS. Nonetheless, conservative fluid management seems prudent in most cases, although fluid restriction sufficient to precipitate acute kidney injury following lung resection also correlates with adverse outcome (see also Chapter 23).[25] Recent advances in fluid management include better understanding of the importance of the endothelial glycocalyx in the formation of edema, and factors that affect the redistribution of colloid and crystalloid from the intravascular space.[26] Administration algorithms have moved away from the traditionally calculated "third space" fluid loss for a procedure and instead advocate for measured replacement of insensible fluid deficits with crystalloid (eg, lactated Ringer solution), and, in the absence of major bleeding or anemia, the use of colloid infusion for subsequent euvolemia maintenance. This strategy rarely translates intraoperatively into more than 1 liter of crystalloid and 1 L of colloid total for most patients.

ANESTHESIA EMERGENCE AND RECOVERY

As outlined above, in formulating an anesthetic plan for thoracic surgery, considerable respect must be paid to a serious complication of emergence whose occurrence is partly under the influence of the anesthesiologist—failure to achieve tracheal extubation. This is particularly important since major pulmonary complications of lung resection surgery are more than twice as likely in the setting of postoperative respiratory failure[27] and highly associated with other markers of adverse outcome, including postoperative mortality (see Table 13–2). Contributors to the generally high risk of respiratory failure after lung resection include "variable" factors amenable to optimization such as inadequate respiratory mechanics (from residual paralysis, suboptimal positioning, and pain-related chest wall splinting), post-extubation upper airway obstruction, and respiratory depression due to residual anesthetic agents, and "fixed" factors such as pre-existing disease, infection, and surgery-related loss of parenchyma, lung contusion, and airway soiling. An effective tracheal extubation strategy must focus on optimizing "variable" factors, including preemergence interventions (airway suctioning, positioning, analgesia, etc), appropriate agent selection throughout surgery (as outlined above), and a logical brief sequence of anesthetic withdrawal and tracheal extubation.[28] Subsequent to tracheal extubation but equally important activities include the *continuous* maintenance of a patent airway and precise monitoring to identify those who will require reintubation.

Chest wall closure and skin suturing identify the final phase of all lung resection surgeries. Routine interventions poorly tolerated at lighter anesthetic depths should occur early during chest closure, such as gastric, throat and endotracheal tube suctioning, and oral and/or nasal airway insertion. Reducing anesthetic depth and neuromuscular block over the 10 to 15 minute closure period is critical to preparation for emergence. Until just prior to extubation, spontaneous respiration is discouraged to avoid hypoventilation and unrecognized CO_2 narcosis, the somnolence from carbon dioxide accumulation that can develop at levels as low as 70 mm Hg.[29] An alternate approach during chest closure is to allow spontaneous respiration assisted by pressure-support mode ventilation; this strategy can prevent gas rebreathing and hypercarbia (from the considerable dead space of the double-lumen tube), while allowing respiratory drive to develop.

Since pain at emergence is extremely difficult to treat without adding acute respiratory depression and interfering with efforts to extubate the patient, the anesthesiologist must be confident that analgesia is established preemergence. If a thoracic epidural catheter has been placed, a common practice is to supplement existing analgesia with an additional 2 mL bolus of 2% preservative-free lidocaine (for an average adult male) 10 to 15 minutes prior to emergence; this represents a modest "insurance policy" against emergence pain that is rarely associated with block-mediated hypotension but allows the patient to be awake and extubated before more pain management decisions are needed.

Prior to emergence, the patient should be moved into a sitting or deck chair position; the flex at the waist and supine head up position raises the chest and displaces the abdominal contents caudad. Practically speaking, such positioning establishes or increases functional residual capacity, which reduces the likelihood of oxygen desaturation through the emergence phase.[28] If the patient is otherwise stable, and tracheal extubation is expected to be a major challenge, transfer from the operating table to the bed prior to awakening (while maintaining adequate monitoring) eliminates this interruption to coordinated breathing. When dealing with a patient with extremely impaired pulmonary function, a near vertical sitting position supported by pillows is essential.

As wound dressing is completed, steps can be coordinated to eliminate residual anesthetic and muscle relaxant drugs while simultaneously positioning the patient. Only a brief period of responsiveness, coordinated strength, and regular breathing pattern with acceptable tidal volume and/or maximum inspiratory pressure should precede prompt tracheal extubation and 100% O_2 by face mask. Among post-extubation options for maintaining a patent airway, the nasopharyngeal trumpet is best tolerated for prolonged periods but must be placed very carefully to minimize any risk of epistaxis.

Patients with severely impaired pulmonary function commonly cannot meet "ideal" tidal volume or maximum inspiratory pressure extubation criteria, and experience and judgement from the anesthesiologist is particularly neccessary in timing endotracheal tube removal for these patients, appreciating that some *will* require reintubation.[28] For patients with severe disease, appropriate responsiveness, strength, and breathing pattern may warrant a trial of tracheal extubation without evidence of deep breaths, since delay increases the chances of CO_2 narcosis in this population.[29] Yang and colleagues found an f/Vt ratio (frequency of breaths per minute divided by the tidal volume in liters) <100 to be highly predictive of successful tracheal extubation in critically ill patients with limited respiratory reserve, but the value of this metric in perioperative patients has not been assessed.[30] Fortunately, such difficult emergence occurrences are infrequent, but the patient with limited respiratory reserve likely has the most to gain from an experienced anesthesia team and avoidance of a prolonged episode of postoperative mechanical ventilation.

To distinguish the stable extubated patient with limited respiratory reserve from one who needs reintubation, beyond clinical appearance and pulse oximetry monitoring, an extremely useful tool is arterial blood gas CO_2 trends. Sequential repeated blood gas determinations immediately following tracheal extubation (eg, every 3 min) identify two main patterns; the first, a steady decrease of CO_2 levels toward the patient's baseline, even if starting from extremely high values (eg, 100 to 120 mm Hg), favorably predicts successful extubation and generally indicates simple ongoing conservative care will be sufficient; the second, where CO_2 levels are stable or rising, is much more concerning and requires further prompt intervention and optimization to avert respiratory failure and tracheal reintubation. Should tracheal reintubation be required, it is important to remember that bag-mask ventilation and oxygenation should avert major problems and allow this to be a controlled event.

REFERENCES

1. Dulu A, Pastores SM, Park B, Riedel E, Rusch V, Halpern NA. Prevalence and mortality of acute lung injury and ards after lung resection. *Chest.* 2006;130(1):73-78.
2. Grichnik KP, D'Amico TA. Acute lung injury and acute respiratory distress syndrome after pulmonary resection. *Semin Cardiothorac Vasc Anesth.* 2004;8(4):317-334.
3. Harpole DH Jr, DeCamp MM Jr, Daley J, et al. Prognostic models of thirty-day mortality and morbidity after major pulmonary resection. *J Thorac Cardiovasc Surg.* 1999;117(5):969-979.
4. Lindstrom I, Nordling S, Nissen AM, Tammilehto L, Mattson K, Knuutila S. DNA copy number changes in lung adenocarcinoma in younger patients. *Mod Pathol.* 2002;15(4):372-378.
5. Kaifi JT, Gusani NJ, Deshaies I, et al. Indications and approach to surgical resection of lung metastases. *J Surg Oncol.* 2010;102(2):187-195.
6. Call S, Rami-Porta R, Obiols C, et al. Repeat mediastinoscopy in all its indications: experience with 96 patients and 101 procedures. *Eur J Cardiothorac Surg.* 2011;39(6):1022-1027.
7. Villamizar NR, Darrabie MD, Burfeind WR, et al. Thoracoscopic lobectomy is associated with lower morbidity compared with thoracotomy. *J Thorac Cardiovasc Surg.* 2009;138(2):419-425.
8. Whitson BA, Groth SS, Duval SJ, Swanson SJ, Maddaus MA. Surgery for early-stage non-small cell lung cancer: a systematic review of the video-assisted thoracoscopic surgery versus thoracotomy approaches to lobectomy. *Ann Thorac Surg.* 2008;86(6):2008-2016; discussion 2016-2008.
9. Gopaldas RR, Bakaeen FG, Dao TK, Walsh GL, Swisher SG, Chu D. Video-assisted thoracoscopic versus open thoracotomy lobectomy in a cohort of 13,619 patients. *Ann Thorac Surg.* 2010;89(5):1563-1570.
10. Fleisher LA, Beckman JA, Brown KA, et al. ACC/AHA 2007 guidelines on perioperative cardiovascular evaluation and care for noncardiac surgery: a report of the American College of Cardiology/American Heart Association Task Force on practice guidelines (writing committee to revise the 2002 guidelines on perioperative cardiovascular evaluation for noncardiac surgery): developed in collaboration with the American Society of Echocardiography, American Society of Nuclear Cardiology, Heart Rhythm

Society, Society of Cardiovascular Anesthesiologists, Society for Cardiovascular Angiography and Interventions, Society for Vascular Medicine and Biology, and Society for Vascular Surgery. *Circulation.* 2007;116(17):e418-e499.
11. Leonovicz BM, Gordon EA, Wass CT. Paraneoplastic syndromes associated with lung cancer: a unique case of concomitant subacute cerebellar degeneration and lambert-eaton myasthenic syndrome. *Anesth Analg.* 2001;93(6):1557-1559, table of contents.
12. Griffiths DF, Williams GT, Williams ED. Duodenal carcinoid tumours, phaeochromocytoma and neurofibromatosis: islet cell tumour, phaeochromocytoma and the von Hippel-Lindau complex: two distinctive neuroendocrine syndromes. *Q J Med.* 1987;64(245):769-782.
13. Zografos GN, Vasiliadis GK, Zagouri F, et al. Pheochromocytoma associated with neurofibromatosis type 1: concepts and current trends. *World J Surg Oncol.* 2010;8:14.
14. Jensen RT, Berna MJ, Bingham DB, Norton JA. Inherited pancreatic endocrine tumor syndromes: advances in molecular pathogenesis, diagnosis, management, and controversies. *Cancer.* 2008;113(7 Suppl):1807-1843.
15. Horlocker TT, Wedel DJ, Benzon H, et al. Regional anesthesia in the anticoagulated patient: defining the risks (the Second Asra Consensus Conference on Neuraxial Anesthesia and Anticoagulation). *Reg Anesth Pain Med.* 2003;28(3):172-197.
16. Chow MY, Liam BL, Thng CH, Chong BK. Predicting the size of a double-lumen endobronchial tube using computed tomographic scan measurements of the left main bronchus diameter. *Anesth Analg.* 1999;88(2):302-305.
17. Vanden Hoek TL, Morrison LJ, Shuster M, et al. Part 12: cardiac arrest in special situations: 2010 American Heart Association guidelines for cardiopulmonary resuscitation and emergency cardiovascular care. *Circulation.* 2010;122(8 Suppl 3):S829-S861.
18. Abe K, Shimizu T, Takashina M, Shiozaki H, Yoshiya I. The effects of propofol, isoflurane, and sevoflurane on oxygenation and shunt fraction during one-lung ventilation. *Anesth Analg.* 1998;87(5):1164-1169.
19. Ishikawa S. Oxygenation may improve with time during one-lung ventilation. *Anesth Analg.* 1999;89(1):258-259.
20. Roze H, Lafargue M, Ouattara A. Case scenario: management of intraoperative hypoxemia during one-lung ventilation. *Anesthesiology.* 2011;114(1):167-174.
21. De Conno E, Steurer MP, Wittlinger M, et al. Anesthetic-induced improvement of the inflammatory response to one-lung ventilation. *Anesthesiology.* 2009;110(6):1316-1326.
22. Grocott HP. Oxygen toxicity during one-lung ventilation: is it time to re-evaluate our practice? *Anesthesiol Clin.* 2008;26:273-280, v.
23. Walker MG, Yao LJ, Patterson EK, et al. The effect of tidal volume on systemic inflammation in acid-induced lung injury. *Respiration.* 2011;81(4):333-42.
24. Jeon K, Yoon JW, Suh GY, et al. Risk factors for post-pneumonectomy acute lung injury/acute respiratory distress syndrome in primary lung cancer patients. *Anaesth Intensive Care.* 2009;37(1):14-19.
25. Martin D, Kushins S, Phillips-Bute B, Onaitis M, Stafford-Smith M. Comparison of post-pneumonectomy outcomes and AKI by AKIN creatinine rise and AKIN oliguria criteria. *Anesthesiology.* 2009;111:A176.
26. Chappell D, Jacob M, Hofmann-Kiefer K, Conzen P, Rehm M. A rational approach to perioperative fluid management. *Anesthesiology.* 2008;109(4):723-740.
27. Stephan F, Boucheseiche S, Hollande J, et al. Pulmonary complications following lung resection: a comprehensive analysis of incidence and possible risk factors. *Chest.* 2000;118(5):1263-1270.
28. Miller KA, Harkin CP, Bailey PL. Postoperative tracheal extubation. *Anesth Analg.* 1995;80(1):149-172.
29. Langford NJ. Carbon dioxide poisoning. *Toxicol Rev.* 2005;24(4):229-235.
30. Yang KL, Tobin MJ. A prospective study of indexes predicting the outcome of trials of weaning from mechanical ventilation. *N Engl J Med.* 1991;324(21):1445-1450.
31. Pruszkowski O, Dalibon N, Moutafis M, et al. Effects of propofol vs sevoflurane on arterial oxygenation during one-lung ventilation. *Bri J Anaesth.* 2007;98(4):539-544.

Extrapleural Pneumonectomy

14

Timothy E. Miller

Key Points

1. In an extrapleural pneumonectomy the lung is removed en bloc, together with parietal and visceral pleura, ipsilateral hemidiaphragm and pericardium, as well as mediastinal lymph nodes.
2. The operation is now reserved almost exclusively for the treatment of mesothelioma. A recent randomized control trial showed no improved survival in patients treated with surgery in the context of trimodal therapy.
3. 2-10% of individuals with prolonged asbestos exposure will develop mesothelioma, but more than 80% of mesothelioma patients have a history of exposure to asbestos.
4. The major anesthetic issues are significant blood loss, hemodynamic instability, difficult fluid therapy, risk of cardiac herniation and high probability of dysrhythmias.

Case Vignette

The patient is a 57-year-old ex-shipyard worker who presents for an extrapleural pneumonectomy after a work-up for dyspnea revealed a malignant pleural effusion positive for mesothelioma. He has no evidence of extrathoracic disease. He has a history of 40 pack-years of smoking but has not smoked in 10 years.

He has no other medical problems and medications include only a multivitamin. Vital signs: BP 135/70, HR 70, room air SpO_2 93%. Routine laboratory examination is unremarkable. Pulmonary function tests are notable for a FEV_1/FVC ratio of 80%, an FEV_1 of 70% predicted, a FVC of 75% predicted, and a DLCO of 50% predicted.

Extrapleural pneumonectomy (EPP) was introduced in the 1940s for the treatment of tuberculous empyema and other pleural space infections.[1] It is a radical surgery that differs from conventional pneumonectomy in that the lung is removed en bloc, together with parietal and visceral pleura, ipsilateral hemidiaphragm and pericardium, as well as mediastinal lymph nodes. In modern times the operation is reserved almost exclusively for the treatment of malignant pleural mesothelioma (MPM). Rarely, it can also be performed for locally advanced lung cancer, or other malignancies and infections confined to a single pleural space.

Table 14-1. Mortality of Extrapleural Pneumonectomy

Investigators	Year	No. of Patients	Operative Mortality (%)
Bamler and Maassenn	1974	17	23
Butchart et al	1976	29	31
Lung Cancer Study Group	1991	20	15
Faber	1994	40	8
Rusch and Venkatramen	1999	115	5
Sugarbaker et al	2004	496	4
Opitz	2006	63	3.2

EPP is a technically difficult operation accompanied by a significant mortality rate, recently estimated at between 3% and 7%.[2-4] This has dramatically improved since the 1970s when mortality was over 30%,[5] with the trend now toward improved operative survival, especially if used as part of a multimodal approach (Table 14–1). Nevertheless, morbidity remains high even in large volume centers with aggressive intervention, exceeding that for pneumonectomy.[4] Accordingly its use remains controversial, and patient selection is imperative. Anesthesia management is challenging and may contribute to safe patient outcomes.

MALIGNANT PLEURAL MESOTHELIOMA

Malignant pleural mesothelioma (MPM) is a rare, locally aggressive tumor of the mesothelial cells that line the pleura. It tends to spread or recur locally, and encases and invades the lung parenchyma in late stages of the disease. MPM is almost universally caused by, and in fact owes its entire existence as a disease entity to its relationship with asbestos. Asbestos is a naturally occurring mineral found all over the world but mainly in Canada, South Africa, Australia, and northern Italy. Due to its extraordinary fire-resistant properties it was used in the construction and shipping industries in the 1940s, during which time an estimated 40% of the US workforce were exposed.[6] The first description of an association between MPM and asbestos exposure was by Wagner in patients exposed to the long, fine asbestos fiber crocidolite in South African mines.[7] All types of asbestos fiber can cause mesothelioma, with crocidolite considered the highest risk. When inhaled, the fibers are too large to be removed by pulmonary macrophages, and over the years they burrow into the serosal surfaces of the pleura, pericardium, and peritoneum. Fortunately only 2% to 10% of individuals with prolonged asbestos exposure will develop MPM, whereas over 80% of MPM patients have a history of exposure to asbestos.[8]

The average latency period following exposure and development of the disease or death is very long—usually a minimum of 20 years—although the range is wide. Cases developing within 15 years of exposure are rare. This is unlike most risk factors, including smoking, when increasing time from stopping exposure to the carcinogen will decrease the risk of malignancy. In 1972, the US Occupational Safety and Health Administration established permissible exposure limits to asbestos, and since then many countries have banned its use completely. The importance and relevance of the latency period is reflected by the increasing incidence of mesothelioma. In the US the current incidence is 3000 cases per year, comprising about 3% of cancer diagnoses, and this is projected to increase until at least 2020.[9]

Typically, patients with MPM present with a pleural effusion, which is often associated with chest wall pain or breathlessness. The chest pain typically progresses relentlessly during the course of the illness. Constitutional symptoms such as weight loss and fatigue can be present, and are often associated with a poor prognosis. Occasionally the disease is found incidentally on a chest x-ray (Figure 14–1). CT scans often demonstrate encasement of the lung by a thickened pleural peel (Figure 14–2).

Diagnosis of MPM is possible from cytological examination of pleural fluid, but findings are often negative despite repeated sampling. The gold standard is thoracoscopy, which yields a diagnosis in 98% of patients.[10]

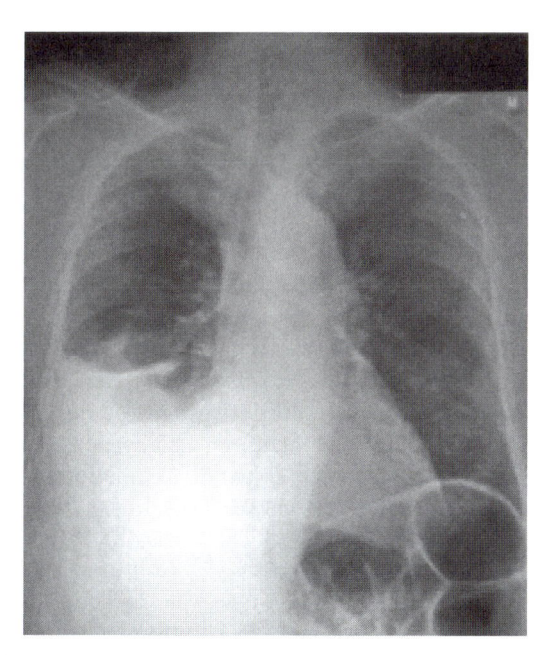

Figure 14–1. Chest radiograph demonstrating the four classic findings of a patient with the clinical diagnosis of pleural mesothelioma: pleural thickening, pleural effusion, decreased thoracic volume, and no shift of the mediastinum to the affected side.

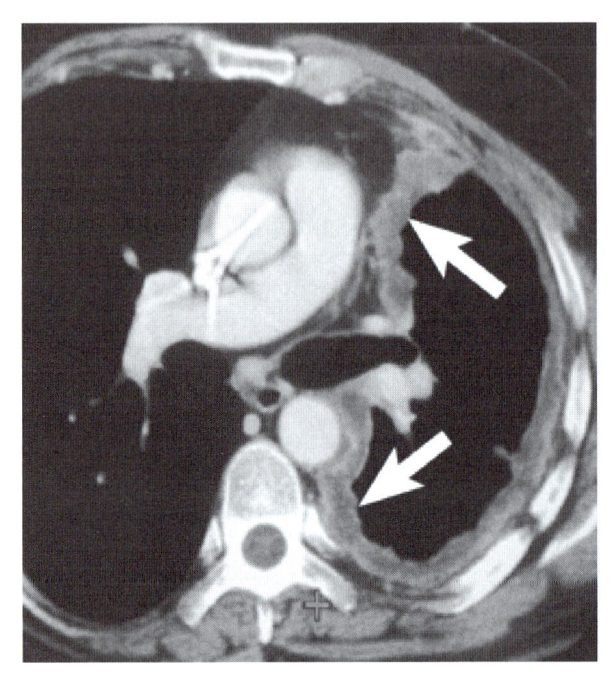

Figure 14–2. Pleural thickening in a 51-year-old man with MPM. Axial contrast-enhanced CT scan shows circumferential and nodular left-sided pleural thickening (arrows). The tumor encases the contracted left hemithorax, having a rind-like appearance.

Treatment

Without treatment, MPM is associated with an extremely poor prognosis: a median survival duration of less than 1 year and a 5-year survival rate of less than or equal to 1%.[11] No single treatment modality dramatically improves this since none reliably results in cure.

The goal of any surgical treatment is complete resection. However, in the case of MPM this is rarely achieved—presumably due to the diffuse spread of MPM throughout the hemithorax, and the difficulty of achieving deep margins. Therefore, treatment has focused on surgery in combination with a multimodality treatment program. Other therapies include systemic or intrapleural chemotherapy, high-dose hemithoracic radiation, and intensity-modulated radiation therapy (IMRT).[12]

The two main surgical options are EPP and pleurectomy/decortication (P/D), which involves resection of the pleura, pericardium and diaphragm when necessary but spares the lung. There are no randomized controlled trials between these techniques, and no established practice guidelines. EPP offers the most complete cytoreduction, and is considered by many to be the best surgical option. However, a recent multicenter retrospective series showed improved 5-year survival after P/D.[13] Previous series have argued against this perspective,[14-16] with Sugarbaker et al finding a median survival of 51 months in selected patients after EPP.[15] The decision to perform P/D is often made intraoperatively, with early disease commonly resected by P/D when it appears macroscopic complete resection can be achieved. Bulky disease is more likely to be approached by EPP, offering significant bias to any comparative retrospective series. An additional benefit of EPP is that it facilitates the administration of postoperative hemithoracic radiation, which is not possible after P/D, and provides excellent local disease control.[17]

The recent mesothelioma and radical surgery (MARS) trial is the first randomized controlled trial to compare EPP versus no EPP in the context of trimodal therapy (chemotherapy, radiotherapy, and further surgery if needed). Although the trial was small with only 50 patients randomized, patients undergoing EPP had shorter median survival (14.4 months vs 19.5 months), and more serious adverse events (10 vs 2), without any gain in quality of life. The authors therefore conclude that EPP within trimodal therapy may offer no benefit, and possibly harm patients. This is almost certain to significantly decrease the number of EPPs performed in the coming years. Further studies are needed to evaluate the role of lung sparing surgery in the future management of mesothelioma.[18]

TECHNIQUE OF EXTRAPLEURAL PNEUMONECTOMY

Step One: Incision

The extrapleural space is usually approached through an extended posterolateral thoracotomy incision in the sixth intercostal space with resection of the sixth rib, although a median sternotomy can be used for a right EPP.

Step Two: Extrapleural Dissection

Combined blunt and sharp extrapleural dissection is performed superiorly toward the apex of the thorax, and then medially down to the azygos vein. Packing the dissected area diminishes blood loss from the numerous small vessels lining the inner thoracic cavity. During this dissection, any internal mammary grafts on the operative side will almost certainly be lost, and there may be traction to the superior vena cava (SVC). Inferiorly the diaphragm is divided and dissected from the underlying peritoneum, taking care to keep the peritoneum intact and prevent peritoneal seeding.

Step Three: Division of the Major Vessels and Bronchus

The pericardium is opened and resected, with the major vessels dissected free. The main pulmonary artery and veins are divided using a vascular stapler. After a complete subcarinal lymph node dissection the main stem bronchus is exposed and divided (Figure 14–3). This can be performed under direct vision with a fiberoptic bronchoscope to assure a short stump that is flush with the carina.[19] The specimen is then removed en bloc, followed by radical mediastinal lymph node dissection.

Step Four: Reconstruction

The bronchial stump is reinforced with a tissue flap, usually from either pericardial fat or a thymic fat pad. The hemithorax is then irrigated with warm saline and

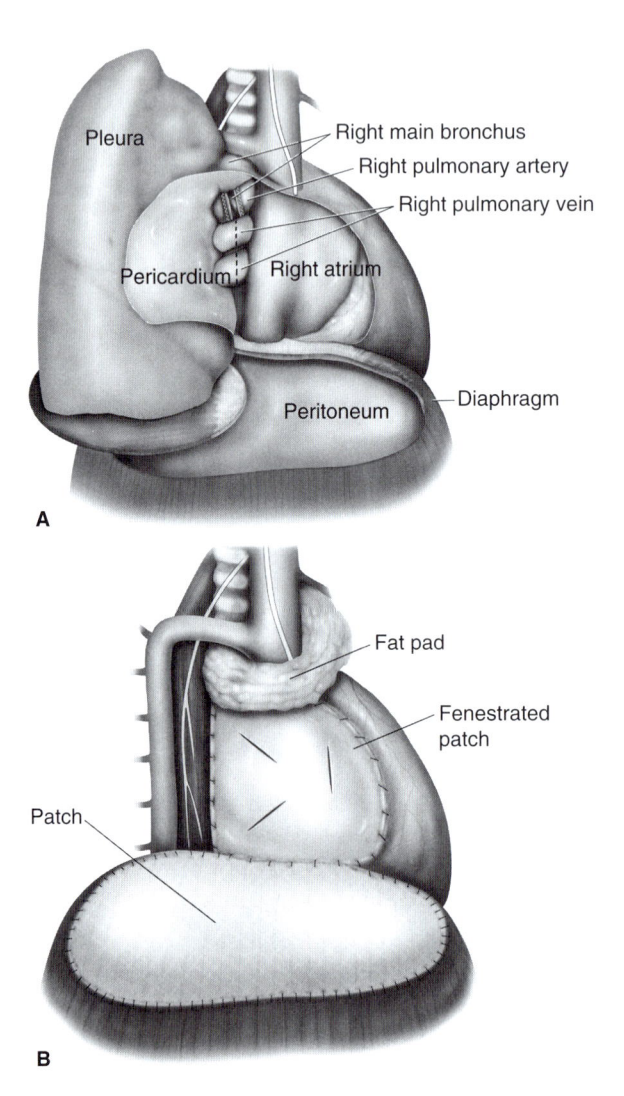

Figure 14-3. **A.** The intrapericardial dissection and isolation of the hilar vessels with subsequent ligation and division of the vessels using endoscopic vascular staplers. **B.** Operative drawing after completion of the pericardial and diaphragmatic reconstruction. The right bronchial stump has been reinforced with a thymic fat pad. The pericardial patch is fenestrated to prevent tamponade.

water to remove residual microscopic tumor. The pericardium and diaphragm are then reconstructed using Gore-Tex patches (Gore-Tex, Inc., Flagstaff, AZ) to prevent any subsequent herniation of the heart or abdominal contents into the empty hemithorax. The pericardial patch must be fenestrated to prevent any constrictive physiology occurring postoperatively. The chest is then closed in the usual fashion once hemostasis has been achieved.

Table 14-2. Suggested Selection Criteria for Extrapleural Pneumonectomy

ECOG* Performance Status 0-1
Predictive postoperative FEV_1 >1 liter
Room air PaO_2 >65 mm Hg
Room air $PaCO_2$ <45 mm Hg
Mean pulmonary artery pressure <30 mm Hg
Left Ventricular Ejection Fraction >45%, with no significant cardiac arrhythmias
No significant renal or liver disease
No previous coronary artery bypass grafts
Epithelial subtype mesothelioma
Stage I or II mesothelioma (International Mesothelioma Interest Group Staging System)

*ECOG = Eastern Cooperative Oncology Group

PATIENT SELECTION

Estimates have suggested that only 1% to 5% of all patients with mesothelioma might be suitable for surgery.[20] Selection of appropriate patients for EPP is crucial, and varies between different centers although the principles remain the same. Table 14–2 lists commonly used patient selection criteria.

Importantly for a patient to be considered for an EPP, they should have a good performance status. This is defined as Eastern Cooperative Oncology Group (ECOG) Performance Status 0-1 (Table 14–3).[21] Patients should have adequate pulmonary function to tolerate a pneumonectomy, with predictive forced expiratory volume in 1 second (FEV_1) greater than 1 liter. All patients with predictive

Table 14-3. Eastern Cooperative Oncology Group (ECOG) Performance Status

Grade	ECOG
0	Fully active, able to carry on all pre-disease performance without restriction
1	Restricted in physically strenuous activity but ambulatory and able to carry out work of a light or sedentary nature, e.g., light house work, office work
2	Ambulatory and capable of all selfcare but unable to carry out any work activities. Up and about more than 50% of waking hours
3	Capable of only limited selfcare, confined to bed or chair more than 50% of waking hours
4	Completely disabled. Cannot carry on any selfcare. Totally confined to bed or chair
5	Dead

FEV_1 less than 2 liters are recommended to undergo radionucleotide ventilation-perfusion scanning to assess the contribution of the diseased lung, and improve the accuracy of the predicted postoperative value. Arterial blood gases are obtained to rule out baseline hypoxia and/or hypercapnia.

Two-dimensional dobutamine echocardiography is necessary to rule out ventricular dysfunction (EF <45%), significant coronary artery disease, and pulmonary hypertension (mean pulmonaryartery pressure >30 mm Hg) that may increase perioperative risks.

Patients potentially suitable for radical surgery have epithelioid tumors of low volume. Studies have consistently demonstrated the significance of epithelial histology in the outcomes of mesothelioma patients.[22] The International Mesothelioma Interest Group (IMIG) developed a new staging system in 1994 based on the TNM system of lung cancer.[23] Stages I and II disease are both N0M0, meaning there is no evidence of regional lymph node or distant metastases respectively. Accurate preoperative staging requires CT, MRI, PET, and often thoracoscopy and mediastinoscopy. Final staging is only possible at surgery.

ANESTHETIC MANAGEMENT

Anesthesia for EPP is challenging with a high rate of perioperative morbidity. There are a number of potential management problems in addition to the standard anesthetic issues for a pneumonectomy. The major additional anesthetic issues are listed in Table 14–4.

Most importantly EPP is associated with significant extra blood loss as small blood vessels are disrupted during the blunt dissection of the pleura. There is also the potential for acute blood loss if major blood vessels are disrupted. This can be accompanied by alterations in preload and cardiac output caused by surgical pressure on the pericardium and great vessels. Therefore, the anesthetic plan needs to be tailored to expect hemodynamic instability and major fluid shifts.

Table 14–4. Major Anesthetic Issues for Extrapleural Pneumonectomy

Potential for significant blood loss during dissection phase
Greater hemodynamic instability due to mechanical disruption of venous return and cardiac output
Greater need for vasopressors and inotropic support
Difficult fluid management issues
Potential for disruption of major blood vessels causing dramatic, acute blood loss
High risk for disruption of ipsilateral internal mammary artery coronary artery bypass grafts
Potential for cardiac herniation or tamponade related to the pericardial patch
High probability of dysrhythmias

Planning—Lines, Monitors, and Equipment

Adequate venous access is essential in these patients. If large-bore peripheral intravenous access cannot be obtained, it is prudent to insert a wide-bore central line for rapid infusion of blood products. Invasive arterial and central venous monitoring are routine. A method of delivering blood products rapidly should be available, and blood should be in the operating room. Pulmonary artery catheters are rarely used, and the data have been shown to be difficult to interpret during pneumonectomy.[24] Transesophageal echocardiography (TEE) should be available to assess right and left ventricular filling and function if needed. Vasoconstricting agents should be available, especially for large tumors and if epidural anesthesia is to be used intraoperatively. It is essential that patients are adequately warmed, so appropriate use of warming devices and fluid warmers is recommended.

Thoracic Epidural Anesthesia

Thoracic epidural anesthesia (TEA) is generally considered the technique of choice for postoperative analgesia after EPP. TEA has a number of potential benefits after thoracic surgery. In a meta-analysis, compared with systemic opioids, TEA was found to decrease the overall incidence of atelectasis, pulmonary infections, and pulmonary complications in thoracic surgery.[25] There are also clear benefits in areas such as pain relief, facilitation of early extubation, and reducing the length of intensive care stay. The superior pain relief is important for effective cough, vigorous physiotherapy, and mobilization in the early postoperative period. This control of postoperative acute pain is important to reduce the incidence of chronic postthoracotomy pain syndrome (see also Chapter 24).[26]

In EPP, the large incision makes the use of TEA even more appealing. However, the sympatholytic effects of epidural local anesthetic may complicate hemodynamic effects during the dissection phase of the operation. Consideration should therefore be given to giving an opioid bolus in the epidural space at induction, and then starting a local anesthetic and opioid infusion once the major dissection has been completed, and the risk of major bleeding has diminished.

Intraoperative Management

There is no evidence that any particular anesthetic technique is superior for EPP. However, it seems sensible to use short-acting agents, and to limit intravenous narcotic use as much as possible to facilitate early extubation. An arterial line should be placed before induction to enable continuous monitoring of blood pressure, particularly in patients with a large tumor burden, and possible impairment of venous return. Induction agents should be used cautiously, often with concomitant administration of vasoconstrictors.

Lung isolation is generally best obtained by intubating the nonoperative bronchus with an appropriately sized double-lumen endotracheal tube (DLT). A left-sided DLT is an alternative for left EPP but it must be pulled back at the time of bronchial cross-clamping, thereby inevitably causing some risk of disruption to the bronchial stump. For this reason most thoracic anesthesiologists place a right-sided DLT (see Chapter 5) for a left pneumonectomy procedure. Bronchial blockers can be used but are more difficult to place, more likely to become dislodged, and there is no ability to oxygenate or suction the operative lung. Whatever technique is used, complete collapse of the operative lung does not usually occur, despite good tube position, due to pleural adhesions caused by the tumor.

Patients undergoing thoracotomy are at risk of gastroesophageal reflux (GER), which may lead to tracheal aspiration in an appreciable proportion of patients. Therefore, prophylactic pharmacologic management of GER should be given preoperatively.[27] The DLT should be positioned with a fiberoptic bronchoscope to prevent the need for repositioning and cuff deflation, and gel lubrication should be applied to the DLT cuff to prevent aspiration past microfolds in the inflated cuff when it comes into contact with the trachea.[28]

During one-lung ventilation (OLV), a protective ventilation strategy should be used to prevent volutrauma, barotrauma, and atelectrauma (low-volume injury). Lung protective strategies include a 3 to 4 mL/kg tidal volume, minimizing PEEP (and a high index of suspicion for auto PEEP), and limiting plateau and peak inspiratory pressures to less than 25 cm H_2O and 35 cm H_2O, respectively. The weight of the tumor in EPP can inhibit compliance of the dependent lung, and mechanical pressure causing changes in compliance require vigilance to prevent high airway pressures or volumes.

During the dissection phase of EPP, hemodynamic management is frequently difficult and complex. Hypotension is common and multifactorial, with disruption of venous return, blood loss, and mechanical pressure on the pericardium and great vessels all contributing. Blood loss during EPP is nearly always at least 1 L and can be significantly more even in experienced hands. Communication with the surgical team is vital to limit changes in hemodynamics whilst proceeding with the dissection. Brief periods of hypotension sometimes need to be tolerated if mechanical compression is necessary for adequate dissection or retraction. Disruptions in venous return should be treated with vasopressors rather than volume. If volume expansion is required, a low threshold for administration of blood is often prudent, whilst at the same time limiting crystalloid use. Early consideration should also be given to fresh frozen plasma if blood transfusion is needed.

After removal of the specimen venous return should improve. Ongoing hypotension is usually related to hypovolemia, and should be corrected with colloids or blood products as indicated. If this is not the case, other complications should be considered before leaving the operating room. Aggressive bolus dosing of the thoracic epidural at this point can complicate the clinical picture. If not used during the case, it is therefore often sensible to start an epidural infusion as soon as the specimen is removed and the patient is hemodynamically stable to limit bolus requirements.

COMPLICATIONS AFTER EXTRAPLEURAL PNEUMONECTOMY

Mortality

There have been several studies recently that have looked at mortality after EPP. The largest of these looked at 496 consecutive patients at a single institution.[4] Four

Table 14–5. Cause of Mortality after Extrapleural Pneumonectomy in 779 Patients

Cause	Number of Patients
Pulmonary embolism	9
ARDS	7
Myocardial infarction	6
Unknown	3
Cardiac arrhythmia	3
Cardiac herniation	2
Sepsis	2
Right ventricular failure	2
Bronchopleural fistula with empyema	2
Renal failure	1
Heparin induced thrombocytopenia	1
Aspiration pneumonia	1
Intraoperative hemorrhage	1
Perforated esophagus	1

smaller current series have looked at 100, 74, 62, and 49 patients, respectively.[3,17,29,30] The combined cause of mortality in these five studies is shown in Table 14–5.

Pulmonary embolism, myocardial infarction and acute respiratory distress syndrome (ARDS) were the three commonest causes, accounting for over 50% of the total mortality. Other cardiac causes of death were lethal cardiac arrhythmias, cardiac herniation, and right ventricular failure.

Cardiac Complications

Cardiac complications that occur most frequently are dysrhythmias, myocardial ischemia and infarction, cardiac tamponade, and right ventricular failure. Other rare but serious complications relating to the pericardial patch include a restrictive physiology pattern when it is too tight, and total or partial cardiac herniation if any dehiscence occurs.

Dysrhythmias

Atrial fibrillation (AF) is by far the most common cardiac (and overall) complication following EPP, with an incidence of approximately 50%.[31] The etiology is multifactorial, with mechanical factors predominating. The increased pulmonary vascular resistance after removal of one lung will naturally lead to right heart distention and right atrial dilatation. Dilation of one or both atria is known to occur in over 50% of patients with chronic AF.[32] In patients with postoperative AF following EPP, echocardiography demonstrates right ventricular dilatation in 75% of patients. Age less than 65 years, preoperative heart rate more than 72 beats per minute, male gender, structural abnormalities of the heart, and right heart stress have also been reported as risk factors.[31,33] Conversely sympathetic blockade with thoracic epidural bupivacaine has a protective effect compared to equi-analgesic epidural narcotics.[34]

However, none of this explains the high incidence of AF in EPP compared to a much lower incidence of 20% in conventional pneumonectomy.[19] The difference is attributed to the extensive pericardial resection that is often required during EPP. A patch reconstruction of the pericardium in right-sided EPP can also irritate the epicardium, and some studies have identified right-sided EPP as an additional risk factor.[4,35]

Isolated intraoperative dysrhythmias are generally triggered by mechanical irritation and do not appear to predict postoperative events. Routine attachment of ECG leads to a defibrillator in order to enable intraoperative synchronized cardioversion has been advocated.[19] Postoperatively anticoagulation should be considered in patients with persistent AF less than 48 hours when the bleeding risk from the raw pleural surface has diminished.

MYOCARDIAL ISCHEMIA

The incidence of myocardial ischemia in EPP is not known, mainly due to the difficulty in defining ischemia. Alterations in the position of the heart during the procedure, and the difficulty in placing the V5 lead correctly in left-sided EPP add to the difficulty. Therefore, if ischemia is suspected the best monitoring tool is TEE. The incidence of myocardial infarction after EPP is 1.5% to 4%.[4,17] Mild elevation in troponin levels can occur and are usually transient.

RIGHT VENTRICULAR FAILURE

Right ventricular (RV) dysfunction and failure can occur after EPP due to the increased pulmonary vascular resistance (and therefore RV afterload) encountered when the entire cardiac output needs to flow through one lung. This has a poor prognosis due to the limited contractile reserves of the RV, and there is increasing evidence for the use of nitric oxide to reduce RV afterload in this setting.[36] Low doses (<10 ppm) given with the mixture of anesthetic gases for the duration of the operation has been described to try and reduce the rise in pulmonary artery pressure on completion of the pneumonectomy.[3]

CARDIAC HERNIATION

Although rare, cardiac herniation is lethal if unrecognized. It is more common after right EPP, and is usually precipitated by an event such as a change in position of the patient, or high-intrathoracic pressures from coughing or obstructed ventilation causing dehiscence of the right-sided pericardial patch. The classic scenario occurs when the patient is turned to the supine position at the end of the procedure, and usually results in ventricular tachycardia followed by fibrillatory arrest. When the heart herniates into the right chest, venous return is severely compromised as both inferior and superior cavae become occluded. If this occurs or there is significant

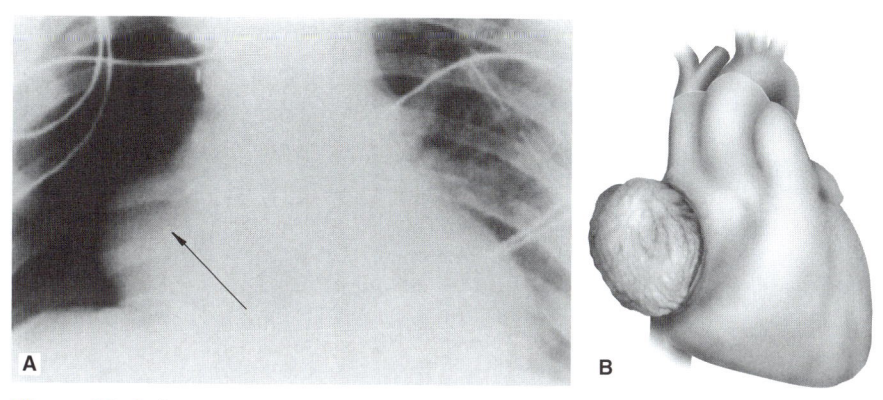

Figure 14–4. **A.** The hemispheric contour from partial cardiac herniation resembles the shape of a snow cone. Clinical awareness of this sign of impending herniation is important, so risk factors known to produce herniation may be modified. **B.** Diagram of partial herniation to demonstrate the "snow cone" appearance.

hypotension at this point, the patient should be immediately returned to the lateral position, followed by clean out of the chest and surgical correction. The surgeon, therefore, must be in the operating room when the patient is turned.

If the diagnosis is less obvious (ie, partial herniation) a portable chest radiograph (Figure 14–4) and TEE can aid decision making. The differential diagnosis includes hypovolemia, restrictive physiology, and tamponade.

Postoperatively if herniation occurs resuscitation can be difficult as closed cardiac compression will not be effective if the heart is empty and out of position. Early consideration should be given to emergency thoracotomy and open cardiac massage, with the only effective treatment being return of the heart to its normal position.

OTHER CARDIAC COMPLICATIONS

The incidence of postoperative cardiac tamponade is 3.6%.[4] Any significant pericardial effusion can be diagnosed by TEE and should be drained. In the absence of a notable effusion, diastolic filling of the right ventricle should be carefully observed to see if a pericardial patch reconstruction is too tight. If this is the case it should immediately be revised.

Less commonly a restrictive physiology pattern can occur postoperatively if the pericardium becomes inflamed. Additionally impaired venous return can result from the diaphragmatic patch compressing the inferior vena cava.

Respiratory Complications

Pulmonary complications frequently occur after EPP and are a significant cause of morbidity and mortality (Table 14–6). Early extubation and mobilization after EPP is the key to reducing pulmonary complications. Of paramount importance

Table 14-6. Pulmonary Complications after Extrapleural Pneumonectomy in 328 Patients[36]

Prolonged intubation	7.9%
Vocal cord paralysis	6.7%
Aspiration	2.7%
ARDS	3.6%
Need for tracheostomy	1.8%
Bronchopleural fistula	0.6%

for this is effective thoracic epidural analgesia with a combination of local anesthetics and opioids. Epidural management should be guided by a 24-hour dedicated pain service. Frequent use of bronchoscopy to clear retained secretions is also recommended. Care should be taken to avoid postoperative fluid excess, especially with crystalloids; and aggressive diuresis may be necessary to prevent pulmonary edema.

Early detection of vocal cord dysfunction is also highly important and is often overlooked. Recurrent laryngeal nerve damage is more common after EPP, especially in patients with extensive mediastinal disease, and places the patient at high risk for aspiration and pneumonia. If a hoarse voice is present postoperatively, the patient should undergo immediate bronchoscopy to inspect the vocal cords under direct vision. If the condition is diagnosed, oral feeding should be stopped and aggressive chest physiotherapy implemented. This is followed by early surgical treatment with vocal cord medialization to prevent any further aspiration, and to restore a functional cough.

Compared to standard pneumonectomy, the extrapleural dissection in an EPP induces rapid filling of the hemithorax within the first few days postoperatively, and before the suture lines have fully healed; thus placing the patient at increased risk of empyema formation. This challenging problem is complicated by the presence of artificial patches in the field. A typical infection prophylaxis regime includes 48 hours of perioperative antibiotics and aggressive intraoperative irrigation of the chest cavity with saline.[37]

Clinical signs of empyema can be difficult to detect, with nonspecific features such as low-grade fevers, lethargy, and fatigue. Closed antibiotic drainage for 5 days can be used to treat empyema without bronchopleural fistula.[4] In more severe cases with bronchial stump disruption open drainage and removal of the pericardial and diaphragmatic patches is recommended. This usually prevents the patient from receiving any adjuvant therapy, thus severely compromising the benefits of surgery.

Thromboembolic Complications

Pulmonary embolism is the leading cause of death after EPP so aggressive measures should be undertaken in the prevention and treatment of deep vein thrombus.

Preoperative noninvasive vascular studies are performed in some centers, with an inferior vena cava filter placed preoperatively if any clots are found.[37] Sequential pneumatic compression devices (SCDs) should be used intraoperatively in all patients. Postoperatively there should be a low threshold for imaging in patients with even mild symptoms. The investigation of any unexplained oxygen desaturations should also include CT of the chest to look for evidence of pulmonary emboli.

Other Complications

Most diaphragmatic patch problems will manifest in the first week, if not earlier. Diagnosis in a left-sided dehiscence is usually made with a postoperative chest radiograph showing the gastric bubble in the hemithorax. Right-sided patch disruptions can be harder to diagnose as the liver is more fixed in position, and an ultrasound or CT scan is often needed to diagnose the problem.

Chylothorax is a rare problem caused by injury to the thoracic duct resulting in lymph leakage into the pneumonectomy space. Conservative therapy with no oral feeding is generally the first choice of management.[38] In refractory cases lymph duct ligation may be required, and more recently percutaneous embolization of the thoracic duct has been described.[39] Table 14–7 lists the most common complications after EPP and their possible causes.

TRIMODALITY THERAPY FOR MESOTHELIOMA

Trimodality therapy for MPM was first reported in 1991 with Sugarbaker and colleagues describing EPP with adjuvant chemotherapy and sequential radiotherapy.[40] The same group have since published the largest series to date with 183 patients having a median survival of 51 months.[15] Other centers have used induction chemotherapy, followed by resection and adjuvant chemotherapy.[41] However, EPP after induction chemotherapy has the additional challenge of dissection through inflamed, obliterated tissue planes and immunosuppression. Chemotherapy regimens usually involve cisplatin with one or two additional agents.

Recent work has studied hyperthermic intraoperative cisplatin (HIOC). In patients with less than 1 cm^3 residual tumor by direct inspection after resection, HIOC is perfused in the chest for 1 hour at 42°C. This permits higher doses to be used than would be tolerated systemically, and the higher temperature increases tumoricidal activity by increasing the metabolic activity of the cells.[19] A cytoprotective agent is usually given at the same time to help protect the kidneys, but renal toxicity remains problematic.[42] However, a recent phase 2 trial of HIOC showed that it can be performed safely, and might enhance local control in the chest.[43]

After recovery from the operation, adjunctive radiotherapy (RT) is usually initiated at 6 to 8 weeks, where a big advantage of EPP over P/D is that removal of the ipsilateral lung decreases any dose restraints. In this setting high-dose hemithoracic radiation following EPP decreases the risk of local recurrence.[44] Nevertheless, the large and irregular target volume and multiple, sensitive normal structures make this strategy complex.

The most appealing RT approach after EPP is intensity-modulated radiation therapy (IMRT). IMRT is an advanced delivery technique that divides the RT treatment

Table 14–7. Complications of Extrapleural Pneumonectomy

Complication	Possible Causes
Hypotension	
Falling hematocrit	Bleeding +/– coagulopathy
Stable hematocrit	Compression of heart or great vessels by tumor/surgical retraction
	Epidural sympathetic blockade +/– ipsilateral sympathetic chain injury
	Myocardial ischemia
	Atrial arrhythmia
	Right heart dysfunction/failure
	Tight pericardial patch
	Diaphragmatic patch compressing IVC
	Pulmonary embolism
	Cardiac herniation
Ventricular arrhythmia	Myocardial ischemia
	Cardiac herniation or malrotation
Respiratory insufficiency	Mediastinal shift
	Post-pneumonectomy pulmonary edema
	Empyema +/– bronchopleural fistula
	Aspiration pneumonitis
Hoarseness/weak cough	Left recurrent laryngeal nerve injury

fields into multiple subfields of varying dose intensities; thereby making it possible to decrease the dose to a critical structure. A tumoricidal dose for gross disease is more than 60 Gy, whereas the normal tissue tolerance of adjacent tissues is much lower; for example 20 Gy for lung tissue and 40 Gy for the heart. IMRT allows target areas including all preoperative pleural surfaces and ipsilateral mediastinal lymph nodes to receive the higher dose of 50 to 60 Gy. Initial results show excellent local control with a local recurrence rate of 13% in 63 patients.[17] However, the toxicity profile can be severe, and it can cause substantial toxicity to the contralateral lung, including fatal pneumonitis.[45] Novel techniques such as helical tomotherapy[46] and/or IMRT with the addition of electrons[47] may have a role in the future.

CONCLUSION

EPP is a technically demanding operation with a high rate of perioperative morbidity. There have been significant decreases in mortality rates over the last 30 years, with improvements in surgical and anesthetic care, along with case selection.

A number of morbid conditions outlined in this review are unique to EPP. Anesthetic management of EPP requires a thorough understanding of the surgical technique and common perioperative problems. Good outcomes, therefore, require EPP to be performed in centers with extensive experience in the perioperative management of these patients, allied with a multidisciplinary approach.

Whilst mesothelioma remains a deadly disease, there is increasing evidence of a survival benefit, especially when used as a part of trimodal therapy with chemotherapy and adjuvant radiotherapy. An aggressive approach can be undertaken with low mortality and acceptable morbidity in carefully selected patients.

REFERENCES

1. Sarot IA. Extrapleural pneumonectomy and pleurectomy in pulmonary tuberculosis. *Thorax*. 1949;4: 173-223.
2. Opitz I, Kestenholz P, Lardinois D, et al. Incidence and management of complications after neoadjuvant chemotherapy followed by extrapleural pneumonectomy for malignant pleural mesothelioma. *Eur J Cardio-Thorac Surg*. 2006;29(4):579-584.
3. Stewart DJ, Martin-Ucar AE, Edwards JG, et al. Extra-pleural pneumonectomy for malignant pleural mesothelioma: the risks of induction chemotherapy, right-sided procedures and prolonged operations. *Eur J Cardio-Thorac Surg*. 2005;27(3):373-378.
4. Sugarbaker DJ, Jaklitsch MT, Bueno R, et al. Prevention, early detection, and management of complications after 328 consecutive extrapleural pneumonectomies. *J Thorac Cardiovasc Surg*. 2004;128(1): 138-146.
5. Butchart EG, Ashcroft T, Barnsley WC, et al. Pleuropneumonectomy in the management of diffuse malignant mesothelioma of the pleura. Experience with 29 patients. *Thorax*. 1976;31(1):15-24.
6. Ismail-Khan R, Robinson LA, Williams CC Jr, Garrett CR, Bepler G, Simon GR. Malignant pleural mesothelioma: a comprehensive review. *Cancer Control*. 2006;13(4):255-263.
7. Wagner J. Diffuse pleural mesothelioma and asbestos exposure in the North West Cape Province. *Br J Ind Med*. 1960;17:260-271.
8. Cugell DW, Kamp DW. Asbestos and the pleura: a review. *Chest*. 2004;125(3):1103-1117.
9. Robinson BWS, Lake RA. Advances in malignant mesothelioma. *N Engl J Med*. 2005;353(15):1591-1603.
10. Boutin C, Rey F. Thoracoscopy in pleural malignant mesothelioma: a prospective study of 188 consecutive patients. Part 1: diagnosis. *Cancer*. 1993;72(2):389-393.
11. Weiner SJ, Neragi-Miandoab S. Pathogenesis of malignant pleural mesothelioma and the role of environmental and genetic factors. *J Cancer Res Clin Oncol*. 2009;135(1):15-27.
12. Ceresoli GL, Gridelli C, Santoro A. Multidisciplinary treatment of malignant pleural mesothelioma. *Oncologist*. 2007;12(7):850-863.
13. Flores RM, Pass HI, Seshan VE, et al. Extrapleural pneumonectomy versus pleurectomy/decortication in the surgical management of malignant pleural mesothelioma: results in 663 patients. *J Thorac Cardiovasc Surg*. 2008;135(3):620-626.
14. Flores RM, Krug LM, Rosenzweig KE, et al. Induction chemotherapy, extrapleural pneumonectomy, and postoperative high-dose radiotherapy for locally advanced malignant pleural mesothelioma: a phase II trial. *J Thorac Oncol*. 2006;1(4):289-295.
15. Sugarbaker DJ, Flores RM, Jaklitsch MT, et al. Resection margins, extrapleural nodal status, and cell type determine postoperative long-term survival in trimodality therapy of malignant pleural mesothelioma: results in 183 patients. *J Thorac Cardiovasc Surg*. 1999;117(1):54-63; discussion -5.
16. Weder W, Kestenholz P, Taverna C, et al. Neoadjuvant chemotherapy followed by extrapleural pneumonectomy in malignant pleural mesothelioma. *J Clin Oncol*. 2004;22(17):3451-3457.
17. Rice DC, Stevens CW, Correa AM, et al. Outcomes after extrapleural pneumonectomy and intensity-modulated radiation therapy for malignant pleural mesothelioma. *Ann Thorac Surg*. 2007;84(5): 1685-1692; discussion 92-93.
18. Treasure T, Lang-Lazdunski L, Waller D, Bliss JM, et al. Extra-pleural pneumonectomy versus no extra-pleural pneumonectomy for patients with malignant pleural mesothelioma: clinical outcomes

of the Mesothelioma and Radical Surgery (MARS) randomised feasibility study. *Lancet Oncol.* 2011;12(8):763-772.
19. Ng J-M, Hartigan PM. Anesthetic management of patients undergoing extrapleural pneumonectomy for mesothelioma. *Curr Opin Anaesthesiol.* 2008;21(1):21-27.
20. British Thoracic Society Standards of Care Committee. Statement on malignant mesothelioma in the United Kingdom.[see comment][erratum appears in *Thorax.* 2001 Oct;56(10):820]. *Thorax.* 2001;56(4):250-265.
21. Oken MM, Creech RH, Tormey DC, et al. Toxicity and response criteria of the Eastern Cooperative Oncology Group. Am J Clin Oncol. 1982;5(6):649-655.
22. Yan TD, Boyer M, Tin MM, et al. Prognostic features of long-term survivors after surgical management of malignant pleural mesothelioma. *Ann Thorac Surg.* 2009;87(4):1552-1556.
23. Rusch VW. A proposed new international TNM staging system for malignant pleural mesothelioma. From the International Mesothelioma Interest Group. *Chest.* 1995;108(4):1122-1128.
24. Wittnich C, Trudel J, Zidulka A, Chiu RC. Misleading "pulmonary wedge pressure" after pneumonectomy: its importance in postoperative fluid therapy. *Ann Thorac Surg.* 1986;42(2):192-196.
25. Ballantyne JC, Carr DB, deFerranti S, et al. The comparative effects of postoperative analgesic therapies on pulmonary outcome: cumulative meta-analyses of randomized, controlled trials. *Anesth Analgesia.* 1998;86(3):598-612.
26. Katz J, Jackson M, Kavanagh BP, et al. Acute pain after thoracic surgery predicts long-term post-thoracotomy pain. *Clin J Pain.* 1996;12(1):50-55.
27. Agnew NM, Kendall JB, Akrofi M, et al. Gastroesophageal reflux and tracheal aspiration in the thoracotomy position: should ranitidine premedication be routine? *Anesth Analg* 2002;95(6);1645-1649.
28. Sanjay PS, Miller SA, Corry PR, et al. The effect of gel lubrication on cuff leakage of double lumen tubes during thoracic surgery. *Anaesthesia.* 2006;61(2):133-137.
29. de Perrot M, McRae K, Anraku M, et al. Risk factors for major complications after extrapleural pneumonectomy for malignant pleural mesothelioma. *Ann Thorac Surg.* 2008;85(4):1206-1210.
30. Aigner C, Hoda MAR, Lang G, et al. Outcome after extrapleural pneumonectomy for malignant pleural mesothelioma. *Eur J Cardio-Thorac Surg.* 2008;34(1):204-207.
31. Neragi-Miandoab S, Weiner S, Sugarbaker DJ. Incidence of atrial fibrillation after extrapleural pneumonectomy vs pleurectomy in patients with malignant pleural mesothelioma. *Interact Cardiovasc Thorac Surg.* 2008;7(6):1039-1042.
32. Xiao HB, Rizvi SAH, McCrea D, et al. The association of chronic atrial fibrillation with right atrial dilatation and left ventricular dysfunction in the elderly. *Med Sci Monit.* 2004;10(9):CR516-520.
33. Hirose M, Takeishi Y, Miyamoto T, et al. Mechanism for atrial tachyarrhythmia in chronic volume overload-induced dilated atria. *J Cardiovasc Electrophysiol.* 2005;16(7):760-769.
34. Oka T, Ozawa Y, Ohkubo Y. Thoracic epidural bupivacaine attenuates supraventricular tachyarrhythmias after pulmonary resection. *Anesth Analgesia.* 2001;93(2):253-259.
35. Harpole DH, Liptay MJ, DeCamp MM Jr, et al. Prospective analysis of pneumonectomy: risk factors for major morbidity and cardiac dysrhythmias. *Ann Thorac Surg.* 1996;61(3):977-982.
36. McNeil K, Dunning J, Morrell NW. The pulmonary physician in critical care. 13: the pulmonary circulation and right ventricular failure in the ITU. *Thorax.* 2003;58(2):157-162.
37. Zellos L, Jaklitsch MT, Al-Mourgi MA, et al. Complications of extrapleural pneumonectomy. *Semin Thorac Cardiovasc Surg.* 2007;19(4):355-359.
38. Tokunaga T, Inoue M, Ideguchi K, et al. Late-onset chylothorax following etrapleural pneumonectomy for mesothelioma. *Gen Thorac Cardiovasc Surg.* 2007;55(2):50-52.
39. Hoffer EK, Bloch RD, Mulligan MS, et al. Treatment of chylothorax: percutaneous catheterization and embolization of the thoracic duct. *Am J Roentgenol.* 2001;176(4):1040-1042.
40. Sugarbaker DJ, Mentzer SJ, DeCamp M, et al. Extrapleural pneumonectomy in the setting of a multimodality approach to malignant mesothelioma. *Chest.* 1993;103(4 Suppl):377S-381S.
41. Buduhan G, Menon S, Aye R, et al. Trimodality therapy for malignant pleural mesothelioma. *Ann Thorac Surg.* 2009;88(3):870-875; discussion 6.
42. Zellos L, Richards WG, Capalbo L, et al. A phase I study of extrapleural pneumonectomy and intracavitary intraoperative hyperthermic cisplatin with amifostine cytoprotection for malignant pleural mesothelioma. *J Thorac Cardiovasc Surg.* 2009;137(2):453-458.

43. Tilleman TR, Richards WG, Zellos L, et al. Extrapleural pneumonectomy followed by intracavitary intraoperative hyperthermic cisplatin with pharmacologic cytoprotection for treatment of malignant pleural mesothelioma: a phase II prospective study. *J Thorac Cardiovasc Surg.* 2009;138(2):405-411.
44. Rusch VW, Rosenzweig K, Venkatraman E, et al. A phase II trial of surgical resection and adjuvant high-dose hemithoracic radiation for malignant pleural mesothelioma. *J Thorac Cardiovasc Surg.* 2001;122(4):788-795.
45. Miles EF, Larrier NA, Kelsey CR, et al. Intensity-modulated radiotherapy for resected mesothelioma: the Duke experience. *Int J Radiat Oncol Biol Phys.* 2008;71(4):1143-1150.
46. Sterzing F, Sroka-Perez G, Schubert K, et al. Evaluating target coverage and normal tissue sparing in the adjuvant radiotherapy of malignant pleural mesothelioma: helical tomotherapy compared with step-and-shoot IMRT. *Radiother Oncol.* 2008;86(2):251-257.
47. Chan MF, Chui CS, Song Y, et al. A novel radiation therapy technique for malignant pleural mesothelioma combining electrons with intensity-modulated photons. *Radiother Oncol.* 2006;79(2):218-223.

Lung Volume Reduction Surgery 15

Alina Nicoara
Joseph P. Mathew

Key Points

1. For the anesthesiologist, lung volume reduction surgery is a challenging procedure and the tailoring of the anesthetic management requires profound knowledge of the pathophysiology of COPD, ventilatory mechanics in awake and anesthetized COPD patients and pain management in thoracic surgery. A variety of different approaches to LVRS have been proposed; these include median sternotomy, thoracosternotomy, standard thoracotomy and video-assisted thoracosopic surgery (VATS) with both unilateral and bilateral approaches.
2. Potential candidates for LVRS undergo extensive evaluation in order to mitigate perioperative risks and contain perioperative complications. Important physiologic variables when evaluating a patient are FEV_1 and DLCO, the RV/TLC ratio, PCO_2 and oxygen use. The ideal operative candidate should have an FEV_1 of 20% to 35% predicted without very severe reductions in DLCO (<20% predicted), a RV/TLV more than 0.67, a PCO_2 less than 45 mm Hg, and no or low level supplemental oxygen use.
3. Intraoperative management is centered on minimizing further insult due to induction of general anesthesia and institution of positive pressure ventilation. Ventilatory management during one-lung ventilation (OLV) aims to balance competitive priorities: maintaining adequate oxygenation, minimizing intrinsic PEEP, minimizing barotrauma and maximizing CO_2 elimination.
4. Intraoperative hypotension may be due to sympathetic blockade from local anesthetics administered through the thoracic epidural catheter, vasodilatory effects of the induction agents, hypovolemia, myocardial ischemia, dynamic hyperinflation or infrequent but possible catastrophic causes such as tension pneumothorax.
5. Tracheal extubation immediately after surgery is an important aim after LVRS in order to minimize the risk of developing or exacerbating an air leak and avoid the deleterious hemodynamic effects of positive pressure ventilation. Adequate pain control achieved with minimal respiratory depression in LVRS patients is vital to the success of the surgical procedure. Inadequate pain control will result in splinting, poor respiratory effort, and inability to cough and clear secretions leading to airway closure, atelectasis, shunting and hypoxemia.

> ### Clinical Vignette
>
> The patient is a 68-year-old male with advanced emphysema who is scheduled for lung volume reduction surgery (LVRS). He is an ex-smoker who has recently undergone preoperative pulmonary rehabilitation. He has concurrent coronary artery disease and hypertension. Medications include aspirin, valsartan and lovastatin.
>
> Vital signs: BP 140/70, HR 72, and room air oxygen saturation 91%.
>
> Laboratory examination is notable for blood urea nitrogen of 30 mg/dL and creatinine of 1.9 mg/dL. Pulmonary function tests reveal a FEV_1 of 0.9 L (30% predicted), FVC of 3.6 L (50% predicted), TLC 7.1L (110% predicted) and DLCO 22% predicted.

Chronic obstructive pulmonary disease (COPD) is characterized by progressive and largely irreversible airflow limitation caused primarily by exposure to tobacco smoke, and less commonly by other noxious stimuli or by $alpha_1$-antitrypsin deficiency. COPD is one of the leading causes of death and disability worldwide. It is expected that by the year 2020, COPD will become the third leading cause of death worldwide.[1]

The main goals of therapy in COPD patients are focused on relieving symptoms, preventing lung function decline, preventing exacerbations of the disease, and improving exercise capacity and quality of life. In spite of the advances in medical therapy, smoking cessation is the single most effective intervention shown to alter the rate of progression of COPD.[2] Supplemental oxygen therapy in patients with severe COPD and hypoxemia has also been shown to have beneficial effects such as prolonged survival, improvement in cardiac function, and improved exercise tolerance.[3]

The failure of medical management of COPD to produce significant impact on outcomes has led to the development of lung volume reduction surgery (LVRS) in the past century. In selected patients with severe emphysema, LVRS was associated with prolonged survival, improvement in exercise capacity and quality of life, and improvement in lung function and dyspnea.[4] Given the high perioperative mortality and morbidity associated with LVRS, the survival benefit depends on adequate patient selection and containment of perioperative complications associated with anesthesia and surgery.

For the anesthesiologist, lung volume reduction surgery is a challenging procedure and the tailoring of the anesthetic management requires profound knowledge of the pathophysiology of COPD, ventilatory mechanics in awake and anesthetized COPD patients and pain management in thoracic surgery. This chapter summarizes the impact of anesthesia and surgery on lung function in COPD patients, preoperative evaluation and criteria for optimal patient selection and intraoperative and postoperative anesthetic management.

PATHOPHYSIOLOGY OF COPD

The cardinal abnormality in COPD is an irreversible reduction in maximal expiratory flow due to chronic bronchitis, emphysema, or both. Chronic bronchitis is defined as cough and sputum production for most days over 3 months for 2 consecutive years. It is thought to result from the innate immune response to inhaled toxic particles and gases, particularly to tobacco smoke, which results in inflammation of the epithelium of the central airways and mucus-producing glands. The airway inflammation is associated with increased mucus production, reduced mucociliary clearance, and increased permeability of the airspace epithelial barrier.[5] While hyperproduction of mucus may not have a significant impact on smokers with normal lung function, in patients with severe COPD it contributes to the further decline of airflow during expiration.

Emphysema is defined as enlargement of the airspaces distal to the terminal bronchioles due to destruction of the alveolar walls. Destruction of the normal lung parenchyma causes a reduction of the elastic recoil resulting in a progressive deterioration of the maximal expiratory airflow. Emphysema may exist in a centrilobular or a panlobular form. The centrilobular (also known as centriacinar) form results from dilatation or destruction of the respiratory bronchioles, is more closely associated with tobacco smoking and has predominantly an upper lobe distribution.[6] The panlobular (also known as panacinar) form, results in more even dilatation and destruction of the entire acinus, is associated with alpha$_1$-antitrypsin deficiency and has predominantly a lower lobe distribution (Figures 15–1, 15–2, 15–3).

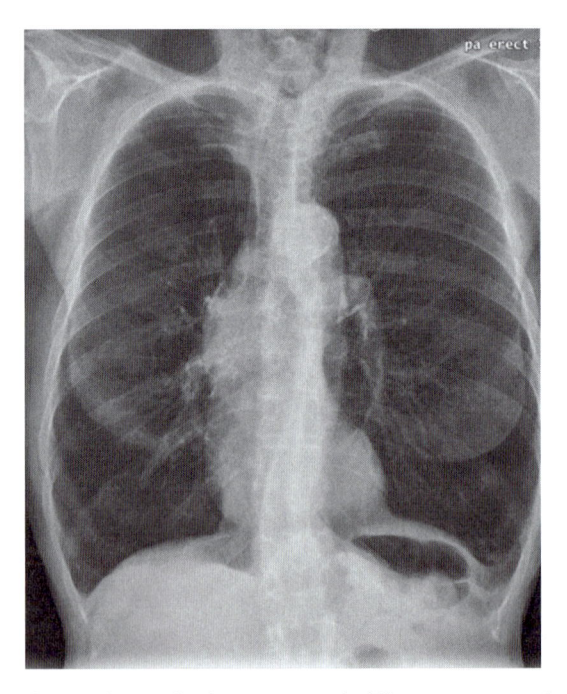

Figure 15–1. A chest radiograph of a patient with diffuse severe emphysema.

Chapter 15 / Lung Volume Reduction Surgery 277

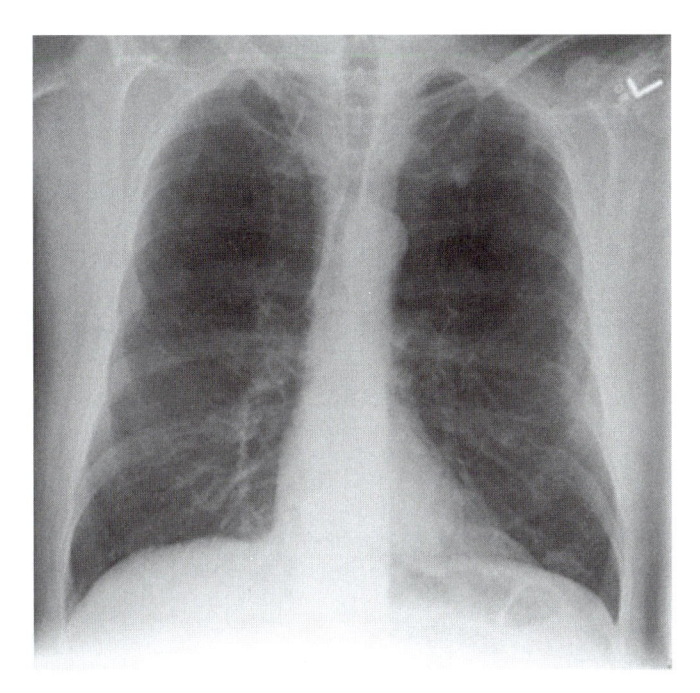

Figure 15-2. A chest radiograph of a patient with severe emphysema and upper lobe predominance.

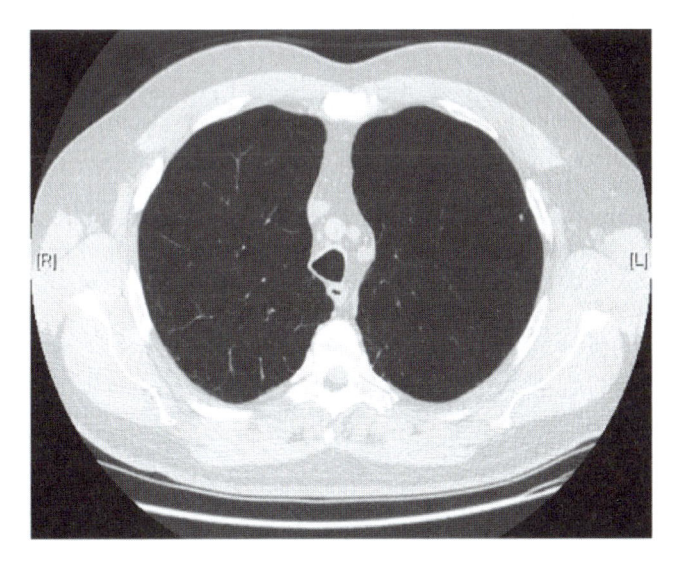

Figure 15-3. A computed tomograph of a patient with pan-lobular emphysema left greater than right.

Table 15-1. Physiologic Classification of the Severity of Chronic Obstructive Pulmonary Disease*

GOLD Staging	COPD Severity	FEV_1/FVC	FEV_1
Stage I	Mild	<0.7	≥80% predicted
Stage II	Moderate	<0.7	<80% predicted
Stage III	Severe	<0.7	<50% predicted
Stage IV	Very severe	<0.7	<30% predicted <50% predicted with chronic respiratory failure

*According to the Global Initiative for chronic obstructive Lung Disease (GOLD).
FEV_1 = forced expiratory volume in 1 second, FVC = forced vital capacity.
Adapted from KF Rabe, S Hurd and A Anzueto et al, Global initiative for chronic obstructive lung disease. Global strategy for the diagnosis, management, and prevention of chronic obstructive pulmonary disease: GOLD executive summary. *Am J Respir Crit Care Med.* 2007; 176(6):532-555. With permission of the American Thoracic Society. Copyright © American Thoracic Society. Official Journal of the American Thoracic Society.

On pulmonary function testing, the expiratory airflow limitation is first identified as a reduction in the ratio of forced expiratory volume in 1 second (FEV_1) to forced vital capacity (FVC). The diagnosis of COPD as established by the Global Initiative for Chronic Obstructive Lung Disease (GOLD) requires an FEV_1/FVC ratio of less than 0.7. Patients are then stratified into four categories from mild to very severe disease based on the severity of FEV_1 impairment[7] (Table 15-1).

Expiratory airflow limitation results in air trapping and hyperinflation with increases in total lung capacity (TLC) and residual volume (RV), and an elevated RV/TLC ratio. As the disease progresses and the recoil of the lungs becomes diminished, the functional residual capacity (FRC) moves rightwards toward the flat portion of the compliance curve of the lungs, to the detriment of pulmonary mechanics. Therefore, the patient with hyperinflation has difficulty with inspiration because the respiratory system moves on a relatively flat portion of its compliance curve and consequently there is increased elastic work of breathing. As COPD progresses, static hyperinflation gets progressively worse, and the operational lung volumes increase toward a threshold that may even result in resting dyspnea.[8] Further elevation in operational lung volumes, superimposed on static hyperinflation occurs during exercise when ventilatory requirements are increased. Due to airflow obstruction and shortened expiratory time during exercise, expiration cannot be completed and inhalation is triggered due to the urge to inspire before FRC is reached. This respiratory pattern leads to "stacking" of breaths and a gradual hyperinflation of the lungs, known as dynamic hyperinflation. Similar exacerbations of hyperinflation occur with increased respiratory rate associated with anxiety and hypoxemia.

The loss of acinar structure and disruption of the alveolar-capillary structure lead to ventilation-perfusion (V/Q) mismatch and impairment of gas exchange. Also, as the hyperinflation develops nonuniformly, the normal parenchyma may become compressed and underexpanded, causing a further increase in the V/Q mismatch. Due to the higher diffusability of carbon dioxide (CO_2), the CO_2 elimination is well-preserved until V/Q abnormalities are severe. As the disease advances, there is an increase in physiologic dead-space secondary to under-perfused alveoli, and the subsequent impairment of CO_2 clearance results in hypercapnic respiratory failure. Also, air trapping and hyperinflation place the diaphragm and other inspiratory muscles at severe mechanical disadvantage, producing alveolar hypoventilation and contributing to hypercapnia. Chronic CO_2 retention occurs slowly and a compensated respiratory acidosis is noted on arterial blood gas analysis. Acute CO_2 retention, however, is a sign of impending respiratory failure and occurs with superimposed respiratory infection and bronchospasm.

Pulmonary hypertension is a frequent complication in the natural history of COPD. It progresses over time and its severity correlates with the degree of airflow obstruction and the impairment of pulmonary gas exchange. However, the rate of progression is slow and the degree of pulmonary hypertension in COPD is of low-to-moderate magnitude, rarely exceeding 35 to 40 mm Hg[9] of mean pulmonary artery pressure. Usually right ventricular function is mildly impaired with preservation of cardiac output. Acute exacerbations in right ventricular afterload in the settings of hypoxia, hypercapnia, or compression of intraalveolar vessels due to dynamic hyperinflation may result in right ventricular failure. Elevated mean alveolar pressure associated with dynamic hyperinflation may compress intraalveolar vessels, increasing pulmonary vascular resistances and right ventricular output impedance. With progressive right ventricular dysfunction, left shifting of the interventricular septum can impair cardiac output further due to ventricular interdependence.[10] Patients with severe COPD and pulmonary hypertension show structural and functional changes in pulmonary muscular arteries and precapillary vessels that explain the irreversible increase of pulmonary vascular resistance. Long-term oxygen therapy may slow down the progression of pulmonary hypertension, however, pulmonary artery pressures rarely return to normal and the structural abnormalities of the pulmonary vessels remain unaltered.[9]

COPD is also associated with high rates of other comorbid illnesses such as cardiovascular disease, malnutrition, peripheral muscle weakness and osteoporosis. Cardiovascular disease is a major cause of death in patients with COPD. There are several reasons for the association between COPD and cardiovascular disease including a major shared risk factor (smoking), use of beta-agonist medications that may stimulate the cardiovascular system, and systemic inflammation.[11,12] Enhanced systemic inflammation may also explain nonpulmonary COPD characteristics such as skeletal muscle dysfunction, cachexia, and malnutrition.[8]

SURGICAL TECHNIQUES FOR LUNG VOLUME REDUCTION SURGERY

Brantigan developed the concept of LVRS in the 1950s when he described resection of 30% of the hyperinflated lung and autonomic denervation through thoracotomy in an attempt to improve expiratory flow.[13] LVRS was not performed widely as it

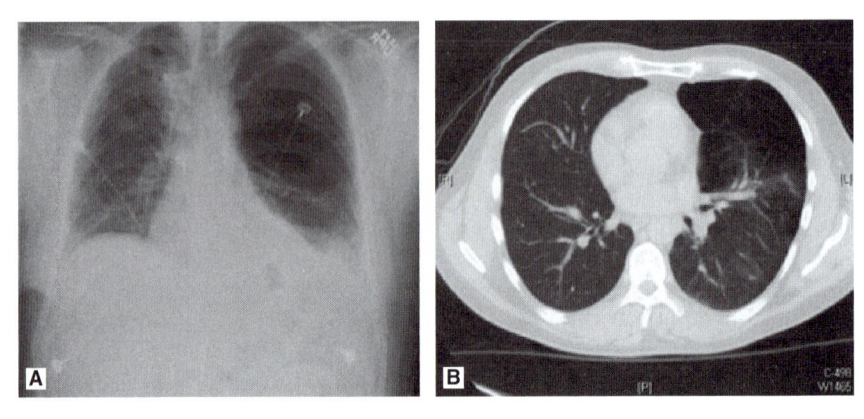

Figure 15–4. A chest radiograph **(A)** and computed tomograph **(B)** of a patient with a left giant bulla for unilateral lung reduction.

was associated with a very high surgical mortality at that time. In 1995, Cooper and colleagues reported dramatic improvements in pulmonary function and no mortality in 20 patients undergoing simultaneous bilateral LVRS using a median sternotomy with resection of 30% of each lung.[14]

Surgical Approach

A variety of different approaches to LVRS have been proposed; these include median sternotomy, thoracosternotomy, standard thoracotomy, and video-assisted thoracosopic surgery (VATS) with both unilateral and bilateral approaches (Figure 15–4). The areas for surgical removal are identified before surgery by computed tomography and radionuclide ventilation-perfusion scanning. Methods for sealing the site of resected lung include the use of staples or laser (neodymium-yttrium aluminum garnet or Nd-YAG).[15]

Median Sternotomy vs VATS

Questions regarding the high perioperative mortality in LVRS patients shown in an analysis of the Medicare claims data (23% at 1 year)[16] and the cost effectiveness and high rehospitalization rates associated with LVRS led to the funding of the National Emphysema Treatment Trial (NETT), the largest randomized trial of LVRS performed to date. The NETT was designed to compare short- and long-term outcomes of best medical therapy for emphysema with best medical therapy plus LVRS. It also included randomized and nonrandomized comparisons of the median sternotomy and VATS for LVRS. This subanalysis showed that functional results as well as morbidity and mortality were comparable for LVRS by VATS or median sternotomy. The VATS approach, however, allowed earlier recovery at a lower cost than median sternotomy.[17] Most studies comparing median sternotomy and VATS have yielded conflicting results. Wisser et al compared median sternotomy versus bilateral VATS in a sequential, nonrandomized study and showed similar postoperative morbidity and mortality and no difference in functional and physiologic results.[18]

In contrast, Roberts et al compared the complications associated with bilateral LVRS through VATS or median sternotomy. They found that although the operating time was greater for the VATS group, the median sternotomy group had a higher incidence of life-threatening complications, longer stay in the intensive care unit, ventilator days, and percent requiring reintubation.[19] In a study predating the NETT, Kotloff et al compared the short-term outcomes following bilateral LVRS performed through median sternotomy (80 patients) and VATS (40 patients). All patients in both groups were extubated at the completion of surgery, but 17.5% of patients in the median sternotomy group and 2.5% in the VATS group subsequently required reintubation at some point during the postoperative course. There was no significant difference in duration of air leaks or length of hospital stay and the functional outcomes achieved with either technique were similar. Thirty-day operative mortality was 4.2% for the median sternotomy group and 2.5% for the VATS group. However, total in-hospital mortality was 13.8% for the median sternotomy group, while it remained 2.5% for the VATS group.[20]

UNILATERAL VS BILATERAL

Bilateral VATS for lung volume reduction is preferred over the unilateral approach. Multiple studies have shown that the bilateral procedure produces greater overall improvement than a unilateral procedure.[21,22] McKenna et al compared unilateral and bilateral VATS procedures and showed that the bilateral procedure provided greater oxygen independence (68% vs 35%), prednisone independence (86% vs 56%), greater improvement in the FEV_1 and an improvement in the perceived degree of dyspnea than the unilateral procedure with comparable mortality and morbidity.[22] However, given the improvement associated with unilateral surgery, unilateral operation may still be offered in some patients who are not candidates for a bilateral operation due to prior thoracic intervention or inappropriate anatomy for bilateral LVR. Similar functional outcome with sustained improvement of FEV_1, 6-minute walk test and gas exchange was shown in other studies.[23,24] The excellent results seen in the postoperative period with the use of bilateral LVRS may not lead to improved long-term survival. A large multi-institutional retrospective study comparing long-term survival in patients undergoing either bilateral or unilateral thoracoscopic lung volume reduction found that there was no significant difference between the two groups in regard to operative mortality or late death at 1 year, 2 years, or 3 years.[25]

STAPLES VS LASER

McKenna et al also showed in a prospective blindly randomized study that patients in whom lung volume reduction surgery is done with staples and buttressing with bovine pericardium have a lower morbidity (fewer delayed pneumothoraces), as well as greater improvement in oxygen independence, lung function, and overall lifestyle and dyspnea scale, than patients treated with contact laser (Nd-YAG).[26]

POSITIONING

Usually, after induction of anesthesia and intubation, the patient is positioned supine with the arms supported above the head utilizing an ether screen. This position offers satisfactory exposure not only for VATS but median sternotomy, as well as anterior/lateral thoracotomy on both sides.[27] For the VATS approach three ports are used on each side, two in the submammary crease and one axillary port. A horseshoe-shaped specimen is removed from the superior portion of the lung avoiding direct tissue handling in order to prevent damage to friable lung tissue with its attendant risk of postoperative air leak.[27]

Mechanisms for Improvement in Respiratory Function after LVRS

The possible mechanisms by which LVRS might provide benefit are not known with certainty. Numerous studies are now available regarding the short-term results of LVRS on pulmonary function, however the results are sometimes conflicting and cover a large range of reported values due to difference in study design, patient selection, surgical technique, presence or absence of pulmonary rehabilitation or pulmonary bronchodilator administration at the time of measurement.

As mentioned above, LVRS results in marked improvement in several parameters characterizing lung function. An overview of the results available in the literature shows that in the majority of patients, LVRS leads to an improvement of FEV_1 accompanied by an increase in the FVC. Moreover, there is a decrease in total lung capacity (TLC) and residual volume (RV).[20,22-24,26,28-31] The improvement in FEV_1 is possibly due to an improvement in elastic recoil, a reduction in expiratory flow limitation and a decrease in dynamic hyperinflation shown by many investigators.[29,32,33] Resection of the emphysematous, nonfunctional lung tissue should also allow the healthier lung tissue to expand and improve expiratory flow by reducing lung compliance, premature airway closure and end-expiratory volume.[34] However, despite improvements in FEV_1, postoperative changes in the FEV_1/FVC ratio are very small or absent, suggesting that FEV_1 increases not only because of an improvement of the expiratory flow but also because of the increase in FVC.[34]

The reports on the changes in resting arterial blood gases are less consistent, ranging from improvements in arterial partial pressure of oxygen (PaO_2) and decreases in arterial partial pressure of carbon dioxide ($PaCO_2$) to little change[28] or even worsening of these parameters.[35] While some studies link the change in oxygenation to an increase in mean alveolar ventilation,[31,36] other studies suggest that the improved oxygenation is due to a reduction in ventilation-perfusion heterogeneity.[35] In a follow-up study on a large cohort of subjects enrolled in the NETT, LVRS was found to increase PaO_2 and decrease self-reported oxygen use at rest and on exertion.[37] Few studies have reported the impact of LVRS on lung diffusing capacity for carbon monoxide (DLCO), however the improvement in DLCO shown appears to be modest.[30,38]

Emphysema leads to an increase in the lung volume at which the respiratory muscles operate, which reduces their mechanical effectiveness and leads to diminished inspiratory muscle force. Due to hyperinflation, muscle fibers have shortened inspiratory muscle pre-contraction length, which diminishes the pressure generated at a given level of tension.[34] Also in patients with chronic inflation, the zone of diaphragmatic apposition, which is the area of the diaphragm immediately apposed to the ribcage, is markedly reduced[32] potentially reducing the ability of the diaphragm to generate adequate inspiratory volume change. Numerous studies have shown an improvement in the respiratory muscle strength and interaction after LVRS as shown in an increase of the diaphragm length,[39] increase in the maximal transdiaphragmatic pressures,[39,40] reduction in maximal inspiratory pressure and reduction in dyspnea.[40]

The reported changes in pulmonary vascular function after LVRS are inconsistent, with some studies showing no change or improvement in pulmonary artery pressures and right ventricular function, and others showing worsening of pulmonary hypertension.[33,41,42] These controversial results are due to possible opposing effects of LVRS on the pulmonary vascular function. Resection of perfused lung can increase the already impaired pulmonary vascular resistance while on the other hand a decrease in vascular resistance might occur through recruitment of vessels in the reexpanding lung tissue or through improvement in elastic recoil, which may increase radial traction on extra-alveolar vessels.[43]

The multiple effects of lung volume reduction surgery are summarized in Table 15–2.

Outcome and Complications

LVRS is associated with higher but acceptable mortality and morbidity than other general thoracic surgical procedures. Awareness and understanding of the potential

Table 15–2. Physiological Effects of Lung Volume Reduction Surgery

Respiratory muscle function
  Increased inspiratory muscle length
  Improved geometry and mechanical effectiveness of inspiratory muscles
  Expiratory derecruitment of abdominal muscles

Lung mechanics
  Improved lung elastic recoil
  Improved airway diameter and lung elastance
  Improved lung homogeneity
  Decreased intrinsic positive end-expiratory pressure

Chest wall mechanics
  Decreased inward recoil at end-expiratory volume

Gas exchange
  Improved alveolar ventilation
  Improved regional ventilation-perfusion relationships
  Increased mixed venous arterial oxygen tension

Pulmonary circulation
  Reduced pulmonary vascular resistance
  Improved right ventricular function

Adapted from Marchand E, Gayan-Ramirez G et al, Physiologic basis of improvement after lung volume reduction surgery for severe emphysema: where are we? *Eur Respir J* 1999;13:686-696. With permission of the European Respiratory Society.

complications associated with LVRS are some of the keys to minimizing their occurrence.[44] Mortality rates associated with LVRS reported in the literature range from 2.5% to 13%.[18,25,31,45] The 90-day mortality rate for LVRS in the NETT for the surgical group overall was 7.9%, much less than the mortality rate reported by Medicare.

Pulmonary complications are the most frequent after LVRS. Pneumonia occurs in about 7% to 14% of the patients. Respiratory failure requiring reintubation occurs in 5% to 10% of the patients, and if postoperative reintubation occurs, more than half of the patients will fail to wean from the ventilator.[44] However, the most common complication after LVRS is prolonged air leak, defined here as an air leak that lasts at least 7 days following the procedure. This complication occurs in approximately 40% to 60% of patients and is associated with a more protracted and prolonged hospital stay. There does not seem to be any significant difference in the incidence of air leak after VATS and median sternotomy procedures.[44] Within the NETT, an air leak occurred at some point in 90% of bilateral LVRS patients; the median duration of an air leak was 7 days, and 12% had a persistent air leak even 30 days postoperatively.[46] Risk factors for post-LVRS air leak include Caucasian race, lower FEV_1 or diffusion capacity, use of inhaled steroids, upper-lobe predominant emphysema and presence of moderate to marked pleural adhesions. Factors such as surgical approach or use of buttressing material at the staple line did not affect the presence or duration of air leak[46] (Figure 15–5).

Cardiac complications are the second most common cause of perioperative morbidity and mortality after lung resection surgery. Major cardiac morbidity, defined as intraoperative or postoperative arrhythmia requiring treatment, myocardial infarction or pulmonary embolus in the 30 days after lung volume reduction surgery, had

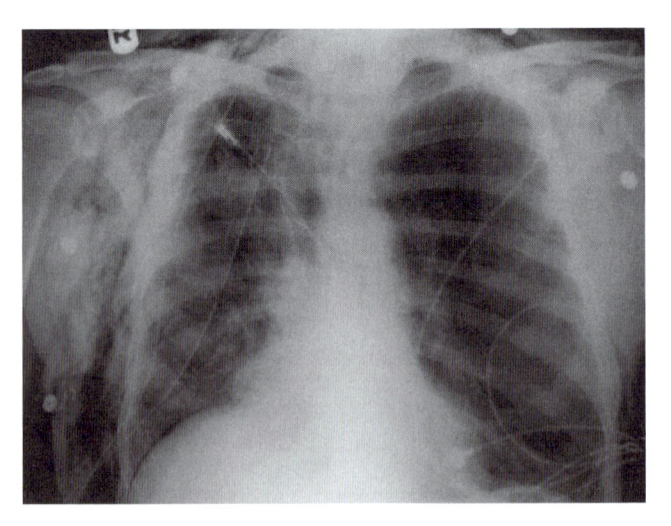

Figure 15–5. A patient with pneumonia and subcutaneous emphysema due to a postsurgical air leak after unilateral lung reduction.

an incidence of 20% in the NETT.[47] The most common cardiac complication is arrhythmia-requiring treatment. Atrial arrhythmias can occur in up to 20% of the patients and are associated with fluid overload, atelectasis and hypoxia.[44]

Bronchoscopic Lung Volume Reduction

Given the potential benefit of LVRS on quality of life, survival and exercise capacity in selected patients with heterogeneous emphysema, several minimally invasive techniques have emerged in order to achieve lung volume reduction without open thoracotomy. Bronchoscopic lung volume reduction (BLVR) allows clinicians to collapse areas of severe emphysema. Several BLVR systems have emerged and are currently under clinical trials. Endobronchial one-way valve systems are deployed into segmental or subsegmental bronchi of emphysematous, hyperinflated lung. They are designed to prevent inspiratory airflow but to allow air and secretions to move from the alveoli to the central airways, therefore resulting in progressive deflation and collapse of the lung distal to the valve.[48,49] Complications include migration of the device, hemoptysis, pneumothorax, postobstructive pneumonia, and failure of the lung to collapse due to collateral ventilation.

The Endobronchial Valve for Emphysema Palliation Trial (VENT) is the first prospective randomized multicenter trial to evaluate endobronchial valves. The preliminary results showed that the procedure has an acceptable safety profile.[34] The study showed that endobronchial-valve treatment induced modest improvements in lung function, exercise tolerance, and symptoms at the cost of more frequent exacerbations of COPD, pneumonia, and hemoptysis after implantation.[50]

The Exhale Airway Stents for Emphysema (EASE) trial, a double-blinded, randomized, sham-controlled device study for patients with emphysema/COPD was designed to evaluate the safety and effectiveness of the Airway Bypass procedure with Exhale Drug-Eluting Stents. The prospectively defined clinical endpoints of the trial were FVC and the modified Medical Research Council (mMRC) dyspnea score, a measure of the impact of breathlessness on quality of life. Early results showed statistically significant improvement only in mMRC dyspnea score.[51]

Fibrin-based glue, with subsequent collapse and remodeling of emphysematous lung, can also achieve occlusion of airways. In an open-label, phase II study of 50 patients with advanced upper lobe emphysema, a fibrinogen-thrombin hydrogel was administered to eight subsegmental sites (four in each upper lobe). Significant improvement was noted in the primary outcome, residual volume to total lung capacity ratio (RV/TLC), and also in secondary outcomes such as improvement in FEV_1, symptom scores, and health-related quality of life.[52]

PREOPERATIVE ASSESSMENT AND PATIENT SELECTION

Potential candidates for LVRS undergo extensive evaluation in order to mitigate perioperative risks and contain perioperative complications. The patient selection criteria are rigorous, involving both functional and radiological assessment with the goals of identifying the patients that are most likely to benefit from the procedure with an acceptable risk, optimizing medical status and customizing perioperative risk reduction strategies. The criteria for lung resection in patients with emphysema have developed over time. Before the NETT there was a high variability in the reported results due to differences in patient population, study design, surgical technique and perioperative management. The NETT, a multi-institutional randomized study sponsored jointly by the National heart, Lung and Blood Institute and the Center for Medicare and Medicaid Services, provided reliable estimates of risk and benefit from LVRS and established criteria selection for patients who will benefit most from lung volume reduction.

Clinical Evaluation

The clinical evaluation of the patients should be focused on identifying the clinical manifestations of the lung disease, presence of comorbid conditions, active cigarette smoking, corticosteroid use, and nutritional status. Medical contraindications include any conditions that increase the perioperative risk or predict a short-life expectancy due to non-emphysema illnesses. Advanced age has also been suggested as a risk factor for an unacceptable outcome.[30,53] Previous studies of the LVRS population showed that patients aged 70 years or older are at risk for an increased perioperative morbidity and mortality[53] or for less postoperative improvement in lung function.[54] Although the NETT did not identify age as a prognostic factor for operative mortality, patients with advanced age were at higher risk for major pulmonary morbidity and cardiovascular complications.[47]

Based on mechanisms of lung function improvement after LVRS, it is expected that the patients that benefit most have clinical manifestations of lung disease consistent with parenchymal destruction typical for emphysema with mild or minimal airway disease. Therefore, a history of recurrent bronchial infection with clinically significant daily sputum production might identify patients with primarily intrinsic disease who would not benefit from lung volume reduction. Prior thoracic surgery, which might lead to the formation of pleural adhesions and pleural or interstitial disease, are viewed as exclusion criteria for LVRS.

Careful assessment for cardiac disease before selection for surgery is also necessary as LVRS carries a significant risk of cardiac stress and intraoperative myocardial infarctions have been reported.[55,56] Coronary artery disease (CAD) is frequent among patients with COPD, as the two diseases share cigarette smoking as a common risk factor and a high prevalence of CAD has been shown angiographically in the LVRS patient population.[57] The evaluation of patients with advanced emphysema for the presence and extent of coronary artery disease presents a clinical challenge, as these patients may have poor functional capacity due to the underlying lung disease. However, keeping in mind that elective pulmonary resection surgery is deemed an "intermediate risk" procedure by the American College of Cardiology (ACC)/American Heart Association (AHA) guidelines on perioperative cardiovascular examination for noncardiac surgery,[58] the medical consultant needs to assess the functional status, severity, and stability of cardiac symptoms in a patient who has CAD or heart failure and proceed with noninvasive testing whenever indicated. Patients who have evidence of significant ischemia on noninvasive testing usually undergo coronary angiography; those who have left main or triple-vessel disease are potential candidates for surgical revascularization, whereas those who have single- or double-vessel disease may undergo PCI with or without stenting or be managed medically. Successful LVRS and coronary artery bypass grafting or LVRS and valve replacement have been performed with improvements in pulmonary function similar to those reported after isolated LVRS procedures.[59-62] A recent myocardial infarction (within the past 30 days) represents a major risk factor for perioperative risk complications. Although in the past it was believed that elective surgery should be delayed for 6 months after a myocardial infarction based on Goldman's original risk index, the ACC/AHA guidelines have decreased this interval to 4 to 6 weeks for a medically stable, fully investigated and optimized patient.[58,63]

Another issue with potential perioperative implications is pulmonary hypertension. The degree of pulmonary hypertension in COPD is usually of low to moderate magnitude, with mean pulmonary artery pressures rarely exceeding 35 to 40 mm Hg,[9] and although right ventricular function is generally preserved, multiple perioperative clinical scenarios (hypoxia, hypercapnia, dynamic hyperinflation) can lead to right ventricular failure. It is accepted that a peak systolic pulmonary artery pressure more than 45 mm Hg or mean pulmonary artery pressure more than 35 mm Hg is a relative contraindication to LVRS.[64] As echocardiography is frequently inaccurate in patients with advanced lung disease and tends to considerably overestimate the degree of pulmonary hypertension[65] a right heart catheterization is sometimes required in order to rule out significant pulmonary hypertension.

As smoking cessation has a significant positive impact on the rate of decline of FEV_1, wound healing and postoperative recovery, candidates for LVRS should be nonsmokers for at least 6 months prior to surgery.[66,67] Patients dependent on high-dose corticosteroids therapy may be at risk for delayed wound healing, prolonged postoperative leaks and infectious complications. Also, these patients may have an important coexisting intrinsic inflammatory airway disease component contributing to their airflow obstruction and therefore may not benefit significantly from LVRS. A daily prednisone dose of more than 20 mg (or equivalent) was one of the exclusion criteria in the NETT.[34] Nutritional status in patients with advanced emphysema is of great concern. Approximately 50% of patients undergoing LVRS for emphysema have a deficient nutritional status identifiable by a low BMI, which is associated with increased postoperative morbidity.[68,69] Although patients with advanced emphysema are rarely overweight, obesity also confers a higher postoperative risk of mortality and morbidity; a BMI greater than 31.1 kg/m² in men and 32.3 kg/m² in women was one of the exclusion criteria in the NETT.[34]

Physiologic Variables

Assessment of the risk for postoperative pulmonary complications is crucial to evaluating the patient with advanced emphysema being considered for LVRS; therefore the selection criteria rely on pulmonary function tests. As shown in the NETT subgroup analysis one of the predictors of major pulmonary morbidity was percent-predicted FEV_1. The criteria vary from series to series, but the majority of the investigators agree patients with an FEV_1 higher than 35% to 45% predicted are not surgical candidates. A higher postbronchodilator FEV_1

would not justify the risks associated with LVRS. Before the NETT, there was no consensus regarding the lower acceptable limit for FEV_1. The NETT defined a group of patients with severe emphysema who should not have surgery because of an exceptionally high risk for death after LVRS with little chance of functional benefit. This group of patients had an FEV_1 less than 20% of the predicted value and either homogenous (diffuse) emphysema on chest computed tomography (CT) or a DLCO less than 20% of predicted. The 30-day mortality in this subgroup of NETT patients was 16%, while 30-day mortality in patients with all three high-risk characteristics reached 25%. Based on this data obtained during interim analysis, the NETT investigators ceased the enrollment of patients with low FEV_1 who had either homogenous emphysema on the chest CT scan or a low carbon monoxide diffusing capacity.[70]

In the analysis of risk factors for operative morbidity and mortality in the NETT patients not considered to be high risk, FEV_1 and DLCO together with age were found to be risk factors for major pulmonary morbidity, defined as tracheostomy, failure to wean from mechanical ventilation, reintubation, pneumonia, and mechanical ventilation for 3 days or more. Other investigators have also suggested that a low DLCO increases the risk of mortality and morbidity with the lower limit varying from 10%[71] to 30%.[72] Another respiratory parameter investigated is the RV/TLC ratio. Analysis of a physiologic model proposed by Fessler and Permutt suggested that an increase in RV/TLC might be the best predictor of improvement in expiratory flow rates after LVRS. In this model the greatest impact of LVRS results from the relatively greater reduction in RV than in TLC with a consequent increase in vital capacity (VC) and an appropriate resizing of the lungs to the chest cavity.[73] A study of LVRS patients based on this physiologic model using multi-variate logistic regression identified the RV/TLC ratio as the only preoperative predictor of improvement in FVC and FEV_1. In these patients, 68% of the change in FEV_1 was attributed to change in FVC. The patients with RV/TLC >0.67 had significantly greater absolute and percent improvements in FEV_1 and FVC and a significantly greater decrease in residual volume (RV).[74] Although post-rehabilitation postbronchodilator TLC more than 100% predicted and RV less than 150% predicted were part of the inclusion criteria, the NETT did not identify lung volume as a predictor of mortality or cardiopulmonary morbidity after LVRS.[47]

Arterial blood gas abnormalities have also been suggested as predictive of a bad outcome with significant controversies surrounding this issue. Data regarding oxygenation are contradictory. Although McKenna et al showed no association between preoperative room air blood gas PaO_2 and postoperative change in FEV_1 or dyspnea score, they reported significantly worse outcome for patients using 4 L of supplemental oxygen at rest before the operation.[54] The NETT excluded patients with oxygen requirement greater than 6 L/min to maintain oxygen saturation more than 90% during exercise.[70]

As patients with COPD have varying degrees of hypercapnia, the data regarding the prognostic value of preoperative $PaCO_2$ on perioperative mortality and morbidity are conflicting. Many investigators have proposed excluding patients with hypercapnia from surgical treatment due to an unacceptable postoperative outcome.

Szekely et al found a $PaCO_2$ greater than 45 mm Hg as a strong predictor of mortality within 6 months and prolonged hospital stay.[75] Other investigators consider a $PaCO_2$ greater than 50 mm Hg[20,76] or 55 mm Hg[71] associated with adverse outcomes. Other studies have shown similar outcomes in patients with hypercapnia ($PaCO_2$ >45 to 55 mm Hg) when compared with patients with normocapnia.[77,78] The NETT data did not reveal hypercapnia to be a predictor of worse outcome, however patients with a $PaCO_2$ greater than 60 mm Hg (55 mm Hg in Denver) were excluded from the trial, by trial design.[47]

The NETT investigators did not identify poor exercise tolerance as a predictor of operative mortality or cardiopulmonary morbidity, however the investigators required a postrehabilitation 6-minute-walk distance of over 140 m as a measure of functional status.[47]

In summary, important physiologic variables when evaluating a patient for LVRS are FEV_1 and DLCO, the RV/TLC ratio, PCO_2 and oxygen use. The ideal operative candidate should have an FEV_1 of 20% to 35% predicted without very severe reductions in DLCO (<20% predicted), a RV/TLV more than 0.67, a PCO_2 less than 45 mm Hg, and no or low level supplemental oxygen use.

Imaging Studies

High-resolution computer tomography (HRCT) is a powerful tool for evaluation of pulmonary emphysema and has become the radiographic study of choice in evaluation potential LVRS patients. CT permits quantitative analysis of the severity of pulmonary emphysema and allows judgment of the heterogeneity of the disease. The NETT has established thoracic imaging as a crucially important tool in the evaluation of patients considered for LVRS. In the NETT, the magnitude and distribution of the emphysema in the participating patients was classified by HRCT as predominantly upper-lobe or non-upper-lobe using a visual scoring scale according to the study protocol.[79]

As mentioned in the section above, an initial report, based on interim analysis of the mortality data by the Data and Safety Monitoring Board, identified an increased risk of surgical mortality in patients with severe obstruction ($FEV_1 \leq 20$% predicted) and either diffuse emphysema on HRCT or a DLCO less than or equal to 20% predicted[79] and ceased enrollment of patients with these characteristics.

In the analysis of patients not at high-risk during a mean follow-up period of 29 months, the only individual base-line factors associated with differences in mortality between the treatment groups were the craniocaudal distribution of emphysema (presence or absence of upper-lobe predominance) and baseline exercise capacity (low or high, with the cutoff point for defining low baseline exercise capacity at the 40th percentile, ie, 25 Watts for women and 40 Watts for men).[70] When patients were divided into four subgroups on the basis of combinations of upper-lobe or non-upper-lobe emphysema and low or high exercise capacity at base line, there was strong evidence of differential effects on the primary endpoints of the NETT (ie, survival and exercise capacity at 24 months). The patients with upper-lobe disease and low baseline exercise capacity had the most survival advantage and improvement in exercise capacity from LVRS. LVRS did not show any survival advantage when compared with medical therapy in patients with upper-lobe disease and high baseline exercise capacity and in patients with non-upper-lobe disease and low baseline exercise capacity, but there was difference in the functional outcome. LVRS resulted in improved exercise capacity and health related quality of life in the patients with upper-lobe predominant disease and high-exercise capacity. In the patients with non-upper-lobe disease and low exercise capacity LVRS resulted only in improvement in the health-related quality of life. Patients who had non-upper-lobe predominant disease and high exercise capacity and underwent LVRS had a higher risk of death than those in the medical therapy group and there was difference in the improvement in the exercise capacity or health-related quality of life compared with the medical group[70,80] (Figure 15–6).

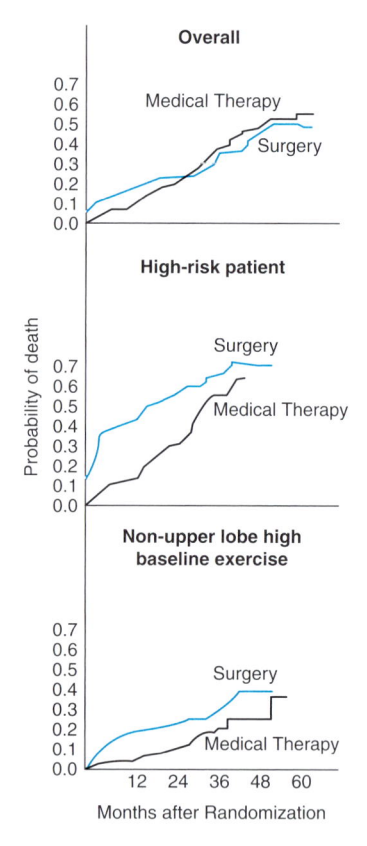

Figure 15–6. Kaplan-Meier estimates of the probability of death as a function of the number of months after randomization in the National Emphysema Treatment Trial (NETT). The study found no overall survival benefit of surgery over medical therapy, and a higher risk of death with surgery in high-risk patients and in patients with non-upper lobe disease and high exercise tolerance. (From: National Emphysema Treatment Trial Research Group. A randomized trial comparing lung-volume-reduction surgery with medical therapy for severe emphysema. *N Engl J Med*. 2003;348(21):2059-2073, with permission. © 2003 Massachusetts Medical Society. All rights reserved.)

A follow-up study sought to identify preoperative predictors of operative mortality, pulmonary and cardiovascular morbidity by using univariate and multivariate logistic regression and found that non-upper-lobe predominant emphysema was a predictor of both operative mortality and cardiovascular morbidity.[47] Extended follow-up of the patients to a median period of 4.3 years compared the differences in survival, exercise capacity, and health-related quality of life between those patients undergoing LVRS and those receiving optimal medical therapy.[4] A survival advantage was noted in the entire surgical group with 0.11 deaths per person-year compared with the medical group in which there were 0.13 deaths per person-year, despite the expected higher earlier postoperative mortality in the LVRS group. Improvement was also more likely in the LVRS than in the medical group for maximal exercise through 3 years and for health-related quality of life through 4 years.[4] In subgroup analysis, the additional follow-up data also confirmed the beneficial effects of LVRS in patients with upper-lobe-predominant emphysema and low post-rehabilitation exercise capacity. After LVRS, this subgroup of patients demonstrated improved survival and exercise throughout 3 years, and health-related quality of life through 5 years. Upper-lobe predominant and high-exercise capacity LVRS patients obtained no survival advantage but were likely to have significant and sustained improvements in exercise capacity and disease-specific quality of life. At 3 years there was no benefit with regard to survival, quality of life, or exercise capacity in the patients with non-upper-lobe emphysema and either high or low exercise capacity.

A summary of the criteria for determination of candidacy for lung volume reduction surgery is presented in Table 15–3.

Preoperative Preparation

Even the ideal candidate for LVRS has a substantial risk for mortality and morbidity after undergoing this elective surgical procedure. Therefore, meticulous perioperative management is paramount, starting with the preoperative preparation of the patient. Pulmonary rehabilitation attempts to optimize functional status and to improve physical and psychological symptoms, and plays a critical role in preparing selected patients for LVRS. In the patients enrolled in the NETT who underwent 6 to 10 weeks of pulmonary rehabilitation pre-randomization, significant improvements in exercise capacity, dyspnea, and health-related quality of life were observed consistently.[81]

Cigarette smoking has a wide range of effects on pulmonary, cardiovascular and immune functions, wound healing, hemostasis, drug metabolism, and mental status, all of which may impact postoperative outcome.[82,83] Also, smoking cessation is the only long-term intervention that has been shown to slow the rate of decline in lung function.[2] Thus, patients considered candidates for LVRS should be nonsmokers for 6 months prior to surgery.[66]

A large proportion of patients with COPD may have partially reversible airways disease and maximal medical therapy with long-acting bronchodilators and mucolytics should be continued, including on the day of the surgery. COPD exacerbations should be treated aggressively and surgery should be delayed at least 4 to 6 weeks after resolution of the exacerbation to allow stabilization.[66] The patients

Table 15–3. Criteria for Determination of Candidacy for Lung Volume Reduction Surgery

Criteria	Good Candidates	Poor Candidates
History and physical examination	Age <75 y Emphysema by clinical evaluation Ex-smoker (>4 mon) Clinically stable on no more than 20 mg prednisone daily Significant functional limitation after 6–12 wk of pulmonary rehabilitation on optimal medical therapy Demonstrated compliance with medical regimen	Age ≥75 y History of recurrent bronchial infections with increased sputum production Cardiovascular comorbidities including significant coronary artery disease, recent MI, CHF, or uncontrolled hypertension or arrhythmias Pulmonary hypertension at rest Nonpulmonary comorbidities causing significant functional limitation (morbid obesity) or that could limit survival (eg, cancer) History of thoracic surgery or chest wall deformity that could interfere with pulmonary resection
Laboratory evaluation	Post-bronchodilator FEV_1 ≤45% predicted for all ages and ≥15% if age ≥70 y Hyperinflation demonstrated by TLC ≥100% predicted and RV ≥150% predicted Postrehabilitation 6MWD >140 m Low postrehabilitation exercise capacity (demonstrated by maximal achieved cycle ergometry watts) HRCT demonstrating bilateral severe emphysema, ideally with upper-lobe predominance	FEV_1 ≤20% predicted and either DLCO ≤ 20% predicted or homogeneous distribution of emphysema on HRCT scan Non-upper-lobe distribution of emphysema with high exercise capacity postrehabilitation (demonstrated by maximal achieved cycle ergometry watts) Significant pleural or interstitial changes on HRCT

CHF = congestive heart failure, DLCO = carbon monoxide diffusing capacity, HRCT = high-resolution computerized tomography, MI = myocardial infarction, RV = residual volume, TLC = total lung capacity, 6MWD = 6-minute-walk distance, FEV_1 = forced expiratory volume in 1 second. Adapted from DeCamp MM, Lipson D, Krasna M et al, The evaluation and preparation of the patient for lung volume reduction surgery. *Proc Am Thorac Soc.* 2008;5:427-431. With permission of the American Thoracic Society. Copyright © American Thoracic Society. Official Journal of the American Thoracic Society.

must be free of respiratory infections for at least 3 weeks before lung volume reduction surgery and must require no antibiotic therapy preoperatively.[84] Despite clear evidence that systemic steroids are indicated only for short courses during COPD exacerbations,[85] the reported use of systemic steroids in stable patients with moderate and severe COPD is high.[86] However, systemic steroids have been linked to possible increased risks for perioperative delayed wound healing and infectious complications and the NETT investigators found that systemic corticosteroid use increased postoperative cardiovascular morbidity.[47] Therefore, systemic corticosteroids should be weaned off or decreased to the lowest possible tolerated dosage before surgery.

As anxiety is associated with tachypnea, dynamic hyperinflation and dyspnea, psychological preparation plays a crucial role in optimizing the overall preoperative status of the patient. Judicious anxiolytic therapy may be necessary in the perioperative period.

PERIOPERATIVE MANAGEMENT

Important advancements in monitoring, anesthetic agents, perioperative pain management, and in understanding of the physiological responses to surgical and anesthetic insults, has provided the anesthesiologist with a clinical armamentarium which allows implementing medical interventions aimed to improve postoperative outcome. More important than the specific agents and techniques used is devising an anesthetic plan tailored to the specific needs and goals of every patient.

Adverse Effects of Anesthesia on Respiratory Function

General anesthesia has multiple adverse effects on respiratory mechanics and blood gas exchange irrespective of the anesthetic agent used or whether the patient is breathing spontaneously or is being mechanically ventilated.[87] By changing the body position from upright to supine in an average healthy subject there is a decrease in the FRC by 0.8 to 1.0 L, with a further decrease by 0.4 to 0.5 L after induction of anesthesia. The decrease seems to be related to loss of respiratory muscle tone, shifting the balance between the elastic recoil force of the lung and the outward forces of the chest wall to a lower chest and lung volume.[87] Compliance of the respiratory system is also decreased during general anesthesia (from 95 to 60 mL/cm H_2O) mostly due to a decrease in the lung compliance.

Atelectasis appears in around 90% of patients who are anesthetized irrespective of the type of surgery. It occurs both during spontaneous breathing and after muscle paralysis, regardless of whether intravenous or inhalational anesthetics are used and involves up to 15% to 20% of the lung, mostly in the dependent areas. In addition to atelectasis, intermittent airway closure may reduce ventilation in the dependent areas of the lungs, resulting in worsening of the V/Q mismatch with increased number of low V/Q units. A three-compartment lung model can thus be constructed to explain oxygenation impairment during anesthesia. The model consists of one compartment with normal ventilation and perfusion, one with airway closure that impedes ventilation, and one of collapsed lung with no ventilation at all resulting in increased intrapulmonary shunt.[87] The alveolar-arterial oxygen gradient (pA-aO_2)

increases during general anesthesia, irrespective of the type of anesthetic agent and mode of ventilation (spontaneous or mechanically ventilated)[82] probably as a result of atelectasis, a greater V/Q mismatch, and attenuation of the hypoxic pulmonary vasoconstriction response. Ventilation of the lungs with pure oxygen might worsen the pA-aO$_2$ by promoting atelectasis through alveolar collapse in the low V/Q units.

Patients with COPD with already impaired gas exchange in the awake state experience further worsening of gas exchange during anesthesia. The mechanisms of gas exchange impairment may be different than in patients with healthy lungs. Patients with COPD develop minimal or no atelectasis during anesthesia, experience only a minor decrease in FRC and a small shunt. There is, however, a large dispersion of V/Q ratios with a further increase in V/Q mismatch and a widened perfusion distribution.[88] The preservation of FRC during anesthesia in patients with COPD might be explained by the chronic airflow obstruction, which leads to air trapping, intrinsic PEEP and loss of lung elastic recoil, and increased stiffness of the chest wall.[82] Carbon dioxide elimination might also be impaired during anesthesia due to increased distribution of ventilation to areas of the lungs with high V/Q ratio.

General anesthetic agents modulate respiratory function though various mechanisms: impaired respiratory drive, decreased muscular tone, and impaired mucociliary clearance at the level of the airways and attenuation of the hypoxic pulmonary vasoconstriction (HPV) reflex. All inhalational agents, opioids, and most intravenous anesthetic agents attenuate hypoxic and hypercapnic ventilatory reflexes in a dose-dependent manner. This effect might be more pronounced and prolonged in patients with COPD.[10] Inhibition of HPV by inhalational anesthesia is well-recognized. Halothane and nitrous oxide clearly inhibit HPV in a dose-dependent manner;[89] however, the newer inhalation anesthetics isoflurane, desflurane, and sevoflurane appear to be neutral toward HPV or at least not cause a significant depression in clinically relevant doses. None of the intravenous anesthetic agents interfere with the HPV response and intravenous anesthesia with propofol has been proposed as means of avoiding HPV modulation, although research published in the last decade has been controversial.[90-92] Other factors such as surgical manipulation, cardiac output, increased pulmonary artery pressure from elevated airway pressure, hypoxia, hypercarbia, heart failure, or preexisting lung disease may overcome HPV and have a greater influence on intrapulmonary shunt.

Prolonged exposure to general anesthesia may alter the immune defenses and gas exchange by depressing the alveolar macrophage function, interfering with surfactant production, slowing of mucociliary clearance and increasing the permeability of the alveolar capillary barrier.[82]

Intra-thoracic procedures produce marked alteration in respiratory function leading to a restrictive pattern of breathing which gradually improves in 4 to 10 days postoperatively. This pulmonary restrictive syndrome is characterized by reduction in lung volumes and alteration in the mechanics of the chest wall and diaphragm. Postoperative atelectasis, increased airway resistance due to low lung volumes, accumulated secretions and bronchospasm, diaphragmatic dysfunction, and respiratory muscle injury may all contribute to increased work of breathing in the postoperative period.[82]

Table 15–4. Effects of Anesthesia on Respiratory Function

1. Lung volume
   Atelectasis in dependent lung areas
   ↓ Functional respiratory capacity (FRC)
   ↑ Closing volume
   ↓ Lung compliance
   In COPD patients: ↑ FRC and ↑ dead space (air trapping) due to incomplete expiratory emptying of the most diseased lung regions

2. Airways
   Bronchodilatation (volatile anesthetic agents)
   ↓ Tonic activity of the muscle controlling the upper airways
   ↓ Bronchial muco-ciliary clearance
   ↑ = Airway resistance

3. Ventilatory control
   ↓ Ventilatory response to hypercarbia
   ↓ Ventilatory response to hypoxia
   ↓ Ventilatory response to acidosis

4. Pulmonary circulation
   ↓ Hypoxic vasoconstrictor response (volatile anesthetic agents)

5. Blood gas exchange
   ↑ $P_{A-a}O_2$ gradient due to mismatch in regional V_A/Q ratios

6. Immune function
   ↓ Bactericidal activity of alveolar and bronchial macrophages
   ↑ Release of pro-inflammatory cytokines

From Licker M, Schweizer A, Ellenberger C, Tschopp JM, Diaper J, Clergue F. Perioperative medical management of patients with COPD. *Int J Chron Obstruct Pulmon Dis.* 2007;2(4):493-515, with permission from Dove Medical Press Ltd.

A summary of the effects of anesthesia on respiratory function is presented in Table 15–4.

Induction and Maintenance of General Anesthesia

Most anesthesia practitioners avoid sedative premedication in order to avoid respiratory depression in this already critically compromised group of patients and prolongation of emergence at the end of the procedure. However, small doses of benzodiazepines can be administered in patients being treated chronically with benzodiazepines or if increased anxiety related to the upcoming surgery results in tachypnea with the potential of dynamic hyperinflation.

Monitoring for LVRS should include standard monitoring as recommended by the American Society of Anesthesiologists Standards for Intraoperative Monitoring and an indwelling arterial catheter for rapid-response hemodynamic monitoring and intermittent blood gas sampling and analysis. Because of the potential for hemodynamic instability on induction of general anesthesia, the intra-arterial blood pressure monitoring should be established prior to induction. Central venous catheters may be employed for administration of vasoactive medication that cannot be administered through a peripheral line. The placement of the central venous catheter should be done after induction of general anesthesia, due to the discomfort that the patient might experience in the Trendelenburg position.[55] More controversial is the use of pulmonary artery (PA) catheters and transesophageal echocardiography (TEE). The routine use of pulmonary artery catheters is not supported by current literature.[93,94] Central venous pressure and PA pressures may be inaccurate secondary to intrinsic and extrinsic positive end-expiratory pressure (PEEP), lateral decubitus position and open chest. In patients with significant coronary artery disease or pulmonary hypertension, pertinent intraoperative assessment of the right and left heart function can be provided by TEE.[55] However, at the conclusion of the surgical procedure attention should be paid to potential upper airway edema from the insertion and intraoperative manipulation of the TEE probe. As the patients undergoing LVRS receive little or no amnestic agents and may receive insufficient anesthetic agents due to potential hemodynamic instability, brain function monitoring may be helpful to target an adequate depth of anesthesia.[82] The intraoperative use of in-line flow-volume loop monitoring may be helpful in detecting the presence of intrinsic PEEP by the failure of the expiratory flow to return to zero before initiation of a new breath.[95]

If thoracic epidural analgesia will be employed for postoperative pain control, a thoracic epidural catheter should be placed before induction of general anesthesia. The spread of the neural blockade should be checked before induction to ensure proper placement and to avoid respiratory failure due to inadequate pain control.

Multiple agents are available for induction and maintenance of anesthesia. The choice of the anesthetic agent used for induction is mostly determined by the medical condition of the patient. Slow, careful titration of the anesthetic agents and vasoactive drugs during induction may provide better hemodynamic stability. Achievement of an adequate depth of anesthesia before laryngoscopy and intubation is paramount, as intubation in an inadequately anesthetized patient can lead to severe bronchospasm.[84] The anesthetic plan for maintenance is formulated with the goal of extubation of the patient at the end of the procedure. Historically, potent inhalational agents have been the agents of choice in providing anesthesia for thoracic surgical cases given their ease of titration and their potent bronchodilator properties. However, patients undergoing LVRS may benefit from a total intravenous anesthesia (TIVA) approach. Although current literature does not support a clear physiologic advantage of using one technique over another in patients with relatively normal lung function, avoiding modulation of HPV with TIVA may be clinically significant in patients with marginal lung function. More importantly though, patients with COPD undergoing LVRS have increased dead space, and therefore the uptake and distribution of the inhalational agents is unpredictable and the end-tidal volatile anesthetic concentration inaccurate.[10] Furthermore, premature airway closing during expiration and air trapping may hinder elimination of the volatile anesthetic, delaying awakening and extubation. The most common drugs used for TIVA are remifentanil and propofol as a continuous infusion, which allow rapid recovery and more predictable emergence at the end of the procedure. The intravenous administration of opioids, with the exception of ultrashort-acting ones, should be limited in order to avoid postoperative respiratory depression. Intermediate-acting muscle relaxants devoid of hemodynamic effects and easily reversible are recommended. As patients with severe COPD may evidence increased sensitivity to neuromuscular blocking agents, the degree of neuromuscular blockade should be monitored.[55] Local anesthetics or a combination of local anesthetic and narcotics may be administered through the thoracic epidural catheter allowing for a smooth emergence in the absence of pain or respiratory depression.

Besides its well-known adverse effects (higher incidence of myocardial ischemia and wound infection, coagulopathy), hypothermia may result in shivering leading to an increased production of carbon dioxide and delayed extubation. Therefore, the use of warming devices is recommended to maintain normothermia.

Hypotension may occur at any time following induction or during maintenance of general anesthesia and may represent a diagnostic dilemma. Causes of hypotension include sympathetic blockade from local anesthetics administered through the thoracic epidural catheter, vasodilatory effects of the induction agents, hypovolemia, myocardial ischemia, dynamic hyperinflation, or infrequent but possible catastrophic causes such as tension pneumothorax. Air trapping and dynamic hyperinflation resulting in decreased venous return is one of the most common causes of hypotension upon institution of positive pressure ventilation. If this is the etiology of hypotension, disconnecting the endotracheal tube from the breathing circuit and allowing the lung volumes to decrease will result in resolution of hypotension. An extreme form of air trapping and auto-PEEP can have a "tamponade" effect on the heart. Such patients show a progressive increase in central venous pressure, pulmonary hypertension, and proportionally increased pulmonary capillary wedge pressures. This results in a low cardiac output state with progressive systemic hypotension and drastic reduction in oxygen delivery to tissues. If the condition is not recognized and corrected rapidly, the patient may expire.[96] In order to correct or avoid auto-PEEP, airflow obstruction should be aggressively corrected by confirming the correct position of the endotracheal tube, removing secretions and administering inhaled bronchodilators. Optimizing the ventilatory parameters by increasing the expiratory time and decreasing the respiratory rate may allow more time for lung deflation. The abrupt development of cardiovascular collapse unresponsive to volume infusion and vasopressor administration and unexplained by auto-PEEP and/or malposition of the endotracheal tube should raise the suspicion of a pneumothorax. Due to positive pressure ventilation, a pneumothorax becomes rapidly a tension pneumothorax and represents a true emergency. This complication needs immediate detection and treatment by aborting the surgical procedure, re-expanding the operative lung, and immediately inserting a chest tube in the contralateral chest.[96]

One-Lung Ventilation in Patients with Severe Chronic Obstructive Pulmonary Disease

Most of the techniques of lung isolation and considerations related to OLV discussed in detail in Chapters 3 and 4 apply to the patients undergoing LVRS.

However, there are some unique aspects related to the ventilatory management of OLV in these patients.

OLV can be accomplished by any of the usual techniques: DLT, single-lumen tube with bronchial blocker or Univent tube. Although increased airflow resistance through a DLT compared with a single-lumen tube or a Univent tube during OLV[97] might worsen auto-PEEP, DLTs tend to be the favored method for lung separation in LVRS by most practitioners. Bronchial blockers are more prone to dislodgement, provide slower deflation of the operative lung due to the small size of the central lumen, and do not permit suctioning of the operative lung. Irrespective of the method used for lung separation, fiberoptic bronchoscopy should be used for confirmation of appropriate positioning.

Because of decreased elastic recoil of the lung and chronic airflow obstruction, the deflation of the operative lung might be delayed; therefore one should proceed with OLV as early as possible in order to maximize the time available for lung deflation. Intraoperative ventilatory management during OLV aims to balance competitive priorities: maintaining adequate oxygenation, minimizing intrinsic PEEP, minimizing barotrauma, and maximizing CO_2 elimination.

Some investigators have found that oxygenation is preserved for a longer period of time in patients with severe emphysema as compared with patients with normal lung function after initiation of OLV.[98] Explanations include: (1) slow deflation of the operative lung after institution of OLV serving as a reservoir of oxygen, (2) preexisting reduced perfusion to the operative lung secondary to altered HPV in the presence of chronic, irreversible disease in the pulmonary vessels, (3) kinked pulmonary vessels in the deflated, operative lung that inhibit perfusion, (4) development of auto-PEEP in the dependent lung with decreased atelectasis formation and preserved FRC.[99] The position of the patient during surgery might also influence the degree of hypoxemia during OLV. Bardoczky et al found a significantly higher PaO_2 and lower $PA\text{-}aO_2$ in patients with mild pulmonary hyperinflation when OLV was performed in the lateral position compared with the supine position. They also found that PaO_2 was significantly greater when OLV was initiated after turning the patients into the lateral decubitus position.[100] These results are conflicting with the study by Fiser et al, who studied OLV in the supine and lateral position and did not find significant changes in PaO_2 during OLV when the position of the patient was changed from supine to lateral decubitus. However, in their study OLV was initiated in the supine position and maintained continuously, even during turning and positioning of the patient.[101]

Most practitioners have adopted the lung-protective ventilatory strategy with small tidal volumes (TV) (5-7 mL/kg when ventilating two lungs and 3-4 mL/kg when ventilating a single lung), peak inspiratory pressure below 35 cm H_2O, inspiratory/expiratory ratio between 1:3 to 1:5, and low respiratory rates. This ventilatory strategy is aimed at preventing dynamic hyperinflation, minimizing the risk of disruption of suture lines or lung tissue and avoiding the intraoperative occurrence of pneumothorax or air leaks. However, it may lead to hypoventilation and hypercapnia. Permissive hypercapnia with $PaCO_2$ levels up to 70 mm Hg may be well-tolerated for short periods of time, assuming a reasonable cardiovascular reserve and in particular right ventricular function.[89] Inotropic support might be required in more compromised patients. Significant respiratory acidosis, however, has numerous potential adverse effects such as increased intracranial pressure, decreased myocardial contractility, pulmonary hypertension, diaphragmatic dysfunction, and cardiac arrhythmias. When significant acidosis develops (pH <7.20) maneuvers should be instituted to maximize minute ventilation, communication should be initiated with the surgeon, and two-lung ventilation should be resumed whenever possible. In this clinical situation when carbon dioxide elimination is impaired, administration of sodium bicarbonate with the aim to normalize the pH value is not recommended as it might worsen the intracellular acidosis. Due to increased dead space, the gradient between the end-tidal CO_2 and $PaCO_2$ is increased and unpredictable, therefore frequent arterial blood gas sampling and analysis is recommended.[10]

PEEP is commonly applied to the ventilated lung to try to improve oxygenation during OLV but is an unreliable therapy and occasionally causes PaO_2 to decrease further. Slinger et al showed that the effects of the application of 5 cm of PEEP on oxygenation during OLV has a variable effect on oxygenation depending on the relation between the plateau end-expiratory pressure and the inflection point of the static compliance curve. When the application of PEEP causes the end-expiratory pressure to increase from a low level toward the inflection point, oxygenation is likely to improve. Conversely, if the addition of PEEP causes an increased inflation of the ventilated lung that raises the equilibrium end-expiratory pressure beyond the inflection point, oxygenation is likely to deteriorate.[102] The application of external PEEP in patients with severe COPD has generally been discouraged due to the potential risk of barotrauma. Because of the heterogenous nature of auto-PEEP, patients with preexisting auto-PEEP have an unpredictable response to application of external PEEP. The increase in total PEEP after application of external PEEP is not consistent and depends on the level of auto-PEEP.[103] However, the application of low level extrinsic PEEP during weaning from mechanical ventilation might improve the lung mechanics and reduce work of breathing by shifting the effort from the patient, who has to exert a certain inspiratory effort in order to overcome the auto-PEEP, to the ventilator.[104] Intraoperative PEEP titration is difficult and may not be feasible as determination of the inflection point or auto-PEEP requires in-line spirometry.

Although there is no unequivocal evidence that one mode of ventilation may be more beneficial than the other, pressure-controlled ventilation (PCV) may diminish the risk of barotrauma by limiting peak and plateau airway pressures. Also, the decelerating flow pattern results in more homogeneous distribution of the tidal volume and improved dead space ventilation.[105] The concern surrounding PCV relates to the impact that inspiratory resistance and auto-PEEP may have on delivered TV leading to unpredictable low TV and unintended hypoventilation.[105]

At the end of the procedure the operative lung is inflated gradually to a peak inspiratory pressure less than 20 cm H_2O in order to prevent disruption of the staple line. During reinflation of the operative lung it is helpful to clamp the lumen serving the dependent lung to limit overdistension and significant hypotension.[89]

Table 15–5. Strategies to Avoid Delayed or Failed Extubation after Lung Volume Reduction Surgery

Terminal "toilet" bronchoscopy
In-line nebulized bronchodilator treatment at end of surgery Deep remifentanil anesthesia during terminal bronchoscopy
Avoid systemic narcotics (except remifentanil) Avoid inhalational agents (use TIVA)
Full reversal of neuromuscular blockade
Dense thoracic epidural blockade at end of surgery
Limit degree of "permissive hypercapnia" during one-lung ventilation (fast surgery), and cautiously increase ventilation during terminal two-lung phase
Avoid hypothermia

From Hartigan PM, Pedoto A. Anesthetic considerations for lung volume reduction surgery and lung transplantation. *Thorac Surg Clin*. 2005;15:143-157. Copyright © Elsevier.

Emergence

Tracheal extubation immediately after surgery is an important aim after LVRS in order to minimize the risk of developing or exacerbating an air leak and avoid the deleterious hemodynamic effects of positive pressure ventilation. Successful extubation however depends on multiple factors: adequate pain control, reversal of neuromuscular blockade, absence of significant bronchospasm and secretions, absence of significant hypercapnia and acidosis, and absence of respiratory depression due to residual anesthetic agents. Strategies for optimization of the patient prior to extubation are presented in Table 15–5.

Due to underlying ventilatory problem in patients with COPD, extubation can be attempted even in the presence of moderate respiratory acidosis. Most patients demonstrate a pattern of recovery from the moderate hypercapnic acidosis within 1 or 2 hours following extubation.[96] Worsening of respiratory acidosis after extubation may resolve by employing noninvasive ventilation. Occasionally, extubation must be delayed due to severe hypercapnic acidosis. Delaying extubation is preferred over aggressive ventilation, which carries the risk of barotrauma and air leaks.[10]

Some investigators recommend changing the DLT to an SLT at the end of the procedure in order to facilitate "toilet" bronchoscopy and reduce airflow resistance in the spontaneously breathing patient prior to extubation. The benefits of this maneuver have to be weighted against the risk of manipulating the airway, taking into consideration the fact that when both lumens of the DLT are used the airflow resistance is only slightly higher compared to an SLT.[97]

As postoperative respiratory failure and tracheal re-intubation carry significant morbidity, LVRS patients have to be monitored very closely after extubation and any deterioration in their respiratory status has to be treated very aggressively.

The patient should be placed in a steep sitting position to facilitate diaphragmatic excursions, nebulized bronchodilators should be administered immediately after extubation, pain control should be optimized and aggressive chest physiotherapy should be initiated promptly.

Pain Management In Lung Volume Reduction Surgery

The importance of adequate pain control in LVRS patients cannot be overstated. Effective, enduring pain control is vital to the success of the surgical procedure. Inadequate pain control in these high-risk patients will result in splinting, poor respiratory effort, inability to cough and clear secretions leading to airway closure, atelectasis, shunting, and hypoxemia. Also, it is paramount that adequate pain control is achieved with minimal respiratory depression.

Common surgical approaches used in LVRS, VATS, and midline sternotomy are usually associated with less acute postoperative pain than a thoracotomy incision. Although comparative studies of various modalities of pain control in LVRS do not exist, some conclusions could be extrapolated from studies on pain control in thoracic surgery. Regional analgesia techniques are widely employed in thoracic surgery due to their narcotic-sparing effects. Thoracic epidural analgesia (TEA) with a continuous infusion of local anesthetics with or without opioids is the favored modality of postoperative pain control after LVRS by most practitioners. TEA provides a better quality pain control compared to parenteral opioids[106] and may reduce the incidence of myocardial infarction in the perioperative period.[107] Good evidence indicates that TEA reduces the incidence of respiratory complications after thoracic surgery. In a meta-analysis, Ballantyne et al showed that, while epidural opioids had only a tendency to reduce pulmonary complications overall when compared with systemic opioids, epidural local anesthetics increased PaO_2 and decreased the incidence of pulmonary infections and pulmonary complications overall.[108] However, there is concern that by blocking the nerve supply to the intercostal muscles, local anesthetics could impair postoperative respiratory function. Gruber et al showed that this does not occur to a clinically significant degree. In a group of 12 patients undergoing LVRS thoracic epidural blockade with bupivacaine 0.25% did not adversely affect ventilatory mechanics, breathing pattern, gas exchange or inspiratory muscle power.[109] Improved gastrointestinal motility and postoperative gut function was observed in patients with thoracic epidural analgesia especially when the splanchnic fibers (T5-T10) were blocked. This may be of importance given the fact that a small number of LVRS patients may develop postoperative ileus, which can be compounded by the use of parenteral opioids and can lead to diaphragmatic dysfunction, respiratory failure and reintubation.

Nonsteroidal anti-inflammatory drugs (NSAIDs) can be used as adjuvants in postoperative pain control. Ketorolac tromethamine (Toradol) is the most potent analgesic in the NSAID class available in an intravenous form in the United States. Given that ketorolac binds to both isoforms of the cyclooxygenase, its potential adverse effects include decreased renal perfusion, inhibition of platelet aggregation, and predisposition to peptic ulcer disease and gastrointestinal bleeding.[110]

Other potential techniques for pain control in LVRS patients include intrathecal morphine, intercostal nerve blockade, paravertebral nerve blockade, and pleural catheters. Paravertebral blockade provides comparable pain relief with epidural analgesia in thoracic surgery, has a better side-effect profile and is associated with a reduction in pulmonary complications.[111] However, local anesthetic toxicity may be of concern due to the bilateral nature of the surgical approach in thoracoscopic LVRS, and due to the fact that a greater amount of local anesthetic is used for paravertebral blockade. Also, one of the possible complications associated with paravertebral blockade is the development of a pneumothorax, which could manifest after the institution of positive pressure ventilation and have extreme consequences.

Irrespective of the technique used, a very clear plan for pain control has to be designed and discussed with the patient, the surgical team and the acute pain service if available.

SUMMARY

When performed on appropriately selected patients, LVRS is associated with prolonged survival, improvement in exercise capacity and quality of life, and improvement in lung function and respiratory symptoms. It is essential that the thoracic anesthesiologist have a clear understanding of the indications and contraindications for surgery, the pathophysiology of COPD, and the management of one-lung ventilation in this high risk group of patients; also paramount to successful patient outcomes is a well-planned and executed plan for postoperative analgesia.

REFERENCES

1. Pauwels R. Global initiative for chronic obstructive lung diseases (GOLD): time to act. *Eur Respir J.* 2001;18(6):901-902.
2. Buist AS, Sexton GJ, Nagy JM, Ross BB. The effect of smoking cessation and modification on lung function. *Am Rev Respir Dis.* 1976;114(1):115-122.
3. Anthonisen NR. Long-term oxygen therapy. *Ann Intern Med.* 1983;99(4):519-527.
4. Naunheim KS, Wood DE, Mohsenifar Z, et al. Long-term follow-up of patients receiving lung-volume-reduction surgery versus medical therapy for severe emphysema by the National Emphysema Treatment Trial Research Group. *Ann Thorac Surg.* 2006;82(2):431-443.
5. Macnee W. Pathogenesis of chronic obstructive pulmonary disease. *Clin Chest Med.* 2007;28(3):479-513, v.
6. Kim WD, Eidelman DH, Izquierdo JL, Ghezzo H, Saetta MP, Cosio MG. Centrilobular and panlobular emphysema in smokers. Two distinct morphologic and functional entities. *Am Rev Respir Dis.* 1991;144(6):1385-1390.
7. Rabe KF, Hurd S, Anzueto A, et al. Global strategy for the diagnosis, management, and prevention of chronic obstructive pulmonary disease: GOLD executive summary. *Am J Respir Crit Care Med.* 15 2007;176(6):532-555.
8. Cooper CB, Dransfield M. Primary care of the patient with chronic obstructive pulmonary disease-part 4: understanding the clinical manifestations of a progressive disease. *Am J Med.* 2008;121(7 Suppl):S33-45.
9. Barbera JA, Peinado VI, Santos S. Pulmonary hypertension in chronic obstructive pulmonary disease. *Eur Respir J.* 2003;21(5):892-905.
10. Hartigan PM, Pedoto A. Anesthetic considerations for lung volume reduction surgery and lung transplantation. *Thorac Surg Clin.* 2005;15(1):143-157.

11. Au DH, Lemaitre RN, Curtis JR, Smith NL, Psaty BM. The risk of myocardial infarction associated with inhaled beta-adrenoceptor agonists. *Am J Respir Crit Care Med.* 2000;161(3 Pt 1):827-830.
12. Danesh J, Whincup P, Walker M, et al. Low grade inflammation and coronary heart disease: prospective study and updated meta-analyses. *BMJ.* 22 2000;321(7255):199-204.
13. Brantigan OC, Mueller E. Surgical treatment of pulmonary emphysema. *Am Surg.* 1957;23(9): 789-804.
14. Cooper JD, Trulock EP, Triantafillou AN, et al. Bilateral pneumectomy (volume reduction) for chronic obstructive pulmonary disease. *J Thorac Cardiovasc Surg.* 1995;109(1):106-116; discussion 116-109.
15. Stirling GR, Babidge WJ, Peacock MJ, et al. Lung volume reduction surgery in emphysema: a systematic review. *Ann Thorac Surg.* 2001;72(2):641-648.
16. Huizenga HF, Ramsey SD, Albert RK. Estimated growth of lung volume reduction surgery among Medicare enrollees: 1994 to 1996. *Chest.* 1998;114(6):1583-1587.
17. McKenna RJ, Jr., Benditt JO, DeCamp M, et al. Safety and efficacy of median sternotomy versus video-assisted thoracic surgery for lung volume reduction surgery. *J Thorac Cardiovasc Surg.* 2004;127(5):1350-1360.
18. Wisser W, Tschernko E, Senbaklavaci O, et al. Functional improvement after volume reduction: sternotomy versus videoendoscopic approach. *Ann Thorac Surg.* 1997;63(3):822-827; discussion 827-828.
19. Roberts JR, Bavaria JE, Wahl P, Wurster A, Friedberg JS, Kaiser LR. Comparison of open and thoracoscopic bilateral volume reduction surgery: complications analysis. *Ann Thorac Surg.* 1998;66(5): 1759-1765.
20. Kotloff RM, Tino G, Bavaria JE, et al. Bilateral lung volume reduction surgery for advanced emphysema. A comparison of median sternotomy and thoracoscopic approaches. *Chest.* 1996;110(6):1399-1406.
21. Hazelrigg SR, Boley TM, Grasch A, Shawgo T. Surgical strategy for lung volume reduction surgery. *Eur J Cardiothorac Surg.* 1999;16 Suppl 1:S57-60.
22. McKenna RJ, Jr., Brenner M, Fischel RJ, Gelb AF. Should lung volume reduction for emphysema be unilateral or bilateral? *J Thorac Cardiovasc Surg.* Nov 1996;112(5):1331-1338; discussion 1338-1339.
23. Argenziano M, Thomashow B, Jellen PA, et al. Functional comparison of unilateral versus bilateral lung volume reduction surgery. *Ann Thorac Surg.* 1997;64(2):321-326; discussion 326-327.
24. Eugene J, Dajee A, Kayaleh R, Gogia HS, Dos Santos C, Gazzaniga AB. Reduction pneumonoplasty for patients with a forced expiratory volume in 1 second of 500 milliliters or less. *Ann Thorac Surg.* 1997;63(1):186-190; discussion 190-182.
25. Naunheim KS, Kaiser LR, Bavaria JE, et al. Long-term survival after thoracoscopic lung volume reduction: a multiinstitutional review. *Ann Thorac Surg.* 1999;68(6):2026-2031; discussion 2031-2022.
26. McKenna RJ, Jr., Brenner M, Gelb AF, et al. A randomized, prospective trial of stapled lung reduction versus laser bullectomy for diffuse emphysema. *J Thorac Cardiovasc Surg.* 1996;111(2):317-321; discussion 322.
27. Vigneswaran WT, Podbielski FJ. Single-stage bilateral, video-assisted thoracoscopic lung volume reduction operation. *Ann Thorac Surg.* 1997;63(6):1807-1809.
28. Flaherty KR, Martinez FJ. Lung volume reduction surgery for emphysema. *Clin Chest Med.* 2000;21(4):819-848.
29. Gelb AF, Zamel N, McKenna RJ, Jr., Brenner M. Mechanism of short-term improvement in lung function after emphysema resection. *Am J Respir Crit Care Med.* 1996;154(4 Pt 1):945-951.
30. Hazelrigg S, Boley T, Henkle J, et al. Thoracoscopic laser bullectomy: a prospective study with three-month results. *J Thorac Cardiovasc Surg.* 1996;112(2):319-326; discussion 326-317.
31. Miller JI, Jr., Lee RB, Mansour KA. Lung volume reduction surgery: lessons learned. *Ann Thorac Surg.* 1996;61(5):1464-1468; discussion 1468-1469.
32. Marchand E, Gayan-Ramirez G, De Leyn P, Decramer M. Physiological basis of improvement after lung volume reduction surgery for severe emphysema: where are we? *Eur Respir J.* 1999;13(3):686-696.
33. Sciurba FC, Rogers RM, Keenan RJ, et al. Improvement in pulmonary function and elastic recoil after lung-reduction surgery for diffuse emphysema. *N Engl J Med.* 1996;334(17):1095-1099.
34. Mamary A, Criner G. Lung volume reduction surgery and bronchoscopic lung volume reduction in severe emphysema. *Respiratory medicine: COPD update.* 2008;4:44-59.
35. Albert RK, Benditt JO, Hildebrandt J, Wood DE, Hlastala MP. Lung volume reduction surgery has variable effects on blood gases in patients with emphysema. *Am J Respir Crit Care Med.* 1998; 158(1):71-76.

36. Tschernko EM, Wisser W, Hofer S, et al. The influence of lung volume reduction surgery on ventilatory mechanics in patients suffering from severe chronic obstructive pulmonary disease. *Anesth Analg.* 1996;83(5):996-1001.
37. Snyder ML, Goss CH, Neradilek B, et al. Changes in arterial oxygenation and self-reported oxygen use after lung volume reduction surgery. *Am J Respir Crit Care Med.* 15 2008;178(4):339-345.
38. Naunheim KS, Keller CA, Krucylak PE, Singh A, Ruppel G, Osterloh JF. Unilateral video-assisted thoracic surgical lung reduction. *Ann Thorac Surg.* 1996;61(4):1092-1098.
39. Lando Y, Boiselle PM, Shade D, et al. Effect of lung volume reduction surgery on diaphragm length in severe chronic obstructive pulmonary disease. *Am J Respir Crit Care Med.* 1999;159(3):796-805.
40. Martinez FJ, de Oca MM, Whyte RI, Stetz J, Gay SE, Celli BR. Lung-volume reduction improves dyspnea, dynamic hyperinflation, and respiratory muscle function. *Am J Respir Crit Care Med.* 1997;155(6):1984-1990.
41. Haniuda M, Kubo K, Fujimoto K, Aoki T, Yamanda T, Amano J. Different effects of lung volume reduction surgery and lobectomy on pulmonary circulation. *Ann Surg.* 2000;231(1):119-125.
42. Haniuda M, Kubo K, Fujimoto K, et al. Effects of pulmonary artery remodeling on pulmonary circulation after lung volume reduction surgery. *Thorac Cardiovasc Surg.* 2003;51(3):154-158.
43. Sciurba FC. Preoperative predictors of outcome following lung volume reduction surgery. *Thorax.* 2002;57 Suppl 2:II47-II52.
44. McKenna RJ, Jr. Complications after lung volume reduction surgery. *Chest Surg Clin N Am.* 2003;13(4):701-708.
45. Kotloff RM, Tino G, Palevsky HI, et al. Comparison of short-term functional outcomes following unilateral and bilateral lung volume reduction surgery. *Chest.* 1998;113(4):890-895.
46. DeCamp MM, Blackstone EH, Naunheim KS, et al. Patient and surgical factors influencing air leak after lung volume reduction surgery: lessons learned from the National Emphysema Treatment Trial. *Ann Thorac Surg.* 2006;82(1):197-206; discussion 206-197.
47. Naunheim KS, Wood DE, Krasna MJ, et al. Predictors of operative mortality and cardiopulmonary morbidity in the National Emphysema Treatment Trial. *J Thorac Cardiovasc Surg.* 2006;131(1):43-53.
48. Hopkinson NS, Toma TP, Hansell DM, et al. Effect of bronchoscopic lung volume reduction on dynamic hyperinflation and exercise in emphysema. *Am J Respir Crit Care Med.* 2005;171(5):453-460.
49. Venuta F, de Giacomo T, Rendina EA, et al. Bronchoscopic lung-volume reduction with one-way valves in patients with heterogenous emphysema. *Ann Thorac Surg.* 2005;79(2):411-416; discussion 416-417.
50. Sciurba FC, Ernst A, Herth FJ, et al. A randomized study of endobronchial valves for advanced emphysema. *The New England Journal of Medicine.* 2010;363(13):1233-1244.
51. http://www.medicalnewstoday.com/articles/171352.php.
52. Criner GJ, Pinto-Plata V, Strange C, et al. Biologic lung volume reduction in advanced upper lobe emphysema: phase 2 results. *Am J Respir Crit Care Med.* 2009;179(9):791-798.
53. Glaspole IN, Gabbay E, Smith JA, Rabinov M, Snell GI. Predictors of perioperative morbidity and mortality in lung volume reduction surgery. *Ann Thorac Surg.* 2000;69(6):1711-1716.
54. McKenna RJ, Jr., Brenner M, Fischel RJ, et al. Patient selection criteria for lung volume reduction surgery. *J Thorac Cardiovasc Surg.* 1997;114(6):957-964; discussion 964-957.
55. Brister NW, Barnette RE, Kim V, Keresztury M. Anesthetic considerations in candidates for lung volume reduction surgery. *Proc Am Thorac Soc.* 2008;5(4):432-437.
56. Hogue CW, Jr., Stamos T, Winters KJ, Moulton M, Krucylak PE, Cooper JD. Acute myocardial infarction during lung volume reduction surgery. *Anesth Analg.* 1999;88(2):332-334.
57. Thurnheer R, Muntwyler J, Stammberger U, et al. Coronary artery disease in patients undergoing lung volume reduction surgery for emphysema. *Chest.* 1997;112(1):122-128.
58. Fleisher LA, Beckman JA, Brown KA, et al. ACC/AHA 2007 Guidelines on Perioperative Cardiovascular Evaluation and Care for Noncardiac Surgery: Executive Summary: A Report of the American College of Cardiology/American Heart Association Task Force on Practice Guidelines (Writing Committee to Revise the 2002 Guidelines on Perioperative Cardiovascular Evaluation for Noncardiac Surgery) Developed in Collaboration with the American Society of Echocardiography, American Society of Nuclear Cardiology, Heart Rhythm Society, Society of Cardiovascular Anesthesiologists, Society for Cardiovascular Angiography and Interventions, Society for Vascular Medicine and Biology, and Society for Vascular Surgery. *J Am Coll Cardiol.* 2007;50(17):1707-1732.

59. Choong CK, Abu-Omar Y, Agarwal A, et al. Concomitant bilateral lung volume reduction surgery and aortic valve replacement: multidisciplinary strategies in achieving a successful outcome. *J Thorac Cardiovasc Surg.* 2009;137(6):1551-1552.
60. Choong CK, Naylor J, Vuylsteke A, et al. Successful combined bilateral lung volume reduction and coronary artery bypass grafting surgery: implications and advantages. *J Thorac Cardiovasc Surg.* 2009;137(6):1552-1554.
61. Schmid RA, Stammberger U, Hillinger S, et al. Lung volume reduction surgery combined with cardiac interventions. *Eur J Cardiothorac Surg.* 1999;15(5):585-591.
62. Whyte RI, Bria W, Martinez FJ, Lewis P, Bolling SF. Combined lung volume reduction and mitral valve reconstruction. *Ann Thorac Surg.* 1998;66(4):1414-1416.
63. Cohn SL. Preoperative cardiac evaluation of lung resection candidates. *Thorac Surg Clin.* 2008;18(1):45-59.
64. Martinez FJ, Flaherty KR, Iannettoni MD. Patient selection for lung volume reduction surgery. *Chest Surg Clin N Am.* 2003;13(4):669-685.
65. Arcasoy SM, Christie JD, Ferrari VA, et al. Echocardiographic assessment of pulmonary hypertension in patients with advanced lung disease. *Am J Respir Crit Care Med.* 2003;167(5):735-740.
66. DeCamp MM, Jr, Lipson D, Krasna M, Minai OA, McKenna RJ, Jr, Thomashow BM. The evaluation and preparation of the patient for lung volume reduction surgery. *Proc Am Thorac Soc.* 2008;5(4):427-431.
67. Yusen RD, Lefrak SS, Trulock EP. Evaluation and preoperative management of lung volume reduction surgery candidates. *Clin Chest Med.* 1997;18(2):199-224.
68. Mazolewski P, Turner JF, Baker M, Kurtz T, Little AG. The impact of nutritional status on the outcome of lung volume reduction surgery: a prospective study. *Chest.* 1999;116(3):693-696.
69. Nezu K, Yoshikawa M, Yoneda T, et al. The effect of nutritional status on morbidity in COPD patients undergoing bilateral lung reduction surgery. *Thorac Cardiovasc Surg.* 2001;49(4):216-220.
70. Fishman A, Martinez F, Naunheim K, et al. A randomized trial comparing lung-volume-reduction surgery with medical therapy for severe emphysema. *N Engl J Med.* 2003;348(21):2059-2073.
71. Yusen RD, Lefrak SS. Evaluation of patients with emphysema for lung volume reduction surgery. Washington University Emphysema Surgery Group. *Semin Thorac Cardiovasc Surg.* 1996;8(1):83-93.
72. Geddes D, Davies M, Koyama H, et al. Effect of lung-volume-reduction surgery in patients with severe emphysema. *N Engl J Med.* 27 2000;343(4):239-245.
73. Fessler HE, Permutt S. Lung volume reduction surgery and airflow limitation. *Am J Respir Crit Care Med.* 1998;157(3 Pt 1):715-722.
74. Fessler HE, Scharf SM, Permutt S. Improvement in spirometry following lung volume reduction surgery: application of a physiologic model. *Am J Respir Crit Care Med.* 1 2002;165(1):34-40.
75. Szekely LA, Oelberg DA, Wright C, et al. Preoperative predictors of operative morbidity and mortality in COPD patients undergoing bilateral lung volume reduction surgery. *Chest.* 1997;111(3):550-558.
76. Keenan RJ, Landreneau RJ, Sciurba FC, et al. Unilateral thoracoscopic surgical approach for diffuse emphysema. *J Thorac Cardiovasc Surg.* 1996;111(2):308-315; discussion 315-306.
77. O'Brien GM, Furukawa S, Kuzma AM, Cordova F, Criner GJ. Improvements in lung function, exercise, and quality of life in hypercapnic COPD patients after lung volume reduction surgery. *Chest.* 1999;115(1):75-84.
78. Wisser W, Klepetko W, Senbaklavaci O, et al. Chronic hypercapnia should not exclude patients from lung volume reduction surgery. *Eur J Cardiothorac Surg.* 1998;14(2):107-112.
79. Patients at high risk of death after lung-volume-reduction surgery. *N Engl J Med.* 11 2001;345(15):1075-1083.
80. Edwards MA, Hazelrigg S, Naunheim KS. The National Emphysema Treatment Trial: summary and update. *Thorac Surg Clin.* 2009;19(2):169-185.
81. Ries AL, Make BJ, Lee SM, et al. The effects of pulmonary rehabilitation in the national emphysema treatment trial. *Chest.* Dec 2005;128(6):3799-3809.
82. Licker M, Schweizer A, Ellenberger C, Tschopp JM, Diaper J, Clergue F. Perioperative medical management of patients with COPD. *Int J Chron Obstruct Pulmon Dis.* 2007;2(4):493-515.
83. Warner DO. Perioperative abstinence from cigarettes: physiologic and clinical consequences. *Anesthesiology.* 2006;104(2):356-367.

84. Tschernko EM. Anesthesia considerations for lung volume reduction surgery. *Anesthesiol Clin North America*. 2001;19(3):591-609.
85. Niewoehner DE, Erbland ML, Deupree RH, et al. Effect of systemic glucocorticoids on exacerbations of chronic obstructive pulmonary disease. Department of Veterans Affairs Cooperative Study Group. *N Engl J Med*. 24 1999;340(25):1941-1947.
86. Barr RG, Celli BR, Martinez FJ, et al. Physician and patient perceptions in COPD: the COPD Resource Network Needs Assessment Survey. *Am J Med*. 2005;118(12):1415.
87. Hedenstierna G, Edmark L. The effects of anesthesia and muscle paralysis on the respiratory system. *Intensive Care Med*. 2005;31(10):1327-1335.
88. Gunnarsson L, Tokics L, Lundquist H, et al. Chronic obstructive pulmonary disease and anaesthesia: formation of atelectasis and gas exchange impairment. *Eur Respir J*. 1991;4(9):1106-1116.
89. Lohser J. Evidence-based management of one-lung ventilation. *Anesthesiol Clin*. 2008;26(2):241-272, v.
90. Beck DH, Doepfmer UR, Sinemus C, Bloch A, Schenk MR, Kox WJ. Effects of sevoflurane and propofol on pulmonary shunt fraction during one-lung ventilation for thoracic surgery. *Br J Anaesth*. 2001;86(1):38-43.
91. Pilotti L, Torresini G, Crisci R, De Sanctis A, De Sanctis C. Total intravenous anesthesia in thoracotomy with one-lung ventilation. *Minerva Anestesiol*. Jul-1999;65(7-8):483-489.
92. Pruszkowski O, Dalibon N, Moutafis M, et al. Effects of propofol vs sevoflurane on arterial oxygenation during one-lung ventilation. *Br J Anaesth*. 2007;98(4):539-544.
93. Buettner AU, McRae R, Myles PS, et al. Anaesthesia and postoperative pain management for bilateral lung volume reduction surgery. *Anaesth Intensive Care*. 1999;27(5):503-508.
94. Triantafillou AN. Anesthetic management for bilateral volume reduction surgery. *Semin Thorac Cardiovasc Surg*. 1996;8(1):94-98.
95. Bardoczky GI, d'Hollander AA, Cappello M, Yernault JC. Interrupted expiratory flow on automatically constructed flow-volume curves may determine the presence of intrinsic positive end-expiratory pressure during one-lung ventilation. *Anesth Analg*. 1998;86(4):880-884.
96. Keller CA, Naunheim KS. Perioperative management of lung volume reduction patients. *Clin Chest Med*. 1997;18(2):285-300.
97. Slinger PD, Lesiuk L. Flow resistances of disposable double-lumen, single-lumen, and Univent tubes. *J Cardiothorac Vasc Anesth*. 1998;12(2):142-144.
98. Aschkenasy SV, Hofer CK, Zalunardo MP, et al. Patterns of changes in arterial PO2 during one-lung ventilation: a comparison between patients with severe pulmonary emphysema and patients with preserved lung function. *J Cardiothorac Vasc Anesth*. 2005;19(4):479-484.
99. Grichnik KP, Clark JA. Pathophysiology and management of one-lung ventilation. *Thorac Surg Clin*. 2005;15(1):85-103.
100. Bardoczky GI, Szegedi LL, d'Hollander AA, Moures JM, de Francquen P, Yernault JC. Two-lung and one-lung ventilation in patients with chronic obstructive pulmonary disease: the effects of position and F(IO)2. *Anesth Analg*. 2000;90(1):35-41.
101. Fiser WP, Friday CD, Read RC. Changes in arterial oxygenation and pulmonary shunt during thoracotomy with endobronchial anesthesia. *J Thorac Cardiovasc Surg*. 1982;83(4):523-531.
102. Slinger PD, Kruger M, McRae K, Winton T. Relation of the static compliance curve and positive end-expiratory pressure to oxygenation during one-lung ventilation. *Anesthesiology*. 2001;95(5):1096-1102.
103. Slinger PD, Hickey DR. The interaction between applied PEEP and auto-PEEP during one-lung ventilation. *J Cardiothorac Vasc Anesth*. 1998;12(2):133-136.
104. Smith TC, Marini JJ. Impact of PEEP on lung mechanics and work of breathing in severe airflow obstruction. *J Appl Physiol*. Oct 1988;65(4):1488-1499.
105. Nichols D, Haranath S. Pressure control ventilation. *Crit Care Clin*. 2007;23(2):183-199, viii-ix.
106. Block BM, Liu SS, Rowlingson AJ, Cowan AR, Cowan JA, Jr., Wu CL. Efficacy of postoperative epidural analgesia: a meta-analysis. *JAMA*. 2003;290(18):2455-2463.
107. Beattie WS, Badner NH, Choi P. Epidural analgesia reduces postoperative myocardial infarction: a meta-analysis. *Anesth Analg*. 2001;93(4):853-858.
108. Ballantyne JC, Carr DB, deFerranti S, et al. The comparative effects of postoperative analgesic therapies on pulmonary outcome: cumulative meta-analyses of randomized, controlled trials. *Anesth Analg*. 1998;86(3):598-612.

109. Gruber EM, Tschernko EM, Kritzinger M, et al. The effects of thoracic epidural analgesia with bupivacaine 0.25% on ventilatory mechanics in patients with severe chronic obstructive pulmonary disease. *Anesth Analg.* 2001;92(4):1015-1019.
110. Koehler RP, Keenan RJ. Management of postthoracotomy pain: acute and chronic. *Thorac Surg Clin.* 2006;16(3):287-297.
111. Davies RG, Myles PS, Graham JM. A comparison of the analgesic efficacy and side-effects of paravertebral vs epidural blockade for thoracotomy–a systematic review and meta-analysis of randomized trials. *Br J Anaesth.* 2006;96(4):418-426.

Pericardial Window Procedures 16

Hilary P. Grocott
Harleena Gulati
G. Burkhard Mackensen

Key Points

1. Patients presenting for pericardial drainage procedures require a thorough, but often urgent, preoperative evaluation in order to understand the etiology of the effusion and any associated hemodynamic instability, such as tamponade.
2. Echocardiography plays a central role in the diagnosis of effusion and pericardial tamponade and can guide drainage.
3. Thoracoscopic procedures and subxiphoid approaches are the most common techniques for definitive drainage of pericardial effusion. However, ultrasound-guided needle pericardiocentesis can be used for emergent drainage in the unstable patient.
4. The anesthetic technique needs to be tailored to the individual patient characteristics, but can be accomplished successfully with inhalational, as well as intravenous induction techniques. The hemodynamic goals of augmented preload with maintenance of afterload, contractility, and heart rate should be targets.

Case Vignette

The patient is a 37-year-old woman with stage 4 breast cancer who presents with increasing shortness of breath, reduced exercise tolerance and intermittent chest discomfort. She has also complained of worsening headaches for the past few weeks. She has a history of receiving Adriamycin chemotherapy, interrupted for reasons unclear to her, and was healthy before her cancer diagnosis 3 years ago. She has been unable to lie flat for 24 hours and has poor venous access. She has steroid induced diabetes. Medications include lansoprazole, iron and lorazepam at night.

Vital signs: BP 90/40, HR 110, room air SaO_2 89%.

Laboratory examination is notable for: hemoglobin 8.2, WBC 5.8, platelets 164, BUN 40, creatinine 1.4, glucose 145.

Chest wall echocardiogram revealed a large pericardial effusion.

She is listed for a pericardial window procedure via thoracoscopy.

Pericardial window procedures allow the drainage of fluid from the pericardial space and are performed with relative frequency by the cardiothoracic surgical team. In order to provide optimal anesthetic management for such patients, a thorough understanding of the associated pathophysiology and the various etiologies of pericardial effusion is essential.

Pericardial tamponade can occur in numerous acute conditions such as penetrating chest trauma, or present in the decompensated state of various subacute processes such as malignant tumors (Table 16–1). Although pericardial effusions can occur in isolation, they often occur in combination with other clinical conditions such as pleural effusions. This can confuse the clinical picture considerably, as symptoms of dyspnea and orthopnea can be secondary to the pleural effusion and/or other pulmonary involvement. Frequently the therapeutic intervention for pericardial effusion involves concomitant pleural drainage.

The clinical presentation and perioperative management strategy of these patients depend upon the rapidity of fluid accumulation. The variable hemodynamic consequences of excessive pericardial fluid accumulation bring special anesthetic considerations that need to be understood in order to adequately care for these patients.[3]

Table 16–1. Etiology of Pericardial Effusion/Pericarditis

Infectious
- Viral
- Bacterial
- Tuberculosis
- Other

Noninfectious
- Traumatic
  - Penetrating
  - Nonpenetrating
  - Aortic aneurysm (leaking into pericardial sac)
  - Post-cardiac surgery
- Malignancy
  - Primary
  - Metastatic
- Acute myocardial infarction
- Post-myocardial infarction (Dressler syndrome)
- Renal insufficiency/uremia
- Myxedema
- Chylopericardium
- Post irradiation
- Idiopathic

Auto-immune
- Rheumatic fever
- Rheumatoid arthritis
- Systemic lupus erythematosus
- Drug induced (procainamide)

Data adapted from Braunwald[1] and Oakley.[2]

The post-cardiac surgical patient represents a unique group presenting for pericardial drainage. The clinical presentation of tamponade in this patient population must frequently be differentiated from cardiogenic shock, either from global left ventricular failure, or from isolated right ventricular failure. In addition, these patients rarely present with the classic signs and symptoms of cardiac tamponade due to the prior pericardial disruption from the preceding cardiac surgical procedure, as well as the likelihood that the fluid in these postoperative patients is hemorrhagic, often with loculated thrombus. The anesthesiologist needs to be familiar with the incidence and common locations of these effusions, in addition to the echocardiographic features of cardiac tamponade in this patient population.[4-6]

PATHOPHYSIOLOGY OF CARDIAC TAMPONADE

The clinical presentation of pericardial effusion is generally dependent upon both the speed of accumulation and the total volume of the pericardial fluid.[7] Spodick, in a recent extensive review, outlined the relationship between the pericardial stretch induced by the accumulating fluid and the subsequent development of increasing intrapericardial pressure.[8] Figure 16–1 demonstrates

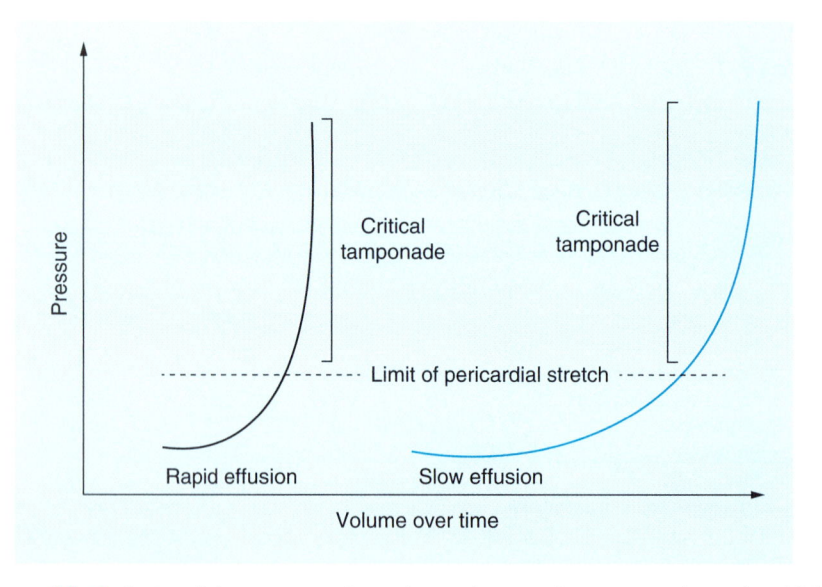

Figure 16–1. Pericardial pressure–volume (or strain–stress) curves are shown in which volume increases slowly or rapidly over time. In the left-hand panel, rapidly increasing pericardial fluid first reaches the limit of the pericardial reserve volume (the initial flat segment) and then quickly exceeds the limit of parietal pericardial stretch, causing a steep rise in pressure, which becomes even steeper as smaller increments in fluid cause a disproportionate increase in the pericardial pressure. In the right-hand panel, a slower rate of pericardial filling takes longer to exceed the limit of pericardial stretch, because there is more time for the pericardium to stretch and for compensatory mechanisms to become activated. (Spodick DH. Acute cardiac tamponade. *N Engl J Med.* 2003;349(7):684-690, with permission. © 2003 Massachusetts Medical Society. All rights reserved.)

the intrapericardial pressure curves in slowly developing effusions versus those that develop more rapidly. These pressure curves represent the impact that an accumulating effusion can exert on diastolic function. In general, cardiac filling is dependent upon the difference between the intracardiac and the intrapericardial pressure; this difference is conventionally defined as the myocardial transmural pressure. As intrapericardial pressure increases, there is a compression of all the cardiac chambers. As the chambers become smaller, the cardiac inflow becomes limited, and with this, there is a corresponding reduction in diastolic compliance. Eventually, there is an equalization of pericardial and cardiac chamber pressures and the myocardial transmural pressure becomes zero (with cessation of both cardiac filling and forward blood flow). The progression to this equalization is dependent upon the relative stretch of the pericardium and the rate of fluid accumulation. This equalization is a dynamic process, fluctuating due to various extracardiac factors such as the influence of pressure changes arising during ventilation.

Ventilation (both spontaneous as well as positive pressure) can have significant consequences on myocardial filling and consequent hemodynamic effects. Respiratory variation in cardiac filling normally occurs due to the influence exerted through the transmission of negative intrathoracic pressure on transmural pressure during spontaneous ventilation.[9,10] During inspiration, transmural pressure and right heart filling transiently increase, at the expense of a shift in the interventricular septum toward the left ventricle. With normal compliance, the pericardial space usually accommodates most of this shift. This accommodation is incomplete, however, and it is normal for a slight fall in systolic pressure to occur during inspiration. Because the right ventricular diastolic volume increases with inspiration, this is transmitted to the left heart after several cardiac cycles, and manifests as an increase in blood pressure following expiration. These two factors combine to produce the minor, yet normal respiratory variation in systolic blood pressure.

The changes in stroke volume (SV) seen during inspiration that manifest as respiratory variation with continuous blood pressure monitoring have also been suggested to be secondary to pleural pressure-induced changes in the capacitance of the pulmonary venous bed. Katz et al concluded that there is a pooling of blood in the pulmonary veins due to the negative pressures occurring during inspiration.[11] Although this may be a contributing factor under normal conditions, others attribute the respiratory-induced changes in stroke volume to the competition of the right heart for the relatively fixed total diastolic volume with the resultant reduction in inspiratory left ventricular filling.[6,7,9,12]

With the development of tamponade, however, and its associated reduction in cardiac chamber compliance, the left heart cannot expand into the constricted pericardial space, resulting in a reduction in forward flow. This results in *pulsus paradoxus*, manifested as a significant reduction in systolic pressure during inspiration. Pulsus paradoxus, defined as an inspiratory systolic arterial pressure reduction more than or equal to 10 mm Hg during spontaneous ventilation, is a hallmark of significant tamponade.[13] The increase and decrease in the arterial pulse volume can often be palpated, but is usually demonstrated by either an invasive arterial pressure monitor or other pulse-contour monitoring device. Concomitant with

Table 16–2. Conditions Where Pulsus Paradoxus May Not Manifest

Aortic insufficiency (severe)
Localized effusion
Severe right ventricular hypertrophy with pulmonary hypertension
Atrial septal defect
Tense ascites
Severe pre-existing arterial hypertension

pulsus paradoxus is either a steady (and often increased) central venous pressure during inspiration.

Although pulsus paradoxus is usually present in the most serious forms of tamponade, it can be notably absent in some (Table 16–2). As a result, when present it is a useful guide to identifying a potentially high-risk patient, but its disparate sensitivity and specificity presents some limitations. Notable absence of pulsus paradoxus, despite significant hemodynamic compromise, can be seen in cases of loculated effusion causing only localized chamber compression (ie, regional pericardial tamponade) that similarly limits filling, independent of respiratory variation. It can also be seen in severe right ventricular hypertrophy (RVH) with pulmonary hypertension, severe preexisting arterial hypertension, atrial septal defects (ASD) and severe aortic insufficiency (AI). Furthermore, the specificity of pulsus paradoxus outside the setting of discreet clinical suspicion has been questioned, as it has also been reported to be present in severe chronic obstructive pulmonary disease (COPD), exacerbations of asthma, obesity, congestive heart failure (CHF) and significant hypovolemia.[3] The differential diagnosis of pulsus paradoxus is outlined in Table 16–3.

DIAGNOSIS OF PERICARDIAL EFFUSION AND TAMPONADE

The clinical signs and symptoms of pericardial tamponade have been well described. However, the general nonspecificity of the clinical presentation leads to the reliance on other diagnostic modalities. The electrocardiogram (EEG) usually demonstrates

Table 16–3. Differential Diagnosis of Pulsus Paradoxus

Pericardial tamponade
Severe chronic obstructive pulmonary disease
Obesity
Congestive heart failure
Asthma
Hypovolemia

tachycardia and may show small voltages, with changes in size due to swinging of the heart within the pericardium (electrical alternans). Auscultation of the heart may reveal muffled heart sounds as well as possible pericardial friction rubs. The finding of a pericardial rub, classically described as being triphasic corresponding to atrial systole, ventricular systole and rapid filling during early diastole, needs to be distinguished from that of a pleural rub, which varies with respiration.[6]

Elevated central venous pressure (CVP) and distension of the jugular veins are frequently seen with tamponade. Although the CVP waveform often demonstrates elevated pressures, it should not be relied upon for diagnosis; as a result, in the acute management of these patients, any delay in therapy should not be undertaken in order to secure central venous access. Though not always reliable, the CVP waveform can be used to differentiate tamponade from constrictive pericarditis: the "square-root" appearance of the waveform is seen in constrictive pericarditis but not with tamponade. The chest x-ray may demonstrate an enlarged cardiac silhouette; the presence of cardiomegaly indicates an effusion of at least 250 mL.[6] Other radiographic studies (such as computerized tomography [CT] and magnetic resonance imaging [MRI]) may also demonstrate pericardial fluid accumulation.

Echocardiography plays a central role in the diagnosis of pericardial effusion.[14-16] Ultrasound evaluation of the heart and surrounding structures adds critical information regarding the intracardiac blood flow velocities, as well as the volume and composition of the pericardial fluid. For example, differentiating circumferential fluid from loculated effusions is particularly important in the post-cardiac surgery patient, as the pericardial space and mediastinum may contain an abundance of loculated thrombus. Normally, there is less than 5 to 10 mL of fluid in the pericardial space, with larger collections being pathologic and easily detected by echocardiography.[17] The amount of pericardial fluid present may be estimated by echocardiography by measuring the distance between the parietal and visceral pericardium (the interpericardial distance). Mild, moderate and large effusions correspond to interpericardial distances of 0.5 cm, 0.5 to 2.0 cm and greater than 2.0 cm respectively.[17] Figure 16–2 demonstrates a circumferential collection of fluid in the pericardial space with Figure 16–3 demonstrating a smaller apical effusion. Localized collections, frequently loculated and thrombotic in nature, can also result in similar hemodynamic sequelae (Figure 16–4). Discriminating between a simple effusion and tamponade depends upon accurate interpretation of both 2-D echocardiographic and Doppler assessments of blood flow.

In addition to direct chamber compression, increases in pericardial pressure can result in collapse of chamber walls during the cardiac cycle. As the right atrium generally has the lowest pressure of the cardiac chambers, it is usually the first to collapse. This is represented by invagination of the right atrial wall during ventricular systole, which represents the period where atrial pressures are lowest.[18] A similar atrial systolic collapse of the left atrium or collapse of the right ventricle during diastole (most notable at the apex) can also occur. In addition to the 2D images which may show variable amounts and distribution of the effusion, Doppler assessments of transmitral flow show characteristic patterns in both the spontaneously breathing and positive pressure ventilation patient.[12,19-21]

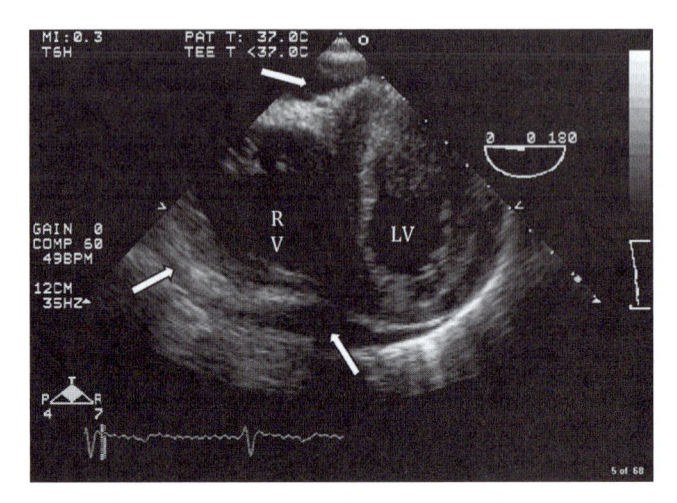

Figure 16–2. A transgastric short-axis transesophageal echocardiographic (TEE) image of a moderately large pericardial effusion. Note the circumferential fluid between the epicardium and the pericardium (arrows). RV = right ventricle; LV = left ventricle.

Quantitative assessment of the transvalvular (ie, tricuspid and mitral) Doppler flow characteristics and its variation with respirations is central to the echocardiographic diagnosis of pericardial tamponade (Figure 16–5).[9] In normal patients, early diastolic filling velocity (E wave) across the tricuspid and pulmonary valves usually increases slightly with inspiration. Correspondingly, early diastolic inflow velocities across the mitral and aortic valves decrease slightly. In patients with

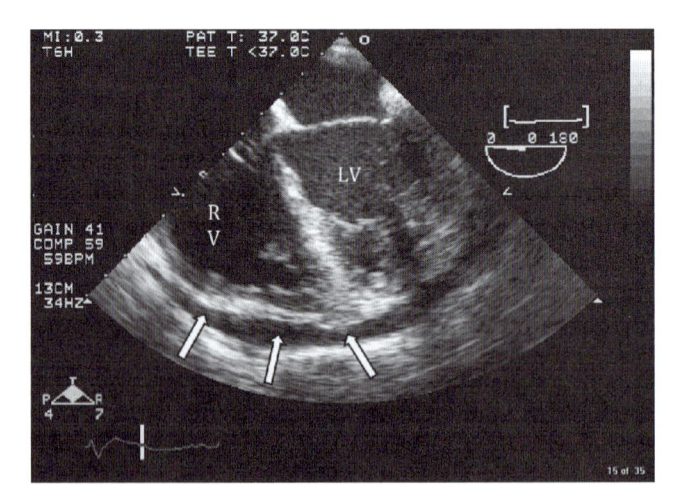

Figure 16–3. A transesophageal echocardiographic (TEE) 4-chamber view of small effusion near the apex of the heart (arrows). RV = right ventricle; LV = left ventricle. (With kind permission from Springer Science+Business Media: Grocott et al[27].)

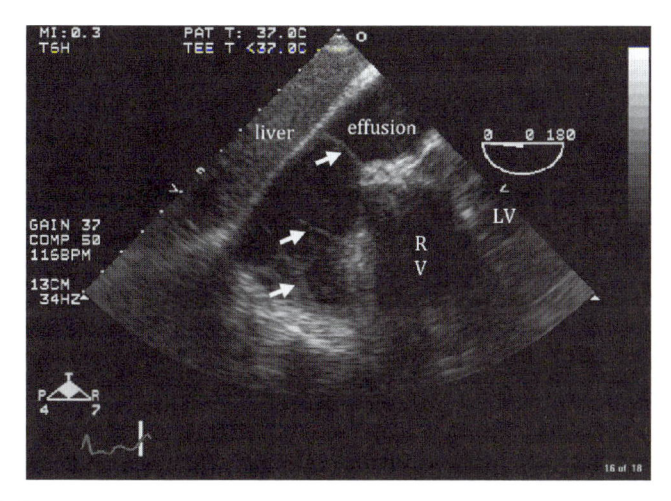

Figure 16–4. A transgastric short-axis transesophageal echocardiographic (TEE) image of a large effusion in a patient 2 weeks following cardiac surgery. Note the fibrinous loculations (arrows) between the pericardial and epicardial surfaces.

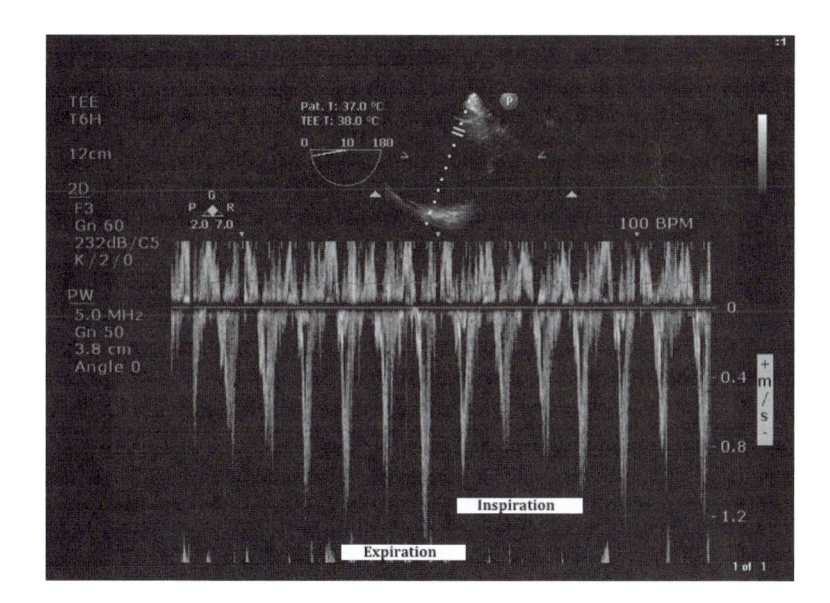

Figure 16–5. A Doppler tracing obtained using transesophageal echocardiography (TEE) of the transmitral flow in spontaneously breathing patients with pericardial tamponade. Note the reduction in velocities that occur during inspiration, highlighting the echocardiographic correlate of pulsus paradoxus. (With kind permission from Springer Science+Business Media: Grocott et al[27].)

tamponade, early filling (E wave) velocities across the tricuspid (and pulmonary) valve increase sharply (up to 80%) while the mitral and aortic velocities decrease. The reduction in transmitral early filling velocity ranges from 25% to 35%.[14,22] The changes in transvalvular flows, and the physiologic reasons behind them, are akin to the blood pressure changes defined by pulsus paradoxus. That is, with spontaneous inspiration, the trans-tricuspid flow increases consequent with the increased venous return due to the negative intrathoracic pressure. The corresponding decreases in stroke volume (accentuated with tamponade) are due to the leftward shift of the interventricular septum, as well as due to the pooling of blood in the pulmonary venous bed.

SURGICAL MANAGEMENT

Numerous approaches have been described to diagnose and treat pericardial effusions. These include needle pericardiocentesis, percutaneous catheter drainage and balloon pericardiotomy, pericardioperitoneal shunt, subxiphoid pericardial window, and pericardial window through either anterolateral thoracotomy or thoracoscopy.[23] Needle pericardiocentesis, best performed with ultrasound guidance, can be used to obtain fluid for diagnostic purposes, and depending on the etiology, definitive drainage. The optimal drainage procedure for non-constrictive effusions is not clear, and varies according to operator preference and familiarity. Choice of drainage procedures is partly dependent on the etiology of the effusion as well as the clinical condition of the patient. Constrictive pericarditis is best treated with pericardiectomy through a sternotomy in order to allow a more thorough removal of a large portion of the diseased pericardium.

The most common surgical approaches involve either subxiphoid access to the pericardial space or a direct intrathoracic technique via either thoracotomy or video-assisted thoracoscopy (VATS). Compared with the subxiphoid window, the advantage of the thoracotomy or a VATS approach is that it allows the fashioning of a pleuropericardial window for continued drainage from the pericardial space into the adjoining pleural space.[24,25] Whereas this may not always address the primary reason for the fluid collection itself, it does prevent the development of an ongoing pericardial effusion and decreases the risk of recurrent tamponade. Any subsequent pleural accumulation, if significant, can be managed via subsequent tube thoracostomy.

ANESTHETIC CONSIDERATIONS

The acuity of presentation, the patient's signs and symptoms, as well as the planned surgical approach are all important considerations when determining the anesthetic management strategy for the patient with pericardial effusion. Most importantly, the perioperative management of the patient with pericardial effusion/tamponade requires a multidisciplinary approach that is based on clear communication amongst the entire operative team.

The preoperative assessment, intraoperative management and immediate postoperative period all require careful consideration. Preoperative assessment of the patient should begin with a focused history and physical examination in order to elicit the etiology of the pericardial effusion (and any concomitant conditions) as well as the severity of the hemodynamic compromise. Although ideally a thorough and complete preoperative evaluation should be undertaken, the time required to do this must be balanced by the overall condition of the patient. Frequently, there is limited time for an extensive evaluation as the urgency of the situation often dictates rapid intervention. An evaluation for the presence of tamponade should be foremost as the preoperative evaluation proceeds. Key symptoms to identify and explore include tachypnea, dyspnea, orthopnea, lightheadedness, and chest pain/pressure. Physical examination should include an evaluation of vital signs and an assessment of any respiratory compromise, including the presence of decreased oxygen saturation and adequacy of air entry on chest auscultation. Tachycardia, hypotension, pulsus paradoxus, and jugular venous distension should be identified, with cardiac auscultation focusing on the presence of any pericardial rubs or muffling of the heart sounds. A brief anesthetic history, list of current medications and any allergies should also be noted.

The extent of preoperative investigations is dependent on the stability of the patient and the urgency of surgery. Laboratory investigations should focus on hematologic (hemoglobin and platelet count), coagulation (INR, aPTT), and biochemical analysis (particularly electrolytes and creatinine level to assess renal function). If conditions allow, a chest x-ray, CT scan or MRI can all be useful, however, an echocardiogram can be essential in confirming the correct diagnosis of pericardial effusion and tamponade.

Pre-induction invasive arterial blood pressure monitoring is essential. Although useful, central venous access is clearly optional and its establishment should not delay urgent pericardial decompression in severely compromised patients. Preparation for induction should include the availability of adequate fluids for resuscitation as well as ready access to vasopressors (such as phenylephrine or norepinephrine boluses and infusions) and inotropic agents (particularly epinephrine).

Several anesthetic approaches can be utilized for patients presenting for a drainage procedure.[3,26,27] Figure 16–6 summarizes the various anesthetic management strategies that can be considered. The patient that presents with significant symptoms and signs of compromise (such as dyspnea in the recumbent position, or overt pulsus paradoxus) needs to be managed with extreme caution. If hemodynamic collapse is imminent, a percutaneous approach to relieve the immediate compromise is warranted, followed by subsequent definitive treatment. On the other hand, the asymptomatic patient who demonstrates no hemodynamic consequence can be managed more conventionally and with considerably more preparation and time. However, a vast number of patients lay between these two clinical extremes.

Local anesthesia, with supplemental sedation (for example with ketamine, which allows the maintenance spontaneous ventilation), may be used for needle pericardiocentesis or subxiphoid windows procedures. Otherwise, general anesthesia is required, usually with concomitant endotracheal intubation. For patients requiring general anesthesia, attention should be paid to maintaining—and usually augmenting—preload, along with the maintenance of afterload, contractility, and heart rate (optimally in sinus rhythm).

```
                      Pericardial Effusion
                              │
                              ▼
                                        Yes
                      Cardiogenic shock ─────▶ Cooperative patient
                                                      │
                                                      │ Yes
                                                      ▼
                              No              Needle pericardiocentesis
                                                      │
                                                      ▼
                                              Is more definitive        No
                                              drainage required? ──────────┐
                              ▼                       │                    │
                      Pulsus paradoxus/evidence       │ Yes                │
                      of tamponade         ◀─────────┘                    │
                         │                                                │
                 Yes ────┴──── No*                                        │
                  │            │                                          │
                  ▼            ▼                                          │
         Suitable for       Conventional i.v. induction                   │
         inhalational induction?                                          │
           │                                                              │
      Yes ─┴─ No                                                          │
       │      │                                                           │
       ▼      ▼                                                           │
  Is positive pressure    i.v. induction                                  │
  ventilation             • after prepping and draping for                │
  hemodynamically           emergency open drainage                       │
  tolerated after         • ± vasoactive therapy                          │
  intubation?             • preparations made for possible                │
                            resuscitation           ◀─────────────────────┘
      │   No
  Yes │────┐
      ▼    ▼
  Continue positive     Continue spontaneous
  pressure ventilation  ventilation ± vasoactive therapy
  ± paralytic agent
```

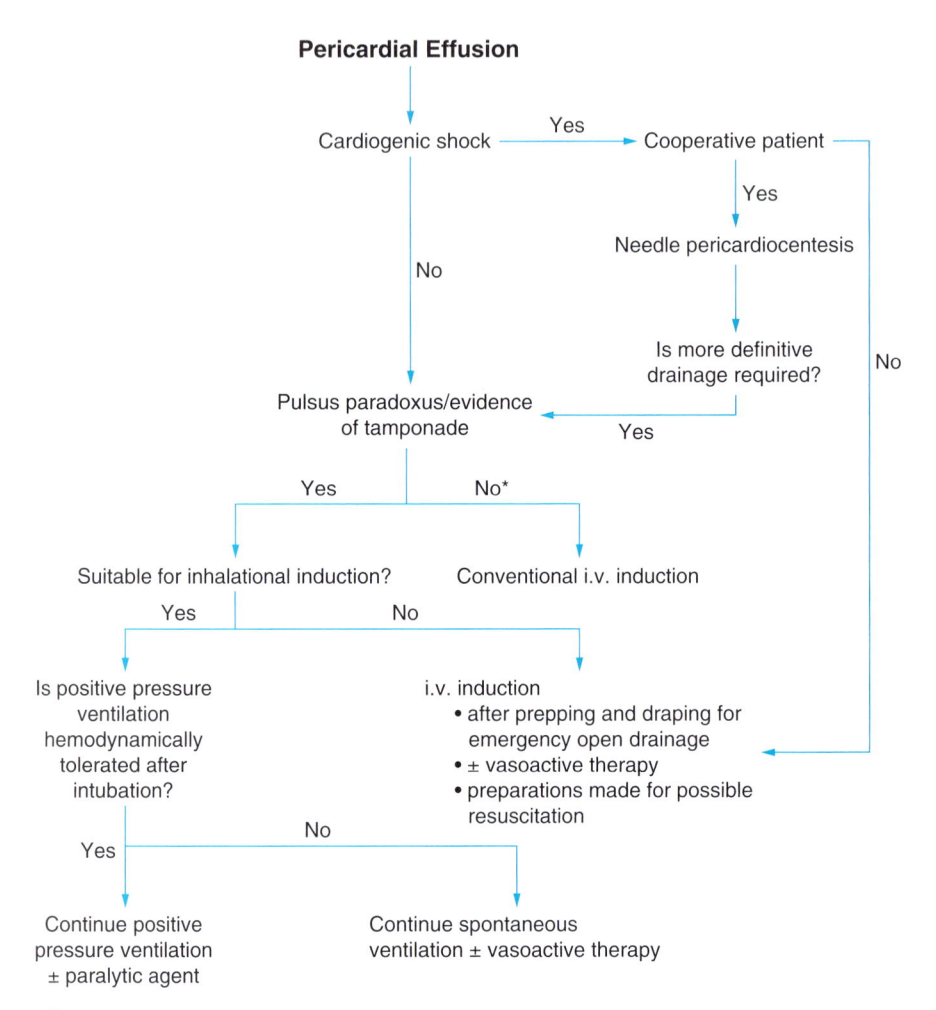

Figure 16-6. Management strategies for patients with varying severity of pericardial effusion/tamponade. *Conditions that might preclude inhalational induction include significant aspiration risk, severe orthopnea, or an uncooperative patient. (With kind permission from Springer Science+Business Media: Grocott et al[27].)

Considerable attention needs to be directed to airway and ventilatory management. Positive pressure ventilation should be avoided when possible, and if and when it is required, it should be instituted cautiously with only the minimal inspiratory pressure required to provide adequate minute ventilation. The combination of positive pressure ventilation, which decreases venous return, as well as the vasodilation and direct myocardial depression caused by the anesthetic agents can result in life-threatening hypotension. When conditions allow, an inhalational induction technique is ideal and should aim to minimize coughing and straining while maintaining spontaneous ventilation; the use of sevoflurane therefore offers many advantages.

Premedication with any agents that can depress respiration should be avoided, as these can prolong induction by reducing minute ventilation. Care should be taken to ensure a deep level of anesthesia before any manipulation of the airway is attempted. Invariably, hypotension from vasodilation occurs and can be treated with a continuous vasopressor infusion as the inhalational induction continues.

Intravenous (IV) induction of anesthesia can be safely accomplished in patients with pericardial effusion who are hemodynamically stable without evidence of tamponade. However, consideration should be given to positioning the patient to allow for surgical preparation and draping, so that the operation can proceed expeditiously once the patient is anesthetized and the airway secured if the hemodynamics deteriorate during induction. This preparation for immediate surgical intervention can also be prudent during inhalational induction, with careful attention not to provide any noxious stimuli to the patient during induction that may lead to coughing and/or apnea.

Once the airway is instrumented, the choice of endotracheal tube is partly dependent upon the surgical technique utilized. Subxiphoid approaches can be accomplished without the need for lung isolation and one-lung ventilation (OLV). However, OLV is usually required for some thoracotomy and VATS approaches. This can be achieved with a double lumen tube, or with a single-lumen endotracheal tube in conjunction with an endobronchial blocker.[28] One of the limitations of thoracoscopy is the difficulty in tolerating OLV encountered occasionally. In this population, the subxiphoid approach may be a better operative choice.

Maintenance of anesthesia can be accomplished with various combinations of inhalational agents, intravenous opioids, propofol, and benzodiazepines. The possibility of a breach of the pleural space, as well as the possibility of preoperative hypoxemia, should preclude the use of nitrous oxide. Muscle relaxants may be utilized if necessary, but ideally only when the patient has been demonstrated able to tolerate positive pressure ventilation. Continuous intravenous infusions of vasopressor or inotropic agents may be required to maintain hemodynamic stability, but should be considered temporizing measures that have their own adverse consequences due to excessive vasoconstriction that may limit overall cardiac output.

Long acting opioids (ie, morphine or hydromorphone) can be given prior to emergence of anesthesia for postoperative analgesia. In addition, consideration should be given to either local anesthetic infiltration of the wound or the performance of regional nerve blocks (ie, intercostal blocks) by the surgeon or anesthesiologist. The decision to extubate at the conclusion of the procedure should depend on the patient's cardiovascular and respiratory status. Similarly, the need for intensive postoperative monitoring is dependent upon the overall status of the patient. Patients may require a period of continuous monitoring in a post anesthesia care unit (PACU) or an intensive care unit (ICU) setting.

SUMMARY

In summary, patients presenting for pericardial drainage procedures require a thorough, but often urgent, preoperative evaluation in order to understand the etiology of the effusion and any associated hemodynamic instability, such as tamponade.

Thoracoscopic procedures and subxiphoid approaches are the most common techniques for definitive drainage of pericardial effusion. However, ultrasound-guided needle pericardiocentesis can be used for emergent drainage in the unstable patient.

The anesthetic technique needs to be tailored to the individual patient characteristics, but can be accomplished successfully with inhalational, as well as intravenous induction techniques. The hemodynamic goals of augmented preload with maintenance of afterload, contractility, and heart rate should be targets.

REFERENCES

1. Braunwald E. *Harrison's Principles of Internal Medicine*. 17th ed. New York: McGraw Hill; 2008:1489.
2. Oakley CM. Myocarditis, pericarditis and other pericardial diseases. *Heart*. 2000;84(4):449-454.
3. Kaplan JA, Bland JW, Jr, Dunbar RW. The perioperative management of pericardial tamponade. *South Med J*. 1976;69(4):417-419.
4. Bommer WJ, Follette D, Pollock M, Arena F, Bognar M, Berkoff H. Tamponade in patients undergoing cardiac surgery: a clinical echocardiographic diagnosis. *Am Heart J*. 1995;130(6):1216-1223.
5. Pepi M, Muratori M, Barbier P, et al. Pericardial effusion after cardiac surgery: incidence, site, size, and haemodynamic consequences. *Br Heart J*. 1994;72(4):327-331.
6. Lange RA, Hillis LD. Clinical practice. Acute pericarditis. *N Engl J Med*. 2004;351(21):2195-2202.
7. Spodick DH. Acute cardiac tamponade. Pathologic physiology, diagnosis and management. *Prog Cardiovasc Dis*. 1967;10(1):64-96.
8. Spodick DH. Acute cardiac tamponade. *N Engl J Med*. 2003;349(7):684-690.
9. Guntheroth WG, Morgan BC, Mullins GL. Effect of respiration on venous return and stroke volume in cardiac tamponade. Mechanism of pulsus paradoxus. *Circ Res*. 1967;20(4):381-390.
10. Morgan BC, Guntheroth WG, Dillard DH. Relationship of pericardial to pleural pressure during quiet respiration and cardiac tamponade. *Circ Res*. 1965;16:493-498.
11. Katz L, Gauchat H. Observations in pulsus paradoxus (with special reference to pericardial effusions) II. Experimental. *Arch Intern Med*. 1924;33:371-393.
12. Reydel B, Spodick DH. Frequency and significance of chamber collapses during cardiac tamponade. *Am Heart J*. 1990;119(5):1160-1163.
13. Shabetai R, Fowler NO, Fenton JC, Masangkay M. Pulsus paradoxus. *J Clin Invest*. 1965;44(11):1882-1898.
14. D'Cruz II, Rehman AU, Hancock HL. Quantitative echocardiographic assessment in pericardial disease. *Echocardiography*. 1997;14(2):207-214.
15. Feigenbaum H, Waldhausen JA, Hyde LP. Ultrasound diagnosis of pericardial effusion. *JAMA*. 1965;191:711-714.
16. Feigenbaum H, Zaky A, Grabhorn LL. Cardiac motion in patients with pericardial effusion. A study using reflected ultrasound. *Circulation*. 1966;34(4):611-619.
17. Whittington J, Borrow L, Skubas N, Fontes M. Pericardial diseases. *Clinical Manual of TEE*. McGraw-Hill; 2005:253-265.
18. Durand M, Lamarche Y, Denault A. Pericardial tamponade. *Can J Anaesth*. 2009;56(6):443-448.
19. Gillam LD, Guyer DE, Gibson TC, King ME, Marshall JE, Weyman AE. Hydrodynamic compression of the right atrium: a new echocardiographic sign of cardiac tamponade. *Circulation*. 1983;68(2):294-301.
20. Kronzon I, Cohen ML, Winer HE. Diastolic atrial compression: a sensitive echocardiographic sign of cardiac tamponade. *J Am Coll Cardiol*. 1983;2(4):770-775.
21. Singh S, Wann LS, Schuchard GH, et al. Right ventricular and right atrial collapse in patients with cardiac tamponade—a combined echocardiographic and hemodynamic study. *Circulation*. 1984;70(6):966-971.

22. Faehnrich JA, Noone RB, Jr, White WD, et al. Effects of positive-pressure ventilation, pericardial effusion, and cardiac tamponade on respiratory variation in transmitral flow velocities. *J Cardiothorac Vasc Anesth.* 2003;17(1):45-50.
23. Moores DW, Dziuban SW, Jr. Pericardial drainage procedures. *Chest Surg Clin N Am.* 1995;5(2):359-373.
24. Georghiou GP, Stamler A, Sharoni E, et al. Video-assisted thoracoscopic pericardial window for diagnosis and management of pericardial effusions. *Ann Thorac Surg.* 2005;80(2):607-610.
25. O'Brien PK, Kucharczuk JC, Marshall MB, et al. Comparative study of subxiphoid versus video-thoracoscopic pericardial "window." *Ann Thorac Surg.* 2005;80(6):2013-2019.
26. Stanley TH, Weidauer HE. Anesthesia for the patient with cardiac tamponade. *Anesth Analg.* 1973;52(1):110-114.
27. Grocott HP, Gulati H, Srinathan S, Mackensen GB. Anesthesia and the patient with pericardial disease. *Can J Anesth.* 2011;58(10):952-966.
28. Grocott HP, Scales G, Schinderle D, King K. A new technique for lung isolation in acute thoracic trauma. *J Trauma.* 2000;49(5):940-942.

Esophageal Cancer Operations

17

Mark F. Berry
Rebecca A. Schroeder

Key Points

1. Esophagectomy is associated with considerable morbidity and mortality despite improvements in surgical technique and perioperative care.
2. The optimal technique in a particular patient depends on specific patient characteristics as well as surgeon- and center-specific experience and preference more than tumor morphology or staging.
3. Multimodal anesthetic management utilizing thoracic epidural analgesia, protective ventilation, prevention of tracheal aspiration, and judicious fluid management helps reduce postoperative morbidity, particularly pulmonary complications and anastomotic leakage.

Case Vignette

A 65-year-old male patient who presents with advanced Barrett esophagus is scheduled to undergo an esophagectomy. He has a long standing history of gastroesophageal reflux, a 20 pack-year history of smoking and consumes 2 to 4 drinks per night.

His only medication is omeprazole.

Vital signs: BP 140/80, HR 80, RA SpO_2 94%.

Laboratory examination is notable only for marginally elevated AST and ALT.
An exercise-stress echocardiogram was normal.

Esophageal cancer is the most common indication for esophagectomy. The incidence of esophageal cancer is increasing and the epidemiology is changing such that adenocarcinoma, which is linked to obesity and gastroesophageal reflux disease, is now more common than squamous cell carcinoma. Mortality following esophagectomy has decreased but still exceeds that of most surgical procedures and long-term survival remains poor. Consequently, it is of critical importance to minimize perioperative morbidity in any manner possible. Esophageal resection can be performed via several different techniques, with the most appropriate technique for any specific individual patient being dependent on both patient and surgeon factors.

ESOPHAGEAL CANCER

Epidemiology

With less than 14,000 new cases annually in the United States, esophageal cancer is relatively uncommon. However, its incidence is steadily increasing and its epidemiology is changing significantly.[1-3] Recent evidence indicates that the incidence among white males has almost doubled while the incidence among blacks has decreased by almost 50%.[1]

Esophageal cancers are differentiated by histologic type and location, but also have many features in common. More than 90% of esophageal cancers in the United States are either adenocarcinomas (57%) or squamous cell carcinomas (37%).[1,3] The distribution of tumor types varies according to race: 64% cases in whites are adenocarcinomas, while among the black population, 82% are of squamous cell origin.[1] Tobacco use and a history of mediastinal radiation are risk factors for both tumor types. Other risk factors for adenocarcinoma include gastroesophageal reflux disease (GERD), obesity, and Barrett esophagus. Barrett esophagus with high-grade dysplasia is considered a premalignant condition as 50% are found to harbor occult malignant disease at the time of biopsy.[4] Additional risk factors for squamous cell carcinoma are conditions that cause chronic esophageal irritation and inflammation such as alcohol abuse, achalasia, esophageal diverticuli, and frequent consumption of extremely hot beverages.[2] Tumor location also distinguishes these two common cell types. Approximately three quarters of all adenocarcinomas are found in the distal esophagus, whereas squamous-cell carcinomas are more evenly distributed throughout the distal two-thirds.[2] Survival rates are similar for patients with either adenocarcinoma or squamous cell carcinoma regardless of treatment modality, suggesting that both cell types share significant physiologic and cellular features.[5] Overall 5-year survival for patients with esophageal cancer remains poor, although some improvement has been achieved with an increase from 5% to 17% over the last four decades.[1]

Clinical Presentation and Workup

The most common presenting symptoms of esophageal cancer are dysphagia (74%) and weight loss (57%) with less common symptoms being heartburn, odynophagia, shortness of breath, chronic cough, hoarseness, and hematemesis.[6] The physical examination is usually unremarkable.[2] A contrast study of the upper gastrointestinal (GI) tract is usually the initial diagnostic study and typically shows a stricture or ulceration when malignancy is present. Upper GI endoscopy is usually part of the initial workup and often shows a friable, ulcerated mass, which is then biopsied for pathologic examination. A computed tomographic (CT) scan of the chest, abdomen, and pelvis with intravenous contrast should be obtained when esophageal cancer is detected to evaluate for distant metastatic disease. Positron-emission tomography

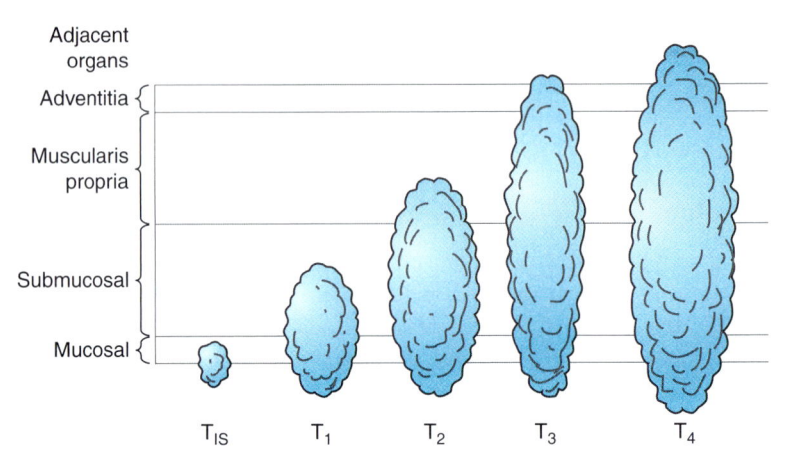

Figure 17–1. Definition of T stage for esophageal cancer.

scans improve staging and will detect previously unsuspected metastatic disease in up to 15% of patients.[7] The extent of loco-regional disease is defined by the depth of tumor invasion and the extent of lymph-node involvement, and may be evaluated with endoscopic ultrasound.[2]

STAGING AND PROGNOSIS

Staging of esophageal cancer has been defined by the American Joint Committee on Cancer Staging System, 6th edition. This system establishes tumor-node-metastasis (TNM) subclassifications in which the primary tumor (T) is defined by depth of invasion (Figure 17–1), lymph node involvement (N) is defined as present or absent, and extent of metastatic disease (M) is noted as none, regional or distant. The current system is described in Tables 17–1A and 17–1B.[8] The likelihood of nodal metastases is almost zero in TIS lesions, but increases with increasing depth of invasion and as many as 50% patients with T1 lesions will have lymph node

Table 17–1A. Esophageal Cancer Staging: Definitions

TIS: in-situ	N0: negative regional nodes	M0: no distant metastases
T1: lamina propria or submucosal invasion	N1: positive regional nodes	M1a: metastases to cervical or celiac nodes
T2: muscularis propria invasion		M1b: other distant metastases
T3: adventitia invasion		
T4: invasion of adjacent tissue		

Data from Greene FL, Page DL, Fleming ID, April F.[8]

Table 17–1B. Esophageal Cancer Staging: Classification System

Stage	Tumor (T)	Node (N)	Metastasis (M)
0	Tis	N0	M0
I	T1	N0	M0
IIA	T2-3	N0	M0
IIB	T1-2	N1	M0
III	T3	N1	M0
	T4	N0-1	M0
IVA	any T	any N	M1a
IVB	any T	any N	M1b

Data from Greene FL, Page DL, Fleming ID, April F.[8]

involvement.[9,10] At the time of diagnosis, approximately 50% of patients have evidence of distant metastatic disease.[1,2]

Survival is related to the stage at diagnosis and subsequent treatment. Current short- and long-term survival rates are listed in Table 17–2.[1,2] In general, patients who undergo complete resection of their cancer have a 5-year disease-free survival of 32%, while for patients with residual disease following surgical resection, overall survival is less than 5%.[11]

Treatment Options

Choice of treatment for esophageal cancer depends heavily on stage and tumor location. However, as outcomes remain poor with all strategies, most remain somewhat controversial and an area of active research.[12] Treatment options include local mucosal therapies, esophagectomy, chemotherapy, and radiation therapy.

Table 17–2. Surgical Treatment of Esophageal Cancer and Long-Term Outcomes

Stage	Surgical Recommendation	Overall 5-Year Survival (in %)
0 I	proceed to surgery (except T3)	37.0
IIA IIB III IVA	induction therapy followed by surgery (except T4)	18.5
IVB	palliative care, possible radiation or chemotherapy	3.0

Data from Horner M, Ries L, Krapcho M, et al.[1] and Enzinger PC, Mayer RJ.[2]

Mucosal treatments such as endoscopic mucosal resection, photodynamic therapy, or radiofrequency ablation are considered for patients with carcinoma *in situ* or high-grade dysplasia but are not appropriate for patients with stage-T1 (or greater) disease due to the likelihood of lymph node involvement. For patients with stage I-III disease who receive surgical treatment, 5-year survival is 28%, compared to 10% for those treated medically.[13] Therefore, primary nonsurgical treatment should be reserved for those who refuse surgery, have unresectable tumors, or are not thought to be surgical candidates for other reasons. Patients with distant metastatic disease (M1b) generally receive palliative treatment with chemotherapy and possibly radiation. To summarize, esophagectomy with chemotherapy and radiation therapy as possible adjuncts should be considered for all patients other than those who are stage T0 or IVb.

Most patients with T1-2 (stage I-II) esophageal cancer without lymph node involvement undergo surgery without other preoperative treatment.[14] Patients with T3, N1, and M1a (stage III or IVa) disease who are resection candidates are considered for induction therapy and then surgery. Use of either induction chemotherapy or radiation alone followed by surgery does not improve survival compared with surgery alone.[11,15,16] However, patients who receive induction chemotherapy *and* radiation therapy followed by surgery may have a modest survival advantage compared with surgery alone.[12,17-20] Postoperative radiation alone may reduce the incidence of local recurrence in those patients who have residual tumor after resection but is not beneficial in the absence of residual disease.[2,21,22] Postoperative chemotherapy has not been shown to have an additive effect on survival compared with surgery alone, although additional therapy may be warranted in patients who have a high likelihood of metastatic disease based on a large number of tumor positive nodes.[23]

Techniques of Esophagectomy

Resection of the esophagus for malignancy is a very complex procedure. The esophagus traverses three body regions or cavities and the anatomy of the esophagus in the posterior mediastinum is such that its accessibility is very different at different positions in the chest. In addition, an appropriate conduit must be prepared in order to reestablish gastrointestinal continuity, and this conduit must be placed in a location such that its blood supply will remain viable. Esophageal resection generally requires access to at least two body cavities, and often requires at least two incisions and patient repositioning intraoperatively. Structures at significant risk include the spleen, trachea, and main stem bronchi as well as major vascular structures in the chest.

The most common surgical techniques used for esophagectomy are listed in Table 17–3. Minimally invasive techniques with either laparoscopy and/or thoracoscopy have been reported for most approaches (except the left thoracoabdominal approach). The final approach chosen for a particular patient depends on surgical experience and preference, institutional tradition and patient characteristics. Relevant factors include stage of disease, associated lesions such as Barrett esophagus or achalasia, other medical comorbidities, pulmonary function, and previous surgical history. In general,

Table 17-3. Characteristics of the Different Esophagogastrectomy Procedures

Procedure	Position	Order of Operation	Location of Anastomosis	One-Lung Ventilation
Three-Incision	1) left lateral 2) supine	1) right thoracic 2) abdominal with left cervical	left cervical	Yes
Transhiatal	supine	abdominal with left cervical	left cervical	No
Ivor-Lewis	1) supine 2) left lateral	1) abdominal 2) right thoracic	right chest	Yes
Left Thoracoabdominal	supine with chest bumped 45°	left thoracoabdominal	left chest	Yes

a proximal and distal disease-free margin of at least 5 cm should be achieved; thus, the location of the tumor is a critical factor in determining the surgical approach.[12,24] Also, as the total number of lymph nodes involved and removed is an important predictor of survival, the transthoracic approaches may be preferred over others that do not provide equivalent access to the relevant nodes.[23,25-27]

Surgeons overwhelmingly choose to use the stomach as the final conduit and the majority of these patients have good or excellent functional results.[28] On the other hand, the colon may be the conduit of choice if the patient has had prior gastric surgery or another disqualifying condition such as diabetic gastroparesis. Its use carries similar morbidity and mortality and provides good long-term eating capability.[29,30]

The optimal location for the esophageal anastomosis after resection (cervical versus intrathoracic) is controversial, although almost 60% are placed in the cervical region.[28] The advantages of a cervical anastomosis include better access for a wider primary esophageal resection, avoidance of highly morbid thoracotomy incisions, and less severe postoperative symptoms of reflux.[12,31] Conversely, advantages of an intrathoracic anastomosis include a lower incidence of anastomotic leak and injury to the recurrent laryngeal nerves as well as a lower risk of postoperative stricture formation.[12,31,32] In the current era, mortality associated with cervical and intrathoracic leaks is similar, although intrathoracic leaks are more likely to require surgical intervention.[12,31,33,34]

Specifics for each surgical technique are described below with advantages and disadvantages listed in Table 17–4. In general, all patients undergo preoperative upper endoscopy to confirm tumor location prior to resection; patients with tumors in the mid-esophagus should have bronchoscopy to rule out airway involvement. A nasogastric (NG) tube should be placed prior to the start of the procedure to assist with esophageal mobilization and is manipulated during the procedure as requested and guided by the surgical team. Also, a jejunostomy feeding tube is

Table 17–4. Advantages and Disadvantages of Specific Esophagogastrectomy Procedures

	Advantages	Disadvantages
Three-Incision (Modified McKeown)	all tumors good nodal access maximal margins ↓ GERD minimally invasive approach possible access to thoracic duct no thoracic anastomosis	thoracic incision ↑ risk pulmonary complications requires intraoperative repositioning ↑ risk of RLN injury
Transhiatal	no thoracic incision no thoracic anastomosis maximal margins possible ↓ risk of GERD	poor access to nodes blunt thoracic dissection ↑ risk RLN injury risk of hemorrhage, dysrhythmia, tracheal injury, hemodynamic instability
Ivor-Lewis	good access to nodes ↓ RLN injury access to thoracic duct possibly no cervical incision	thoracic anastomosis thoracic incision not good for tumors in proximal third of esophagus
Thoracoabdominal		only for tumors beyond 30–35 cm very large incision ↑ rate of residual + margins ↑ risk of GERD due to low thoracic location of anastomosis

RLN = recurrent laryngeal nerve, GERD = gastroesophageal reflux disease

placed at the end of the procedure, as there is often a delay in the return of normal eating during the postoperative period.

THREE-INCISION ESOPHAGECTOMY (MCKEOWN)

The three-incision esophagectomy or modified McKeown approach combines left cervical, right thoracic, and abdominal incisions (Figure 17–2A). This approach is especially useful for tumors of the mid and upper esophagus and for tumors where a long Barrett segment is present. The patient is initially positioned in the left lateral decubitus position for a right thoracotomy or thoracoscopy. One-lung ventilation (OLV) is instituted for the thoracic portion of the case. The esophagus is mobilized from the thoracic inlet to the esophageal hiatus and a lymph node dissection performed. Azygous vein and recurrent laryngeal nerve injury are significant risks during this portion of the procedure. The thoracic incisions are closed after placement of a chest tube and the patient is repositioned in the supine position with a roll under the scapula to extend the neck, and the head turned to the right to maximally expose

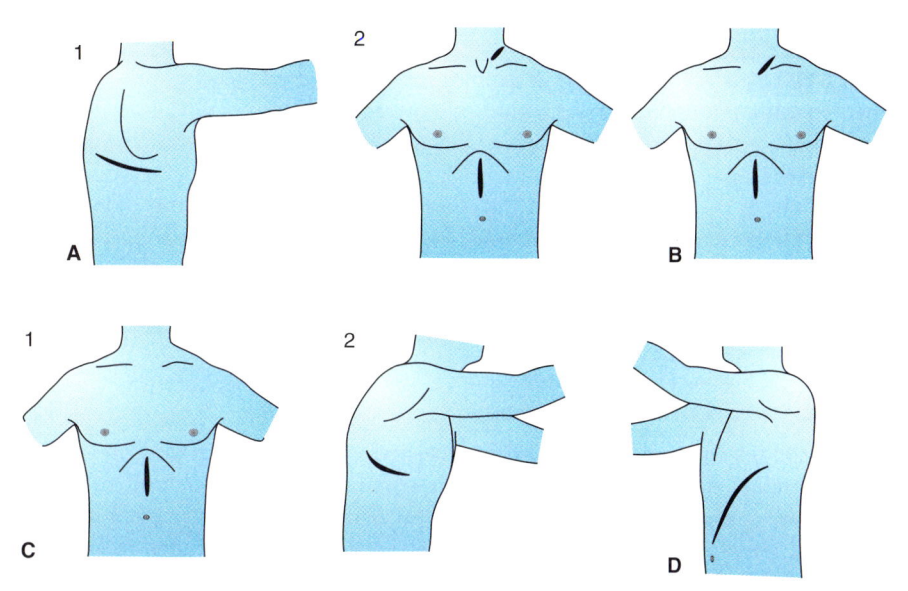

Figure 17–2. Incisions used for esophagectomy. **A.** Three-Incision; **B.** Transhiatal; **C.** Ivor-Lewis; **D.** Left Thoracoabdominal.

the left neck. An upper midline laparotomy or laparoscopy is then performed and the esophageal hiatus is mobilized.

The third and final incision, a left cervical incision, is then made and the cervical esophagus is dissected free in the neck. The recurrent laryngeal nerve is again at significant risk at this point. The nasogastric tube is partially withdrawn and the cervical esophagus is divided. A suture or a rubber drain is fastened to the distal end of the divided esophagus and the distal esophagus is withdrawn through the esophageal hiatus into the abdominal incision. The prepared gastric conduit is then pulled back through the hiatus and up into the neck with care to avoid torsion. The cervical anastomosis is then performed and the NG tube is guided through the anastomosis under direct supervision by the surgical team.

TRANSHIATAL ESOPHAGECTOMY

The transhiatal esophagectomy combines left cervical and abdominal incisions. (Figure 17–2B) This approach is probably ideal for patients with Barrett and high-grade dysplasia where lymph node dissection is not as critical for staging purposes. The abdominal portion of this procedure is performed as described above for the three-incision technique. The hiatus is dilated, and the surgeon's hand is inserted into the mediastinum to bluntly dissect the esophagus free from other intrathoracic structures. A cervical incision is then made, and the esophagus is dissected in a similar manner from the neck into the chest but with special care to avoid injury to the recurrent laryngeal nerve. After complete esophageal mobilization, the esophagus is divided and the anastomosis is performed in the neck as described above for the three-incision technique.

Ivor-Lewis Esophagectomy

The Ivor-Lewis esophagectomy resembles the modified McKeown approach, but involves only two incisions: right thoracic and upper abdominal. (Figure 17–2C) Although it also requires OLV, the Ivor Lewis begins with the patient in the supine position for laparotomy or laparoscopy for preparation of the gastric conduit. The gastric tube is then advanced into the chest as far as possible and the abdomen is closed. The patient is then repositioned in the left lateral decubitus position for right thoracotomy or thoracoscopy. In the chest, the esophagus is mobilized and divided. The gastric conduit is pulled further into the chest and the anastomosis performed. The thoracotomy or thoracoscopy incisions are closed after placement of a chest tube.

Left Thoracoabdominal Esophagectomy

The left thoracoabdominal approach can be performed with acceptable morbidity and mortality, but is only considered for patients with tumors limited to the distal esophagus, and even in those cases is associated with high rates of residual disease.[35] This approach necessitates OLV, and the patient is positioned in the right lateral decubitus position but with the abdomen rolled back approximately 45°. A thoracoabdominal incision is made along the 7th intercostal interspace across the costal margin, and the diaphragm is taken down circumferentially from the chest wall (Figure 17–2D). Esophageal and gastric mobilization and resection are performed as described for the Ivor-Lewis technique but with reconstruction of the diaphragm prior to closure.

Anesthetic Management for Esophagectomy Procedures

Anesthetic care is an important component of the multidisciplinary approach to management of esophagectomy patients that has been shown in clinical studies to improve perioperative. Good results have been achieved with multimodal care plans utilizing thoracic epidural analgesia, early extubation, early mobilization, and a restrictive approach to fluid management.[36,37] Other anesthetic concerns include preoperative assessment, the need for OLV, management of intraoperative events including dysrhythmias, hemorrhage and airway injury, and use of protective ventilation strategies. In addition, it is important to be aware of the specific surgical plan, as each approach to esophagectomy has its own requirements and implications for the anesthesia care team.

General Considerations

In general, patients presenting for esophagectomy for malignant disease have significant comorbidities and these will guide preoperative assessment and the need for invasive monitoring to a greater degree than the procedure itself. Invasive arterial blood pressure monitoring is routinely used both for blood gas sampling during OLV and for continuous blood pressure measurement during procedures that may involve significant dysrhythmias or sudden changes in cardiac output or blood loss. Central venous pressure monitoring is not routinely used, but if necessary, should be placed in the great veins on the right-hand side in cases in which a cervical anastomosis is planned.

Prior to surgical incision, an NG tube should be placed and left either to intermittent low suction or to gravity drainage. In cases of an obstructing lesion, most surgeons will still request an NG tube be placed in the proximal esophagus to assist with the cervical dissection. As discussed above, prior to stapling or dividing the distal esophagus, the NG tube should be withdrawn either into the pharynx or as specifically directed by the surgical team, and then advanced through the esophageal anastomosis, again under direct surgical supervision. When the tube is in final position, it should be firmly secured to avoid displacement during extubation or patient transfer or movement. It is also helpful to place a reference mark on the tube itself so that it can be easily determined if its position has changed.

Airway, Ventilation, and Extubation

As noted above, all surgical approaches to esophagectomy other than transhiatal require OLV, and this can be accomplished with a bronchial blocker or use of a double-lumen endotracheal tube. Esophagectomy surgery is marked by a significant inflammatory response, and as such, lung protective strategies may contribute to decreasing postoperative pulmonary morbidity.[38,39] While it is also true that very low-volume ventilation also causes lung injury, esophagectomy patients ventilated with a tidal volume of 5 mL/kg during OLV had lower indices of inflammation and were extubated earlier than those who received 9 mL/kg.[39] It seems prudent therefore to continue to recommend a reduced tidal volume, in line with current thinking on lung protection strategies. In addition, peak and plateau inspiratory pressures should be minimized as much as possible and inspired oxygen concentration should be kept as low as possible to avoid oxygen toxicity (this is particularly important in patients who have received induction chemotherapy) as well as to minimize the remote risk of fire in the event of an airway injury.[40]

Timing of extubation has been a point of controversy in recent times. In the past, it was routine practice to leave patients intubated following esophagectomy to avoid the possibility of trauma to the anastomosis should reintubation become necessary. However, more recent retrospective reviews support immediate extubation.[41,42] In these series, use of thoracic epidural analgesia and restrictive fluid management have been associated with successful early extubation. Conversely, other studies have suggested increased mortality rates in patients who were extubated early.[43] However, it seems that early extubation is safe when it is part of a management plan that involves early mobilization, pulmonary toilet and optimal analgesia.[41]

Fluid Management

Strategies guiding perioperative fluid management must balance the maintenance of perfusion pressure and oxygen delivery to vital organs and the intended surgical conduit while at the same time avoiding peripheral and pulmonary edema.[40] Erring to either extreme is problematic, as hypovolemia results in hypoperfusion of the mesentery, while fluid overload impairs anastomosis and wound healing, and exacerbates cardiac or respiratory dysfunction.

Debates have raged for decades over the optimal amount and type of fluid to administer. Recent investigations have suggested that relative crystalloid restriction may improve outcome in major gastrointestinal surgery.[44-47] Furthermore, fluid restriction has been part of several multimodal management strategies that have been successful in decreasing pulmonary morbidity.[41,48] However, difficulty arises from the fact that there is no common definition for exactly what constitutes "restrictive." Goal-directed therapy using noninvasive measures of cardiac output has been successfully employed for abdominal surgery, but has not been specifically investigated for esophageal resection.[49,50] Nevertheless, attempts to synthesize what data do exist seem to warrant the conclusion that, in general, liberal strategies contribute to less positive outcomes, but that goal-directed therapy may be better than either an empiric liberal or restrictive approach.

Intraoperative Complications

Cardiac dysrhythmias occur in up to 65% patients undergoing esophagectomy.[51,52] These occur most commonly during transhiatal procedures during the blunt dissection portion of the case and are well-tolerated most of the time. Most are atrial tachydysrhythmias, but more than 50% of these are of combined atrial and ventricular origin. Interestingly, in a closely monitored observational study, there was no correlation between the incidence of dysrhythmias and that of hypotension, but there was a strong correlation between hypotension and the duration of manipulation.[51]

Other serious intraoperative events that must be considered are the risks of hemorrhage and airway injury. While massive bleeding is rare, it may require rapid conversion from a minimally invasive to an open technique, or even an emergent change in patient position to facilitate surgical exposure of the involved vessel. In general, if severe bleeding occurs in the mid- or upper-esophagus, it may require conversion to a right thoracotomy for approach to the azygous vein, and if from the lower third of the esophagus, a left thoracotomy may be required to access a bleeding esophageal branch from the aorta. Fortunately, such vascular injuries occur in less than 2% of transhiatal esophagectomy cases.[53] Similarly, airway injury is rare (<1% cases) and often minor.[54] These injuries are mostly limited to the distal membranous trachea or proximal bronchi, and are usually detected by the smell of inhaled anesthetic in the field or a feeling of airflow by the surgeon with each ventilator-delivered breath. It is rare that an injury is large enough to be detected by loss of ventilator volume unless very low-fresh gas flows are being used. If an airway injury is detected, it may require deflation of the endotracheal tube cuff and advancement of the tube past the injury with manual guidance by the surgeon. If the injury is large, a right thoracotomy may be required to access the carina for surgical repair. In any case of airway injury, it is crucially important to extubate the patient immediately postoperatively and avoid reintubation to prevent pressure on or manipulation of the suture line.

Pain Management

Adequate pain control is of paramount importance in augmenting postoperative recovery and rehabilitation following esophagectomy and there is evidence as well as general consensus that thoracic epidural analgesia (TEA) is the optimal technique to achieve this. In addition to superior pain control, TEA may also exert a positive effect on immune function and the stress response to surgery, decrease pulmonary complications, and decrease the risk of anastomotic leak.[55] Indeed, lack of TEA has been associated with increased morbidity and an increased risk of developing post-thoracotomy pain syndrome.[56] However, a systematic review has indicated that paravertebral blocks may also be a good choice for esophagectomy patients and may have a lower incidence of side effects.[57]

Immediate and Long-Term Outcomes Following Esophagectomy

Even with advances in surgical technique, anesthetic and critical care, esophagectomy continues to be a source of significant morbidity and mortality in both the immediate perioperative period and for long-term survivors. Estimates of perioperative mortality range from 8.8% to 14% with major and total morbidity measured at 25% and 50%, respectively.[6,15,31,33,58-68] Patients undergoing esophageal surgery have long hospital stays and prolonged overall recovery periods, and this is more than double when significant complications occur.[31,62,64,69] It is perhaps for these reasons that surgery is pursued for only 34% potentially resectable stage I, II, and III esophageal cancers.[13]

Interestingly, clinical studies have shown that surgical and center experience is much more important in determining ultimate outcome than choice of procedure. Prospective trials have failed to demonstrate any significant differences in short- or long-term survival or quality of life between transthoracic and transhiatal esophagectomies, although some evidence suggests that the transhiatal approach has a slightly lower rate of perioperative complications and these patients may achieve better activity levels postoperatively.[59-61,69-71] However, centers and surgeons that perform high volumes of esophageal surgery report mortality rates that are significantly lower for both transhiatal and transthoracic procedures than those reported in multicenter studies or national databases.[12,15,31,72,73] In fact, it appears that the mortality rate for low versus high volume centers and surgeons may differ by as much as 50%. Interestingly, high volume is defined as greater than 12 or 5 cases/year for centers and surgeons respectively, and low volume as less than 5 or 2 cases/year, again for centers and surgeons, respectively.[61,74-76] Similarly, improvements reported in long-term surgical outcomes are significantly better for high volume centers and surgeons, with some centers reporting recent mortality rates as low as 1%.[15,62,72,77-80] Specialty training also appears to have a significant effect on outcome, with surgeons without specialty training having 37% to 50% higher mortality than those with specialty training.[64,74,81]

Minimally invasive esophagectomy can be performed by experienced surgeons with low conversion rates and a median reported hospital stay of 7 days.[65,82] These techniques may result in less morbidity and mortality and shorter postoperative recovery times, but they continue to have initially longer operative times, and morbidity and mortality rates as high as 46% and 6%, respectively.[67,82,83] The improved results seen with minimally invasive techniques are probably due not only to the differences in surgical approach, but also to the fact that they are being performed by experienced and highly trained esophageal surgeons at high volume centers.

Morbidity Following Esophagectomy

A summary of complications following esophagectomy is listed in Table 17–5. Risk factors for major morbidity are pulmonary disease, older age, black race, congestive heart failure, coronary artery disease, peripheral vascular disease, malnutrition, decreased functional status, hypertension, insulin-requiring diabetes, higher American Society of Anesthesiology Physical Status Classification, and use of tobacco or steroids.[58,60,64] Preoperative predictors of mortality based on multivariable analysis include higher Charlson score (a measure of comorbid

Table 17–5. Perioperative Complications Following Esophagogastrectomy[6, 15, 31, 33, 58-61, 64-68, 86, 87]

Complication	Incidence (in %)
Technical	
anastomotic stricture	19-48
anastomotic leak	6-14
vocal cord palsy	2-14
wound infection	5.3-12
fascial dehiscence	2-5
delayed gastric emptying	1.8-3.7
chylothorax	0.8-9
Pulmonary Complications (total)	28.5-29.7
pneumonia	8-26
reintubation	6-17
respiratory failure	1.8-16
aspiration	7
atelectasis requiring bronchoscopy	4.50
Miscellaneous	
deep venous thrombosis	0.9-2
myocardial infarction	0.7-1.2
pulmonary embolism	0.7-1.7
atrial fibrillation	14-17.5
renal failure	0.9-3.4

conditions), older age, renal dysfunction, diabetes, alcohol abuse, decreased functional status, intraoperative transfusion, and ascites.[58,63] Tumor location and histology are also important, with squamous cell carcinomas and upper third esophageal tumors being associated with worse outcomes.[84,85] As noted above, undergoing surgery at a center where less than 12 esophagectomies are performed per year is also a risk factor for postoperative mortality.[63] Finally, neoadjuvant therapy has been variably identified as a predictor of significant morbidity and mortality in the postoperative period.[58,64]

Considering the overall poor prognosis for esophageal cancer patients, the impact of surgical complications on survival and quality of life cannot be overstated.[12,88] However, surgical technique and perioperative care have implications beyond immediate perioperative survival. Improved long-term survival and quality of life are often directly related to avoidance of postoperative complications.[89] Measures that have been successful in reducing perioperative morbidity include aggressive preoperative conditioning, minimizing intensive care unit stay, aggressive pain management, early ambulation, involvement of a dedicated intensivist in the perioperative care team and an overall multidisciplinary, multimodal approach to management.[15]

Anastomotic Complications: Stricture and Leak

Anastomotic leaks occur in 6% to 14% patients following esophagectomy surgery and have traditionally been associated with extremely high mortality. However, with improvements in surgical technique and critical care, mortality rates as low as 3.3% have been achieved.[33,90,91] Clinical features commonly associated with leaks include fever, leukocytosis, pleural effusion, and sepsis, although small leaks are often identified in asymptomatic patients.[92] Many leaks (57%) can be managed nonoperatively, although operative alternatives include stent placement, primary anastomotic repair, anastomotic tissue reinforcement (muscle flap), and esophageal diversion.[93,94] Early leaks (within 5 days) and those associated with gastric tip necrosis (incidence 2%-3%) are most likely to require surgical treatment.[91,92]

Respiratory Complications

Respiratory complications are the most common cause of death following esophagectomy.[31] Risk of pneumonia appears to be highest in those approaches that involve a thoracotomy incision. Reducing pulmonary complications with the use of epidural analgesia and aggressive use of bronchoscopy for clearance of pulmonary secretions appears to reduce perioperative mortality.[95] Other strategies include careful assessment of swallowing abnormalities and risk of aspiration by cineradiography or fiberoptic endoscopy before initiating oral intake.[31]

Chylothorax

Chylothorax occurs in up to 9% patients who have undergone esophagectomy.[68] Conservative management is not often pursued as this usually results in nutritional and immunologic depletion and an increased risk of infectious complications. Early intervention with thoracic duct ligation is generally successful and avoids these complications.[96] Thoracic duct ligation in the course of a thoracic procedure may be considered as a prophylactic measure.

Vocal Cord Paralysis

The incidence of recurrent laryngeal nerve injury manifesting as early postoperative hoarseness is reportedly as high as 36% following esophagectomy. Such injuries also occur in 4.5% to 14% patients who have a cervical anastomosis.[15,68] Hoarseness is generally transient and resolves in 2 to 12 weeks. Patients with persistent vocal cord paralysis require cord medialization procedures, as long-term persistent hoarseness is associated with debilitated performance status, as well as swallowing and pulmonary dysfunction.[97] Patients with evidence of aspiration should undergo early cord medialization, as this has been shown to decrease the incidence of pneumonia and need for bronchoscopy.[98]

Anesthesia for Post-Esophagectomy Patients

It is not uncommon for a patient to require general anesthesia for additional procedures (eg, for anastomotic dilation) following esophagectomy. In such cases, it is crucial to remember that these patients are at significant risk for aspiration, and that aspiration, even when minor, can result in aspiration pneumonitis, lung abscess, or respiratory failure. (Figure 17–3) Post-esophagectomy patients should be managed with a rapid

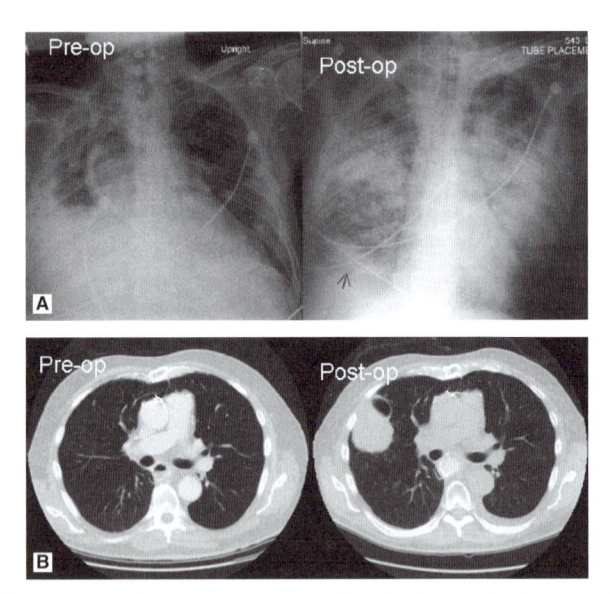

Figure 17–3. Radiographic consequences of aspiration on induction of general anesthesia in post-esophagectomy patients. **A.** 83-year-old male patient s/p esophagogastrectomy developed new bilateral pulmonary opacities after aspirating on induction of general anesthesia for pulmonary decortication. **B.** 65-year-old male patient s/p esophagectomy who aspirated gastric contents on induction of general anesthesia for a partial nephrectomy and developed a right-sided lung abscess.

sequence technique with cricoid pressure when undergoing induction of general anesthesia. It is important to remember, however, that if the patient had a cervical anastomosis, the cricoid cartilage may no longer overlie the esophagus, and cricoid pressure may not, therefore, occlude its lumen. Minimizing the time period during which aspiration may occur is thus of the utmost importance. Also important is pharmacologic prophylaxis with a non-particulate antacid. Metoclopramide, H_2-blockers and proton-pump inhibitors should also be considered. If aspiration occurs, patients should undergo immediate bronchoscopy with suction removal of all visible evidence of aspirated material and lavage of the airways. Prophylactic use of antibiotics and steroids remains controversial. The planned surgical procedure should be cancelled (depending on the urgency of the case), and a minimum period of observation in a monitored setting is mandatory. If any respiratory symptoms develop, the patient should be admitted to an intensive care unit for observation.

REFERENCES

1. Horner M, Ries L, Krapcho M, et al. SEER Cancer Statistics Review, 1975-2006, National Cancer Institute. Bethesda, MD, http://seer.cancer.gov/csr/1975_2006/, based on November 2008 SEER data submission, posted to the SEER web site, 2009.
2. Enzinger PC, Mayer RJ. Esophageal cancer. *N Engl J Med.* 2003;349(23):2241-2252.
3. Pennathur A, Luketich JD. Resection for esophageal cancer: strategies for optimal management. *Ann Thorac Surg.* 2008;85(2):S751-S756.
4. Nigro JJ, Hagen JA, DeMeester TR, et al. Occult esophageal adenocarcinoma: extent of disease and implications for effective therapy. *Ann Surg.* 1999;230(3):433-438; discussion 438-440.
5. Chang DT, Chapman C, Shen J, Su Z, Koong AC. Treatment of esophageal cancer based on histology: a surveillance epidemiology and end results analysis. *Am J Clin Oncol.* 2009;32(4):405-410.
6. Daly JM, Fry WA, Little AG, et al. Esophageal cancer: results of an American College of Surgeons Patient Care Evaluation Study. *J Am Coll Surg.* 2000;190(5):562-572; discussion 572-563.
7. Downey RJ, Akhurst T, Ilson D, et al. Whole body 18FDG-PET and the response of esophageal cancer to induction therapy: results of a prospective trial. *J Clin Oncol.* 2003;21(3):428-432.
8. Greene FL, Page DL, Fleming ID, April F, eds. *AJCC Cancer Staging Manual.* 6th ed. New York: Springer-Verlag; 2003.
9. Nigro JJ, Hagen JA, DeMeester TR, et al. Prevalence and location of nodal metastases in distal esophageal adenocarcinoma confined to the wall: implications for therapy. *J Thorac Cardiovasc Surg.* 1999;117(1):16-23; discussion 23-15.
10. Rice TW, Zuccaro G, Jr, Adelstein DJ, Rybicki LA, Blackstone EH, Goldblum JR. Esophageal carcinoma: depth of tumor invasion is predictive of regional lymph node status. *Ann Thorac Surg.* 1998;65(3):787-792.
11. Kelsen DP, Winter KA, Gunderson LL, et al. Long-term results of RTOG trial 8911 (USA Intergroup 113): a random assignment trial comparison of chemotherapy followed by surgery compared with surgery alone for esophageal cancer. *J Clin Oncol.* 2007;25(24):3719-3725.
12. D'Amico TA. Surgery for esophageal cancer. *Gastrointest Cancer Res.* 2008;2(4 Suppl):S6-S9.
13. Paulson EC, Ra J, Armstrong K, Wirtalla C, Spitz F, Kelz RR. Underuse of esophagectomy as treatment for resectable esophageal cancer. *Arch Surg.* 2008;143(12):1198-1203; discussion 1203.
14. Ajani JA, Barthel JS, Bekaii-Saab T, et al. Esophageal cancer. *J Natl Compr Canc Netw.* 2008;6(9):818-849.
15. Orringer MB, Marshall B, Chang AC, Lee J, Pickens A, Lau CL. Two thousand transhiatal esophagectomies: changing trends, lessons learned. *Ann Surg.* 2007;246(3):363-372; discussion 372-364.
16. Arnott SJ, Duncan W, Gignoux M, et al. Preoperative radiotherapy for esophageal carcinoma. *Cochrane Database Syst Rev.* 2005(4):CD001799.
17. Graham AJ, Shrive FM, Ghali WA, et al. Defining the optimal treatment of locally advanced esophageal cancer: a systematic review and decision analysis. *Ann Thorac Surg.* 2007;83(4):1257-1264.

18. Fiorica F, Di Bona D, Schepis F, et al. Preoperative chemoradiotherapy for oesophageal cancer: a systematic review and meta-analysis. *Gut.* 2004;53(7):925-930.
19. Kaklamanos IG, Walker GR, Ferry K, Franceschi D, Livingstone AS. Neoadjuvant treatment for resectable cancer of the esophagus and the gastroesophageal junction: a meta-analysis of randomized clinical trials. *Ann Surg Oncol.* 2003;10(7):754-761.
20. Chirieac LR, Swisher SG, Ajani JA, et al. Posttherapy pathologic stage predicts survival in patients with esophageal carcinoma receiving preoperative chemoradiation. *Cancer.* 2005;103(7):1347-1355.
21. Fok M, Sham JS, Choy D, Cheng SW, Wong J. Postoperative radiotherapy for carcinoma of the esophagus: a prospective, randomized controlled study. *Surgery.* 1993;113(2):138-147.
22. Teniere P, Hay JM, Fingerhut A, Fagniez PL. Postoperative radiation therapy does not increase survival after curative resection for squamous cell carcinoma of the middle and lower esophagus as shown by a multicenter controlled trial. French University Association for Surgical Research. *Surg Gynecol Obstet.* 1991;173(2):123-130.
23. Peyre CG, Hagen JA, DeMeester SR, et al. Predicting systemic disease in patients with esophageal cancer after esophagectomy: a multinational study on the significance of the number of involved lymph nodes. *Ann Surg.* 2008;248(6):979-985.
24. Barbour AP, Rizk NP, Gonen M, et al. Adenocarcinoma of the gastroesophageal junction: influence of esophageal resection margin and operative approach on outcome. *Ann Surg.* 2007;246(1):1-8.
25. Peyre CG, Hagen JA, DeMeester SR, et al. The number of lymph nodes removed predicts survival in esophageal cancer: an international study on the impact of extent of surgical resection. *Ann Surg.* 2008;248(4):549-556.
26. Greenstein AJ, Litle VR, Swanson SJ, Divino CM, Packer S, Wisnivesky JP. Effect of the number of lymph nodes sampled on postoperative survival of lymph node-negative esophageal cancer. *Cancer.* 2008;112(6):1239-1246.
27. Wolff CS, Castillo SF, Larson DR, et al. Ivor Lewis approach is superior to transhiatal approach in retrieval of lymph nodes at esophagectomy. *Dis Esophagus.* 2008;21(4):328-333.
28. Enestvedt CK, Perry KA, Kim C, et al. Trends in the management of esophageal carcinoma based on provider volume: treatment practices of 618 esophageal surgeons. *Dis Esophagus.* 2010;23(2):136-144.
29. Cerfolio RJ, Allen MS, Deschamps C, Trastek VF, Pairolero PC. Esophageal replacement by colon interposition. *Ann Thorac Surg.* 1995;59(6):1382-1384.
30. Kolh P, Honore P, Degauque C, Gielen J, Gerard P, Jacquet N. Early stage results after oesophageal resection for malignancy—colon interposition vs gastric pull-up. *Eur J Cardiothorac Surg.* 2000;18(3):293-300.
31. Atkins BZ, Shah AS, Hutcheson KA, et al. Reducing hospital morbidity and mortality following esophagectomy. *Ann Thorac Surg.* 2004;78(4):1170-1176; discussion 1170-1176.
32. Okuyama M, Motoyama S, Suzuki H, Saito R, Maruyama K, Ogawa J. Hand-sewn cervical anastomosis versus stapled intrathoracic anastomosis after esophagectomy for middle or lower thoracic esophageal cancer: a prospective randomized controlled study. *Surg Today.* 2007;37(11):947-952.
33. Alanezi K, Urschel JD. Mortality secondary to esophageal anastomotic leak. *Ann Thorac Cardiovasc Surg.* 2004;10(2):71-75.
34. Urschel JD. Esophagogastrostomy anastomotic leaks complicating esophagectomy: a review. *Am J Surg.* 1995;169(6):634-640.
35. Forshaw MJ, Gossage JA, Ockrim J, Atkinson SW, Mason RC. Left thoracoabdominal esophagogastrectomy: still a valid operation for carcinoma of the distal esophagus and esophagogastric junction. *Dis Esophagus.* 2006;19(5):340-345.
36. Brodner G, Pogatzki E, Van Aken H, et al. A multimodal approach to control postoperative pathophysiology and rehabilitation in patients undergoing abdominothoracic esophagectomy. *Anesth Analg.* 1998;86(2):228-234.
37. Low DE, Kunz S, Schembre D, et al. Esophagectomy—it's not just about mortality anymore: standardized perioperative clinical pathways improve outcomes in patients with esophageal cancer. *J Gastrointest Surg.* 2007;11(11):1395-1402; discussion 1402.
38. Kooguchi K, Kobayashi A, Kitamura Y, et al. Elevated expression of inducible nitric oxide synthase and inflammatory cytokines in the alveolar macrophages after esophagectomy. *Crit Care Med.* 2002;30(1):71-76.
39. Michelet P, D'Journo XB, Roch A, et al. Protective ventilation influences systemic inflammation after esophagectomy: a randomized controlled study. *Anesthesiology.* 2006;105(5):911-919.

40. Ng JM. Perioperative anesthetic management for esophagectomy. *Anesthesiol Clin.* 2008;26(2):293-304, vi.
41. Lanuti M, de Delva PE, Maher A, et al. Feasibility and outcomes of an early extubation policy after esophagectomy. *Ann Thorac Surg.* 2006;82(6):2037-2041.
42. Yap FH, Lau JY, Joynt GM, Chui PT, Chan AC, Chung SS. Early extubation after transthoracic oesophagectomy. *Hong Kong Med J.* 2003;9(2):98-102.
43. Bartels H, Stein HJ, Siewert JR. Early extubation vs late extubation after esophagus resection: a randomized, prospective study. *Langenbecks Arch Chir Suppl Kongressbd.* 1998;115:1074-1076.
44. Nisanevich V, Felsenstein I, Almogy G, Weissman C, Einav S, Matot I. Effect of intraoperative fluid management on outcome after intraabdominal surgery. *Anesthesiology.* 2005;103(1):25-32.
45. Brandstrup B, Tonnesen H, Beier-Holgersen R, et al. Effects of intravenous fluid restriction on postoperative complications: comparison of two perioperative fluid regimens: a randomized assessor-blinded multicenter trial. *Ann Surg.* 2003;238(5):641-648.
46. Holte K, Foss NB, Andersen J, et al. Liberal or restrictive fluid administration in fast-track colonic surgery: a randomized, double-blind study. *Br J Anaesth.* 2007;99(4):500-508.
47. Joshi GP. Intraoperative fluid restriction improves outcome after major elective gastrointestinal surgery. *Anesth Analg.* 2005;101(2):601-605.
48. Kita T, Mammoto T, Kishi Y. Fluid management and postoperative respiratory disturbances in patients with transthoracic esophagectomy for carcinoma. *J Clin Anesth.* 2002;14(4):252-256.
49. Venn R, Steele A, Richardson P, Poloniecki J, Grounds M, Newman P. Randomized controlled trial to investigate influence of the fluid challenge on duration of hospital stay and perioperative morbidity in patients with hip fractures. *Br J Anaesth.* 2002;88(1):65-71.
50. Button D, Weibel L, Reuthebuch O, Genoni M, Zollinger A, Hofer CK. Clinical evaluation of the FloTrac/Vigileo system and two established continuous cardiac output monitoring devices in patients undergoing cardiac surgery. *Br J Anaesth.* 2007;99(3):329-336.
51. Malhotra SK, Kaur RP, Gupta NM, Grover A, Ramprabu K, Nakra D. Incidence and types of arrhythmias after mediastinal manipulation during transhiatal esophagectomy. *Ann Thorac Surg.* 2006;82(1):298-302.
52. Sedrakyan A, Treasure T, Browne J, Krumholz H, Sharpin C, van der Meulen J. Pharmacologic prophylaxis for postoperative atrial tachyarrhythmia in general thoracic surgery: evidence from randomized clinical trials. *J Thorac Cardiovasc Surg.* 2005;129(5):997-1005.
53. Parekh K, Iannettoni MD. Complications of esophageal resection and reconstruction. *Semin Thorac Cardiovasc Surg.* 2007;19(1):79-88.
54. Hulscher JB, ter Hofstede E, Kloek J, Obertop H, De Haan P, Van Lanschot JJ. Injury to the major airways during subtotal esophagectomy: incidence, management, and sequelae. *J Thorac Cardiovasc Surg.* 2000;120(6):1093-1096.
55. Michelet P, Roch A, D'Journo XB, et al. Effect of thoracic epidural analgesia on gastric blood flow after oesophagectomy. *Acta Anaesthesiol Scand.* 2007;51(5):587-594.
56. Cense HA, Lagarde SM, de Jong K, et al. Association of no epidural analgesia with postoperative morbidity and mortality after transthoracic esophageal cancer resection. *J Am Coll Surg.* 2006;202(3):395-400.
57. Davies RG, Myles PS, Graham JM. A comparison of the analgesic efficacy and side-effects of paravertebral vs epidural blockade for thoracotomy—a systematic review and meta-analysis of randomized trials. *Br J Anaesth.* 2006;96(4):418-426.
58. Bailey SH, Bull DA, Harpole DH, et al. Outcomes after esophagectomy: a ten-year prospective cohort. *Ann Thorac Surg.* 2003;75(1):217-222; discussion 222.
59. Chang AC, Ji H, Birkmeyer NJ, Orringer MB, Birkmeyer JD. Outcomes after transhiatal and transthoracic esophagectomy for cancer. *Ann Thorac Surg.* 2008;85(2):424-429.
60. Rentz J, Bull D, Harpole D, et al. Transthoracic versus transhiatal esophagectomy: a prospective study of 945 patients. *J Thorac Cardiovasc Surg.* 2003;125(5):1114-1120.
61. Connors RC, Reuben BC, Neumayer LA, Bull DA. Comparing outcomes after transthoracic and transhiatal esophagectomy: a 5-year prospective cohort of 17,395 patients. *J Am Coll Surg.* 2007;205(6):735-740.
62. Dimick JB, Wainess RM, Upchurch GR, Jr, Iannettoni MD, Orringer MB. National trends in outcomes for esophageal resection. *Ann Thorac Surg.* 2005;79(1):212-216; discussion 217-218.
63. Ra J, Paulson EC, Kucharczuk J, et al. Postoperative mortality after esophagectomy for cancer: development of a preoperative risk prediction model. *Ann Surg Oncol.* 2008;15(6):1577-1584.

64. Wright CD, Kucharczuk JC, O'Brien SM, Grab JD, Allen MS. Predictors of major morbidity and mortality after esophagectomy for esophageal cancer: a Society of Thoracic Surgeons General Thoracic Surgery Database risk adjustment model. *J Thorac Cardiovasc Surg.* 2009;137(3):587-595; discussion 596.
65. Luketich JD, Alvelo-Rivera M, Buenaventura PO, et al. Minimally invasive esophagectomy: outcomes in 222 patients. *Ann Surg.* 2003;238(4):486-494; discussion 494-485.
66. Bizekis C, Kent MS, Luketich JD, et al. Initial experience with minimally invasive Ivor Lewis esophagectomy. *Ann Thorac Surg.* 2006;82(2):402-406; discussion 406-407.
67. Luketich JD, Schauer PR, Christie NA, et al. Minimally invasive esophagectomy. *Ann Thorac Surg.* 2000;70(3): 906-911; discussion 911-902.
68. Swanson SJ, Batirel HF, Bueno R, et al. Transthoracic esophagectomy with radical mediastinal and abdominal lymph node dissection and cervical esophagogastrostomy for esophageal carcinoma. *Ann Thorac Surg.* 2001;72(6):1918-1924; discussion 1924-1915.
69. de Boer AG, van Lanschot JJ, van Sandick JW, et al. Quality of life after transhiatal compared with extended transthoracic resection for adenocarcinoma of the esophagus. *J Clin Oncol.* 2004;22(20):4202-4208.
70. Hulscher JB, van Sandick JW, de Boer AG, et al. Extended transthoracic resection compared with limited transhiatal resection for adenocarcinoma of the esophagus. *N Engl J Med.* 2002;347(21):1662-1669.
71. Goldminc M, Maddern G, Le Prise E, Meunier B, Campion JP, Launois B. Oesophagectomy by a transhiatal approach or thoracotomy: a prospective randomized trial. *Br J Surg.* 1993;80(3):367-370.
72. Davies AR, Forshaw MJ, Khan AA, et al. Transhiatal esophagectomy in a high volume institution. *World J Surg Oncol.* 2008;6:88.
73. Griffin SM, Shaw IH, Dresner SM. Early complications after Ivor Lewis subtotal esophagectomy with two-field lymphadenectomy: risk factors and management. *J Am Coll Surg.* 2002;194(3):285-297.
74. Dimick JB, Goodney PP, Orringer MB, Birkmeyer JD. Specialty training and mortality after esophageal cancer resection. *Ann Thorac Surg.* 2005;80(1):282-286.
75. Birkmeyer JD, Siewers AE, Finlayson EV, et al. Hospital volume and surgical mortality in the United States. *N Engl J Med.* 2002;346(15):1128-1137.
76. Birkmeyer JD, Stukel TA, Siewers AE, Goodney PP, Wennberg DE, Lucas FL. Surgeon volume and operative mortality in the United States. *N Engl J Med.* 2003;349(22):2117-2127.
77. Hofstetter W, Swisher SG, Correa AM, et al. Treatment outcomes of resected esophageal cancer. *Ann Surg.* 2002;236(3):376-384; discussion 384-375.
78. Law S, Wong KH, Kwok KF, Chu KM, Wong J. Predictive factors for postoperative pulmonary complications and mortality after esophagectomy for cancer. *Ann Surg.* 2004;240(5):791-800.
79. Liu JF, Wang QZ, Ping YM, Zhang YD. Complications after esophagectomy for cancer: 53-year experience with 20,796 patients. *World J Surg.* 2008;32(3):395-400.
80. Ruol A, Castoro C, Portale G, et al. Trends in management and prognosis for esophageal cancer surgery: twenty-five years of experience at a single institution. *Arch Surg.* 2009;144(3):247-254; discussion 254.
81. Leigh Y, Goldacre M, McCulloch P. Surgical specialty, surgical unit volume and mortality after oesophageal cancer surgery. *Eur J Surg Oncol.* 2009;35(8):820-825.
82. Decker G, Coosemans W, De Leyn P, et al. Minimally invasive esophagectomy for cancer. *Eur J Cardiothorac Surg.* 2009;35(1):13-20; discussion 20-11.
83. Biere SS, Cuesta MA, Van Der Peet DL. Minimally invasive versus open esophagectomy for cancer: a systematic review and meta-analysis. *Minerva Chir.* 2009;64(2):121-133.
84. Abunasra H, Lewis S, Beggs L, Duffy J, Beggs D, Morgan E. Predictors of operative death after oesophagectomy for carcinoma. *Br J Surg.* 2005;92(8):1029-1033.
85. Alexiou C, Khan OA, Black E, et al. Survival after esophageal resection for carcinoma: the importance of the histologic cell type. *Ann Thorac Surg.* 2006;82(3):1073-1077.
86. Orringer MB, Marshall B, Iannettoni MD. Eliminating the cervical esophagogastric anastomotic leak with a side-to-side stapled anastomosis. *J Thorac Cardiovasc Surg.* 2000;119(2):277-288.
87. Dresner SM, Lamb PJ, Wayman J, Hayes N, Griffin SM. Benign anastomotic stricture following transthoracic subtotal oesophagectomy and stapled oesophago-gastrostomy: risk factors and management. *Br J Surg.* 2000;87(3):362-373.
88. Rizk NP, Bach PB, Schrag D, et al. The impact of complications on outcomes after resection for esophageal and gastroesophageal junction carcinoma. *J Am Coll Surg.* 2004;198(1):42-50.

89. Ando N, Ozawa S, Kitagawa Y, Shinozawa Y, Kitajima M. Improvement in the results of surgical treatment of advanced squamous esophageal carcinoma during 15 consecutive years. *Ann Surg.* 2000;232(2):225-232.
90. Martin LW, Swisher SG, Hofstetter W, et al. Intrathoracic leaks following esophagectomy are no longer associated with increased mortality. *Ann Surg.* 2005;242(3):392-399; discussion 399-402.
91. Sarela AI, Tolan DJ, Harris K, Dexter SP, Sue-Ling HM. Anastomotic leakage after esophagectomy for cancer: a mortality-free experience. *J Am Coll Surg.* 2008;206(3):516-523.
92. Page RD, Shackcloth MJ, Russell GN, Pennefather SH. Surgical treatment of anastomotic leaks after oesophagectomy. *Eur J Cardiothorac Surg.* 2005;27(2):337-343.
93. Crestanello JA, Deschamps C, Cassivi SD, et al. Selective management of intrathoracic anastomotic leak after esophagectomy. *J Thorac Cardiovasc Surg.* 2005;129(2):254-260.
94. Hunerbein M, Stroszczynski C, Moesta KT, Schlag PM. Treatment of thoracic anastomotic leaks after esophagectomy with self-expanding plastic stents. *Ann Surg.* 2004;240(5):801-807.
95. Whooley BP, Law S, Murthy SC, Alexandrou A, Wong J. Analysis of reduced death and complication rates after esophageal resection. *Ann Surg.* 2001;233(3):338-344.
96. Merigliano S, Molena D, Ruol A, et al. Chylothorax complicating esophagectomy for cancer: a plea for early thoracic duct ligation. *J Thorac Cardiovasc Surg.* 2000;119(3):453-457.
97. Baba M, Natsugoe S, Shimada M, et al. Does hoarseness of voice from recurrent nerve paralysis after esophagectomy for carcinoma influence patient quality of life? *J Am Coll Surg.* 1999;188(3):231-236.
98. Bhattacharyya N, Batirel H, Swanson SJ. Improved outcomes with early vocal fold medialization for vocal fold paralysis after thoracic surgery. *Auris Nasus Larynx.* 2003;30(1):71-75.

Bronchopleural Fistula: Anesthetic Management

18

Angela Truong
Dam-Thuy Truong
Dilip Thakar
Bernhard Riedel

Key Points

- Bronchopleural fistula is a direct communication between the bronchial tree and the pleural cavity causing an air leak from the lung. In pneumothorax, the communication is peripheral, between a ruptured bleb or alveolar duct and the pleural cavity.
- Anesthesia for patients with a BPF is based on two important techniques central to thoracic anesthesia: effective lung isolation and ventilation of an open airway.
- Prompt lung isolation is essential during anesthetic management in order to minimize the risk of ventilating the pleural cavity and soiling the contralateral lung.

Clinical Vignette

A 72-year-old man with a history of T_3N_2 supraglottic squamous cell carcinoma, treated with chemoradiotherapy, was found to have a large tumor in the right lower lobe of the lung. Computed tomography (CT)–guided biopsy showed poorly differentiated squamous cell carcinoma. He underwent a right pneumonectomy with mediastinal lymph node dissection and a rotational serratus anterior muscle flap.

Following surgery, he remained intubated and ventilated overnight in the intensive care unit (ICU) and was extubated the following morning. On postoperative day 3 he developed refractory hypoxemia and respiratory failure requiring re-intubation and mechanical ventilation. The following week was characterized by deterioration in his clinical state—with low-grade fever, copious tracheal secretions, and persistent drainage of purulent pleural fluid from a chest tube. Serial chest radiographs and a CT scan revealed an increasing air level and decreasing pleural fluid level in the right pleural cavity, with consolidation of the left lower lobe. Fiber-optic bronchoscopy demonstrated purulent material trickling from a 3-mm-diameter bronchopleural fistula (BPF) in the bronchial stump.

> **Clinical Vignette (Continued)**
>
> A small open-window thoracostomy was created, and the pleural cavity was drained and thoroughly irrigated, and then packed daily. The patient received intravenous antibiotic therapy based on sensitivity analysis of blood and pleural fluid cultures; enteral feeding via a percutaneous gastrostomy tube; tight glucose control with insulin; and pressure control ventilation using permissive hypercapnea to maintain low mean airway pressures.
>
> Over the next 4 weeks, the infection process was eradicated and the patient's clinical status improved. The BPF did not close spontaneously, however, as evidenced by a persistent air leak through the thoracostomy tube. This necessitated a return to the operating room for bronchoscopic assessment of the fistula, possible closure of the fistula with fibrin glue and, if needed, thoracotomy for BPF closure.

Bronchopleural fistula is a direct communication between the central bronchial tree and the pleural cavity which results from disruption of a bronchial stump or tracheobronchial anastomosis, causing an air leak from the lung. This contrasts with a pneumothorax, in which the communication is peripheral, between a ruptured bleb or alveolar duct and the pleural cavity. When the fistula or sinus tract of a BPF extends to the skin of the chest wall it is termed a bronchopleural-cutaneous fistula. Although rare, BPF represents a challenging management problem; it is associated with high rates of morbidity and mortality and poses formidable challenges during anesthetic management because of the risks of life-threatening loss of ventilation, tension pneumothorax, and contamination of the remaining lung through the fistula.

Incidence

Bronchopleural fistula is relatively rare, with an overall reported incidence following pulmonary resection between 1.5% and 20%.[1,2] About two-thirds of cases occur as a postoperative complication of pulmonary resection, by far the most common cause of BPF. Other less common causes of BPF include necrotizing lung infections, persistent spontaneous pneumothorax, chemotherapy or radiotherapy (for lung cancer), and tuberculosis (Table 18–1). The incidence is higher with pneumonectomy than with lobectomy, since the lobes remaining after lobectomy may offer stabilization and protection to the bronchial stump. Left-sided pneumonectomy is less vulnerable than right-sided pneumonectomy because the bronchial stump is smaller and usually located just under the aortic arch, deriving some protection from it.

Etiology

The destruction of a bronchial wall that leads to BPF may result from a variety of etiologies; including surgical causes, anesthetic-related causes, and medical causes (Table 18–1).

Table 18–1. Etiology of Bronchopleural Fistula

Surgical causes
  Bronchial stump dehiscence following lung resection
  Blunt or penetrating trauma to the chest
  Transbronchial biopsy
  Thoracentesis
Anesthetic-related causes
  Traumatic endotracheal and endobronchial intubation
  Tracheobronchial injury caused by an intubating stylet or light wand
  Bronchial perforation caused by an endotracheal tube exchanger
Medical causes
  Infection (empyema, lung abscess, tuberculosis)-induced necrotizing changes
  Inflammatory diseases
  Necrotizing lung cancer following chemotherapy or radiotherapy
  Persistent spontaneous pneumothorax

BPF after Lung Resection: Pathophysiology, Risk Factors, and Types

An understanding of the pathophysiology and risk factors involved in BPF development is essential for its prevention and successful management. Not a distinct disease entity, BPF is rather a pathological process following lung resection. Necrosis of the wall between the bronchial system and the pleural cavity results from the complex interaction of three factors: trauma, infection, and poor wound healing. Each factor can potentiate the harmful effects of the other factors. For instance, infection not only contributes directly to the occurrence of BPF, but can also impede wound healing and render the affected area more vulnerable to trauma during subsequent airway manipulation.

Bronchopleural fistula is classified as acute or chronic, and each has a distinct presentation and treatment. Acute BPF classically occurs within the first week following lung resection, resulting from sudden dehiscence of the bronchial stump suture line. Acute BPF is essentially related to surgical technique, and infection and serious coexisting medical conditions play lesser roles. In contrast, chronic BPF, which may take weeks or months to develop, can occur after lung resection or be associated with nonsurgical conditions such as empyema or lung abscess. It usually occurs in patients with severe chronic debilitating comorbid conditions, and infection plays a primordial role.

The risk factors associated with development of BPF can be classified as preoperative, intraoperative, or postoperative. Preoperative factors include immunosuppression, prolonged corticosteroid therapy, preexisting infection such as active tuberculosis with pathogen-positive sputum, neoadjuvant radiotherapy/chemotherapy, chronic debility, malnutrition, and uncontrolled diabetes mellitus. Intraoperative or surgical risk factors include pneumonectomy, especially right-sided pneumonectomy, a long bronchial stump, and poor surgical technique that results in faulty stump closure and/or compromised blood supply to the bronchial

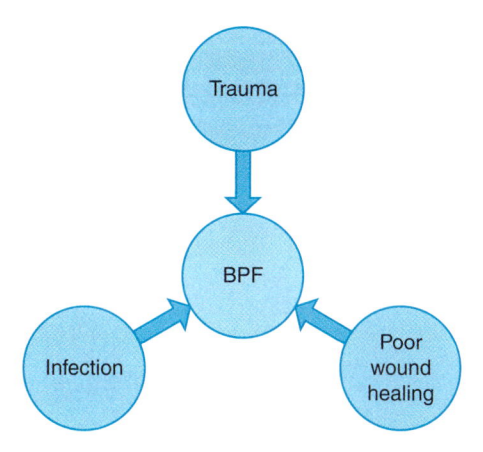

Figure 18–1. Graphical representation of factors that play central roles in BPF formation.

stump. Postoperative factors include prolonged mechanical ventilation, atelectasis, pneumonia, empyema, re-intubation and frequent tracheobronchial suctioning, and residual tumor at the stump.[3,4] Importantly, these risk factors usually contribute to BPF formation through a combination of trauma, infection, and poor wound healing (Figure 18–1).

CLINICAL PRESENTATION

The clinical signs of BPF are determined by the size of the BPF and whether the BPF is acute or chronic in origin. When the fistula is small (of the order of a few millimeters, Figure 18–2), the predominant symptoms are cough, particularly when the patient is lying on the side of the fistula, and severe shortness of breath. A delay in cavity filling after pneumonectomy is also noted. When empyema is present, infectious symptoms dominate. When the fistula is large, formed by sudden massive dehiscence of the bronchial stump, copious expectoration of pleural fluid may be noted. This may result in sudden catastrophic flooding of the airway, and possibly even death by asphyxia due to the large communication between the fluid-filled pleural cavity and the tracheobronchial tree. If the patient is still intubated, positive pressure ventilation with a massive leak through a large BPF will cause severe loss of alveolar ventilation, resulting in acute hypoxia, hypercarbia, and respiratory acidosis. If the correct diagnosis of BPF is not made, desperate attempts to increase positive pressure ventilation will paradoxically worsen the hypoventilation by further increasing the air leak and enlarging the fistula. Furthermore, if a functioning chest tube is not in place, the air leak will quickly result in tension pneumothorax and cardiovascular collapse.

The onset is much more insidious in chronic BPF, with a relatively slow accumulation of purulent material in the pleural cavity and gradual erosion into the bronchial system. The clinical picture often consists of low-grade fever, fatigue, generalized

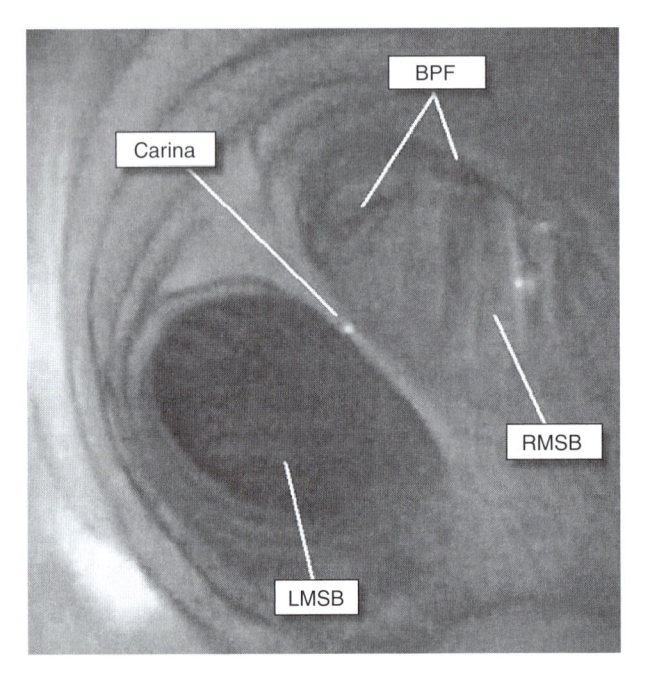

Figure 18–2. Bronchoscopy showing two small BPFs in the bronchial stump. Abbrev: RMSB, right main stem bronchus; LMSB, left main stem bronchus.

malaise, and cough with purulent or blood-tinged sputum. Hemoptysis, fetid breath, and subcutaneous emphysema are less frequently observed. The clinical picture may be very difficult to differentiate from similar nonspecific symptoms associated with other complications observed during the postpneumonectomy period.

Diagnosis

The diagnosis of BPF is made by clinical examination, diagnostic imaging techniques, nuclear scintigraphy, and bronchoscopy, which is universally accepted as the "gold standard."

Even though the clinical presentation of BPF is often nonspecific, a high index of suspicion based on the combination of suggestive signs and symptoms should alert clinicians to the potential diagnosis of BPF. In a simple bedside test that has been used to confirm the diagnosis of BPF, methylene blue is injected into the pleural space of a patient with a suspected BPF and the diagnosis confirmed through expectoration of blue-tinged sputum. Diagnostic imaging studies more often used for the detection of BPF include chest x-ray and CT. Bronchography and sinography may also be performed.

In the immediate period following lung resection, chest radiograph and CT scan normally show progressive accumulation of fluid in the postpneumonectomy space coupled with decreasing amounts of air. Because of the large empty space left

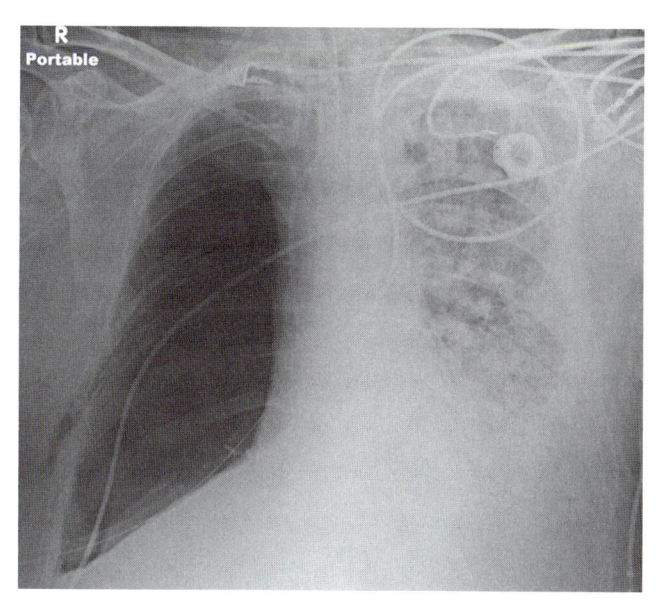

Figure 18–3. Chest x-ray showing postpneumonectomy pneumonitis and tension pneumothorax with mediastinal shift as a result of a BPF.

behind after pneumonectomy, there is normally an accompanying gradual elevation of the ipsilateral hemidiaphragm and a slight shift of the mediastinum toward the side of surgery. In cases of BPF, these trends are reversed: air accumulation increases and fluid level decreases in the postpneumonectomy pleural space, air-fluid level drops by more than 2 cm, and mediastinal shift is absent or a previously shifted mediastinum returns to the unaffected side.[5-7] In severe cases, a tension pneumothorax may develop within the postpneumonectomy space, with accompanying mediastinal shift (Figure 18–3). In the immediate postoperative period, these radiographic findings are particularly valuable in making an early diagnosis of BPF in an otherwise asymptomatic patient.[8]

It is much more challenging to directly identify the fistula tract on CT scan (Figures 18–4 and 18–5), especially when the BPF is very small or has an extremely tortuous path. Visualization of the fistula tract on CT scan can be facilitated by special techniques such as spiral CT with thin sections and three-dimensional reconstruction.[9] Bronchography or radiography of the bronchial system after intrabronchial instillation of a radio-opaque contrast medium allows visualization of the fistula. Similarly, if a bronchopleural cutaneous fistula is present, sinography or fistulography can be performed by injection of contrast dyes percutaneously into the fistula skin opening to outline the contour of the sinus tract.

When the BPF is too small to be detected by CT scan, ventilation radionuclide scintigraphy studies of a tracer gas such as Xe-133 or Tc-99m DTPA[10,11] or nitrous oxide[12] may aid diagnosis. Nitrous oxide is inhaled by the patient and, after gaining

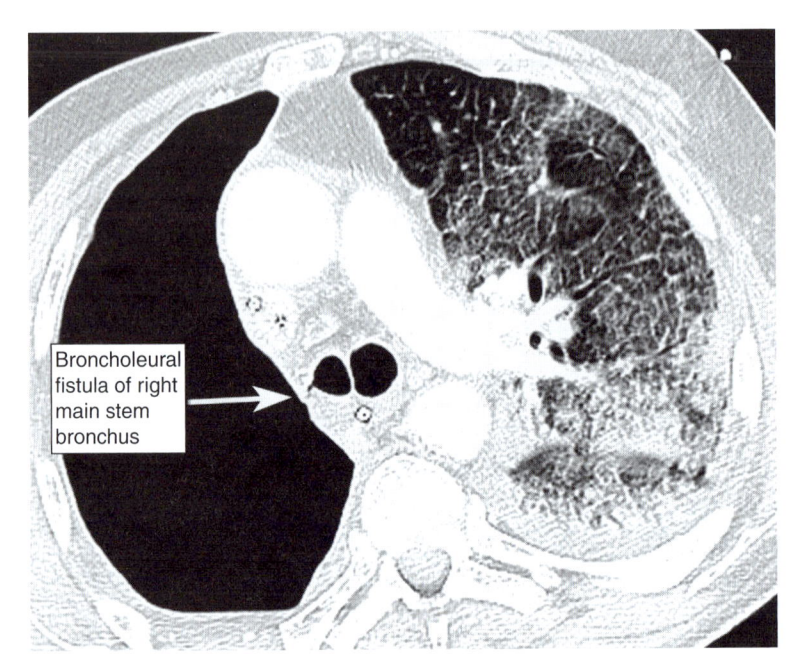

Figure 18–4. CT scan identifying a BPF tract in the main stem bronchial stump following pneumonectomy for mesothelioma.

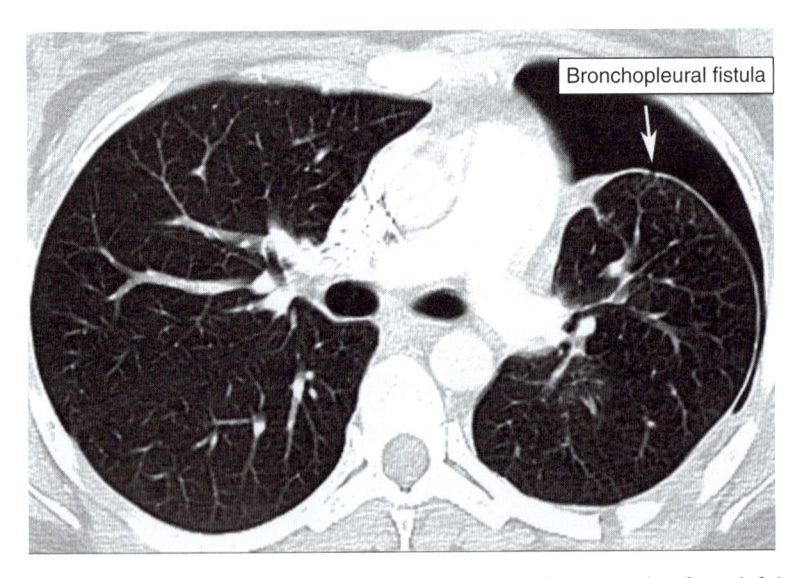

Figure 18-5. CT scan identifying a peripheral BPF in a patient 2 weeks after a left lower lobectomy, potentially related to cystic rupture of a subpleural metastasis.

access to the pleural cavity through the BPF, is then detected by gas analyzer connected to the chest tube.

While these investigations are all valuable, fiber-optic bronchoscopy is generally considered the optimum tool for establishing a definitive diagnosis, because it allows proper evaluation of the stump, localization of the fistula, determination of fistula size, exclusion of tuberculosis or other infectious etiologies, and visual assessment of the viability of the stump (Figure 18–2). If bronchoscopic findings are inconclusive, methylene blue may be instilled into the bronchial stump during bronchoscopy. If the dye is subsequently seen trickling into the pleural space, the diagnosis of BPF is confirmed. Bronchoscopy also plays a role in therapeutic intervention, allowing introduction of a sealant into the fistulous tract.

Assessment of Air Leak Severity

In most clinical settings, the air leak can be assessed by observing the appearance of bubbles from the chest tube during the respiratory cycle. If the air leak is small, bubbles appear only during inspiration. In larger air leaks, bubbling is continuous during both inspiration and expiration. Some commercially available pleural drainage systems include air leak meters that allow a rudimentary quantification of the air leak (see Chapter 22, Figure 18–3). To obtain a more precise estimate of the leak, a semiquantitative assessment can be made by measuring the difference between delivered and exhaled tidal volumes using a spirometer attached to the ventilator, or a tight-fitting face mask in extubated patients. Similarly, the amount of air leak can be measured with a spirometer attached directly to the chest tube.[13]

Anesthetic Problems Associated with BPF

A logical goal-oriented approach is used to develop an anesthetic plan that is appropriate to the surgical needs and the medical conditions of the patient. Anesthesia for patients with a BPF is based on two important techniques central to thoracic anesthesia: techniques of lung isolation and techniques of ventilation of an open airway.

Care should be taken to avoid complications associated with the fistula, since pleural cavity contents have free access to the bronchial system with potential for soiling with septic material into the "normal" contralateral lung or for flooding of the tracheobronchial tree by pleural fluid, resulting in catastrophic asphyxiation. A patient with BPF may not show any symptoms when awake and breathing spontaneously, but spillage of even small amounts of potentially septic material can cause severe lung damage. Under general anesthesia with mechanical ventilation, the tidal volume delivered may be lost through the low resistance fistula, resulting in severe hypoventilation, hypercarbia, acute respiratory acidosis, and hypoxemia. Furthermore, if a chest tube is not in place, then positive pressure ventilation may cause pneumothorax that can rapidly progress to a life-threatening tension pneumothorax with resultant cardiovascular collapse.

MANAGEMENT

Therapeutic success has been variable, and the lack of consensus suggests that no optimal therapy is available; rather, current therapeutic options seem to be complementary, and treatment needs to be individualized.

Since infection and trauma constitute two major causative factors of BPF, it is essential to observe meticulous aseptic and atraumatic techniques, especially during airway manipulation. Caution must be exercised to avoid further barotrauma from mechanical ventilation, and if sterility techniques are not adhered to, the chest tube, while indispensable for draining the infected pleural space, can serve as a conduit for introduction of more serious infections. Furthermore, since BPF is often associated with severe predisposing factors such as sepsis, uncontrolled diabetes mellitus, and multisystem organ failure, it is essential to ensure that underlying conditions are optimally managed during the perioperative period.

The first step to managing the actual BPF is to perform a bronchoscopy and drain the chest cavity. Depending on the dimension of the fistula and the timeframe of onset (acute vs chronic), the fistula can be managed by using a variety of surgical and/or medical procedures. Surgical therapy (eg, Clagett procedure, direct repair, or thoracoscopy) is traditionally the treatment of choice, but interest is increasing in bronchoscopic application of various glues, coils, and sealants. Location and size of the fistula may indicate the potential benefits of an endoscopic approach, which may serve as a temporary bridge in high-risk patients, allowing the patient's clinical status to improve.

Acute BPF

Acute BPF usually manifests within the first week after lung resection. The cause is primarily surgical, with a sudden and often complete dehiscence of the bronchial stump, and it may be associated with suboptimal surgical technique. In such cases, the onset is often very sudden and dramatic, with rapid onset of extreme shortness of breath and catastrophic cardiovascular collapse secondary to tension pneumothorax on the affected side. A chest tube, if not already in place, must be inserted as soon as possible not only to relieve tension pneumothorax but also to drain the pleural fluid to minimize the risk of bronchial and lung contamination. In life-threatening emergencies, the tension pneumothorax can be drained expeditiously by either large-bore needle puncture or reopening of the old chest tube site. At times, emergency reopening of the thoracotomy incision may be life saving. During these critical situations, the goals of anesthetic care are centered on resuscitation and hemodynamic support, allowing the patient to be transported to the operating room for emergency thoracotomy and BPF closure.

Attention must be paid to protecting the healthy lung from contamination and sudden flooding by the pleural contents. Postural drainage achieved by positioning the patient with the affected side dependent and head elevated may help prevent such aspiration. If these maneuvers are insufficient because of large volume output from the open bronchus, emergent intubation should be carried out, with placement of a double-lumen tube (DLT) to isolate the affected lung. In difficult airway situations, intubation of the contralateral lung with a single-lumen cuffed endotracheal tube in a mainstem bronchus may provide an acceptable means to secure the airway. Generally, patients presenting with acute BPF do not have severe comorbid conditions, provided that the healthy lung has not been flooded with pleural fluid (which can lead to aspiration pneumonitis). Once the surgical problem is recognized and addressed in a timely manner by reoperation, the prognosis is usually excellent.

Chronic BPF

BPF is essentially a pathological process and not a distinct and specific disease entity in itself. It is a manifestation of the patient's underlying serious lung condition, which leads to poor wound healing and fistula formation. Infection remains the chief reason for development of chronic BPF and plays a key role in its continued presence in chronically ill and debilitated patients. For this reason, the underlying factors that contribute to poor wound healing must be vigorously treated. Efforts to improve the patient's overall medical condition include optimizing nutritional status through parenteral or enteral feeding, preventing thromboembolism through prophylaxis, and managing poorly controlled diabetes to prevent hyperglycemia.

Underlying lung pathologies that can predispose to the formation of a BPF weeks to months following pneumonectomy include severe infections such as pneumonia, empyema, and acute respiratory distress syndrome (ARDS). Efforts to surgically close the fistula without first addressing the underlying causes will ultimately fail. Reversible causes for airway obstruction are treated with bronchodilators, and secretions are cleared with careful suctioning and chest physiotherapy. The empyema associated with chronic BPF is often thick-walled and multiloculated, and drainage by chest tube is usually inadequate, necessitating thorough washing out of the infected pleural space and packing with antibiotic solution. Often a pedicle flap is needed ultimately to fill up the cavity. The main principle of the surgical management of BPF with empyema is centered on elimination of the pleural space.

Treatment of concomitant ARDS in the ICU aims to optimize the patient's oxygenation while providing adequate minute ventilation. The goal involves limiting flow through the fistula in order to create an environment conducive to healing. Ventilatory management, therefore, centers on decreasing the amount of ventilatory support needed, thereby limiting barotrauma and promoting healing of the BPF. Strategies include limiting peak and mean airway pressures, early weaning from positive pressure support, decreasing the need for positive end-expiratory pressure ventilation (PEEP), permissive hypercapnia, and early extubation. This can be accomplished by restricting tidal volume (3-4 mL/kg if only one lung is present), minimizing inspiratory time, avoiding PEEP (both applied and auto-PEEP), and reducing the number of positive pressure breaths by using pressure support instead of total ventilatory support.

Even though the DLT is the technique of choice for lung isolation in the operating room, one-lung ventilation (OLV) is not usually desirable for prolonged stay in the ICU because the collapsed lung is vulnerable to infection. In the majority of cases, therefore, ventilation of a patient with a chronic BPF in the ICU is through a single-lumen tube (SLT), using the mode of ventilation that produces the lowest peak and mean airway pressures to avoid barotrauma and still ensure adequate oxygenation and CO_2 removal. Other methods have been developed to decrease air loss through the BPF. These include application of positive pressure to the pleural space during inspiration to oppose the air leak and placement of unidirectional valves in the chest tube. Unfortunately, the presence of purulent material in the chest cavity quickly disables the proper functioning of these devices.

If conventional ventilation fails, high-frequency ventilation may be used; it has been approved by the US Food and Drug Administration for the management of BPF. The advantages offered by high-frequency ventilation include a lower mean airway pressure to decrease the incidence of barotrauma to the lungs and tracheobronchial tree; improvement of cardiac output by reducing intrathoracic pressure, allowing increased venous return; and improving oxygenation through reduction in the shunt fraction and alveolar-arterial PO_2 gradient. These effects promote improved perfusion to the bronchial stump, thereby promoting healing and closure of the BPF.

While isolated reports claim success using various modalities of high-frequency ventilation in this setting, this is not consistent. In other reports, high-frequency ventilation has not been proven to achieve better results than conventional ventilation, particularly in patients with severe lung pathology and bilateral lung disease. This may be explained by the finding that as frequency increases, expiratory time decreases, auto-PEEP quickly occurs and mean airway pressure rises rapidly, thereby defeating the theoretical advantages of high-frequency ventilation in reducing airway pressures. In these circumstances, high-frequency ventilation may worsen oxygenation and CO_2 retention as compared to conventional ventilation techniques. For any particular clinical situation, therefore, trial periods of conventional ventilation and high-frequency ventilation are warranted, observing mean airway pressures, oxygenation, and CO_2 removal to decide which technique is most suitable. In cases of severe refractory ARDS, the last resort is the use of extracorporeal membrane oxygenation as a means of providing cardiac and pulmonary support. It is important to recognize that, in these rare situations, extracorporeal membrane oxygenation is used to manage life-threatening ARDS and not to treat the BPF per se.

Endoscopic Management of BPF

Bronchoscopy has been increasingly recognized as an essential step in the diagnostic evaluation of most respiratory diseases. It is particularly useful in BPF not only for diagnostic purposes but also as an invaluable modality of treatment. Bronchoscopy for BPF is utilized in three different settings, as follows:

1. Diagnosis: As soon as a BPF is suspected in the postoperative period following lung resection, bronchoscopy is performed to confirm the presence of a BPF,

estimate the size of the fistula, and evaluate the general conditions and viability of the bronchial stump.

2. Endoscopic closure: Bronchoscopy is done to follow the progressive course of a BPF during conservative management in the ICU. In general, the size of the communication dictates whether the patient is a candidate for instillation of a sealant material such as fibrin glue to close the fistula. If the opening is 3 mm or less, bronchoscopically instilled sealant material is usually successful. A BPF larger than 8 mm diameter requires surgical closure. The fistula must be directly visualized and trials of occlusion must convincingly show a cessation or appreciable decrease in the leak before the sealant is applied to the fistula. A large number of sealant compounds are available, and as yet no consensus exists on which provides the best results.

3. Surgical closure: Bronchoscopy is routinely performed prior to and on completion of a definitive surgical closure of a BPF.

Bronchoscopy can be performed under topical anesthesia or general anesthesia. Topical anesthesia for awake bronchoscopy is similar to that used during awake laryngoscopy and endotracheal intubation, with added topicalization of the bronchial system distal to the carina. An effective technique consists of the combination of ultrasonic nebulization (5 mL of 4% lidocaine nebulized with high O_2 flow at 8-10 L/min) followed by more distal spraying under direct visualization during fiberoptic bronchoscopy.[14] To promote delivery of the droplets to the distal bronchi, the patient is encouraged to take deep inspirations to generate a high inspiratory flow rate that will carry the droplets into the distal small airways. In severely debilitated patients unable to take deep breaths, the distal airways can be topicalized adequately through the fiberoptic bronchoscope by spraying lidocaine through the suction port either directly or through an epidural catheter inserted through it. As a general rule, meticulous airway topicalization is all that is needed, and other more invasive techniques such as superior laryngeal nerve blocks and transtracheal injection are usually redundant, since they are linked with increased risk for potential complications and minimal effects on the distal airways.

The choice of general anesthesia techniques for bronchoscopy depends on three considerations: (1) risk of pulmonary aspiration of gastric contents, (2) risk of contamination of the airway and the lungs through the fistula, and (3) risk of air leak and loss of alveolar ventilation. If the risk of gastric aspiration is minimal, the pleural cavity has been thoroughly drained, and the air leak is small, then a laryngeal mask airway (LMA) can be safely used. The important advantage is that an LMA allows room to maneuver the adult fiberoptic bronchoscope and offers unobstructed access to the bronchial stump and the fistula. If the risk of aspiration of gastric contents is high, a standard rapid sequence intubation with a single-lumen cuffed endotracheal tube should be considered. The endotracheal tube should be large enough for easy passage and maneuvering of the bronchoscope. In rare cases in which the BPF causes an unacceptable air leak or the risk of lung contamination from pleural fluid is high, a DLT is necessary for lung isolation. Maneuvering the adult bronchoscope through the relatively narrow tracheal lumen of the DLT is more difficult than maneuvering it through the LMA.

In the large majority of cases, bronchoscopy is relatively uneventful. In some high-risk patients, however, bronchoscopy may cause severe bronchoconstriction due to reactive airways and inadequate topicalization. Similarly, airway manipulation can lead to hemodynamic compromise with tachycardia, hypertension, and hypoxemia, resulting in myocardial ischemia. Finally, exaggerated suctioning of the distal airways may lead to diffuse alveolar collapse and atelectasis.

Operative Management of BPF

Optimal anesthetic management of patients requiring surgical closure of a BPF through a thoracotomy involves three important objectives: optimal management of the thoracostomy tube, proper positioning of the patient, and successful lung isolation.

1. Optimal management of the thoracostomy tube: The chest tube plays a vital role in prevention of a life-threatening pneumothorax during positive pressure ventilation under general anesthesia. It is, therefore, imperative to assure that the chest tube is well positioned in the pleural cavity. In many cases of BPF, the chest tube becomes obstructed by the thick purulent material of an empyema. If there is any doubt concerning the patency of the chest tube, the tube should be changed before induction of anesthesia. The chest tube must be kept on continuous suction up to the moment just before induction in order to keep the pleural cavity as empty as possible. After induction and before institution of positive pressure ventilation, the suction should be discontinued to limit the loss of ventilation through the fistula. To avoid the possibility of tension pneumothorax, the chest tube should never be clamped. During manual ventilation of the patient, it is important to carefully observe the amount of bubbling as different levels of inspiratory pressure are applied. This helps in estimating the size of the leak at each level. Obviously, the larger the air leak, the greater is the need for lung isolation using a DLT to prevent inadequate ventilation.

2. Positioning prior to induction: Even though a chest tube may have been in place for several days, it should never be assumed that the pleural cavity is empty and that there is no risk of bronchial contamination. If, as often happens, a collection of pus becomes loculated in the pleural cavity, the chest tube becomes ineffective. It is imperative, therefore, that the patient is properly positioned prior to induction. The head up, lateral decubitus position with the affected side down minimizes the risk of contamination of the tracheobronchial tree and lungs by pleural cavity contents.

3. Lung isolation: In the operating room, insertion of a DLT is the method of choice for securing the airway for the surgical repair of a BPF, like any other thoracotomy. Awake fiberoptic intubation with a DLT tube with the endobronchial lumen placed in the unaffected side is the safest way of managing BPF. Importantly, introduction of the DLT under direct vision with a fiberoptic bronchoscope avoids inadvertent trauma and prevents further injury to the bronchial stump and fistula. The advantage of maintaining spontaneous ventilation is that tension pneumothorax is prevented.

Some important considerations should be taken into account. If awake fiberoptic intubation is elected, it is important that airway topicalization be meticulous, since the DLT is more bulky, more difficult to insert, and involves greater irritation of the bronchus than a SLT; not only the upper part of the trachea must be topicalized, but also the areas deeper into the bronchial tree below the carina. Judicious intravenous sedation may be used sparingly, since it is imperative to maintain spontaneous breathing at all times until the DLT is successfully placed and its position carefully checked with fiber-optic bronchoscopy. Furthermore, it is advisable to use a DLT large enough to be secured in place to avoid movement and dislodgment during repeated surgical manipulations of the stump.

On rare occasions when a patient is unwilling or unable to undergo awake intubation, the DLT may be placed under inhalational anesthesia with the patient breathing spontaneously. Use of a volatile agent such as sevoflurane, which allows rapid induction with minimal airway irritation, is preferred. It is still advisable to topicalize the airway in order to abolish airway reflexes, which may still be present with inhalational anesthesia alone. In case of difficulty inserting a DLT with direct laryngoscopy, a special video laryngoscope for DLT (Airtraq yellow) can be used.

The most common ventilatory technique consists of one-lung ventilation with collapse of the affected lung (obviously not needed in cases of previous pneumonectomy). Should continuous positive airway pressure be needed for the affected lung, then the level of this pressure must be maintained below the critical pressure needed to cause air leak through the BPF. Similarly, the DLT can be ventilated via independent two-lung ventilation, using two ventilators and settings appropriate for each lung. In rare cases, high-frequency ventilation can be used. As in any other thoracotomy, the lung can be isolated with an SLT and a bronchial blocker.

Thoracic epidurals are not used for postoperative pain management because of the risk of infection. Delivery of local anesthetics to the surgical site through a regulated infusion pump and intercostal nerve blocks can supplement the use of intravenous narcotics.

PROGNOSIS

BPF is a serious condition in terms of mortality and associated costs. Depending on the series, mortality rates vary from 25% to 79%.[15] In acute bronchial stump dehiscence, fatality is associated with aspiration of pleural contents, causing either fatal asphyxia or pneumonitis. In chronic BPF, sepsis and ARDS are the main causes of death. Even if the patient ultimately recovers, the many weeks or months spent in the ICU and hospital carry considerable costs in human suffering and financial burden. The prevention of BPF is, therefore, essential.

PREVENTION

Prevention of BPF should focus on addressing the risk factors that predispose the patient to this complication. Because lung resection, especially right pneumonectomy, constitutes one of the highest risk surgeries for the development of BPF, careful selection of patients for resection is of utmost importance. Once a patient is deemed suitable for pneumonectomy, attention should be given to optimization of his overall medical condition prior to surgery. This entails treating all underlying infections, optimizing lung function, and aggressively treating comorbid conditions such as congestive heart failure and uncontrolled diabetes mellitus. For debilitated malnourished patients, the preoperative improvement of nutritional status can promote wound healing and prevent formation of a BPF.

Anesthesia and surgery providers must pay attention to maintaining strict intraoperative aseptic technique at all times. Instrumentation of the airway during intubation and placement of invasive monitoring catheters should be done with care to prevent infection. Surgical techniques are important in maintaining stump integrity and preventing stump dehiscence. It is important to meticulously appose the cartilaginous layer of the resected bronchus to the membranous layer and to preserve adequate blood supply to the stump. In high-risk patients, the surgeon may fill the hemithorax with saline solution before surgical closure and ask the anesthesiologist to provide a high inflation airway pressure of 40 cm H_2O transiently in order to detect potential bronchial stump leaks. The surgeon can place a sealant such as Gelfoam on the stump as a preventive measure. A prophylactic muscle flap must also be considered to stabilize the bronchial stump.

In the postoperative period, it is essential to extubate the patient as early as possible in order to avoid the detrimental effects of positive pressure ventilation. In cases in which the patient's respiratory status requires continued ventilatory support after pneumonectomy, the goals include limiting inflation pressures to diminish the risk of barotrauma and using aseptic technique during tracheal suctioning to prevent infection.

SUMMARY

Although rare, BPF represents a challenging management problem and is associated with high rates of morbidity and mortality. This complication is best managed by reducing the risk factors that predispose to BPF formation and in patients with an existing BPF using meticulous perioperative management strategies to reduce the risks of life-threatening loss of ventilation, tension pneumothorax, and contamination of the remaining lung through the fistula.

REFERENCES

1. Sirbu H, Busch T, Aleksic I, Schreiner W, Oster O, Dalichau H. Bronchopleural fistula in the surgery of non-small cell lung cancer: incidence, risk factors, and management. *Ann Thorac Cardiovasc Surg.* 2001;7(6):330-336.
2. Cerfolio RJ. The incidence, etiology, and prevention of postresectional bronchopleural fistula. *Semin Thorac Cardiovasc Surg.* 2001;13(1):3-7.
3. Sato M, Saito Y, Fujimura S, et al. Study of postoperative bronchopleural fistulas—analysis of factors related to bronchopleural fistulas. *Nippon Kyobu Geka Gakkai Zasshi*, 1989;37(3):498-503.
4. Sonobe M, Nakagawa M, Ichinose M, Ikegami N, Nagasawa M, Shindo T. Analysis of risk factors in bronchopleural fistula after pulmonary resection for primary lung cancer. *Eur J Cardiothorac Surg.* 2000;18(5):519-523.

5. Lauckner ME, Beggs I, Armstrong RF. The radiological characteristics of bronchopleural fistula following pneumonectomy. *Anaesthesia*. 1983;38(5):452-456.
6. Lams P. Radiographic signs in post pneumonectomy bronchopleural fistula. *J Can Assoc Radiol*. 1980;31(3):178-180.
7. Kim EA, Lee KS, Shim YM, et al. Radiographic and CT findings in complications following pulmonary resection. *Radiographics*. 2002;22(1):67-86.
8. Chae EJ, Seo JB, Kim SY, et al. Radiographic and CT findings of thoracic complications after pneumonectomy. *Radiographics*. 2006;26(5):1449-1468.
9. Westcott JL, Volpe JP. Peripheral bronchopleural fistula: CT evaluation in 20 patients with pneumonia, empyema, or postoperative air leak. *Radiology*. 1995;196(1):175-181.
10. Zelefsky MN, Freeman LM, Stern H. A simple approach to the diagnosis of bronchopleural fistula. *Radiology*. 1977;124(3):843-844.
11. Nielsen KR, Blake LM, Mark JB, DeCampli W, McDougall IR. Localization of bronchopleural fistula using ventilation scintigraphy. *J Nucl Med*. 1994;35(5):867-869.
12. Mulot A, Sepulveda S, Haberer JP, Alifano M. Diagnosis of postpneumonectomy bronchopleural fistula using inhalation of oxygen or nitrous oxide. *Anesth Analg*. 2002;95(4):1122-1123.
13. Benumof J. Anesthesia for emergency thoracic surgery. *Anesthesia for Thoracic Surgery*. 2nd ed. Philadelphia: Saunders; 1995:626-631.
14. Sanchez A, Iyer, R, Morrison, D. Preparation of the patient for awake intubation. *Benumof's Airway Management*. 2nd ed. Philadelphia: Mosby; 2007:263-277.
15. Wright CD, Wain JC, Mathisen DJ, Grillo HC. Postpneumonectomy bronchopleural fistula after sutured bronchial closure: incidence, risk factors, and management. *J Thorac Cardiovasc Surg*. 1996;112(5):1367-1371.

Anesthesia for Lung Transplantation

19

Wendy L. Pabich
Mihai V. Podgoreanu

Key Points

1. Preoperative respiratory assessment should include pulmonary function tests, ventilation/perfusion (V/Q) scans, and an arterial blood gas. The patient's ability to tolerate one-lung ventilation can be determined by V/Q scan, and if both lungs are being transplanted the lung with less perfusion should be transplanted first.
2. Cardiac function should be assessed with particular attention paid to evaluation of right ventricular (RV) function. Elevated pulmonary arterial pressures can precipitate RV failure, and may greatly influence the decision to attempt transplantation with or without CPB.
3. The newly transplanted lung should be ventilated with as low a FiO_2 as possible, ideally room air, to minimize damage by oxygen free radicals. Barotrauma to the new lung can be avoided by keeping inspiratory pressures less than 25 cm H_2O and PEEP less than 10 cm H_2O.
4. Hemodynamic instability or refractory hypoxemia may deem cardiopulmonary bypass necessary and typically occurs at one of three critical phases of the operation: (a) after pulmonary artery clamping during the first transplant; (b) after perfusing the first allograft but before starting the second lung; and, (c) after pulmonary artery clamping during the second transplant.

Case Vignette

The patient is a 45-year-old man who is listed for bilateral sequential lung transplantation due to idiopathic pulmonary fibrosis. He has undergone pulmonary rehabilitation and now continuously uses oxygen at the rate of 4 L/min. His PA pressures are 68/25. Recently his respiratory symptoms have worsened significantly and he has thus been moved to the active transplant list.

He has mild esophageal reflux disease and is otherwise well.

He takes famotidine and albuterol by mouth and is on an epoprostenol (Flolan) infusion.

Vital signs: 105/60, HR 95, SpO_2 on 4 L/min oxygen 91%.

Laboratory values are normal.

BACKGROUND

Providing anesthesia for lung transplantation (LT) is considered by many to be the *coup de maître* of cardiothoracic anesthesia. Some say it involves the most complex manipulation of cardiothoracic physiology, particularly when cardiopulmonary bypass (CPB) is not used. Many anesthetic considerations for LT are in fact similar to those for other thoracic and cardiovascular procedures; however, this chapter highlights the unique clinical elements involved in perioperative management of LT recipients and the implications for their future anesthetic care. Because LT is performed infrequently in clinical practice, typically with little opportunity for preoperative preparation and consultation, a thorough understanding of end-stage lung disease pathophysiology and its specific pharmacological and technical implications is required to minimize associated major morbidity and mortality.

Indications for LT include 4 primary diagnostic groupings of end-stage pulmonary disease: (1) *obstructive lung disease* (chronic obstructive pulmonary disease [COPD], with or without alpha-1-antitrypsin deficiency, due to chronic bronchitis and/or emphysema, and bronchiectasis); (2) *restrictive lung disease* (idiopathic pulmonary fibrosis [IPF], sarcoidosis, obliterative bronchiolitis); (3) *cystic fibrosis* or *immunodeficiency disorders* (hypogammaglobulinemia); and (4) *pulmonary vascular disease* (idiopathic pulmonary arterial hypertension, Eisenmenger syndrome). In 2007, patients with IPF comprised the single largest group of adult LT recipients (27%), while emphysema was the most common diagnosis among LT recipients before 2007.[1,2] Cystic fibrosis (CF) remains the principal indication for LT in pediatric patients older than 5 years, whereas in infants and preschool children the most common indications are idiopathic pulmonary arterial hypertension and congenital heart disease (see Figures 19–1 to 19–4).[3]

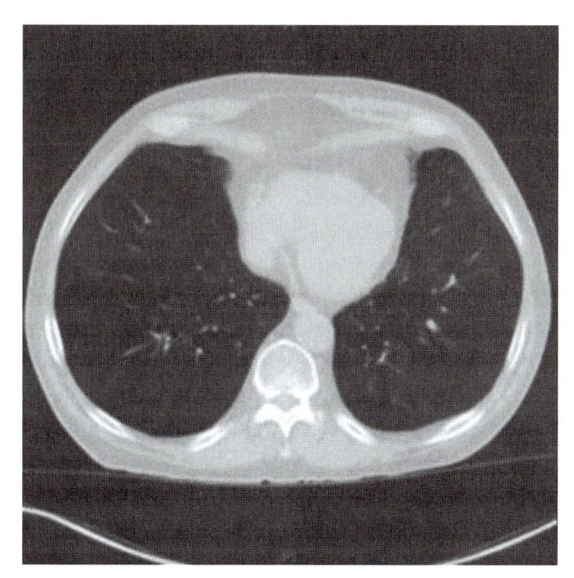

Figure 19-1. Pretransplant chest computed tomography of a patient with panlobular emphysema.

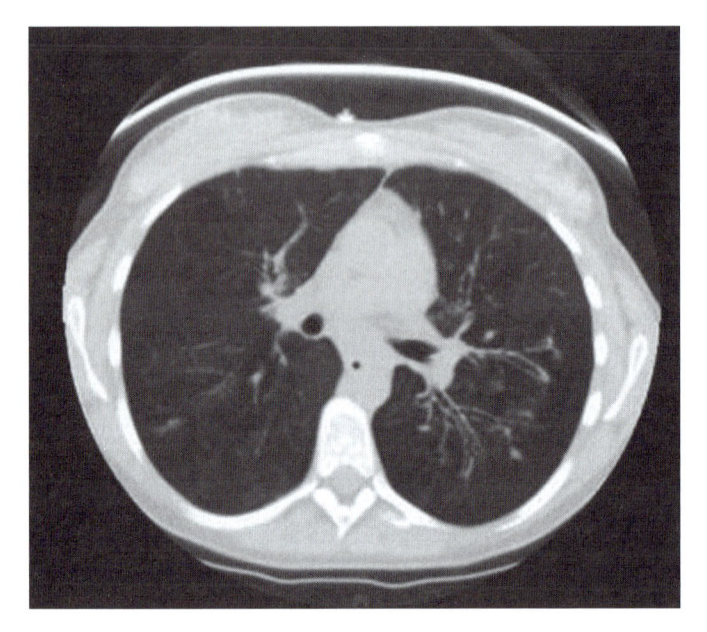

Figure 19–2. Pretransplant chest computed tomography of a patient with cystic fibrosis. Note the cystic bronchiectasis with peribronchial wall thickening.

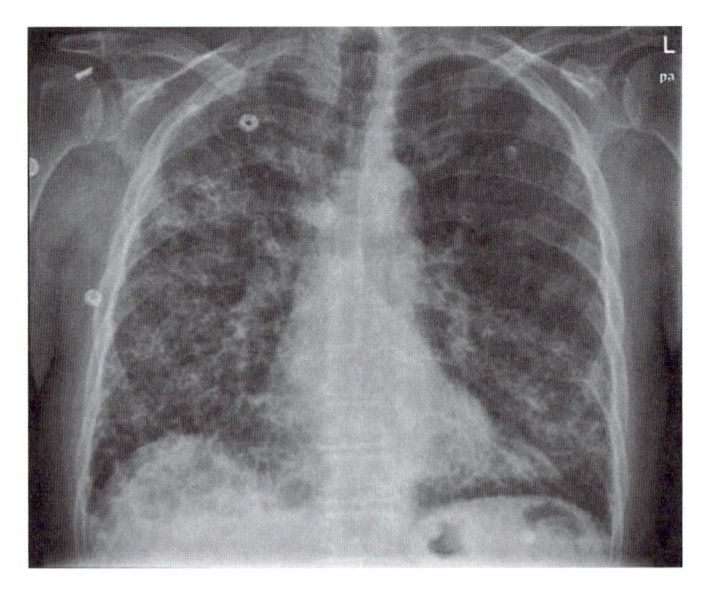

Figure 19–3. Pretransplant chest radiograph of a patient with extensive bilateral pulmonary fibrosis. The patient underwent bilateral lung transplantation.

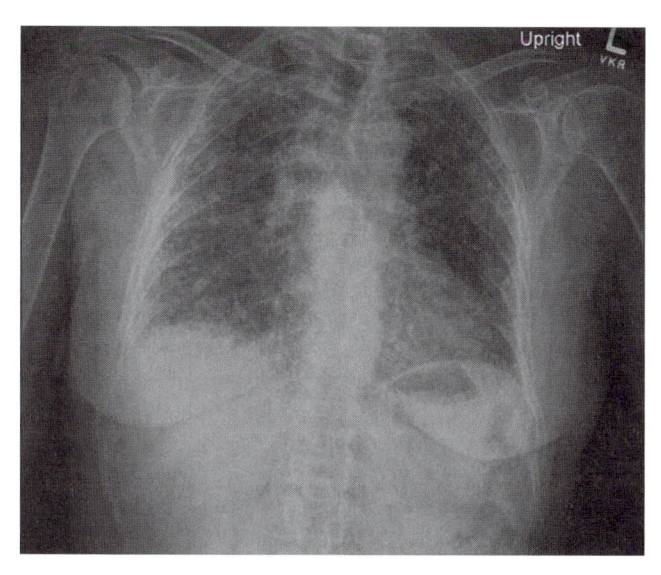

Figure 19–4. Pretransplant chest radiograph of a patient with extensive pulmonary fibrosis, right greater than left. The underwent single right lung transplantation.

The 2005 implementation of the Lung Allocation Score (LAS) system, designed to assign a relative priority score to distribute cadaveric lungs to appropriate recipients, marks the most significant change in LT in the last decade. The LAS includes measures for urgency of need for transplant and posttransplant likelihood of survival, with higher scores representing higher urgency and a greater potential transplant benefit. Adoption of the LAS system has resulted in substantial reductions in both the number of active wait-listed lung candidates and median waiting time.[2] Despite the fact that over time candidates with increasingly higher LAS scores have been receiving transplants, overall recipient survival has continued to improve by era (currently 79% at 1 year; 52% at 5 years), although this has largely been driven by improvements in 1-year survival. Recipient age has also increased consistently over time, most strikingly in patients older than 60 years (35% in 2008).[1] The total number of pediatric LTs also appears to be increasing (93 procedures in 2007), the majority of which are being performed in adolescent patients (12-17 years old).

The recipient's underlying disease process is the major determinant in selecting 1 of the 4 types of transplant procedures generally available: single-lung transplantation, bilateral lung transplantation, transplantation of lobes from living related donors, and combined procedures.

Single-Lung Transplantation

Patients whose transplanted lung will receive most of the ventilation and perfusion, as in the case of IPF or COPD, typically undergo single-lung transplantation

(SLT). Single-lung transplantation extends the limited supply of donor organs to more patients and is characterized by a decreased need for CPB, but it provides less lung function as a buffer for late complications. The procedure, which involves a pneumonectomy of the native lung followed by implantation of the lung allograft is most often performed via a standard posterolateral thoracotomy. Typically, the lung that is more affected (see Figure 19–1) based on preoperative ventilation/perfusion (V/Q) scanning or the site contralateral to a previous thoracotomy is chosen for transplant. If both lungs are equally affected, some centers will preferentially transplant the left lung because it is technically easier to access the pulmonary veins and main stem bronchus on the left side.

Bilateral Lung Transplantation

Bilateral orthotopic lung transplantation (BOLT) is most often performed as two sequential SLTs. The principal indication for BOLT is suppurative lung disease that would result in contamination of the transplanted lung by the native lung (such as in CF or generalized bronchiectasis), although the proportion of BOLT has risen for each of the 4 major indications since 1994. The number of bilateral lung transplantations being performed has steadily increased in past decades, from a trivial percentage of total lung transplants in 1990 to more than two-thirds of the 2708 LTs performed in 2007.[1] Bilateral sequential SLT procedures can be performed with or without CPB. The decision of whether or not to attempt the procedure without CPB depends upon disease severity, but emergent CPB may be required if the patient develops refractory hypoxemia during one-lung ventilation (OLV) or experiences hemodynamic instability during pulmonary artery clamping or surgical manipulation. The most commonly used surgical approach for this procedure is via a single clamshell incision (transverse thoracosternotomy), but sequential thoracotomies or median sternotomy may occasionally be used as well. A less invasive surgical approach involving limited bilateral thoracotomy guided by thoracoscopic visualization has yielded positive early results, does not preclude the use of CPB and may particularly benefit patients with impaired wound healing due to long-term glucocorticoid therapy.[4]

Double-lung transplantation *(en bloc)* using a tracheal anastomosis, although still performed, is falling out of favor because it requires CPB and because the tracheal anastomosis is more susceptible to postoperative complications than the bronchial anastomoses in BOLT.[5]

Living Donor Lung Transplantation

In some selected recipients, LT may be performed using lung tissue from 2 blood-group-compatible living donors. Use of CPB is optional for SLT unless significant pulmonary hypertension or severe hypoxemia is present. For a bilateral lobe transplant, the donor lobes are implanted in a manner similar to a bilateral sequential cadaveric LT, except that CPB is always used to avoid passing the entire cardiac output through a single donor lobe. Living donor-related lobar lung transplantation is only performed in specialized centers. Although it is thought to

Table 19-1. Potential Advantages and Disadvantages for Living Donor Lung Transplant

Advantages	Disadvantages
Potentially better short-term results due to less ischemic time and more careful lung preparation	Risk of evaluation process to donors
	Operative morbidity and mortality to donor
Immunosuppression may need to be less aggressive due to better tissue matching	
	Long-term morbidity to donor such as exercise limitation, less pulmonary reserve with infection or trauma, possible pulmonary hypertension in later years
Avoidance of a long wait at a medical center far from the patient's home	
Shorten the waiting time for others on the lung transplant	Psychological issues before and after transplant for donor and recipient
Donor and recipient satisfaction with recipient survival and improvement in quality of life	

be more beneficial in the pediatric population, the numbers of these transplants have fallen dramatically in recent years.[3] It should be reserved for patients who are judged unlikely to survive until cadaveric lungs become available. However, intubated patients and those undergoing retransplantation have a significantly high risk of mortality.[6] There is an ongoing debate about the ethical issues concerning transplantation from living donors, particularly regarding the added risk of potential complications in the donor patients, although several reports suggest that donor morbidity has been minimal.[7] Table 19-1 outlines the potential advantages and disadvantages of living donor LT.

Combined Procedures

Combined heart-lung transplantation is typically reserved for patients with idiopathic pulmonary arterial hypertension, unrepairable congenital heart disease (with Eisenmenger syndrome), or left ventricular failure (see Figure 19-5). It is performed much less frequently than other kinds of transplantation (only 86 procedures in 2007)[1] and obviously requires use of CPB.

The increased age of acceptable LT recipients has resulted in a higher incidence of concurrent cardiac disease. In well-selected patients, LT may thus be performed simultaneously with valvular or coronary artery bypass graft surgery. The cardiac procedure is usually performed first regardless of whether CPB is planned for LT, and offers a survival benefit compared to LT alone.[8]

Combined lung/liver transplantation may be beneficial in some patients with coexisting severe lung and liver disease, which can be present in CF. This particular

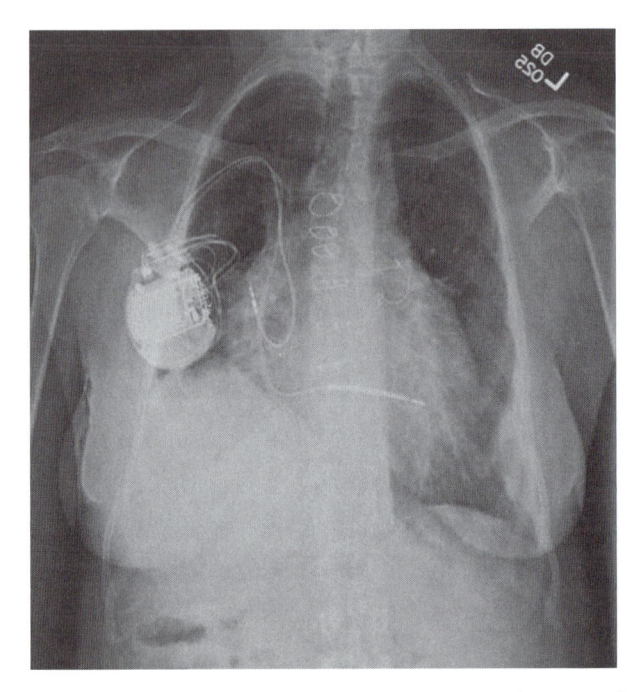

Figure 19–5. Pretransplant chest radiograph of a patient with repaired congenital heart disease but with progressive heart failure. Note the cardiomegaly, prominent right heart border and enlarged pulmonary arteries consistent with known pulmonary arterial hypertension. A heart-lung transplant is planned due to the combination of cardiac and pulmonary disease.

procedure provides a unique challenge to the anesthesiologist with regard to fluid management because the goal of such management in lung transplants typically involves restricting fluids to minimize pulmonary edema, whereas liver transplants are associated with massive transfusion and administration of fluids. The organs are typically transplanted in tandem, with the LT occurring first.

PREOPERATIVE EVALUATION AND PREPARATION

Most LT patients undergo an extensive evaluation to define their clinical condition and suitability for LT before being listed as potential transplant recipients. Preoperative workups should be easily accessible to the anesthesia team because surgery most often occurs at odd hours. Because LT candidates may experience long waits, it is important to assess any potential changes in baseline functional status since the patient's last workup by the transplant service. Anesthetic evaluation should include such routine details as fasting status, previous response to anesthesia, cardiopulmonary assessment, and airway examination, followed by a discussion about anesthetic management and risks, including death and intraoperative recall and use of postoperative thoracic epidural analgesia.[9]

The preoperative respiratory assessment should at least include pulmonary function tests, V/Q scans, and an arterial blood gas measurement. The patient's ability to tolerate OLV can be determined by V/Q scan. If both lungs are being transplanted, the more diseased lung (with less perfusion) should be transplanted first. The likelihood of requiring CPB increases if the non-operative lung has little perfusion or the room air partial pressure of oxygen (PaO_2) is less than 45 mm Hg.

Cardiac function should be assessed with particular attention to evaluating right ventricular (RV) function. Preoperative tests should include an electrocardiogram, a 24-hour Holter monitor, a transthoracic echocardiogram, and left and right cardiac catheterization (to evaluate coronary disease, left and right ventricular function, and pulmonary circulation). Pulmonary arterial pressures (PAP) may be elevated in severe lung disease and can precipitate RV failure when they exceed two-thirds of systemic arterial pressures. This can greatly influence the decision to attempt transplantation with or without CPB. Mean pulmonary arterial (PA) pressures greater than 40 mm Hg and pulmonary vascular resistance greater than 5 Wood units predict an increased likelihood that CPB will be necessary.

Patients with severe pulmonary hypertension may develop right-to-left intracardiac shunting and should be evaluated for a history of embolic events. Understandably, particular care should be taken to avoid injecting any intravascular air in these patients. The presence of a patent foramen ovale or any other intracardiac shunts should be routinely assessed preoperatively by transthoracic echocardiogram in all LT candidates. Severe pulmonary hypertension can also cause vocal cord dysfunction due to impingement of the left recurrent laryngeal nerve by the enlarged pulmonary arteries, placing these patients at an increased risk for aspiration.

Patients with CF may have associated hepatic dysfunction; therefore, liver function tests should be obtained. Many CF patients also experience malabsorption of fat-soluble vitamins from the gastrointestinal tract. Consequently, preoperative coagulation studies should be obtained, and vitamin K should be administered as necessary. Furthermore, CF and bronchiectasis patients are likely to be resistant or allergic to antibiotics and may require preoperative desensitization.

The need for additional preoperative laboratory tests should be dictated by the individual patient's disease. Preoperative hematocrit, white blood cell count, and chemistry panels should be obtained and corrected as necessary. Polycythemia may be present secondary to chronic hypoxemia, requiring special laboratory assessment. Blood group, histocompatibility antigens, and panel-reactive antibodies are routinely assessed to assist with donor matching, perioperative immunosuppression, additional preoperative treatments to reduce alloreactivity (plasmapheresis, intravenous immunoglobulin), and overall risk stratification.

Immunosuppressive induction and antibiotics may be started preoperatively, with the patient receiving the first doses orally. Preoperative sedation should be used cautiously because benzodiazepines and narcotics can exacerbate preexisting hypercarbia and hypoxia, particularly in patients with COPD. Conversely, preoperative anxiety and

Table 19–2. Suggested Intraoperative Monitors for Lung Transplant

Radial and femoral arterial lines • Radial arterial lines may kink, dampen or become dysfunctional with positioning or during surgery • Femoral artery cannulation (preinduction) to allow emergent institution of CPB if required
Continuous cardiac output oximetric pulmonary artery catheter • Placement may be difficult due to right ventricular dysfunction and pulmonary hypertension • Pull back during pulmonary artery anastomosis
Transesophageal echocardiogram • Intraoperative assessment of biventricular function • Evaluation of intracardiac shunts (patent foramen ovale) • Assessment of pulmonary arterial and venous anastomoses
Fiberoptic bronchoscope • Accurate double lumen tube placement and lung isolation • Assess bronchial anastomoses
Ventilatory measurements • Peak and mean airway pressures, lung volumes, positive end-expiratory pressure, pressure support, inspiratory-expiratory ratio • Two separate ventilators may be needed for differential lung ventilation • Nitric oxide concentration
Bispectral index

the accompanying catecholamine surge may worsen RV dysfunction in patients with pulmonary hypertension.[5]

In addition to the American Society of Anesthesiologists standard monitors, Table 19–2 lists suggested monitoring for LT to enable quick diagnosis and treatment of expected intraoperative hemodynamic and respiratory instability during one-lung ventilation (OLV) and pulmonary artery clamping.

Large-caliber peripheral venous access should be obtained to treat intravascular volume losses as they occur. Care should be taken to ensure that access remains unobstructed with standard arm positioning for a clamshell incision; antecubital lines are prone to obstruction. Central line placement before anesthetic induction may prove difficult in patients unable to lie supine without sedation and/or worsening of baseline hypoxia. Strict asepsis should be respected with all line placement given the anticipated immunosuppression in these patients. Blood products should be cross-matched and available in the operating room. At our institution, placement of thoracic epidural catheters for postoperative analgesia is deferred until the patient arrives to the intensive care unit postoperatively.

Although the recipient is prepared for surgery as soon as a potential donor has been identified, induction of anesthesia is postponed until the donor lungs have been inspected and approved by the retrieval team and confirmed with the transplant coordinator.

INTRAOPERATIVE MANAGEMENT

Lung transplant candidates are usually critically ill with severe cardiopulmonary disease, yet the nature of the transplant operation is to induce further dysfunction with OLV, surgical manipulation, intravascular volume loss, sudden change in ventilatory function, severe acid-base abnormalities, and difficulties with oxygenation.[10] Several periods are particularly critical in the intraoperative management of LT and will be discussed in greater detail below. These include induction of anesthesia, initiation of positive pressure ventilation, establishment and maintenance of OLV, pulmonary artery clamping and unclamping, and reperfusion of the pulmonary allograft. However, unanticipated problems often occur, and the anesthesiology team must be ready to react quickly and treat sudden changes in multiple physiological functions. Full cardiopulmonary bypass (CPB) support and a perfusion team are always on standby throughout the procedure.

Anesthetic Induction and Maintenance

Both denitrogenation and achievement of an amnestic end-tidal level of inhaled anesthetic are significantly slower in patients with end-stage lung disease due to increased V/Q mismatch and thus may prolong the period of vulnerability to recall at the beginning of the procedure.[5]

Rapid-sequence or modified rapid-sequence induction is usually indicated, as the procedure is typically urgent and patients may not have been fasting. Agents with minimal cardiac depressant effects are preferred, including etomidate and narcotics, but hypnotic agents, including ketamine, propofol, and midazolam, have also been used.[11] Attention to hemodynamic changes with slow titration of induction agents is critical for a safe induction, but profound hypotension and ventricular depression can occur and is counteracted with small fluid boluses, inotropes, and pulmonary vasodilators.[5] Patients with end-stage lung disease are in general at least moderately hypovolemic due to preoperative diuretics and increased insensible losses from the increased work of breathing. Although intraoperative fluid restriction is of paramount importance in the overall management of LT, as the resultant pulmonary edema can compromise allograft function,[12] judicious preoperative fluid boluses may attenuate the hemodynamic effects of anesthetic induction and positive-pressure ventilation. In patients with severe pulmonary hypertension, induction should begin only with an available surgeon in the operating room and typically after femoral arterial cannulation to facilitate emergent CPB in the case of cardiac arrest.[9]

Once the position is verified via fiberoptic bronchoscopy, rapid airway control should be accomplished using either a double-lumen endotracheal tube (DLT) or a single-lumen tube with an endobronchial blocker, depending on institutional practices. A DLT is preferred at our institution because it facilitates better lung isolation, suctioning, application of continuous positive airway pressure (CPAP) to the non-ventilated lung, and permits independent lung ventilation. Further, a left-sided DLT is preferred because the position of the bronchial lumen should not interfere with surgical access to the left main stem bronchus. A single-lumen tube is sufficient in situations when use of CPB is planned electively.

Anesthesia can be maintained with an inhaled agent such as isoflurane, although, as stated above, end-stage lung disease may impact the uptake of inhaled agents. Total intravenous anesthesia may be more predictable, and it better preserves hypoxic pulmonary vasoconstriction that is otherwise blunted with inhaled anesthetics. Moreover, to avoid cardiac depression from volatile anesthetics, many centers rely on a narcotic-based "cardiac anesthetic," which provides improved hemodynamic stability. One note of caution concerning narcotic-based techniques is that initiation of CPB, removal of the native lung, and reperfusion of the transplanted lung are all critical in the pharmacokinetic profiles of narcotics. All narcotics are subject to a decrease in plasma concentration when CPB is initiated. Fentanyl concentrations decrease the most due to binding to the CPB circuit. The lungs also provide a significant "first pass" effect on narcotics, with approximately 60% of sufentanil and 75% of fentanyl undergoing uptake.[13] The implication of this pharmacokinetic profile is that when the native lung is removed, a significant dose of narcotic is also removed. Plasma levels of narcotics will further decrease upon reperfusion of the newly transplanted lung due to the same "first pass" effect. At a time of hemodynamic instability associated with allograft reperfusion, volatile agents may be below the minimum alveolar concentration required to produce amnesia, and a reduction in plasma concentration of narcotics may increase susceptibility to intraoperative awareness or recall. As such, narcotics should be redosed and used in combination with benzodiazepines, volatile agents (if tolerated), or propofol infusion for maintenance of anesthesia.[5] Paralysis will be necessary throughout the procedure and long-acting neuromuscular blocking agents are ideal.

Positioning for the procedure depends upon the type of operation performed and can determine the optimal choice for sites of invasive monitoring. Single-lung transplantation can be done either with the patient supine or in lateral decubitus. Bilateral lung transplantation is often performed with the patient in the supine position with the arms above the head for transsternal bilateral thoracotomy. Once the patient is positioned, airway access can become difficult and intravenous and arterial lines in the upper extremities can be easily occluded. Pressure points should be carefully checked and padded.

After intubation, a transesophageal echocardiography (TEE) probe should be inserted. This allows for direct assessment of dynamic changes in cardiac function (particularly in the right ventricle), preload optimization, evaluation for intracardiac shunts (eg, patent foramen ovale), intracardiac air/assisting with de-airing maneuvers, calculation of PA pressures, and postoperative assessment of vascular anastomotic sites for stenosis, torsion, or kinking. Continuous intraoperative TEE monitoring allows for early recognition of critical events and informs therapeutic interventions.[14]

Intraoperative normothermia should be aggressively maintained unless CPB is planned electively because hypothermia can worsen pulmonary hypertension and coagulopathy and delay extubation.

Mechanical Ventilation

Initiation of positive-pressure ventilation in patients with end-stage lung disease can be associated with many complications. High airway pressure in patients with restrictive lung disease and in those with COPD-associated blebs can lead directly to *barotrauma* (pneumothorax, pneumomediastinum, or air leakage through bronchial anastomoses) or indirectly to *volutrauma* (lung hyperinflation and circulatory collapse). The risk for these complications can be minimized by adequate selection of ventilator settings based on the patient's preoperative values because most of these patients have adapted to levels outside the normal range. Tolerating such "permissive hypercapnia" reduces the adverse effects of mechanical ventilation, although it should be noted that hypercapnia can exacerbate pulmonary hypertension.[9] Although the general benefits of limiting tidal volume and airway pressures have been proven in all thoracic surgical patients including LT patients, based on current evidence, there does not appear to be a clear advantage of one ventilation mode over another (ie, volume-controlled versus pressure-controlled ventilation).[15]

Patients who have severe airflow obstruction are also at increased risk of dynamic hyperinflation during positive pressure ventilation. This results in residual positive end-expiratory pressure (auto-PEEP) and can lead to severe hypotension and even cardiac arrest caused by lung overinflation that results in reduced venous return and direct compression of the heart. In such patients, ventilation settings should maximize expiratory time, avoid extrinsic PEEP, and even include periods of circuit disconnect/apnea if hypotension persists.[9]

Maneuvers to improve oxygenation during OLV include increased fraction of inspired oxygen (FiO_2), titrating PEEP, intermittent reinflation, CPAP to the nonventilated lung, recruitment maneuvers, and fiberoptic-guided suctioning of secretions. Irreversible hypoxemia that develops during OLV can be managed by clamping the pulmonary artery to eliminate the shunt through the deflated, unventilated lung. Further refractory hypoxemia, hemodynamic instability, and/or compromised surgical access at this stage are indications for CPB, which will be discussed later.

Surgical dissection during OLV may be complicated by adhesions from previous thoracic surgery or vascular collaterals. The phrenic and vagus nerves must be safeguarded, and the recurrent laryngeal nerve must be avoided on the left side.

Pulmonary Artery Clamping

As discussed above, clamping of the pulmonary artery that supplies the nonventilated lung improves V/Q matching, oxygenation, and ABG values. The ensuing significant increase in PA pressures is usually well tolerated in patients with normal baseline values but may quickly precipitate RV dysfunction and failure in patients with pre-existing pulmonary hypertension. This results in a vicious cycle—due to ventricular interdependence, RV dilation leads to impaired left ventricular (LV) filling, LV failure, RV ischemia, and further dysfunction. Signs of RV dysfunction include elevated right atrial pressures and new or worsened tricuspid valve regurgitation associated with a dilated and hypocontractile RV on intraoperative TEE. Treatment involves judicious use of pulmonary vasodilators and inotropes. Vasodilators such as nitroglycerin, sodium nitroprusside, and nicardipine can be used to treat pulmonary hypertension, although care must be taken to avoid causing simultaneous systemic hypotension. Gas exchange and V/Q mismatch can generally be worsened by administration of vasodilators through blunting of hypoxic pulmonary vasoconstriction, although this is less of an issue in this setting, where the PA supplying the deflated lung is clamped. Inhaled nitric oxide (iNO) at concentrations up to 20 ppm is usually effective in decreasing the PAP and reducing the RV workload without negatively affecting the systemic circulation.

Right heart failure can be treated with inotropes such as epinephrine (0.02-0.1 mcg/kg/min), dopamine (2-10 mcg/kg/min), norepinephrine (0.05-0.2 mcg/kg/min), milrinone (0.375-0.5 mcg/kg/min), or a combination of agents. Fluid loading should be used cautiously because RV function may deteriorate rapidly. Initiation of CPB should be considered after adequate heparinization if the patient remains hemodynamically labile despite pharmacologic intervention.

Pulmonary Artery Unclamping and Reperfusion

Once the native lung is extracted and the donor lung implanted, three anastomoses are performed in their posterior-anterior anatomic sequence: bronchus, pulmonary artery, and pulmonary veins-left atrium. The ischemic period ends when the vascular clamps are removed, but arterial oxygenation will not improve until ventilation is resumed. The pulmonary artery should not be unclamped until ventilation of the newly transplanted lung is possible, as perfusion of the unventilated lung would cause profound hypoxia. The newly transplanted lung should be ventilated with as low an FiO_2 as possible (ideally room air) to minimize damage by oxygen free radicals. Barotrauma to the new lung can be avoided by keeping inspiratory pressures below 25 cm H_2O and PEEP below 10 cm H_2O. In SLT recipients, it may be beneficial to ventilate the lungs independently, and the appropriate ventilators should be made available. If oxygenation is marginal, an alveolar recruitment maneuver can be performed. This procedure has been shown to effectively increase arterial oxygenation, promote lung homogeneity, and minimize shear forces. The recruitment strategy typically consists of pressure-controlled ventilation; an increase in inspiratory time to 50%; and a sequential increase in positive inspiratory pressure/PEEP to 40/20, held for 10 breaths, and returned to baseline, which usually includes a PEEP of 8 cm H_2O. However, the hemodynamic effects of recruitment maneuvers can be significant and may be minimized if more selective lobar recruitment maneuvers are performed.[15]

Reperfusion injury results in increased alveolar-arterial gradients, poor lung compliance, and pulmonary edema. It may appear within minutes to hours after reperfusion. Limiting lung volumes and PEEP can lessen the risk of reperfusion injury and primary graft dysfunction (PGD). Methylprednisolone (500 mg) is administered at the time of each lung reperfusion to help prevent acute allograft rejection.

Although unclamping the pulmonary artery should decrease pulmonary vascular resistance and lessen RV afterload, RV dysfunction can persist if allograft perfusion is suboptimal. Moreover, unclamping can result in air emboli that can travel to the coronary circulation, pointing to the importance of thoroughly de-airing the pulmonary artery and left atrium upon completion of the pulmonary vein anastomoses. The right coronary artery is most likely to be affected due to its anterior location in the supine patient, leading to an increased likelihood of RV ischemia. Although these changes are usually transient, increased vasopressor and inotropic support may be necessary.

Intraoperative TEE is essential at this stage to assess ventricular function, assist with de-airing maneuvers, and thoroughly evaluate all pulmonary vascular anastomoses to identify any hemodynamically significant obstructions that require immediate repair. Unrecognized anastomotic stenoses or kinks could precipitate pulmonary venous congestion, elevated PAP, and further right heart dysfunction, as well as allograft dysfunction. Similarly, intraoperative bronchoscopy is performed at the end of the procedure to inspect the bronchial anastomotic sites for stenoses and areas of limited focal necrosis. The bronchial anastomosis has been the most vulnerable site for complications, primarily due to the disruption in bronchial blood supply to the donor lung such that the donor bronchus is dependent upon retrograde bronchial blood flow through the pulmonary circulation.

Cardiopulmonary Bypass

Although CPB is obligatory in pediatric recipients, patients with severe pulmonary vascular disease, and in bilateral living lobar LT and combined heart-lung transplant, the need for CPB in other patient categories has generally been difficult to predict preoperatively and varies with recipient disease (Table 19–3). Though rarely indicated in recipients with obstructive lung disease, several series have reported the use of CPB in 17% to 41% of patients with restrictive lung disease.[16-18] In the case of SLT, preoperative pulmonary function tests and resting oxygenation have poor discriminatory capability, but preoperative hemodynamic profiles may be helpful. In particular, patients with severe pulmonary hypertension are more likely to require CPB. As discussed, pulmonary vascular resistance always increases with clamping of the pulmonary artery; a more severe increase is seen in patients with restrictive versus obstructive disease, but the need for CPB is ultimately determined by the degree of change in cardiac index. In patients with restrictive disease, CPB has usually been necessary if the reduction in cardiac index exceeded 1 to 1.5 L/min/m^2.[16,17]

Unlike SLT, in the case of adult bilateral lung transplantation, the preoperative hemodynamic profile is a poor predictor of need for CPB.[16,18] Rather, CPB is triggered by hemodynamic instability or refractory hypoxemia typically occurring at 1 of 3 critical phases of the operation: (1) after PA clamping during the first transplant; (2) after perfusing the first allograft but before starting the second lung; and (3) after PA clamping during the second transplant. In several series of patients without pulmonary vascular disease, CPB was instituted in 23% to 32% cases at one of these time points.[16,18]

Table 19–3. Indications for Extracorporeal Assistance During Lung Transplantation

Elective
• Significant pre-existing pulmonary hypertension and/or hypoxemia that preclude the use of one-lung ventilation (eg, primary pulmonary hypertension, idiopathic pulmonary fibrosis)
• Baseline pulmonary arterial pressure >2/3 of systemic arterial pressure
• Living-related bilateral lobar lung transplant
• Combined heart-lung transplant
Emergent
• Deterioration of native lung function during one-lung ventilation
• Intractable hypoxemia
• Markedly increased arterial to alveolar pCO_2 ratio
• Acute pulmonary edema unresponsive to therapy
• Acute cardiac decompensation (usually right heart failure following clamping of the pulmonary artery)
• Reduction of >30% in cardiac output during trial of PA clamping
• Doubling of pulmonary vascular resistance
• Increase in systolic PA pressure to >80% of systemic arterial pressure
• Severe wall motion abnormalities with RV distension and septal bulging on TEE
• Vasodilation leading to refractory hypotension
Advantages of extracorporeal membrane oxygenation (ECMO) over cardiopulmonary bypass (CPB)
• Easier insertion
• Avoidance of full heparinization
• Shorter surgical time
• Ability to extend into early postoperative period

Data modified from Grichnik KP, Stafford-Smith M. Anesthetic considerations for lung transplant and thoracic aortic surgery. In: Reves JH, Reeves S, Abernathy JH (eds.). *Atlas of Cardiothoracic Anesthesia*, 2nd edition. New York: Current Medicine Group, Springer, 2009.

Although elective use of CPB for BOLT in patients with COPD does not appear to have adverse effects on early graft function or clinical outcomes,[19] these conclusions should not be extrapolated to SLT, to diseases other than COPD, or to different operative scenarios, such as emergent use of CPB.

POSTOPERATIVE MANAGEMENT

Early postoperative care focuses on ventilatory support, hemodynamic management, immunosuppression, detection of early rejection, and prevention or treatment of infection. If independent lung ventilation is not necessary, the DLT should be exchanged intraoperatively for a single-lumen endotracheal tube at the end of the procedure after suctioning the stomach to prevent any aspiration of gastric contents into the newly transplanted lung(s). The patient is transferred intubated to the intensive care unit where mechanical ventilation continues with minimal FiO_2 and low-level

PEEP. Exceptions are patients undergoing SLT for COPD or emphysema, where PEEP should not be used because it tends to overinflate the more compliant lung.[20]

With an overall incidence variously reported between 10% and 25%, postoperative respiratory failure resulting from PGD is responsible for more than half of early mortality following LT. Recipient, donor, and therapy-related risk factors for PGD include: recipient body mass index greater than 25 kg/m^2 and female sex; primary or secondary pulmonary hypertension; idiopathic or secondary pulmonary fibrosis: donor age greater than 45 years and donor head trauma; SLT; increased ischemic time; intraoperative hemorrhage or cardiovascular complications; and use of CPB in patients with severe RV dysfunction.[21-23] Ischemia-reperfusion injury is the main cause of PGD, with an incidence between 10% and 15%. To standardize the definition of PGD, a grading system has been proposed based on the PaO_2/FiO_2 ratio,[24] which strongly correlates with poor early outcomes.[25] Management of PGD is supportive, including independent lung ventilation and, *in extremis,* extracorporeal membrane oxygenation (ECMO). The role of inhaled nitric oxide (iNO) in improving hemodynamics and ventilation-perfusion matching and reducing the incidence of ischemia-reperfusion injury and pulmonary edema in LT remains controversial.[26-28] The usual recommended concentration of iNO is 10 to 20 ppm. Methemoglobinemia is a potential side effect of iNO and occurs in about 6% of patients. Nebulized epoprostenol (prostacyclin) has been proposed as an alternative to iNO with comparable results.[26,29]

ECMO is reserved for severe, life-threatening primary graft failure (selected grade 3) in patients who do not respond to maximal conventional treatment and a trial of iNO.[30-33] ECMO is a supportive measure to optimize gas exchange during lung function recovery while avoiding the detrimental effects of aggressive mechanical ventilation and persistent severe hypoxemia, and it has been associated with a survival rate of 42% in one series of patients with PGD.[31] Available evidence suggests that ECMO should be initiated within 24 hours of onset of severe PGD and should not be prolonged given the substantial morbidities associated with its use: bleeding, renal failure, neurologic problems, hypotension, and sepsis.[31] When the patient does not require hemodynamic support, veno-venous ECMO should be used instead of veno-arterial ECMO. Retransplantation for PGD is associated with very poor outcomes and is usually avoided.

Some degree of pulmonary edema almost invariably occurs after LT due to increased vascular permeability and severed lymphatic drainage. To minimize lung water, pulmonary capillary wedge pressure should be kept as low as possible; ie, it should be kept consistent with adequate urine output, oxygen delivery, and systemic blood pressure. Combinations of vasopressor, inotropic, and diuretic drugs should be used as needed to achieve this balance. In a retrospective study, elevated central venous pressure (>7 mm Hg) was positively correlated with duration of mechanical ventilation and higher rates of intensive care unit utilization, hospitalization, and 2-month mortality.[34] It remains unclear, though, whether a strategy aimed at maintaining central venous pressure <7 mm Hg would improve outcomes in LT or whether a high central venous pressure was merely a marker of severity of illness. A recent study reported a positive association between volume of intraoperative colloid (predominantly gelatin) and early lung allograft dysfunction, independent of known confounders such as use of CPB, pulmonary artery, and central venous pressures.[12] The optimal choice of fluid for volume replacement post-LT remains unknown. Our institution favors the use of blood products to achieve a target hemoglobin level of 10 mg/dL, supplemented with colloid instead of crystalloid solutions if further volume replacement is necessary.

Differential diagnosis of persistent postoperative hypotension following LT includes the usual culprits (intravascular volume depletion, blood loss, acute myocardial injury, dysrhythmias, and auto-PEEP), but a high index of suspicion should be maintained for tension pneumothorax, pneumopericardium, and pericardial tamponade, which have all been described in LT patients.[35] Excessive postoperative bleeding is particularly troublesome in patients undergoing heart-lung transplant and is usually due to the aortopulmonary collaterals in the chest wall and adhesions from previous thoracic surgeries, as well as impaired liver function from longstanding congestion and poor RV function. Myocardial injury can result from intraoperative coronary artery air embolism, cardiac manipulation during the procedure, postoperative coronary artery embolism of small thrombi from the left atrial pulmonary venous anastomosis, or preexisting coronary artery disease. Atrial dysrhythmias (primarily flutter and fibrillation) are common postoperatively in LT recipients (40%) and respond to conventional treatments, but methods to prevent their occurrence have not been studied.[36] Pulmonary embolism should also be included in the differential diagnosis because LT recipients, like other patients undergoing major surgery, are at increased thromboembolic risk.[37]

Following completion of a V/Q scan and a surveillance bronchoscopy in the early postoperative period, patients without any evidence of ventilatory or hemodynamic instability quickly progress toward weaning from mechanical ventilation. Exceptions are recipients with pulmonary hypertension, especially after SLT, in whom ventilation, sedation, and neuromuscular blockade are usually continued for 1 to 2 days because of their extremely labile oxygenation and hemodynamics during this period.

Weaning from mechanical ventilation can be hindered if the phrenic or recurrent laryngeal nerves have been injured during the procedure. The reported incidence of diaphragmatic paralysis following LT ranges from 3% to 30%, with even higher incidence following heart-lung transplantation (40%).[38,39] A low threshold for tracheostomy is adopted in these patients to facilitate weaning from mechanical ventilation and usually results in longer duration of hospitalization but it is not associated with serious long-term sequelae.[39]

A thoracic epidural catheter for postoperative pain control is placed once the potential need for CPB and heparinization has passed and after appropriate coagulation status has been confirmed. At our institution, the catheter is placed while the patient is still intubated in lateral decubitus. Analgesia can be obtained using epidural narcotics with or without local anesthetics.

Extreme care must be taken throughout the postoperative period to avoid aspiration, which can be catastrophic in these patients. Since both gastroesophageal reflux and gastroparesis are common in LT recipients, early aggressive surgical treatment of reflux (fundoplication) is routinely performed at our institution and has been shown to prevent chronic allograft dysfunction.[40]

Immunosuppression in LT recipients is typically started preoperatively while induction doses of cyclosporine and/or azathioprine and boluses of methylprednisolone

(500-1000 mg) are given intraoperatively prior to reperfusion of each graft. Immunosuppression is continued postoperatively usually using a 3-drug maintenance regimen consisting of cyclosporine or tacrolimus, azathioprine or mycophenolate mofetil, and prednisone. Transbronchial lung biopsies have a high sensitivity for detecting acute rejection or *Cytomegalovirus* (CMV) infection in LT recipients but are inconsistent in diagnosing chronic rejection.

Broad-spectrum antibiotics are routinely continued perioperatively in order to suppress any potential pathogens isolated from either donor or recipient. Absent specific culture results, empiric coverage with 1.5 g of cefuroxime taken 3 times daily is initiated until cultures become available. If fungal species are isolated in early specimens, empiric fluconazole (for *Candida* species) and either itraconazole or nebulized amphotericin B (for *Aspergillus* species) should be added to the regimen.

ANESTHESIA AFTER LUNG TRANSPLANTATION

Important physiologic changes occur following LT, some of them specific to the type of procedure or to the pretransplant lung pathology. General physiologic changes after LT include denervation of the transplanted lung associated with bronchial hyperresponsiveness; impaired cough reflex and mucociliary clearance,

Table 19–4. Anesthetic Considerations for Nonthoracic Procedures after Lung Transplantation

Airway
- Bronchial constrictions/stents at prior anastomotic lines
- Do not blindly advance single or double-lumen ETT into the bronchial anastomosis
- Impaired mucociliary transport: need assistance clearing secretions
- Denervated lungs with reduced cough reflex, potential recurrent laryngeal nerve injury: aspiration risk

Altered physiologic variables
- Diabetes, hypertension, hyperlipidemia, renal insufficiency (posttransplant medical regimen)
- Possible diaphragmatic paralysis, reduces functional reserve capacity

Immunosuppression
- Increased infection risk
- Increased risk of lymphoproliferative disease such as B-cell lymphoma and other malignancies
- Continue immunosuppressive regimen perioperatively

Potential for lung injury
- Disrupted lung lymphatics: increased risk for pulmonary edema
- Lung protective strategy: low tidal volume, low PEEP, minimize FiO_2
- Limit intraoperative fluid administration

Potentially difficult vascular access

Modified with permission from Grichnik KP, Stafford-Smith M. Anesthetic considerations for lung transplant and thoracic aortic surgery. In: Reves JH, Reeves S, Abernathy JH (eds.). *Atlas of Cardiothoracic Anesthesia*, 2nd edition. New York: Current Medicine Group, Springer, 2009.

which increase the risk of aspiration and respiratory infections; and a constellation of gastroesophageal disorders including oropharyngeal dysphagia, gastroesophageal reflux, and gastroparesis. As discussed above, diaphragmatic paralysis may occur in up to 30% of transplant recipients, most commonly in those receiving heart-lung transplants. Implications for future anesthetics include the potential for cardiac denervation, increased infectious risk, immunosuppressant toxicity and medication interaction, as well as the potential for airway strictures, aspiration, and difficulty in clearing secretions (Table 19–4).

REFERENCES

1. Christie JD, Edwards LB, Aurora P, et al. The registry of the international society for heart and lung transplantation: twenty-sixth official adult lung and heart-lung transplantation report-2009. *J Heart Lung Transplant.* 2009;28(10):1031-1049.
2. US Department of Health and Human Services HRaSA, Healthcare Systems Bureau, Division of Transplantation, Rockville, MD. *2008 Annual Report of the U.S. Organ Procurement and Transplantation Network and the Scientific Registry of Transplant Recipients: Transplant Data 1998-2007.*
3. Aurora P, Edwards LB, Christie JD, et al. Registry of the international society for heart and lung transplantation: twelfth official pediatric lung and heart/lung transplantation report-2009. *J Heart Lung Transplant.* 2009;28(10):1023-1030.
4. Fischer S, Struber M, Simon AR, et al. Video-assisted minimally invasive approach in clinical bilateral lung transplantation. *J Thorac Cardiovasc Surg.* 2001;122(6):1196-1198.
5. Miranda A, Zink R, McSweeney M. Anesthesia for lung transplantation. *Semin Cardiothorac Vasc Anesth.* 2005;9(3):205-212.
6. Starnes VA, Bowdish ME, Woo MS, et al. A decade of living lobar lung transplantation: recipient outcomes. *J Thorac Cardiovasc Surg.* 2004;127(1):114-122.
7. Bowdish ME, Barr ML, Schenkel FA, et al. A decade of living lobar lung transplantation: perioperative complications after 253 donor lobectomies. *Am J Transplant.* 2004;4(8):1283-1238.
8. Patel VS, Palmer SM, Messier RH, et al. Clinical outcome after coronary artery. revascularization and lung transplantation. *Ann Thorac Surg.* 2003;75(2):372-377; discussion 377.
9. Myles PS. Aspects of anesthesia for lung transplantation. *Semin Cardiothorac Vasc Anesth.* 1998;2:140-154.
10. Rosenberg AL, Rao M, Benedict PE. Anesthetic implications for lung transplantation. *Anesthesiol Clin North America.* 2004;22(4):767-788.
11. Myles PS, Weeks AM, Buckland MR, et al. Anesthesia for bilateral sequential lung transplantation: experience of 64 cases. *J Cardiothorac Vasc Anesth.* 1997;11(2):177-183.
12. McIlroy DR, Pilcher DV, Snell GI. Does anaesthetic management affect early outcomes after lung transplant? An exploratory analysis. *Br J Anaesth.* 2009;102(4):506-514.
13. Stoelting RK. *Pharmacology and Physiology in Anesthetic Practice.* Philadelphia, PA: Lippincott-Raven; 2005.
14. Serra E, Feltracco P, Barbieri S, et al. Transesophageal echocardiography during lung transplantation. *Transplant Proc.* 2007;39(6):1981-1982.
15. Lytle FT, Brown DR. Appropriate ventilatory settings for thoracic surgery: intraoperative and postoperative. *Semin Cardiothorac Vasc Anesth.* 2008;12(2):97-108.
16. de Hoyos A, Demajo W, Snell G, et al. Preoperative prediction for the use of cardiopulmonary bypass in lung transplantation. *J Thorac Cardiovasc Surg.* 1993;106(5):787-795; discussion 795-796.
17. Hirt SW, Haverich A, Wahlers T, et al. Predictive criteria for the need of extracorporeal circulation in single-lung transplantation. *Ann Thorac Surg.* 1992;54(4):676-680.
18. Triantafillou AN, Pasque MK, Huddleston CB, et al. Predictors, frequency, and indications for cardiopulmonary bypass during lung transplantation in adults. *Ann Thorac Surg.* 1994;57(5):1248-1251.
19. Szeto WY, Kreisel D, Karakousis GC, et al. Cardiopulmonary bypass for bilateral sequential lung transplantation in patients with chronic obstructive pulmonary disease without adverse effect on lung function or clinical outcome. *J Thorac Cardiovasc Surg.* 2002;124(2):241-249.

20. Yonan NA, el-Gamel A, Egan J, et al. Single lung transplantation for emphysema: predictors for native lung hyperinflation. *J Heart Lung Transplant.* 1998;17(2):192-201.
21. Kuntz CL, Hadjiliadis D, Ahya VN, et al. Risk factors for early primary graft dysfunction after lung transplantation: a registry study. *Clin Transplant.* 2009;23(6):819-830.
22. Meyers BF, de la Morena M, Sweet SC, et al. Primary graft dysfunction and other selected complications of lung transplantation: a single-center experience of 983 patients. *J Thorac Cardiovasc Surg.* 2005;129(6):1421-1429.
23. Chatila WM, Furukawa S, Gaughan JP, et al. Respiratory failure after lung transplantation. *Chest.* 2003;123(1):165-173.
24. Christie JD, Carby M, Bag R, et al. Report of the ISHLT Working Group on primary lung graft dysfunction part II: definition. a consensus statement of the International Society for Heart and Lung Transplantation. *J Heart Lung Transplant.* 2005(10);24:1454-1459.
25. Whitson BA, Nath DS, Johnson AC, et al. Risk factors for primary graft dysfunction after lung transplantation. *J Thorac Cardiovasc Surg.* 2006;131(1):73-80.
26. Khan TA, Schnickel G, Ross D, et al. A prospective, randomized, crossover pilot study of inhaled nitric oxide versus inhaled prostacyclin in heart transplant and lung transplant recipients. *J Thorac Cardiovasc Surg.* 2009;138(6):1417-1424.
27. Date H, Triantafillou AN, Trulock EP, et al. Inhaled nitric oxide reduces human lung allograft dysfunction. *J Thorac Cardiovasc Surg.* 1996;111(5):913-919.
28. Meade MO, Granton JT, Matte-Martyn A, et al. A randomized trial of inhaled nitric oxide to prevent ischemia-reperfusion injury after lung transplantation. *Am J Respir Crit Care Med.* 2003;167(11):1483-1489.
29. Fiser SM, Cope JT, Kron IL, et al. Aerosolized prostacyclin (epoprostenol) as an alternative to inhaled nitric oxide for patients with reperfusion injury after lung transplantation. *J Thorac Cardiovasc Surg.* 2001;121(5):981-982.
30. Bermudez CA, Adusumilli PS, McCurry KR, et al. Extracorporeal membrane oxygenation for primary graft dysfunction after lung transplantation: long-term survival. *Ann Thorac Surg.* 2009;87(3):854-860.
31. Fischer S, Bohn D, Rycus P, et al. Extracorporeal membrane oxygenation for primary graft dysfunction after lung transplantation: analysis of the Extracorporeal Life Support Organization (ELSO) registry. *J Heart Lung Transplant.* 2007;26(5):472-477.
32. Shargall Y, Guenther G, Ahya VN, et al. Report of the ISHLT Working Group on primary lung graft dysfunction part VI: treatment. *J Heart Lung Transplant.* 2005;24(10):1489-1500.
33. Dahlberg PS, Prekker ME, Herrington CS, et al. Medium-term results of extracorporeal membrane oxygenation for severe acute lung injury after lung transplantation. *J Heart Lung Transplant.* 2004;23(8):979-984.
34. Pilcher DV, Scheinkestel CD, Snell GI, et al. High central venous pressure is associated with prolonged mechanical ventilation and increased mortality after lung transplantation. *J Thorac Cardiovasc Surg.* 2005;129(4):912-918.
35. Lasocki S, Castier Y, Geffroy A, et al. Early cardiac tamponade due to tension pneumopericardium after bilateral lung transplantation. *J Heart Lung Transplant.* 2007;26(10):1069-1071.
36. Nielsen TD, Bahnson T, Davis RD, et al. Atrial fibrillation after pulmonary transplant. *Chest.* 2004;126(2):496-500.
37. Kroshus TJ, Kshettry VR, Hertz MI, et al. Deep venous thrombosis and pulmonary embolism after lung transplantation. *J Thorac Cardiovasc Surg.* 1995;110(2):540-544.
38. Ferdinande P, Bruyninckx F, Van Raemdonck D, et al. Phrenic nerve dysfunction after heart-lung and lung transplantation. *J Heart Lung Transplant.* 2004;23(1):105-109.
39. Sheridan PHJ, Cheriyan A, Doud J, et al. Incidence of phrenic neuropathy after isolated lung transplantation. The Loyola University Lung Transplant Group. *J Heart Lung Transplant.* 1995;14(4):684-691.
40. Cantu Er, Appel JZr, Hartwig MG, et al; J. Maxwell Chamberlain Memorial Paper. Early fundoplication prevents chronic allograft dysfunction in patients with gastroesophageal reflux disease. *Ann Thorac Surg.* 2004;78(4):1142-1151; discussion.

Thoracic Trauma Management

Brendan L. Howes
Mark L. Shapiro

Key Points

1. Frequent causes of immediate death must be ruled out during the *primary survey*. These include (1) critical airway obstruction, (2) tension pneumothorax, (3) open pneumothorax, (4) massive hemothorax, and (5) cardiac tamponade.
2. Adequate management of rib fracture pain using multimodal analgesia is critical in preventing further morbidity and mortality.
3. Delayed repair of aortic transection can be associated with improved mortality, and endovascular stent grafting may become the technique of choice for definitive treatment of BTAI.

Clinical Vignette

This 22-year-old male was the unrestrained passenger of a pickup truck who suffered a head-on collision at high speed. The patient was ejected and suffered severe facial and chest trauma. He was found conscious upon arrival of the emergency medial team but soon deteriorated, requiring tracheal intubation at the scene.

He has multiple facial and chest contusions, is wearing a Philadelphia collar and is positioned on a trauma board. A CXR in the ED showed opacification of the entire left hemithorax. A chest tube was placed which was followed by brisk 2 liter blood loss. He is moved to the OR for emergency thoracotomy.

Trauma is the most common cause of death in the United States for persons between the age of 1 and 44 years, and thoracic trauma accounts for 25% to 50% of all trauma-related mortality.[1,2] Patients with thoracic trauma may be managed conservatively in many cases, but the 10% that require urgent or emergent thoracotomy can present tremendous challenges to the anesthesiologists and intensivists involved in their care.[2] In particular, members of the trauma care team must simultaneously manage profound hemodynamic instability from massive hemorrhagic or obstructive shock, significant metabolic and acid/base abnormalities, and complex intra- and extrathoracic airway and pulmonary pathology. The complexity and severity of these injuries mandate that the trauma anesthesiologist possess expertise in massive resuscitation, invasive monitoring and line placement, and advanced airway management techniques and equipment. Airway management is further complicated by concerns for associated cervical spine injury and by the fact that the trauma patient is considered to have a full stomach, necessitating a rapid sequence induction and intubation if not already intubated. Thoracic injuries can require prolonged stays in the intensive care unit (ICU) with significant morbidity, including the need for prolonged mechanical ventilation and invasive monitoring. The anesthesiologist may also play a significant role as a pain management consultant and as such must be familiar with a variety of analgesic strategies.

BLUNT VERSUS PENETRATING TRAUMA

The mechanism of chest injury has important implications for the likelihood of specific organ injury, type of injury present, and its management. Blunt injury can be associated with significant injury to the heart, lungs, great vessels, and esophagus and involves three major mechanisms: *compression* between osseous structures, *direct energy transfer* from the impact, and *deceleration*.[3] Compression injury can occur whenever the heart, aorta, or innominate artery is trapped and crushed between the sternum and the thoracic spine as seen when the steering wheel or seatbelt impacts the chest of the driver in a motor vehicle crash (MVC). This mechanism, along with high-speed side impact crashes, is also a significant cause of direct energy transfer injury to intrathoracic organs. Compression and direct energy transfer may result in pulmonary and/or myocardial injury in addition to chest wall injuries. Finally, sudden deceleration may result in injury to the heart or aorta, usually occurring at one of several points of fibrous attachment of the heart and major vessels. The most frequent of these is aortic disruption originating at the attachment of the ligamentum arteriosum; however, sites of other clinically significant attachments include the junctions of the vena cava and the pulmonary veins with the atria, the aortic valve annulus, the origins of the great vessels from the aortic arch, and the aortic hiatus (Figure 20–1).[4] Penetrating trauma can be subdivided into high- and low-velocity mechanisms, also referred to as high- and low-energy transfer wounds. Most knife and small-caliber handgun injuries are considered low-energy transfer wounds, while shotgun and rifle injuries are considered medium- to high-energy and high-energy transfer wounds, respectively. In addition to the direct tissue injury caused by the specific pathway of penetrating objects, high-velocity injuries can be associated with significant damage to surrounding tissues caused by a large energy dissipation into surrounding tissues.[5] The severity of this process of "cavitation" is directly proportional to (1) the surface area of the point of impact, (2) the density of the tissue impacted, and (3) the velocity of the missile at the moment of impact.[6] Cavitation injury is most likely to be significant in water-bearing tissues such as the central nervous system (CNS), liver, and spleen, while tissues such as lung and muscle are less susceptible.

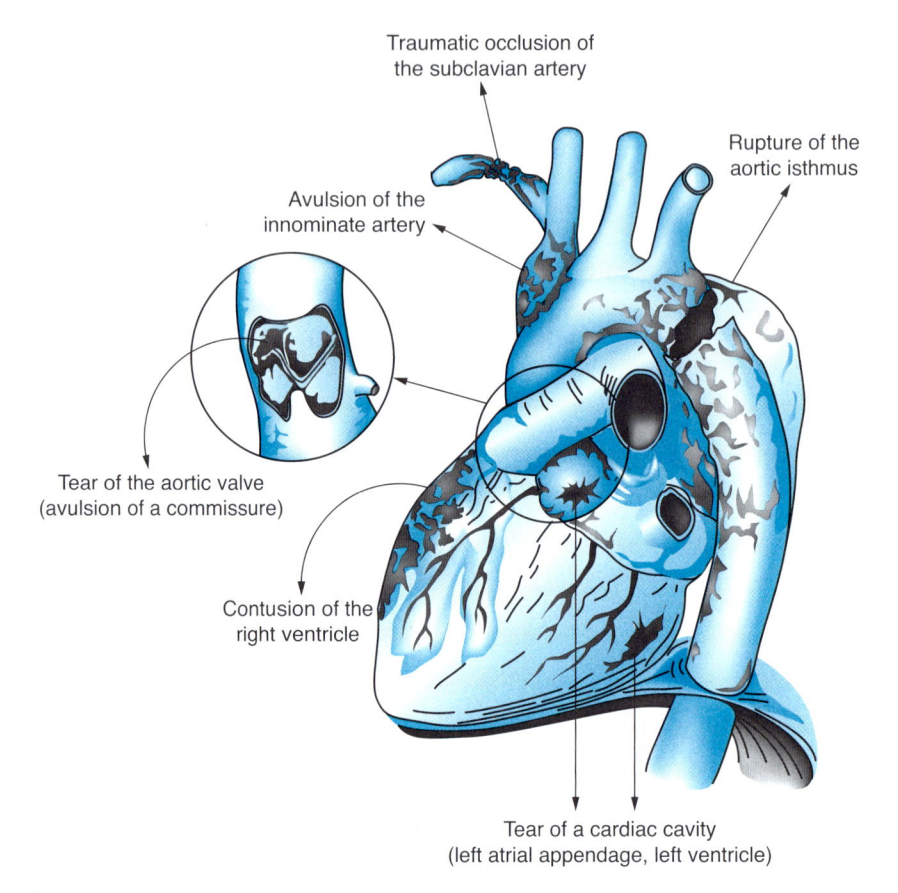

Figure 20-1. Common sites of blunt injury to the heart and aorta. (Reproduced with permission from Pretre R, Chilcott M. Blunt trauma to the heart and great vessels. *N Engl J Med*. 1997 Feb 27;336(9):628, with permission. Copyright © Massachusetts Medical Society. All rights reserved.)

Blast Injury

A growing concern related to the increasing incidence of terrorist attacks is the use of explosives and bombs and the resulting blast injuries. While there is concern that terrorists will gain access to biological and nonconventional weapons of mass destruction, the majority of terrorist attacks both overseas and in the United States to date have involved the detonation of explosive devices.[7] In addition to the threat from terrorist attacks, trauma physicians may also care for patients injured by explosions resulting from industrial accidents. The detonation of a conventional bomb results in the creation of a blast wave consisting of two parts: (1) a shockwave of high pressure resulting from the chemical reaction of the explosion, the peak amplitude of which is termed the *blast overpressure,* which is closely followed by (2) a blast wind, consisting of air in rapid motion outward from the source of explosion.[5,7] Blast overpressure of 35 psi can result in significant pulmonary injury, while pressures above 65 psi are usually fatal.[5] The peak amplitude decreases exponentially with increasing distance from the explosion, whereas the blast waves in confined spaces such as buildings or buses can be amplified due to the complex effects of reflected and standing waves.[8] So-called *enhanced-blast* explosive devices are associated with a different and potentially more dangerous overpressure pattern—the primary blast from these devices distributes the explosives into a larger area and then triggers a secondary explosion. This dual-stage explosion results in a prolonged duration of the overpressurization phase and greatly increases the total energy released.[7] As the outwardly directed energy dissipates, the blast wind returns to the source of the explosion, resulting in *underpressurization*, which can also result in significant injury.

Blast injuries are caused by one of four mechanisms related to the explosion: primary, secondary, tertiary, and quaternary effects. Primary effects are direct results of the overpressurization and underpressurization, which occur as a result of the blast wave. Tympanic membrane rupture, pulmonary injury (including contusion, hemorrhage, pneumothorax, and hemothorax), and rupture of the abdominal viscera, usually the colon, are the most common injuries caused by primary blast effects. Secondary effects include penetrating injury related to the release of fragments that are part of the device itself or released from the environment as a result of the blast. Tertiary effects include blunt and/or penetrating injuries that result from persons or objects being thrown by the blast wind or from collapse of structures. Finally, quaternary effects include burns, asphyxiation, and exposure to toxic substances.[7]

TRIAGE AND INITIAL MANAGEMENT

Patients with thoracic trauma should initially be evaluated according to the guidelines of the American College of Surgeons Advanced Trauma Life Support protocol.[9] Briefly, as for most trauma patients, this initial treatment consists of the primary survey, followed by resuscitation, secondary survey, diagnostic evaluation, and definitive treatment. While these are often presented as discrete or "stepwise" elements, they frequently occur simultaneously.[10] It is during the primary survey that the "ABCDEs" are evaluated: *A*irway (with special considerations and precautions for cervical spine injury), *B*reathing, *C*irculation, *D*isability (or neurologic status), and *E*xposure (removal of clothes) and *E*nvironment (temperature control). A major goal of the primary survey in the patient with thoracic trauma is the *early diagnosis of hypoxia* and any of 5 major injuries which may cause immediate death, including (1) critical airway obstruction, (2) tension pneumothorax, (3) open pneumothorax, (4) massive hemothorax, and (5) cardiac tamponade (Table 20–1). To accomplish the primary survey, the entire thorax including the back must be exposed and examined in a systematic fashion.

Of particular concern to all members of the trauma team is the potential need for emergent thoracotomy, either in the emergency department (ED) or operating suite. The goals and indications for this "resuscitative thoracotomy" include (1) immediate treatment of pericardial tamponade, (2) control of massive intrathoracic hemorrhage, (3) control of bronchopleural fistula or bronchovenous

Table 20–1. Life-Threatening Injuries Which Must Be Diagnosed in the Primary Survey

- Critical airway obstruction
- Tension pneumothorax
- Open pneumothorax
- Massive hemothorax
- Cardiac tamponade

air embolism (which accounts for up to 25% deaths), (4) performance of open cardiac massage, and (5) occlusion of the descending thoracic aorta to redistribute limited cardiac output to the brain and myocardium.[10] On the other hand, many patients with thoracic trauma may be managed with a tube thoracostomy or with a more controlled thoracotomy in the operating suite after initial stabilization. We will review these varied management strategies, together with the anesthetic and perioperative concerns for these patients by examining specific thoracic injuries that may be diagnosed in the primary and/or secondary surveys.

Pleural Space Injuries—Pneumothorax

Pneumothorax is a common result of thoracic trauma and patients may have no signs or symptoms (occult, *simple* pneumothorax) or may be in overt respiratory failure and circulatory shock (*tension* pneumothorax). Pneumothorax can develop whenever there is disruption of the visceral pleura causing a communication between the airways and the pleural space. This can result in the passage of air into the pleural space, typically through a "one-way valve" mechanism in which air enters the pleural space with inspiration but is not expelled from the chest with exhalation. A one-way valve created through a chest wall injury that communicates with the pleural space will also result in the accumulation of air in the pleural space. Both injuries can result in sequestration of air and positive pressure in the ipsilateral hemithorax leading to varying degrees of lung consolidation, tracheal deviation, jugular venous distension (JVD), hypotension, and mediastinal shift toward the contralateral hemithorax. In addition to the ipsilateral lung volume loss, gas exchange may also be significantly impaired by mediastinal compression of the contralateral lung, with the combined mechanisms leading to critical respiratory failure. Impedance to venous return by the increased thoracic pressure and vena caval compression may result in hemodynamic embarrassment.

Clinical signs and symptoms of pneumothorax include chest pain, dyspnea, tachycardia and hypotension, subcutaneous emphysema, JVD, tracheal deviation away from the affected side, *hyperresonance* to percussion and absence of breath sounds or chest rise on the affected side. Chest x-ray (CXR) findings may include tracheal and mediastinal deviation to the contralateral side along with downward displacement of the diaphragm and widening of the intercostal spaces on the ipsilateral side. Treatment of clinically significant pneumothorax should not be delayed for a confirmatory radiographic study. A tension pneumothorax may be temporized with decompression by needle thoracostomy. This has classically been performed by placing a needle or 14 gauge angiocatheter through the second intercostal space in the midclavicular line; however, some argue that a safer technique involves placement through the fifth intercostal space in the midaxillary line, as this may be associated with a lower likelihood of injury to the great vessels.[10]

Definitive management of a pneumothorax usually requires tube thoracostomy. The procedure, while not technically difficult, does require considerable training and experience as significant complications are possible including transdiaphragmatic, extrapleural, or interlobar fissure placement, lung parenchymal injury, and rarely cardiac injury.[10] In most cases, tension pneumothorax will be adequately resolved with chest tube placement. If there is persistent severe air leak or failure of the affected lung to re-expand, the airways should be examined with bronchoscopy to evaluate for bronchopleural fistula, which would likely be associated with decreased tidal volumes and decreased oxygen saturation (SpO_2) despite increasing levels of suction in the pleural drainage system used to drain the ipsilateral hemithorax.

Anesthetic considerations should include a high degree of suspicion for occult pneumothorax in any trauma patient. While many argue that occult pneumothorax can be managed conservatively, there is the possibility of a simple pneumothorax being converted to a tension type upon intubation and initiation of positive pressure ventilation.[2] Strong consideration should be given to placement of a chest tube prior to the initiation of positive pressure ventilation whenever circumstances permit. The diagnosis of de novo tension pneumothorax may be difficult during general anesthesia, but it should always be suspected if there is unexplained hypotension, hypoxia, absent or diminished breath sounds on one side, or a sudden increase in airway pressure. Intraoperative management should include immediate placement of a chest tube or needle thoracostomy if tube thoracostomy is not feasible. Patients with a persistent air leak in the setting of pneumothorax already treated with tube thoracostomy may require surgical repair of a bronchopleural fistula. If performed with video-assisted thoracic surgery (VATS) airway management will require one-lung ventilation. In addition to the usual considerations for lung isolation, the technique may be complicated by facial and cervical spine injuries in the trauma patient. These considerations may dictate which device can be used successfully (ie, placement of a double-lumen endotracheal tube vs use of a bronchial blocker through a single-lumen endotracheal tube already in place). In all cases of pneumothorax, nitrous oxide and positive end-expiratory pressure (PEEP) should be avoided until the injury has been definitively controlled (ie, with tube thoracostomy). Care must be taken to maintain adequate intravascular volume status to avoid a critical decrease in central venous return and attendant hemodynamic compromise.

Pleural Space Injuries—Open Pneumothorax

The open pneumothorax or "sucking chest wound" is caused by a full-thickness injury to the chest wall without a "one-way valve" effect. Theoretically, if the diameter of the defect exceeds two-thirds of the tracheal diameter, the negative pleural pressure associated with inspiration will cause air to preferentially enter the chest via the wound instead of through the trachea. Tension pneumothorax is unlikely in this case because the large size of the injury allows two-way gas exchange between the atmosphere and the pleural space; however, adequate ventilation and oxygenation will quickly become impossible, as air is no longer exchanged between the alveoli and the atmosphere through the trachea.

The open pneumothorax is managed by placement of an occlusive dressing (usually with petrolatum gauze) secured on 3 of the 4 sides. The remaining unsecured side of the dressing allows air in the pleural space to exit the chest, but air will no longer preferentially enter the chest via low resistance pathway and will instead pass normally through the upper airway and trachea. Patients with an open pneumothorax can be safely intubated and placed on positive pressure ventilation prior to placement of a chest tube or surgical repair of the wound.

Pleural Space Injuries—Hemothorax

Similar to a pneumothorax, the signs and symptoms caused by the collection of blood within the thorax can vary greatly. A small hemothorax may be asymptomatic and must be at least 200 mL to create blunting of the costophrenic angle on an upright chest film. A larger hemothorax on the other hand, will likely have similar signs and symptoms to a tension pneumothorax including varying degrees of respiratory failure and cardiovascular collapse. Physical findings of hemothorax include decreased or muffled breath sounds and dullness to percussion on the affected side.

Massive hemothorax is defined as the accumulation of more than 1500 mL of fluid within the pleural space. These are usually caused by large lacerations to the pulmonary parenchyma or injury to intercostal or great vessels. Up to 60% patient's blood volume can accumulate in one hemithorax, so it must be appreciated that profound hemodynamic instability and intravascular volume loss can be accounted for by this injury alone. Indications for thoracotomy include an initial output of 1500 mL or more of blood at the time of chest tube placement or the continued output of 200 mL or more from the chest tubes for 2 to 3 consecutive hours. In stable patients who have less severe hemorrhage, management with VATS can be successful in up to 80% patients.[11] Common indications include retained hemothorax and entrapped lung; many trauma surgeons advocate for the VATS to be performed on post-trauma day 3.

Lung laceration, intercostal vessel bleeding, and great vessel injuries are etiologic in the majority of injuries associated with hemothorax requiring surgery. The source of the hemorrhage will dictate the definitive treatment and therefore the anesthetic considerations. If VATS or thoracotomy is required, the management may include considerations for lung isolation, whereas for embolization procedures, as in the case of intercostal arterial bleeding for example, conventional ventilation with a single-lumen endotracheal tube will likely be sufficient. As with any trauma associated with major hemorrhage, large bore intravenous access and direct arterial blood pressure monitoring should be obtained immediately. Central venous access and invasive hemodynamic monitoring may also be useful for the management of resuscitation in some cases, especially in the presence of severe coexisting cardiopulmonary disease. If available, consideration should be given to the use of autotransfusion techniques. Hemorrhagic shock should not be treated primarily with vasopressors, sodium bicarbonate, or continued crystalloid infusion, but with cross-matched packed red blood cells (PRBCs) or O-negative blood to maintain adequate oxygen-carrying capacity.

Chest Wall—Rib, Clavicle, and Sternum Injuries

Rib fractures are present in at least 10% patients who present with trauma, and in up to 94% who are associated with serious injuries including pneumothorax, hemothorax, and lung contusion.[12] Injuries of multiple ribs, first and second rib fractures, and injuries of the clavicle and scapula are usually associated with high-energy mechanisms of injury and should raise awareness of the possibility of serious associated intra-abdominal and thoracic injuries including aortic transection and great vessel disruption.

In the absence of flail-chest physiology (see next section), the most significant consequences of rib and sternal fractures are usually related to severe pain and the associated effects on pulmonary function (Table 20–2). Particularly in the elderly, inadequate pain management can lead to significant morbidity and mortality, usually from pneumonia because of impaired coughing and clearance of secretions. In one series, mortality in patients 65 years or older increased by 19% for each rib fracture while the risk of pneumonia increased by 27%.[13]

Management of rib fracture pain can be achieved with a number of analgesic modalities including systemic administration of opioids, intercostal nerve blocks, single-injection or continuous paravertebral blocks, intrapleural administration of local anesthetics, and continuous epidural catheters (Figure 20–2). The use of parenteral opioids in the management of rib fracture pain is well described, and its main advantage is absence of any need for a regional analgesic intervention and the associated risks of bleeding, infection, or pneumothorax. However, the usual problems of respiratory and CNS depression related to their administration and the relative inferiority to regional techniques limit the utility of systemic opioids for the treatment of multiple rib fractures. If a regional technique is not feasible (coagulopathy, localized or systemic infection, limitation of patient positioning, etc), patients can be managed adequately with an intravenous (IV) narcotic either as a

Table 20–2. Adverse Effects of Rib Fracture Pain

- Impaired cough and clearance of secretions
  - Increased incidence of pneumonia and sepsis
- Atelectasis
  - Hypoxia
  - Reduced functional residual capacity
- Increased work of breathing from chest wall instability
  - Increased myocardial O_2 demand

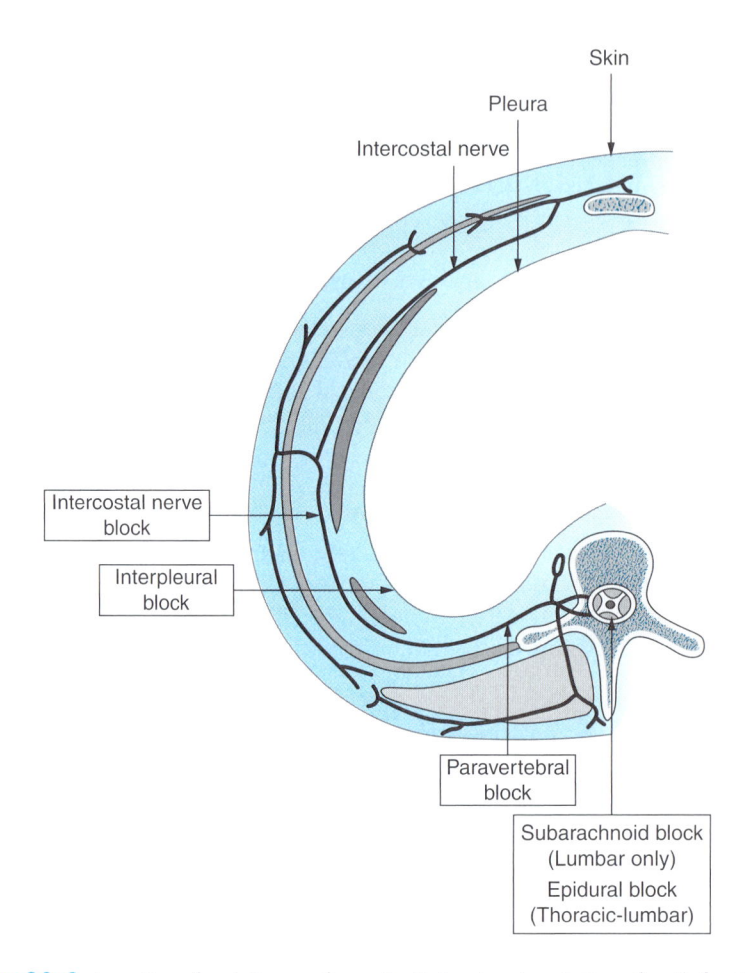

Figure 20–2. Locations for delivery of anesthetic/analgesic solutions for rib fractures.

continuous infusion, intermittent IV dosing, or in the form of a patient-controlled analgesia (PCA) technique.[14]

Intercostal nerve blocks (ICNB) are a simple and universally practiced technique for the management of rib fractures. The main disadvantage of intercostal nerve blocks is the brief duration of pain control, but there are also limitations due to the chest wall sensory anatomy and the technique itself. Because of sensory contributions from segments adjacent to the injury, multiple levels must be injected to achieve adequate sensory block. Further, firm palpation of the chest wall necessary during the technique may cause intolerable pain. However, the 6 to 12 hour duration of this block may be used as a "bridging" technique until a more definitive continuous technique can be initiated. The blocks may also be placed internally by the surgeon at the completion of the operation if the patient requires thoracotomy.

Continuous thoracic paravertebral blockade (TPB) is effective for unilateral analgesia and may be technically easier to place than a continuous epidural catheter, depending upon the preference and skill of the practitioner. In a prospective, controlled pilot study, patients with unilateral multiple level rib fractures treated with continuous TPB achieved equivalent pain relief as patients treated with thoracic epidurals.[15] While there was a slight increase in the incidence of pneumonia in the TPB group, there was no difference in outcome. Continuous TPB may be associated with fewer hemodynamic changes, but increased serum levels of local anesthetic and systemic toxicity are possible.[14]

The infusion of a local anesthetic solution into the pleural space with a percutaneously placed catheter was first described by Kvalheim and Reiestad in 1984.[16] The use of intrapleural analgesia (IPA) was then described for patients with multiple rib fractures by Rocco et al in 1987.[17] Although the mechanism of analgesia is incompletely understood, the technique probably results in a unilateral, multi-level ICNB.[14] While the technique may result in analgesia equivalent to that achieved with systemic opioids or epidural techniques, there are multiple limitations and drawbacks to the technique. In particular, because the anesthetic solution tends to settle in dependent portions of the chest, upper chest wall injuries will likely have poor coverage in the ICU patient with the head of the bead ideally elevated to 30 degrees. There is also the concern that accumulation of the solution on the diaphragm could result in impaired diaphragmatic function and respiratory compromise. Further, there is the possibility of inadvertent removal of the solution by an ipsilateral chest tube that may be in place. IPA can result in high plasma concentrations of local anesthetics that could lead to systemic toxicity. Given these and numerous other problems with the technique, IPA cannot be considered a first-line measure, especially given the efficacy and safety of the other regional techniques described.[14]

Perhaps the most effective and universally accepted analgesic modality for multiple rib fractures is continuous thoracic epidural analgesia (TEA) with local anesthetics, with or without the addition of opioids. In addition to analgesia which is superior to that achieved with systemic opioids and IPA,[18,19] TEA results in superior pulmonary function including improvement in functional residual capacity, dynamic lung compliance, arterial PO_2, and airway resistance.[20] There is also the possibility of immune modulation as suggested by a TEA-induced decrease in plasma levels of interleukin (IL)-8, which may contribute to the development of acute lung injury (although this has not been directly correlated with clinical benefit).[18] There is evidence that patients treated with TEA may require a shorter duration of mechanical ventilation, shorter ICU stays, and shorter hospitalizations.[14] TEA is not appropriate for all trauma patients and contraindications include coagulopathy, infection or significant tissue injury at the intended insertion site, coexisting cardiac disease such as mitral or aortic stenosis, increased intracranial pressure, and ongoing hemodynamic instability. It is incumbent upon the practitioner to rule out associated intra-abdominal trauma as TEA may mask symptoms from these injuries. The addition of opioids to the epidural solution can result in pruritus, nausea, vomiting, urinary retention, and rarely respiratory suppression. In general, all of these side effects are less severe when compared with IV opioid administration.

The specific analgesic modality used in a given patient depends on many variables including the anesthesiologist's preference and skill set, the preference of the thoracic or trauma surgeon, and the limitations of the institution's infrastructure and nursing capabilities. It is important to recognize that the optimal method of analgesia for patients with multiple rib fractures remains a matter of significant controversy, and no single modality can be recommended in all situations. For any patient with acute pain resulting from chest wall injury, multimodal analgesia including the above methods with the addition of nonsteroidal anti-inflammatory drugs (NSAIDs), low-dose ketamine infusion, transcutaneous electrical nerve stimulation (TENS), anticonvulsant drugs, and pain specialist consultation should be considered early during the course of treatment.

Chest Wall—Flail chest

When two or more adjacent ribs are fractured in two or more places, anteriorly and posteriorly, a so-called flail segment can develop. Flail chest may develop in as many as 20% patients hospitalized for blunt chest trauma.[21] The injured portion of the chest wall will demonstrate paradoxical movement with inspiration—that is, the segment will move *inward with inspiration*, and *outward with exhalation*. This pattern of movement occurs because the flail segment becomes mechanically separated from the chest wall and its movement becomes dependent upon the changes in pleural pressure present during spontaneous respiration. If the segment is large enough, pulmonary function may be impaired as a result of this counterproductive motion. However, the pulmonary decline is probably more frequently related to the injury to the lung or chest wall itself (pulmonary contusion, hemothorax, or pneumothorax) and its associated pain. Management of the flail chest thus no longer focuses primarily on surgical stabilization of the segment (see discussion on rib stabilization below), but instead is concerned with the management of the associated pain and lung injury which can result in decreased FRC and vital capacity (VC) and significant V/Q mismatch. Indeed, the management should be similar to that of any patient with multiple rib fractures (see previous discussion), assuming that the segment is not so large that its negative impact on spontaneous ventilation necessitates endotracheal intubation and mechanical ventilation. The management of the patient with flail chest may ultimately be determined by the extent and severity of coexisting injuries. In the setting of multiple severe intrathoracic or intracranial injuries, the patient will likely remain intubated and mechanically ventilated until these injuries are addressed or stabilized. Conversely, in the absence of other significant injuries, the patient may be successfully managed with parenteral narcotics or TEA,[5] and the use of noninvasive positive pressure ventilation (NIPV), which avoids the complications of endotracheal intubation and is showing promise for those patients who still require supportive ventilation.[21]

Historically, reduction and fixation for rib fractures have met with resistance and failure. Traditional management since the early trials of rib traction and wiring has yielded more complications and morbidity than success and relief. Fortunately for some patients, industry has revisited the patient with flail chest and revised the stabilization approach to the fractured rib segments. Formerly, Kirschner wires were subject to fracture and therefore would add to morbidity rather than prevent complications. Newer devices attempt to be specific to ribs and even specific to rib size and side of the chest.[22-25]

Indications for rib stabilization include intractable pain leading to failure to liberate from mechanical ventilation, repeated trauma (as in hemothoraces), and chest wall instability leading to intubation, pneumonia, and failure to thrive.[26-28] Newer techniques and devices have shown promise and several trauma centers have ongoing trials looking at length of stay (LOS), duration of mechanical ventilation, ICU stay, and amount of narcotic use.[29] Many investigations are underpowered and retrospective in their analysis, but a few prospective studies exist that demonstrate significant improvement in LOS, and decreased duration of mechanical ventilation.

In summary, the approach to surgical rib stabilization has been revitalized and appears to improve patient comfort and decrease morbidity, even expedite patient throughput. Time will tell however, if this procedure holds up to the scrutiny of critical review.

PULMONARY CONTUSION

Pulmonary contusion is a common consequence of thoracic trauma, and it may result in significant morbidity and mortality, usually due to the severe hypoxemia. The contusion may arise from any of the common injury mechanisms including deceleration forces, direct energy transfer, or from a shockwave associated with blast injury. The severity of contusions correlates closely with the overall severity of the chest trauma.[5] The pathologic changes include hemorrhage and edema, which can result in complete consolidation of the lung parenchyma. This leads to varying degrees of hypercarbia and hypoxia due to decreased pulmonary compliance and increased pulmonary shunt fraction. The severity of the alveolar hemorrhage and parenchymal injury generally peaks during the first 24 hours after the injury, and the injury usually resolves within 7 days.[30]

Pulmonary contusion should be considered in any trauma patient with dyspnea, hypoxia, cyanosis and tachycardia. Unfortunately, the contusion(s) may not be radiologically apparent upon initial presentation, but they will usually be evident on CXR within the first 6 hours after the injury. Computed tomography (CT) may be more sensitive than CXR in the diagnosis of early contusion.[10]

The management of pulmonary contusion is frequently supportive, including the administration of supplemental oxygen and successful pain management with the goals of maintaining pulmonary toilet and minimizing atelectasis. This may be accomplished by any of the analgesic modalities described above (see Chest Wall—Rib, Clavicle, and Sternum Injuries). In severe injury, pulmonary function may decline to an extent necessitating intubation and mechanical ventilation. Antibiotics and steroids should not be used *routinely*.[30] In the absence of pneumonia and/or the development of the acute respiratory distress syndrome (ARDS), patients are likely to make a complete recovery, although long-term morbidity manifesting as dyspnea related to persistently decreased FRC is possible.[31] This decrease in FRC may make adequate pre-oxygenation prior to anesthetic induction difficult. Approximately 3% patients with pulmonary contusions develop pulmonary pseudocysts, cavitary lesions which are frequently asymptomatic but rarely are complicated by infection, bleeding, or rupture requiring surgical intervention.[32] Anesthetic management of these patients will likely include the need for lung isolation and arterial line placement for arterial blood gas (ABG) analysis. Optimal fluid management for patients with acute pulmonary contusion is controversial, but a balanced approach with judicious crystalloid administration to optimize intravascular volume status makes physiologic sense, as the injury is associated with increased lung water accumulation and excessive administration of crystalloid may exacerbate the pulmonary injury and further impair gas exchange.

PULMONARY LACERATION

Pulmonary laceration can result from penetrating trauma, blunt shearing forces, missile injury associated with a gunshot wound, blast, or explosion, or from the exposed portions of fractured ribs or clavicles. The most common finding from the primary survey and CXR is a hemopneumothorax. Hemorrhage associated with pulmonary laceration is usually self-limited and can be managed definitively with tube thoracostomy.[10] Approximately 10% patients will require thoracotomy, and up to 20% will require anatomic lung resection (lobectomy or pneumonectomy), a procedure which has been associated with a high mortality. Nonanatomic resection, including tractotomy or wedge resection may be associated with a significantly improved mortality and should be considered the operation of choice in non-hilar injuries.[33]

DIAPHRAGMATIC INJURY

Traumatic diaphragmatic rupture (TDR) is a fairly uncommonly diagnosed injury associated with severe thoracoabdominal trauma. It occurs in 0.5% to 8% patients hospitalized for motor vehicle crashes and is found in approximately 5% blunt trauma victims who undergo laparotomy.[34] It is also present in 10% to 15% victims of penetrating lower thoracic trauma.[35] The injury is more likely to be diagnosed on the left side for 2 major reasons: (1) the liver probably provides some degree of protection to the right hemidiaphragm, especially in blunt injury, and (2) victims of stab wounds are usually attacked by right-handed assailants who are more likely to penetrate the victim's chest or abdomen on the left side.[36] Diaphragmatic rupture can occur as a result of three major mechanisms in blunt trauma: (1) the abdominal to thoracic pressure gradient may exceed the normal maximum value of 100 cmH_2O, especially if the patient gasps against a closed glottis at the time of impact, (2) thoracic compression and distortion during the trauma can result in large shearing forces causing tears in the diaphragm's musculoaponeurotic structure, and (3) the patient may have congenital abnormalities leading to areas of relative weakness in the diaphragm.[37] A defect in the diaphragm may allow the herniation of abdominal structures into the pleural space, usually the stomach, omentum, transverse colon, or portions of the small bowel. Respiratory and hemodynamic compromise can follow if a significant volume of viscera becomes sequestered in the thorax, leading to a clinical picture similar to that seen with hemothorax or tension pneumothorax.

Diagnosis of diaphragmatic injury is frequently delayed and the initial CXR may be misinterpreted as representing an elevated diaphragm related to phrenic nerve injury, a "pseudodiaphragm" formed by the wall of a herniated viscus, a loculated hemopneumothorax, gastric dilatation, or subpulmonary hematoma. The delay of diagnosis may be associated with an increase in mortality.[35] As such, the diagnosis of TDR requires a high degree of clinical suspicion in any patient with penetrating injuries below the fifth intercostal space, osseous injuries associated with high energy mechanisms (clavicle, sternum, scapulae, first or second ribs, pelvic, or thoracolumbar spine fractures), or with associated high speed blunt abdominal injuries.[37] If there is no contraindication, a nasogastric tube should be placed as this may appear coiled in the stomach *above* the diaphragm on the CXR. If CXR findings are inconclusive and TDR is still suspected, further diagnostic studies including inspiratory and expiratory films (which can better detect the visceral herniation), contrast studies, or even diagnostic laparoscopy may be required. CT with reconstructed images may be the study of choice for the diagnosis of TDR.[36]

Anesthetic management for patients with known TDR should be similar to those patients with hemothorax and/or tension pneumothorax as similar pulmonary and cardiovascular considerations apply. In addition, it seems prudent to minimize or avoid entirely the use of positive pressure mask ventilation whenever possible, as this may result in entrainment of air into the stomach and proximal small intestine, possibly worsening the compression of intrathoracic organs by the herniated abdominal contents. Rapid sequence induction and intubation may be necessary for this reason and to decrease the risk of pulmonary aspiration of gastric contents. Placement of a gastric tube prior to induction should be considered to decompress the herniated visceral organs, perhaps reducing the risk of aspiration and potentially mitigating the adverse effects of the herniated contents on cardiopulmonary function. Re-expansion pulmonary edema is possible in the setting of rapid decompression of the affected lung and should be suspected if there is sudden hypoxia at the time of thoracic decompression. If thoracotomy or VATS (for chronic diaphragmatic hernias) is required for surgical correction of the TDR, one-lung ventilation may be necessary.

LARYNGEAL AND TRACHEOBRONCHIAL TRAUMA

Injuries to the larynx and tracheobronchial tree are relatively uncommon but can result in immediate death from airway obstruction, and complex injuries can present tremendous challenges for airway and ventilatory management. The incidence of this rare injury is difficult to estimate, but may occur in 3% to 6% patients with penetrating neck injuries, less than 1% patients with penetrating thoracic trauma, and from 0.5% to 2% patients with blunt trauma to the neck or chest.[38] Eighty percent of tracheobronchial injuries occur within 2.5 cm of the carina, but complex injuries may involve multiple areas of the larynx and/or tracheobronchial tree. Clinical symptoms and signs of significant airway injury may include dyspnea and respiratory distress, dysphonia or hoarseness, hemoptysis, pneumothorax, and subcutaneous and/or mediastinal emphysema. Persistent air leak after otherwise successful chest tube placement (as indicated by continuous bubbling in the water seal chamber of the drainage system, or worsening SpO_2 when suction intensity is increased), or failure of the lung to re-expand with suction are possible in the setting of significant airway injury. The CXR and cervical spine films obtained during the primary survey are important in the diagnosis of tracheobronchial injury as cervical mediastinal emphysema and pneumothorax will be seen in 60% and 70% patients, respectively. CT images of the cervical spine (perhaps obtained to evaluate cervical spinal cord injury) are sensitive for diagnosing laryngeal injuries. CT of the chest may be helpful in the diagnosis of tracheobronchial injury, but a negative study does not obviate the need for flexible fiberoptic bronchoscopy (FOB) if there is still a high suspicion of airway injury. While FOB is considered the definitive study for the diagnosis of tracheobronchial disruption, both in the acute and late stages of evaluation, the modality may still fail to diagnose the injury in up to 6% injuries.[38]

Laryngeal trauma can result from a "clothesline" injury mechanism, with a narrow and focused band of energy causing compression of the cervical portion of the trachea against the vertebral bodies. Shear and deceleration forces can injure the trachea at points of relative airway fixation, such as at the cricoid cartilage and the carina, leading to tears and even complete transection of the airway. The sudden widening of the thorax that occurs during antero-posterior compression of the thoracic cage may produce enough bilateral traction on the trachea to cause an injury at the level of the carina. Finally, the airways may rupture as a consequence of sudden thoracic compression in association with a closed glottis at the time of blunt impact. This usually results in linear tears either at the junction of the membranous and cartilaginous portions of the trachea or between cartilaginous rings.[38]

Successful airway management is both the most critical and potentially challenging aspect of the management of patients with laryngeal or tracheobronchial trauma. FOB is perhaps the most useful modality for initial airway examination and intubation. Assuming a significant degree of patient cooperation, the bronchoscope can be introduced into the airway of the trauma patient and used both for evaluation of the location and extent of injury and for directly visualized intubation across injured or transected portions of the airway. This can be accomplished with topical anesthesia if necessary and without any requirement for extension of the neck in patients with actual or suspected cervical spine injury. Adequate control of the airway may necessitate lung isolation, depending upon the location of the injury. This may be accomplished with either a double-lumen endotracheal tube or a single-lumen tube combined with a bronchial blocker. Some argue that double-lumen endotracheal tubes should be avoided as they are stiffer and larger than conventional tubes and may worsen or extend the airway injury. With either technique, bronchoscopic skill and precision are required to ensure that the airway is controlled and the area of injury is successfully traversed and isolated by the tracheal or bronchial tube prior to the initiation of positive pressure ventilation.

Surgical management of the airway may be necessary, and this situation demands close cooperation and communication between the surgeon and anesthesiologist. This may involve a tracheostomy in the setting of laryngeal injury, or for more distal tracheal injury, a sterile endotracheal tube may need to be inserted directly by the surgeon through the operative field. Jet ventilation through small caliber tubes may also be effective as their smaller diameter creates less interference in the operative field during the repair.[38] Cardiopulmonary bypass (CPB) may be necessary in the setting of extremely complex airway injuries or if coexisting cardiac or great vessel injury necessitate its use. The main limitation of CPB is the requirement of profound systemic anticoagulation, which will likely be contraindicated in the patient with multiple injuries or intracranial trauma. Thus, careful and skillful management of the airway by the anesthesiologist and surgeon is usually required if early repair of airway injury is necessary. Indeed, immediate and definitive repair of airway injuries is almost always required as delayed intervention may increase the risk of pulmonary or mediastinal infection and bronchial stenosis.[5]

CARDIAC TRAUMA

The heart can be injured by blunt or penetrating injuries, or by a combination of these mechanisms as may occur with a blast injury. Penetrating cardiac injuries can be caused by relatively low-energy mechanisms such as knife stab wounds, or by high-energy mechanisms in the case of gunshot wounds (GSWs). Complete penetration of the heart and pericardial sac usually results in immediate death from hemorrhage at the scene, whereas patients may survive the initial injury if the pericardium is intact thereby limiting the rate of exsanguination. Blunt cardiac injury (BCI), formerly referred to as myocardial or cardiac contusion, is most commonly caused by a MVC, but any trauma to the chest wall including that resulting from falls, assaults with blunt implements, blast injury, or even cardiopulmonary resuscitation (CPR) can cause injury to the heart. It is estimated that 20% MVC-related fatalities are caused by injury to the heart, and 50% patients will die before arrival to the hospital.[39] Injuries can include cardiac rupture, valvular or septal rupture, damage to coronary arteries, or nonspecific myocardial injury manifesting only as electrophysiologic (rhythm or conduction) disturbances noted on electrocardiography (ECG). Patients may present with no signs or symptoms during the primary survey or may be in overt cardiogenic shock. Patients with blunt cardiac injury will usually have other signs of significant thoracic trauma, but the absence of other findings on the physical exam does not rule out the possibility of significant BCI. Conversely, the presence of an isolated sternal fracture does not warrant further work-up for BCI in the absence of other clinical signs or symptoms.[40]

Cardiac rupture is the most severe form of penetrating injury and is usually fatal at the scene within seconds or minutes of the injury. The chambers most commonly ruptured (in descending order of frequency) are the right atrium, right ventricle, left atrium, and left ventricle.[4] If there is concomitant rupture of the pericardium, the patient will usually exsanguinate rapidly in the field. The patient may survive to hospital admission if the pericardium remains intact, although if there is significant accumulation of pericardial blood the victim will likely develop pericardial tamponade. It should be noted that volumes as small as 15 to 30 mL can be associated with clinically evident tamponade. Stab wounds are likely to be associated with tamponade, which is protective and associated with improved survival, whereas GSWs usually pierce the pericardial sac and result in uncontrolled bleeding into the chest. Pericardial tamponade should be suspected in any victim of blunt or penetrating thoracic trauma with hypotension unresponsive to rapid volume resuscitation, and should be rapidly diagnosed in the primary survey. The diagnosis is frequently made as part of the focused assessment with sonography for trauma (FAST) exam (using subxiphoid or parasternal views) which can approach 100% sensitivity and specificity by experienced practitioners.[41] The diagnosis may also be suggested by persistently elevated central venous pressures (CVP) in the setting of persistent hypotension. The findings of Beck's triad (hypotension, muffled heart sounds, and distended neck veins) are present in only 10% victims, while Kussmaul's sign (swelling of neck veins with inspiration) and pulsus paradoxus (decrease in systolic blood pressure upon inspiration) are similarly unreliable.[10] Unstable patients with pericardial tamponade should undergo immediate subxiphoid pericardial window with local anesthesia either in the ED or OR. Median sternotomy may be necessary if hemorrhage is difficult to control through the pericardial window. The utility of pericardiocentesis is highly controversial, as the procedure may be both unhelpful diagnostically and of little therapeutic value, especially if the fluid collection is not continuous with the entire pericardial space.

Valvular injuries occur in approximately 2% patients with documented BCI.[42] The aortic valve is the most frequently injured, and injury usually results from a sudden increase in aortic pressure associated with thoracic compression. The sudden increase in pressure can cause laceration or avulsion of any of the three aortic valve cusps. Aortic valvular trauma may cause severe acute pump failure or may present in the days or weeks following the initial trauma with only angina or syncope. The mitral valve apparatus may also be injured when thoracic compression coincides with early systole and may result in tearing of the mitral valve leaflets or rupture of a papillary muscle or chordae tendinae. If the resulting mitral regurgitation is severe, cardiac failure and flash pulmonary edema may ensue, and a holosystolic murmur at the apex will likely be present. Injuries to the tricuspid valve may occur, but are much less frequent and less likely to be of immediate hemodynamic consequence. Definitive diagnosis of valve injury resulting from BCI will likely require either transesophageal echocardiography (TEE) or cardiac catheterization, neither of which may be feasible during the initial stabilization and evaluation of the trauma patient. The majority of injuries can be managed conservatively until other associated injuries have been addressed and stabilized.

Septal injuries are present in approximately 5% to 7% patients who die from blunt trauma. Ventricular septal injuries are more common than traumatic atrial septal ruptures, and they usually occur in the muscular portion of the septum near the cardiac apex.[39] Significant injuries can result in left-to-right shunting or hemodynamic compromise that may require urgent repair, whereas smaller injuries frequently can be allowed to heal primarily. Physical findings may include a systolic thrill and/or a harsh holosystolic murmur heard best at the left sternal edge; echocardiography or cardiac catheterization will confirm the diagnosis. If penetrating cardiac injury (of any type) represents a significant concern, TEE should be performed prior to leaving the OR.

Injuries to the coronary arteries are rare, occurring in less than 2% patients with BCI, but can be life-threatening and associated with significant myocardial ischemia.[42] The most commonly involved vessels (in descending order of frequency) are the left anterior descending (LAD), right coronary (RCA), and circumflex coronary arteries. Vessel obstruction may be caused by traumatic rupture of an existing plaque, de novo thrombosis, spasm or contusion of the vessel, or even laceration or dissection. Patients may demonstrate any of the usual signs and symptoms of myocardial ischemia including angina, ST segment elevation, and varying degrees of cardiac failure depending on the extent of the coronary distribution involved. Most patients can be managed medically while associated traumatic injuries are addressed, but severe ischemia may mandate urgent percutaneous coronary intervention (PCI) with stenting or angioplasty or even surgical coronary bypass grafting or vessel repair.

Perhaps the most common yet diagnostically challenging clinical entity associated with BCI is otherwise unexplained sinus tachycardia. The incidence of BCI depends upon the diagnostic criteria used, but may be present in up to one-third of patients with blunt chest trauma.[39] Injury to the myocardium can be associated with hemorrhage, edema, inflammation, and even myocyte necrosis, all of which may result in ECG changes, elevation of cardiac enzymes such as troponin I and CK-MB (which are probably unhelpful in making the diagnosis or guiding therapy), or regions of impaired contractility. Blunt cardiac injury must be differentiated from the distinct clinical phenomenon of *commotio cordis* which is caused by blunt impact to the precordium occurring either 15 to 30 milliseconds prior to the peak of the T wave, or during the QRS complex, leading to ventricular fibrillation or complete heart block, respectively. The impact is *not* associated with demonstrable contusion of the myocardium and the effects are related to the precise timing of the impact and its associated disruption of normal electrical activity of the heart.[3]

ECG is a simple and inexpensive test that should be performed in all patients suspected of having BCI. The most frequent findings are sinus tachycardia, followed by premature atrial and ventricular contractions. Other abnormalities in descending order of frequency include nonspecific T-wave changes, atrial fibrillation or flutter, ST segment elevation or depression, conduction delays, ventricular arrhythmias, and new Q waves.[42] Of note, ventricular fibrillation and pulseless ventricular tachycardia are extremely rare, but obviously require immediate treatment with defibrillation. A normal ECG in a hemodynamically stable patient with minor thoracic trauma and no preexisting cardiac disease effectively rules out significant BCI, and these patients do not require further cardiac telemetry unless other injuries necessitate continuous monitoring.[42] Asymptomatic patients with a history of cardiac disease may develop delayed ECG changes and should therefore be monitored with telemetry for 24 hours with serial 12-lead ECGs. Echocardiography (transthoracic or transesophageal) is indicated for patients with ongoing hemodynamic instability. New symptoms (angina or shock) in the setting of ECG changes necessitate ICU admission and monitoring for at least 24 hours and evaluation with echocardiography which may show segmental wall motion abnormalities (SWMAs).[39]

The measurement of cardiac enzymes such as creatinine kinase (CK), creatinine kinase myocardial type B fraction (CK-MB), and Troponin I and T as a screening tool for BCI is based on the rationale that myocyte injury caused by blunt trauma should be associated with their release into the serum. Historically, CK and CK-MB were the most frequently measured enzymes, but they have been shown to be nonspecific and of little to no value in the screening of patients for BCI.[39,42,43] Troponins T and I, on the other hand, are highly specific for myocyte injury, and while some consider them to be useful in screening for myocardial contusion, practice guidelines do not recommend that cardiac enzymes be obtained *routinely*.[40] However, the combination of a normal admission ECG and normal troponin levels after 4 to 6 hours makes the likelihood of BCI in asymptomatic patients highly unlikely.[43]

Given the variation and severity of injuries resulting from BCI, anesthetic management can be understandably complex. Large bore intravenous access should be obtained immediately and blood products and rapid infusion devices must be prepared as soon as possible in anticipation of a massive resuscitation, especially in the patient with myocardial rupture. The use of pulmonary artery catheterization (PAC) may be useful to monitor the progress of the resuscitation and in the diagnosis of pericardial tamponade. TEE may be necessary for accurate assessment of volume status, however, as BCI may be associated with reduced ventricular compliance, thereby complicating the interpretation of cardiac filling pressures as measured by PAC. TEE may also have the added benefit of diagnosing valvular injury that may not have been detected in the primary survey. Diagnosis of significant aortic or mitral regurgitation with TEE may improve the anesthesiologist's ability to maintain hemodynamic stability by guiding the optimization of heart rate, intravascular volume, and afterload. Blunt trauma victims with coexisting right ventricular myocardial injury and pulmonary trauma (pulmonary contusion, hemothorax, or pneumothorax) resulting in pulmonary hypertension are at increased risk for right heart failure; inhaled nitric oxide (NO) or a combination of epinephrine and nitroglycerine infusions may be required to maintain adequate right ventricular function. Patients with myocardial injury are also at increased risk for the development of arrhythmias. No single anesthetic technique is less likely to exacerbate this problem, but the immediate ability to defibrillate or pace, either with externally placed pads or internal paddles, must be available at all times. The use of catecholamines, which may exacerbate or induce arrhythmias in patients with injured myocardium, may not be avoidable in patients with hypotension and shock.

GREAT VESSEL TRAUMA

Significant trauma to the aorta and aortic arch vessels can result from all traumatic mechanisms including those associated with blunt, penetrating, and blast injuries. Victims of penetrating injuries to the thoracic vessels often die in the field immediately due to their injury; however, patients may occasionally survive if the hematoma is sufficiently contained. Thus, early evaluation with CXR is extremely important for the early recognition of radiographic signs of blunt traumatic aortic injury (BTAI) that may be present. Rapid control of hemorrhage is critical in unstable patients with penetrating injuries to the thoracic vessels. As such, victims of *penetrating* thoracic trauma with massive hemorrhage who arrive in the emergency department *with signs of life* (pupillary activity, respiratory effort, or narrow complex QRS activity) are likely candidates for resuscitative thoracotomy (RT) in the ED.[10] Conversely, victims of *blunt* thoracic trauma are unlikely to be considered candidates for RT, as those who do undergo RT rarely survive.

Bleeding from arch vessels, most commonly originating at the base of the innominate artery, is usually contained by local tissues but can rarely result in massive hemorrhage into the pericardial or pleural spaces. Great vessel injury leading to common carotid artery occlusion may result in cerebral ischemia and varying degrees of neurological deficit, which may or may not be detectable at presentation. Injury to most minor thoracic veins is usually not clinically devastating, but the hemorrhage may create a widened mediastinum on CXR necessitating further work-up for aortic transection (see below). Notable exceptions include injuries to the azygos or pulmonary veins, which may cause massive intrapleural hemorrhage.[4] Injuries to the proximal pulmonary arteries, terminal pulmonary veins, or the vena cava have a mortality rate approaching 75%.[5]

The majority (70%) of injuries to the thoracic aorta occur as a result of blunt trauma sustained in MVCs; however, falls from higher than 30 ft (9 meters), motorcycle crashes, and automobile-pedestrian collisions may also be associated with BTAI (Table 20–3). While the injury occurs in less than 1% MVCs,

Table 20–3. Factors Associated with Thoracic Aortic Injury

Accident factors
- High speed MVC
- Head-on or patient-side impact
- Significant intrusion of the vehicular wall into the passenger compartment
- Death of another passenger in the vehicle
- Falls from >30 ft

Signs and symptoms
- Sharp pain radiating to the back
- Hoarseness
- Unequal upper extremity blood pressures
- Paraplegia or paraparesis

Associated injuries
- Presence of scapula, clavicle, or first or second rib fractures

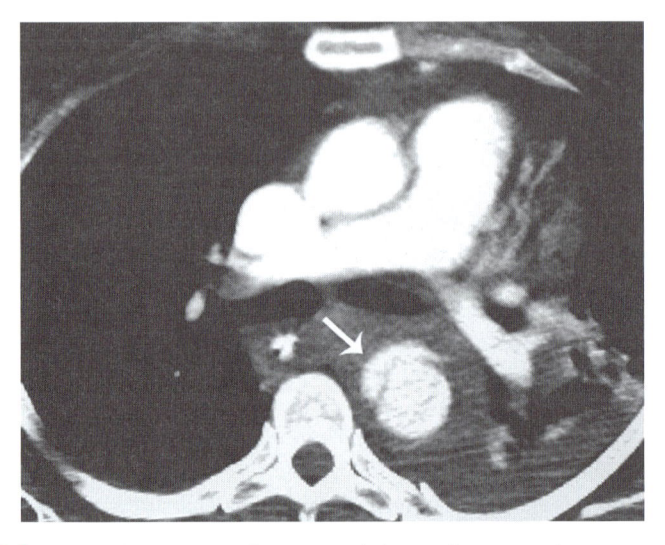

Figure 20–3. Aortic disruption in the proximal descending aorta. (Image courtesy of Mark L. Shapiro, MD.)

it represents the cause of death in up to 15% MVC victims.[44] Approximately 80% patients will die at the scene, and a majority of those who survive to hospital admission will die without a definitive procedure.[45] It was formerly thought that head-on crashes were the most likely to result in aortic transection, but it is now recognized that any MVC with significant energy transfer, regardless of directionality or side of impact may be associated with aortic transection.[10] The mechanism of the injury is probably related to shearing forces resulting from rapid deceleration. These forces usually cause a tear just distal to the takeoff of the left subclavian artery which represents the junction of the relatively mobile aortic arch with the comparably fixed descending aorta (Figure 20–3).[4] While the tear occurs at this aortic *isthmus* in around 90% cases, between 3% and 10% transections may originate in the ascending aorta, aortic arch, or distal descending aorta.[44] In addition to the shearing forces resulting from sudden deceleration, it is also possible that a "water-hammer" effect from simultaneous occlusion of the aorta coinciding with a sudden increase in blood pressure, along with pinching of the vessel between osseous structures during the thoracic compression may contribute to the injury.[45] The injury is characterized by complete *disruption* of all three layers of the aorta; this should be distinguished from *aneurysmal* disease, which involves variable amounts of weakening and expansion of the layers of the aorta. When all three layers are completely disrupted, the patient will usually die within minutes at the scene. However, the hemorrhage may be contained in the form of a pseudoaneurysm, permitting survival for transport and definitive treatment.

Plain CXR is the most important initial study in the evaluation of suspected aortic transection. Suggestive findings include mediastinal widening, an obscured aortic knob, downward deviation of the left mainstem bronchus, rightward deviation of the normal path of the nasogastric tube, and opacification of the aortopulmonary window.[10,45] However, up to 44% patients may have a normal mediastinal appearance on CXR, leading to the recommendation that the diagnosis should be further investigated whenever there is a high suspicion based on the mechanism or circumstances of the injury (Table 20–3).[45] While angiography was considered the gold standard diagnostic modality as recently as 10 years ago, helical CT is currently considered the test of choice.[45,46] Helical CT has a sensitivity approaching 100% and is considered to have an excellent negative predictive value.[47]

Perhaps the most important recent development in the management of blunt aortic injury is a shift in management strategy from emergent surgical repair to one of hemodynamic stabilization followed by delayed repair, either with an open technique or endovascular stent grafting. This strategy is particularly applicable to patients with other life-threatening injuries, such as intracranial trauma, exsanguinating abdominal or pelvic injuries, or severe lung injury, all of which may significantly complicate open repair.[48] The primary goal of this hemodynamic management strategy centers upon lowering cardiac contractility (dP/dt), thereby decreasing the intra-aortic shear forces present at the site of injury. The increasing preference for delayed repair has also been driven by the high morbidity and mortality historically associated with emergent open repair. In a 20-year meta-analysis of over 1700 patients, overall mortality was 32%, and 19% patients for whom a "clamp-and-sew" technique was employed developed paraplegia.[49] Despite this high mortality, there has classically been a sense that patients with contained aortic ruptures represent "ticking time-bombs." However, in a prospective study involving 71 patients with proven BAI, there were no cases of in-hospital aortic rupture when a strategy to keep the heart rate less than 100 bpm and the systolic blood pressure near 100 mm Hg was used. Infusions of either labetalol or esmolol with or without the addition of nitroprusside were used to achieve the hemodynamic goals.[50] It should be noted that sodium nitroprusside is contraindicated in patients with significant intracranial injury due to its potent cerebrovasodilatory effects.

Patients who do require urgent or delayed open surgical repair will present significant perioperative anesthetic and hemodynamic challenges. Whenever possible, the heart rate and systolic blood pressure should be kept below 100 bpm and 110 mm Hg, respectively, to reduce shear stress at the site of the transection. This is probably best achieved with short-acting, titratable agents such as esmolol, which will effectively lower contractility (dP/dt). If patients are more stable and rapid titratability is not as important, the decrease in blood pressure and contractility may also be achieved with labetalol, either intermittently or as an infusion. Monitoring with PAC may be useful both for optimization of filling pressures and to ensure adequate oxygen delivery by measurement of mixed venous oxygen saturation (SvO_2). Lung isolation with selective ventilation of the right lung will be required for surgical access through a left posterolateral thoracotomy at the fourth intercostal space. This may not be well-tolerated by patients with significant pulmonary contusion, and maintenance of adequate oxygenation may be very difficult. For descending aortic injuries, the arterial line should be placed in the right radial artery, whereas placement in the left radial artery may be necessary if repair of an ascending aortic injury will require clamping of the inominate artery. Repair of arch injuries will necessitate full cardiopulmonary bypass (CPB) and hypothermic circulatory arrest. In the traditional "clamp-and-sew" technique utilized in the repair of descending aortic injuries, proximal and distal control of the injury is achieved with two clamps, and an interposition graft is placed as quickly as possible to bridge the defect. This technique is associated with rates of paraplegia as high as 19%,[49] so most centers employ some degree of active bypass to provide perfusion to the distal aorta during clamping of the injured segment. This can be achieved by one of two techniques: (1) bypassing oxygenated blood from the left atrium to the femoral artery with a simple centrifugal pump, or (2) venoarterial bypass with a pump oxygenator, either through direct cannulation of the pulmonary artery or by placing a right atrial catheter via the femoral vein. Both techniques require only minimal systemic heparinization or the use of heparin-coated tubing.[45]

While still not widely accepted as the standard of care, endovascular repair of aortic injuries with placement of stent grafts is becoming more popular, and the technique can greatly simplify the intraoperative management of patients with aortic trauma. There is no requirement for lung isolation and if necessary the procedure can even be performed under local anesthesia. Thoracotomy is not necessary, greatly minimizing concerns for post-operative pain. Of importance to the patient with head injury and concern for increased ICP, the procedure can also be performed with the head of the bed elevated. In addition to simplifying management, outcomes are also improved with this technique. In a recent meta-analysis comparing open with endovascular repair, mortality was reduced from 15.2% in the open-repair group to 7.6% in the group treated with endovascular repair, while paraplegia was similarly reduced from 5.6% to 0%.[51] Patients undergoing endovascular stent grafting still require meticulous management of heart rate and blood pressure as described for patients requiring open repair. Invasive hemodynamic monitoring with a PAC may still be useful despite the greatly simplified operative requirements to ensure adequate oxygen during controlled hypotension.

REFERENCES

1. National Center for Injury Prevention and Control. Available at: http://webappa.cdc.gov/sasweb/ncipc/leadcaus10.html Atlanta, GA. Accessed June 30, 2009.
2. Moloney JT, Fowler SJ, Chang W. Anesthetic management of thoracic trauma. *Curr Opin Anaesthesiol.* 2008;21(1):41-46.
3. Orliaguet G, Ferjani M, Riou B. The heart in blunt trauma. *Anesthesiology.* 2001;95(2):544-548.
4. Pretre R, Chilcott M. Blunt trauma to the heart and great vessels. *N Engl J Med.* 1997;336(9):626-632.
5. Gerhardt MA, Gravlee GP. Anesthesia considerations for cardiothoracic trauma. In: Smith CE, ed. *Trauma Anesthesia.* Cambridge, New York: Cambridge University Press; 2008:279-299.
6. American College of Surgeons. Committee on Trauma. Appendix 3: biomechanics of injury. *Advanced Trauma Life Support Program for Doctors: ATLS.* 7th ed. Chicago, IL: American College of Surgeons; 2004:315-335.
7. DePalma RG, Burris DG, Champion HR, Hodgson MJ. Blast injuries. *N Engl J Med.* 2005;352(13):1335-1342.

8. Champion HR, Holcomb JB, Young LA. Injuries from explosions: physics, biophysics, pathology, and required research focus. *J Trauma.* 2009;66(5):1468-1477; discussion 1477.
9. American College of Surgeons. Committee on Trauma. *Advanced Trauma Life Support Program for Doctors: ATLS.* 7th ed. Chicago, IL: American College of Surgeons; 2004.
10. Herzig D, Biffl WL. Thoracic trauma. In: Fink MP, ed. *Textbook of Critical Care.* 5th ed. Philadelphia, PA: Elsevier Saunders; 2005:2077-2087.
11. Casos SR, Richardson JD. Role of thoracoscopy in acute management of chest injury. *Curr Opin Crit Care.* 2006;12(6):584-589.
12. Ziegler DW, Agarwal NN. The morbidity and mortality of rib fractures. *J Trauma.* 1994;37(6):975-979.
13. Bulger EM, Arneson MA, Mock CN, Jurkovich GJ. Rib fractures in the elderly. *J Trauma.* 2000;48(6):1040-1046; discussion 1046-1047.
14. Karmakar MK, Ho AM. Acute pain management of patients with multiple fractured ribs. *J Trauma.* 2003;54(3):615-625.
15. Mohta M, Verma P, Saxena AK, Sethi AK, Tyagi A, Girotra G. Prospective, randomized comparison of continuous thoracic epidural and thoracic paravertebral infusion in patients with unilateral multiple fractured ribs—a pilot study. *J Trauma.* 2009;66(4):1096-1101.
16. Reiestad F, Kvalheim L. Continuous intercostal nerve block for postoperative pain relief. *Tidsskr Nor Laegeforen.* 1984;104(7):485-487.
17. Rocco A, Reiestad F, Gudman J, McKay W. Intrapleural administration of local anaesthetics for pain relief in patients with multiple rib fractures: preliminary report. *Reg Anesth.* 1987;12(1):10-14.
18. Moon MR, Luchette FA, Gibson SW, et al. Prospective, randomized comparison of epidural versus parenteral opioid analgesia in thoracic trauma. *Ann Surg.* 1999;229(5):684-691; discussion 691-682.
19. Luchette FA, Radafshar SM, Kaiser R, Flynn W, Hassett JM. Prospective evaluation of epidural versus intrapleural catheters for analgesia in chest wall trauma. *J Trauma.* 1994;36(6):865-869; discussion 869-870.
20. Dittmann M, Keller R, Wolff G. A rationale for epidural analgesia in the treatment of multiple rib fractures. *Intensive Care Med.* 1978;4(4):193-197.
21. Davignon K, Kwo J, Bigatello LM. Pathophysiology and management of the flail chest. *Minerva Anestesiol.* 2004;70(4):193-199.
22. Vecsei V, Frenzel I, Plenk H Jr. A new rib plate for the stabilization of multiple rib fractures and thoracic wall fracture with paradoxical respiration. *Hefte Unfallheilkd.* 1979;138:279-282.
23. Labitzke R, Schmit-Neuerburg KP, Schramm G. Indications for thoracotomy and rib stabilization in thoracic trauma in the aged. *Chirurg.* 1980;51(9):576-580.
24. Sales JR, Ellis TJ, Gillard J, et al. Biomechanical testing of a novel, minimally invasive rib fracture plating system. *J Trauma.* 2008;64(5):1270-1274.
25. Vu KC, Skourtis ME, Gong X, Zhou M, Ozaki W, Winn SR. Reduction of rib fractures with a bioresorbable plating system: preliminary observations. *J Trauma.* 2008;64(5):1264-1269.
26. Cacchione RN, Richardson JD, Seligson D. Painful nonunion of multiple rib fractures managed by operative stabilization. *J Trauma.* 2000;48(2):319-321.
27. Nirula R, Allen B, Layman R, Falimirski ME, Somberg LB. Rib fracture stabilization in patients sustaining blunt chest injury. *Am Surg.* 2006;72(4):307-309.
28. Pettiford BL, Luketich JD, Landreneau RJ. The management of flail chest. *Thorac Surg Clin.* 2007;17(1):25-33.
29. Tanaka H, Yukioka T, Yamaguti Y, et al. Surgical stabilization of internal pneumatic stabilization? a prospective randomized study of management of severe flail chest patients. *J Trauma.* 2002;52(4):727-732; discussion 732.
30. Cohn SM. Pulmonary contusion: review of the clinical entity. *J Trauma.* 1997;42(5):973-979.
31. Kishikawa M, Yoshioka T, Shimazu T, Sugimoto H, Sugimoto T. Pulmonary contusion causes long-term respiratory dysfunction with decreased functional residual capacity. *J Trauma.* 1991;31(9):1203-1208; discussion 1208-1210.
32. Crestanello JA, Samuels LE, Kaufman MS, Thomas MP, Talucci R. Posttraumatic pulmonary pseudocyst. *J Trauma.* 1998;44(2):401-403.
33. Cothren C, Moore EE, Biffl WL, Franciose RJ, Offner PJ, Burch JM. Lung-sparing techniques are associated with improved outcome compared with anatomic resection for severe lung injuries. *J Trauma.* 2002;53(3):483-487.

34. Al-Refaie RE, Awad EM, Mokbel EM. Blunt traumatic diaphragmatic rupture: a retrospective observational study of 46 patients. *Interact Cardiovasc Thorac Surg.* 2009;9(1):45-49.
35. Mihos P, Potaris K, Gakidis J, et al. Traumatic rupture of the diaphragm: experience with 65 patients. *Injury.* 2003;34(3):169-172.
36. Sorensen VJ. Diaphragmatic injuries. In: Karmy-Jones R, Nathens A, Stern E, eds. *Thoracic Trauma and Critical Care.* Norwell, MA: Kluwer Academic Publishers; 2002:261-266.
37. Stene JK, Grande CM, Bernhard WN, Barton CR. Perioperative anesthetic management of the trauma patient: thoracoabdominal and orthopaedic injuries. In: Stene JK, Grande CM, eds. *Trauma Anesthesia.* Baltimore, MD: Williams & Wilkins; 1991:177-249.
38. Wood DE. Tracheobronchial trauma. In: Karmy-Jones R, Nathens A, Stern E, eds. *Thoracic Trauma and Critical Care.* Norwell, MA: Kluwer Academic Publishers; 2002:109-123.
39. Biffl WL, Moore EE. Blunt cardiac injury. In: Karmy-Jones R, Nathens A, Stern E, eds. *Thoracic Trauma and Critical Care.* Norwell, MA: Kluwer Academic Publishers; 2002:281-288.
40. Pasquale M, Fabian TC. Practice management guidelines for trauma from the Eastern Association for the Surgery of Trauma. *J Trauma.* 1998;44(6):941-956; discussion 956-947.
41. Rozycki GS, Feliciano DV, Schmidt JA, et al. The role of surgeon-performed ultrasound in patients with possible cardiac wounds. *Ann Surg.* 1996;223(6):737-744; discussion 744-736.
42. Elie MC. Blunt cardiac injury. *Mt Sinai J Med.* 2006 Mar;73(2):542-552.
43. Sybrandy KC, Cramer MJ, Burgersdijk C. Diagnosing cardiac contusion: old wisdom and new insights. *Heart.* 2003;89(5):485-489.
44. Navid F, Gleason TG. Great vessel and cardiac trauma: diagnostic and management strategies. *Semin Thorac Cardiovasc Surg.* 2008;20(1):31-38.
45. Neschis DG, Scalea TM, Flinn WR, Griffith BP. Blunt aortic injury. *N Engl J Med.* 2008;359(16):1708-1716.
46. Demetriades D, Velmahos GC, Scalea TM, et al. Diagnosis and treatment of blunt thoracic aortic injuries: changing perspectives. *J Trauma.* 2008;64(6):1415-1418; discussion 1418-1419.
47. Mirvis SE, Shanmuganathan K, Buell J, Rodriguez A. Use of spiral computed tomography for the assessment of blunt trauma patients with potential aortic injury. *J Trauma.* 1998;45(5):922-930.
48. Fabian TC, Richardson JD, Croce MA, et al. Prospective study of blunt aortic injury: multicenter trial of the American Association for the Surgery of Trauma. *J Trauma.* 1997;42(3):374-380; discussion 380-373.
49. von Oppell UO, Dunne TT, De Groot MK, Zilla P. Traumatic aortic rupture: twenty-year metaanalysis of mortality and risk of paraplegia. *Ann Thorac Surg.* 1994;58(2):585-593.
50. Fabian TC, Davis KA, Gavant ML, et al. Prospective study of blunt aortic injury: helical CT is diagnostic and antihypertensive therapy reduces rupture. *Ann Surg.* 1998;227(5):666-676; discussion 676-667.
51. Tang GL, Tehrani HY, Usman A, et al. Reduced mortality, paraplegia, and stroke with stent graft repair of blunt aortic transections: a modern meta-analysis. *J Vasc Surg.* 2008;47(3):671-675.

Anesthesia for Pediatric Thoracic Surgery

21

Laura K. Diaz
Arjunan Ganesh
Katherine Grichnik
John B. Eck

Key Points

1. Infants with unilateral lung disease are best oxygenated with the healthy lung in the nondependent position given the soft, compressible nature of their ribcage, the relationship of FRC to residual volume, and less significant hydrostatic pressure gradient between the right and left lungs. This is contrary with what is usually seen in the adult population.
2. The choice of induction technique (spontaneous breathing versus positive pressure ventilation) during airway foreign body retrieval should be dictated by the location of the foreign body and by the risk of advancing that object to a location in the respiratory tree that either obstructs ventilation or is not easily retrievable.
3. The anesthetic management for a patient presenting with an anterior mediastinal mass is both complex and hazardous, particularly during induction of anesthesia. Maintenance of spontaneous ventilation is often preferred. The availability of a rigid bronchoscope, the ability to reposition the patient easily, and in some cases circulatory support (ECMO) assistance may be indicated for large and/or very symptomatic mediastinal masses.

Clinical Vignette

A 2-month-old infant was diagnosed prenatally with a right-sided congenital cystic adenomatoid malformation. He is scheduled for a surgical resection via right thoracotomy. He just completed a 14-day course of antibiotics for pulmonary infection.

Vital signs Wt: 3.6 kg, BP 74/42, HR 135, RR 40, SpO_2 96% on 0.2 L/min oxygen. CT scan reveals multiple 2 to 3 cm cystic lesions in the right upper lobe, some with air/fluid levels.

Thoracic surgery in the pediatric population presents additional challenges to the routine problems encountered in adult patients presenting with thoracic disease. This chapter will review the key knowledge necessary to care for these patients and will use one condition (congenital cystic adenomatous malformations) as an example of the general issues to consider for intrathoracic surgery in an infant. In addition, the chapter will provide a discussion of two other conditions that may result in a pediatric thoracic surgical procedure: foreign body in the airway and anterior mediastinal mass.

OVERVIEW

Conditions Necessitating Thoracic Surgery

Conditions that present in the first year of life may include lesions of the respiratory tree, lung, vasculature, and diaphragm.[1] Examples include tracheal stenosis and malacia (both congenital and secondary to prolonged intubation), pulmonary sequestration, pulmonary hypoplasia (associated with a number of intrauterine problems), congenital diaphragmatic hernia, tracheoesophageal fistula, esophageal atresia, coarctation of the aorta and patent ductus arteriosus. Conditions that more commonly arise after the first year of life include primary or metastatic tumors (especially lymphoblastic lymphoma, Hodgkin lymphoma and neuroblastoma), severe infection (consolidated pneumonia, abscess and empyema), arteriovenous malformation, pectus excavatum and kyphoscoliosis. Finally, a common cause for an emergent thoracic procedure is a foreign body in the airway.

Anatomic Differences

There are several key differences between adult and pediatric airway anatomy.[2] The first is the large head relative to the body, with a more prominent occiput in infants and young children (Figure 21–1). Due to this anatomic configuration, the neck may be slightly flexed when supine and can lead to difficulty with airway manipulation and intubation. Secondly, pediatric patients have a relatively large tongue compared to the size of the oropharynx, which can also lead to difficulty with intubation. Further, the laryngeal structures are distinct: the larynx itself is situated in more anterior and cephalad position compared to the adult (C2-3 compared to C4-5). The epiglottis is large, long and can appear U-shaped, often necessitating the use of a straight laryngoscope blade to lift it for vocal cord visualization (Figure 21–2). The narrowest portion of the funnel shaped larynx is below the vocal cords at the level of the cricoid cartilage. Finally, the trachea and neck are proportionally shorter in infants and small children relative to adult anatomy.

Preoperative Assessment

As in adults, an assessment of the presenting problem, a family history, current medications, history of gastroesophageal reflux, drug, food, and/or environmental allergies and a review of systems for coexisting medical problems are necessary.

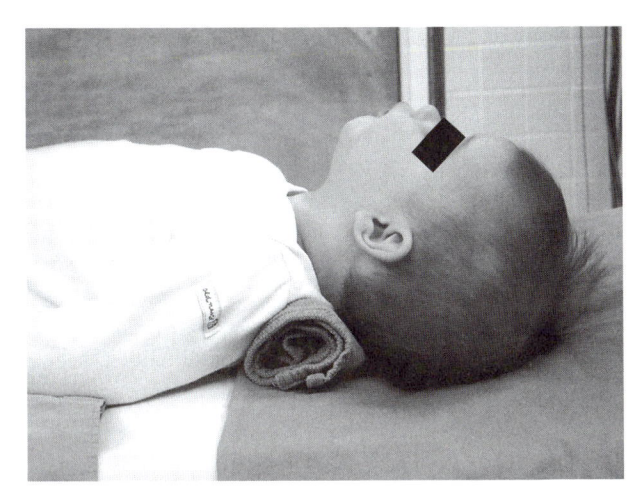

Figure 21-1. A child being positioned for an anesthetic. Note the size of the head relative to the body. A roll under the shoulders may avoid flexion at the neck and maintain a patent airway. (Courtesy of Scott Tolle.)

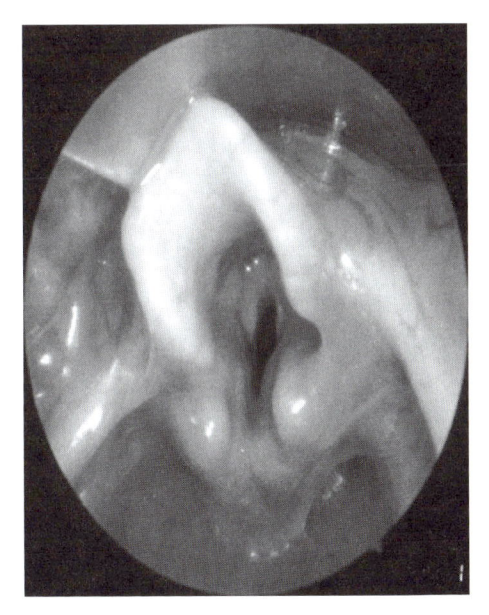

Figure 21-2. The glottic opening of an infant. Note the relatively long epiglottis. (Courtesy of A. Inglis, MD.)

For infants, the birth history along with any significant perinatal medical history, including the existence of coexisting syndromes or chromosomal abnormalities should be reviewed.

Recent or ongoing upper respiratory infections should be reviewed carefully as they are common in children and may increase the risk of perioperative oxygen desaturation, laryngospasm or bronchospasm, and postoperative croup.[3] Surgery is often deferred until several weeks after an infectious process has resolved; however, some thoracic surgical conditions may include concurrent, frequent infections (eg, congenital cystic adenomatous malformations [CCAM]) that necessitate proceeding with the surgical intervention in the face of a respiratory illness. Extra vigilance for airway-related complications is important in that circumstance.

Physical examination of the infant or child should emphasize evaluation of the airway, cardiovascular system, state of hydration, and potential sites of vascular access. Difficulties with mouth opening or neck extension should be noted. Vital signs should also include measurement of baseline hemoglobin-oxygen saturation, and pulses should be assessed in all extremities. Laboratory studies, including a complete blood count and platelet count, should be reviewed and any abnormalities should be noted. A chest radiograph should also be obtained and reviewed for any evidence of mediastinal shift, pulmonary herniation, or inferior displacement of the hemidiaphragm.

Imaging

Infants and children presenting for thoracic surgery will most likely have had multiple types of imaging studies, which should be examined prior to an anesthetic. In addition to a chest radiograph, computed tomography (CT), magnetic resonance imaging (MRI) and/or arteriography may have been performed. Echocardiography, ventilation to perfusion scanning, and pulmonary function testing may be indicated for some conditions. The anatomic location of the lesion to be surgically corrected should be understood, along with its blood supply and relationship to nearby key anatomic structures.

One-Lung Ventilation for Pediatrics

Although major pediatric intrathoracic surgery has traditionally been performed using a single-lumen endotracheal tube and manual lung compression by the surgeon, the advent of video-assisted thoracic surgery (VATS) has led to the more widespread use of one-lung ventilation (OLV) for major thoracic procedures. A VATS approach may be preferred as it provides better cosmetic results, probably decreases postoperative pain, and limits future development of scoliosis or musculoskeletal deformity sometimes seen after open thoracotomy.[4] Although several techniques for lung isolation have been described in children,[5-20] due to the small size of the infant's trachea and bronchi, only some of these techniques can be used in the smallest patients. Similar to the adult population, there are several important considerations for both the establishment of OLV and management of oxygenation, ventilation, and perfusion during OLV.[1]

Endobronchial Intubation

The first step is to control the airway in a manner that facilitates OLV. One technique is to use a single-lumen endotracheal tube (ETT) with deliberate mainstem intubation of the bronchus on the contralateral side of the planned surgery.[21] Right bronchial intubation is straightforward, but to intubate the left bronchus, the bevel of the tube is rotated 180 degrees while the patient's head is turned to the patient's right.[22] Selective bronchial intubation may also be accomplished using a fiberoptic bronchoscope or fluoroscopy to guide the ETT into the desired bronchus. Cuffed ETTs may also be used, but care should be taken to ensure that the distance from the proximal cuff to the tip of the ETT is shorter than the length of the bronchus.[23] A variation on this technique is the independent intubation of both bronchi.[24,25] Problems with endobronchial intubation techniques include possible obstruction of the right upper lobe bronchus, inability to provide an adequate seal with partial inflation of the operative lung, and inability to evacuate secretions from the operative lung. The primary risk related to endobronchial intubation is endobronchial injury resulting from a relatively large endotracheal tube relative to the size of the bronchus.

Endobronchial Blockers

Multiple options also exist for the use of balloon-tipped endobronchial blockers that pass either beside or through the endotracheal tube. The usual limitation is the relative size of the bronchial blocker compared to the endotracheal tube. The Fogarty embolectomy catheter (Edwards Lifesciences, Irvine, CA; Arrow International, Reading, PA) is the most commonly used catheter for bronchial blockade[8,26,27] in small infants, but the Arndt blocker (Cook Critical Care, Bloomington, IN) has also been occasionally used in this age group.[27,28] The advantages of bronchial blockers include the ability to achieve lung isolation, intermittently ventilate both lungs (by deflating the blocker), and aspirate blood and secretions from the operative side when blockers with end-holes are used.

The Fogarty embolectomy catheter set includes a wire stylet that can be curved at the distal end to help direct the catheter's tip into the appropriate bronchus. The blocker may be inserted through or beside the ETT. A fiberoptic scope may be used to guide the blocker into the appropriate bronchus. In one case report, an endobronchial blocker was coupled to the fiberoptic scope intratracheally in an interesting approach that helped successfully achieve OLV in a 3-kg infant.[28] Fluoroscopy may also be used to assist in blocker placement. In small children, the Arndt blocker has been placed successfully using fluoroscopy with the ETT then being placed beside the blocker.[27]

Dislodgment is the most common problem associated with bronchial blockers. This can be corrected intraoperatively using either fiberoptic or fluoroscopic guidance. Another problem associated with blockers is the potential for bronchial rupture or injury.[29] Thus, lung isolation in small infants requires the services of a team experienced in these techniques.

Table 21-1. Endotracheal Tube Selection for One-Lung Ventilation in Children

Age (yr)	ETT (ID)[a] (mm)	BB (F)[b]	Univent[c]	DLT (F)[d]
0.5-1	3.5-4.0	5		
1-2	4.0-4.5	5		
2-4	4.5-5.0	5		
4-6	5.0-5.5	5		
6-8	5.5-6	6	3.5	
8-10	6.0 cuffed	6	3.5	26
10-12	6.5 cuffed	6	4.5	26-28
12-14	6.5-7.0 cuffed	6	4.5	32
14-16	7.0 cuffed	7	6.0	35
16-18	7.0-8.0 cuffed	7	7.0	35

ETT = endotracheal tube, ID = internal diameter, F = French size, DLT = double-lumen tube, BB = bronchial blocker.
[a]Sheridan Tracheal Tubes, Kendall Healthcare, Mansfield, MA
[b]Arrow International Corp., Redding, PA
[c]Fuji Systems Corporation, Tokyo, Japan
[d]#26F, Rusch, Duluth, GA; 28-35 Fr, Mallinckrodt Medical, Inc., St. Louis, MO
Reproduced with permission from Hammer GB, Fitzmaurice BG, Brodsky JB. Methods for single-lung ventilation in pediatrics patients. *Anest Analg.* 1999;89:1426.

Dual-Lumen Endotracheal Tubes

Dual-lumen endotracheal tubes (DLT) offer the advantage of superb airway control but have a large cross-sectional area and are therefore mostly useful in larger children. The smallest cuffed DLT is size 26 French, which may be used in children as young as 8 years old. 28 French and 32 French DLTs are usually suitable for children aged 10 and older[1] (Table 21-1). With DLT use, one must be aware of the increased resistance to airflow with OLV. Excessive positive-pressure ventilation may cause barotrauma resulting in pneumothorax, pneumomediastinum, or interstitial emphysema. This usually occurs in the ventilated, dependent lung but occasionally occurs in the non-dependent lung upon re-expansion.

Principles of OLV

The general principles of OLV in adults apply to pediatrics as well. General anesthesia, muscle relaxants, lateral position, and dependent lung compression often cause a decrease in functional residual capacity of both lungs and atelectasis in the dependent lung. Hypoxic pulmonary vasoconstriction that normally minimizes V/Q mismatch may be limited by inhaled anesthetics and other vasodilating drugs.[1]

The approach to OLV in infants requires an understanding of the physiological differences between adults and very small children. Positioning these patients in the lateral decubitus position can significantly worsen V/Q matching compared to an adult. In adults with unilateral lung disease, oxygenation is better with the healthy lung dependent and the diseased lung nondependent due to a relative increase in perfusion of the dependent lung.[30] However, in infants the situation is reversed: oxygenation is improved when the healthy lung is nondependent and the diseased lung is dependent.[31] Several variables may account for this problem. The rib cage is soft and compressible, FRC is close to residual volume (leading to airway closure), abdominal hydrostatic pressure is proportionally less, and there is a reduced hydrostatic pressure gradient between the nondependent and dependent lungs. Airway closure may also occur with tidal volume ventilation.[1,32] Further, pediatric patients have relatively higher oxygen requirements (6-8 mL/kg/min of oxygen in an infant vs 2-3 mL/kg/min in an adult) and are thus at high risk of hypoxemia during lateral positioning and OLV. OLV techniques used in children should therefore ideally include the option of providing oxygen to the operative lung.[33]

Pain Management for Thoracic Surgery

The amount of pain that an infant or child may experience is dependent on the surgical incision, the location and extent of the operation, and concurrent disease states. In general, as in adults, pain management may be achieved with intravenous medications (opiates and non-opioids), regional or peripheral nerve infiltration with local anesthetic, and neuraxial blockade.

The use of intravenous opioids will be influenced both by the surgical approach and adjunctive use of regional anesthesia techniques. In neonates and infants, the authors prefer to titrate narcotic dosage according to respiratory effort after reversal of the neuromuscular blockade at the conclusion of the operation. Bupivacaine 0.25% (maximum 1 mL/kg) may also be infiltrated into incision sites to assist with postoperative pain management.

Thoracic Epidural Analgesia for pediatrics

More extensive thoracic surgical procedures may be treated with a more aggressive analgesic plan, usually including the use of regional anesthetic techniques. Thoracic epidural analgesia is a logical choice for thoracic procedures and is frequently used in the pediatric population. A primary advantage of epidural analgesia in neonates and infants is the decreased need for intravenous opioids,[34] thus decreasing the likelihood of apnea, bradycardia, and occasionally, respiratory arrest.[35] Epidural analgesia following thoracotomies may also improve the chances of successful postoperative extubation.[36]

Thoracic epidural catheters may be placed at the level of the incision in the older child or via a caudal approach in the younger child. The caudal approach was first described in a 3-phase study in which cadaveric and animal trials were performed before the technique was attempted on neonates undergoing biliary surgery.[37]

Feasibility, safety, and efficacy of thoracic epidural catheters inserted via the caudal route were well demonstrated. The technique starts with the identification of the sacral hiatus and advancement of an 18-gauge intravenous catheter (18-gauge Tuohy or Crawford needles may also be used) through the sacrococcygeal membrane into the epidural space. The epidural space may be expanded with normal saline, after which a 20-gauge catheter is advanced to the desired level (the distance to the desired level is measured before advancing the catheter). The importance of radiographic confirmation of the epidural catheter's tip following insertion was emphasized in a retrospective study.[38]

Stimulating epidural catheters have also been successfully placed using the technique described by Tsui and colleagues.[39,40] The stimulating epidural catheter (Arrow International Inc., Reading, PA) is flushed with normal saline and then inserted via an 18-gauge intravenous catheter initially placed in the epidural space. An electric current of 1 to 10 mA is applied through the catheter as it is advanced cephalad. The level of muscle twitch indicates the level of the catheter; therefore, neuromuscular blockade cannot be used at the time of catheter placement.

Recently, ultrasound has been used to locate the tip of caudally advanced epidural catheters.[41,42] Ultrasound has the advantage of being noninvasive and can be used in small infants in whom there is a clear window for visualization due to incomplete ossification of the posterior elements of the spinal canal.

Direct placement of a thoracic epidural catheter may also be attempted; however, it is less frequently done due to the risk of spinal cord injury. In a prospective multicenter study in France, no complications related to direct thoracic epidural catheter placement were noted in children,[43] but data gathered from the same group suggested that thoracic epidural catheters should be placed by experienced anesthesiologists. In a recent study, ultrasound guidance for placement of lumbar and thoracic epidural catheters was compared to traditional loss-of-resistance technique.[44] The group concluded that, in experienced hands, ultrasound reduces both the duration of catheter placement and the incidence of bony contacts.

Perhaps the most important decision is when to place the epidural catheter relative to the induction of general anesthesia. In an older, sedated child, direct placement of the catheter may be indicated with the child being his/her own monitor for neural symptoms. Direct placement of a thoracic epidural catheter in an anesthetized person is still controversial. However, caudal placement is generally considered safe in the anesthetized child.

A combination of local anesthetics, epidural opioids, and alpha-2 agonists may be used to provide optimal analgesia.[45] Use of epidural local anesthetic solution alone necessitates a higher rate of infusion to obtain adequate analgesia.[46] Close attention must be paid to local anesthetic infusion in order to avoid toxicity. The recommended maximal infusion rates for bupivacaine are 0.4 mg/kg/h in older infants and 0.2 to 0.25 mg/kg/h in neonates.[47] The addition of opioids to epidural solutions may also reduce the risk of local anesthetic toxicity by allowing less local anesthetic to be used.[47] In a prospective randomized double-blind study, the addition of fentanyl 2 mcg/mL to an epidural solution of bupivacaine 1 mg/mL was shown to improve analgesia when compared to bupivacaine 1 mg/mL alone in infants up to 6 months of age undergoing thoracotomy.[48]

Safety concerns have been raised regarding elevated concentrations of bupivacaine[49,50,51] during prolonged (>48 hour) infusions in neonates and infants. In a recent study of infant patients who received continuous epidural ropivacaine infusion in the dose of 0.2 to 0.4 mg/kg/h for up to 72 hours, plasma concentrations of bound and unbound ropivacaine were found to be below toxic levels.[52] This, coupled with a better safety profile regarding cardiotoxicity and resuscitation from overdose[53,54] makes ropivacaine a wiser choice compared to bupivacaine in young infants.

Patients who are treated with continuous epidural analgesia, particularly after a thoracotomy, are often monitored in an intensive care unit. Monitoring should include the following measures:

- Continuous ECG and pulse oximetry
- Recording of hourly vital signs, including heart and respiratory rate, blood pressure, and oxygen saturation
- Pain assessment at least every 4 hours
- Monitoring epidural catheter insertion site every 12 to 24 hours
- Setting alarms to detect bradycardia, bradypnea, and apnea

In addition to the above, rescue analgesic medication should be ordered for breakthrough pain along with naloxone to treat opioid-induced respiratory depression. A bag and mask, along with an oxygen source, must be available at the bedside to treat signs and symptoms of respiratory depression.

Potential complications include local anesthetic toxicity related to intravascular administration or prolonged infusions at high rates, epidural hematoma and/or abscess formation, meningitis, superficial cellulitis, and abnormal catheter location during insertion. When assessing or monitoring for local anesthetic toxicity, physicians and nurses must remember that an infant or young child will not report any symptoms and may only manifest restlessness or agitation.[47]

SPECIFIC CONDITIONS

Examples of several types of intrathoracic conditions requiring surgical intervention in infants and children are now presented. Congenital cystic adenomatous malformations are presented as a specific example of an intrathoracic lesion requiring thoracoscopy/thoracotomy in an infant. In addition, several intrathoracic conditions common to older pediatric patients (foreign body in the airway and anterior mediastinal mass) are reviewed.

CONGENITAL CYSTIC ADENOMATOUS MALFORMATIONS

Congenital cystic adenomatous malformations (CCAMs) were initially described by Ch'in and Tang in 1949.[55] CCAMs are predominantly a unilateral lesion, derived from an abnormality in the formation of parenchymal lung tissue that results in adenomatous overgrowth of terminal bronchiolar structures and formation of cystic structures of various sizes (Table 21–2). CCAMs

Table 21–2. Characteristics of CCAMs

Abnormal proliferation of bronchiolar-like tissue
Lack of normal alveoli
Bilateral lung involvement rare
Usually arises from one lobe of the lung
Usually communicates with tracheobronchial tree
Usual blood supply from pulmonary circulation
Cyst diameter can range from <1 mm to >10 cm
Presence of mucous secreting cells
Absence of inflammation

communicate with the bronchopulmonary tree, resulting in air trapping, and may have normal arterial blood supply. This contrasts with bronchopulmonary sequestrations (BPS), which are composed of a nonfunctioning mass of tissue lacking connection to the tracheobronchial tree, and in which blood is supplied by an anomalous systemic artery. Although the overall incidence of CCAMs is low (approximately 1 in 25,000 births),[56] CCAMs remain the most common pediatric cystic thoracic lesion, accounting for approximately 25% congenital lung malformations. Hybrid lung masses that appear to demonstrate clinicopathological characteristics typical of both CCAMs and sequestration lesions have also been described.[57,58]

CCAMs are categorized by clinical or pathological criteria (Table 21–3). Adzick and colleagues classified CCAMs based on a combination of ultrasound and gross anatomical features,[59] with prognosis determined by the size of the mass and the resultant degree of physiological derangement. Polyhydramnios (secondary to esophageal compression), mediastinal shift, and lung hypoplasia can occur with large masses. Interventions in utero to decompress the lesion via thoraco-abdominal or thoraco-amniotic shunting or resection of the mass may be indicated. Alternatively, resection may be performed using an ex utero intrapartum therapeutic approach. Postpartum, even in asymptomatic infants and children, resection of the mass is warranted due to the risk of infection and/or malignant transformation.[60-65]

Diagnosis and Timing of Surgery

Most infants with a CCAM are diagnosed prenatally[66] by ultrasound imaging or fetal magnetic resonance imaging. One must differentiate CCAMs from congenital diaphragmatic hernias.[67,68] Even if regression is anticipated and the chest radiograph is normal, a postnatal CT should be performed, as small lesions frequently are often still present.[69] Doppler imaging or angiography can confirm the origin of blood supply to the lesion.

The indication and timing for surgery is controversial. In addition to recurrent infection, the risk of spontaneous pneumothorax and the chance of malignant transformation are often cited as reasons to pursue early surgical resection of a

Table 21-3. Classification of CCAMs by Clinical or Pathological Criteria

Bale[1] (1979)	*Term or older infant*: Primarily cystic lesion, recurrent infections, associated anomalies rare	*Near-term infant*: Severe respiratory distress at birth, cystic-solid lesion, emergent surgical intervention often required	*Premature infant*: Primarily solid lesion, other anomalies common, rarely survive
Stocker et al[2] (1977)	*Type I:* Macrocystic; Single or multiple large cysts >1 cm in diameter, mediastinal shift in >75% cases, tachypnea, grunting, difficulty feeding, repeated infections. Occasional pulmonary hypoplasia/pulmonary hypertension. Usually affect a single lobe; good prognosis.	*Type II:* Microcystic: Multiple evenly spaced cysts rarely > than 1.2 cm in diameter; rare mediastinal shift. High incidence of stillbirth and early death.	*Type III:* Grossly solid: Cysts rarely >0.5 cm in diameter. Mediastinal shift in all cases. Severe respiratory distress after birth with death in 1-5 hours.
Adzick et al[3] (1985)	*Macrocystic:* Single or multiple cysts >5 mm	*Microcystic:* Smaller echogenic cysts <5 mm	

Adapted from Bale PM. Congenital cystic malformation of the lung. A form of congenital bronchiolar ["adenomatoid"] malformation. *Am J Clin Pathol*. 1979;71:411-420; Stocker JT, Madewell JE, Drake RM. Congenital cystic adenomatoid malformation of the lung. Classification and morphologic spectrum. *Hum Pathol*. 1977;8:155-171; Adzick NS, Harrison MR, Glick PL, et al. Fetal cystic adenomatoid malformation: prenatal diagnosis and natural history. *J Pediatr Surg*. 1985;20:483-488.

known lesion.[70] A review of childhood pulmonary neoplasms by Hancock et al revealed that 8.6% were associated with previously documented cystic lesions.[18] Further, early resection may encourage compensatory lung growth.

Most surgeons recommend that lobectomy and resection of a CCAM be performed between 1 and 6 months of age[70] in an attempt to balance the desire for early resection against the risks of anesthesia in a neonate.[71,72] Truitt et al recommended observation of asymptomatic patients until ages 12 to 18 months, with VATS resection of the lesion to be performed at that time.[73] In Aspirot's series, 75% patients requiring more than 24 hours of postoperative mechanical ventilation were younger than 3 months old.[36]

Preoperative Assessment

It is likely that surgery will be performed in the face of a concurrent infection due to the frequent occurrence of infections in patients with a CCAM. Infants diagnosed prenatally should undergo a CT scan within the first months of life to confirm the presence and size of the CCAM as well as to determine the appropriate timing for surgical resection. Preoperative assessment should also include echocardiography (if fetal echocardiography was not previously performed) to rule out cardiac disease or compromise. The usual fasting guidelines indexed to patient age are appropriate. A thorough review of the planned procedure, the invasive monitoring necessary, the anticipated need for ICU care and potential complications must be discussed in detail with the parents. Premedication should similarly be used in an age appropriate manner, titrated (or eliminated) based on the degree of respiratory compromise an infant may have at baseline.

Surgery

CCAM resection is via open thoracotomy or a minimally invasive VATS. Knowledge of the surgical approach and the possibility of conversion to an open thoracotomy are critical, as the VATS approach often mandates a OLV technique. OLV may be poorly tolerated in smaller or sicker patients. As such, invasive monitoring may be warranted in this patient subgroup. Pain management strategies will likewise differ depending on the planned surgical approach.

Monitoring, Induction, and Maintenance

The standard monitors include pulse oximetry probes placed on both upper and lower extremities, oscillometric blood pressure measurement, and a 3- or 5-lead electrocardiogram. In neonates, a pulse oximetry probe that suddenly ceases to function may portend hypotension and/or poor peripheral perfusion. Thus, the presence of a second pulse oximetry probe is extremely useful in differentiating between probe failure and a physiological change. Accurate temperature monitoring is also critical and may be accomplished via the use of rectal, esophageal, or nasopharyngeal temperature probes. Placement of an arterial catheter facilitates monitoring of arterial blood gases for optimization of ventilatory parameters.

A standard anesthetic induction for an infant, utilizing either an intravenous or inhalation technique is appropriate, with the caveat to avoid nitrous oxide. The placement of two intravenous lines is recommended to allow for intraoperative administration of blood and/or inotropes, if necessary. In more critically ill infants with mediastinal shift secondary to CCAM, it may be desirable to preserve spontaneous ventilation until lung isolation has been achieved to avoid worsening mediastinal shift and cardiorespiratory collapse.[66] OLV will usually be indicated so one must plan for the occurrence of hypoxia and hypercarbia.

Risks

Aspirot et al noted significantly fewer perioperative complications in asymptomatic versus symptomatic patients. For this reason, discussions with parents should reflect the potentially increased risk and possible need for prolonged mechanical ventilatory support for children who have large masses or ongoing infections.[36] Ideally, all but the sickest neonates can be tracheally extubated in the operating room at the conclusion of the procedure or shortly thereafter. In a review by Tsai and colleagues of 105 asymptomatic infants who underwent surgical resection of either CCAM or BPS, 103 were tracheally extubated immediately after the surgical procedure.[74] There was no associated mortality in this patient group, but a 6.7% morbidity rate was seen due to residual air leakage and need for transfusion.[74] Therefore, postoperative chest films should be obtained in all patients to rule out pneumothorax or hemothorax. Recovery in an intensive care setting is appropriate, especially for infants with indwelling epidural catheters.

FOREIGN BODY IN THE AIRWAY

Most anesthesiologists will be faced with the need to anesthetize a child for a foreign body in the airway. This often occurs in children under the age of three years—in part due to the use of the mouth to explore nonfood substances in addition to normal food intake and their tendency to be in motion while eating.[75] Further, the immaturity or lack of molar teeth can lead to the ingestion of large pieces of food. Commonly aspirated items include grapes, seeds, and small pieces of meat. More dangerous are dried foods capable of swelling (raisins) or small objects such as buttons or balloons, which can cause complete tracheal obstruction. Foreign body aspirations in children most often occur in the right mainstem bronchus (Table 21–4), due to the angle of the right mainstem bronchus relative to the left mainstem bronchus from the trachea[76] (Figure 21–3). One should further recognize that the aspirated object may not be associated with an acute event, resulting in the possibility of concurrent lung or mucosal inflammation, infection and/or chronic bronchial obstruction. As such, either intermittent or chronic airway edema and bronchospasm may be present. A preoperative bronchodilator may be indicated to improve the chances of successful object retrieval. The most

Table 21–4. Location of Aspirated Foreign Bodies in Children

Anatomic Location	Percent
Larynx	3
Trachea	13
Right mainstem bronchus	52
Right middle bronchus	1
Right lower lobe bronchus	6
Left mainstem bronchus	18
Left lower lobe bronchus	5
Bilateral airways	2

Reprinted with permission from Eren S, Balci AE, Dikici B, Doblan M, Eren MS. Foreign body aspiration in children: experience of 1160 cases. *Ann Trop Paediatr Int Child Health.* 2003 Mar;23(1):31-37(7). http://www.maney.co.uk/journals/atp and http://www.ingentaconnect.com/content/maney/atp

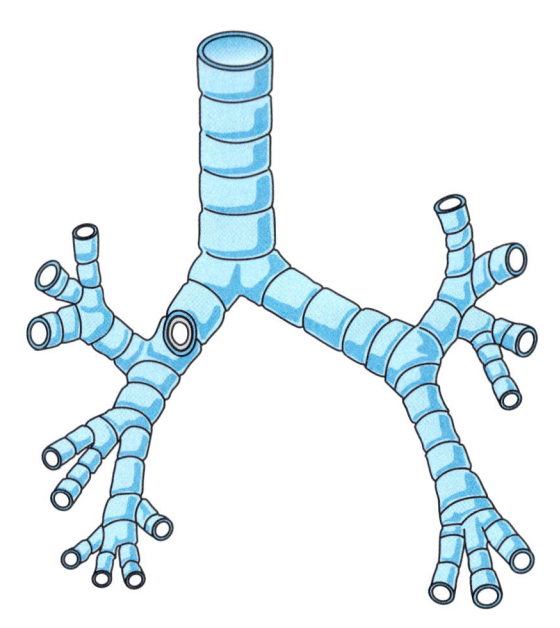

Figure 12-3. The normal anatomy of the tracheobronchial tree with a foreign body in the right mainstem bronchus. The right mainstem bronchus is at a less acute angle relative to the trachea than the left mainstem bronchus. Therefore, aspirated foreign objects are much more likely to be a located in the right airways than the left.

important preoperative management step is communication with the surgeon or invasive pulmonologist including a shared understanding of where the object is, the anticipated degree of difficulty in extraction, and what steps would be necessary in the event of complete airway obstruction.

Anesthetic Induction and Airway Management

The induction of anesthesia must be carefully planned with the need for airway manipulation to retrieve the foreign body.[77] A flexible bronchoscopy may initially be considered to diagnose and perhaps extricate the object, usually in a pulmonary suite. However, the anesthesiologist is most often faced with the need to induce anesthesia and control respiration while creating ideal conditions for the placement of a rigid bronchoscope. The first choice is the type of induction, with the decision about whether to keep a child spontaneously breathing or use positive pressure ventilation. In part, this decision is dictated by the location of the foreign body and, with positive pressure ventilation, the risk of advancing that object to a place in the respiratory tree that it either obstructs ventilation or is not easily retrievable. Conversely, one must be cautious about the risk of a child coughing during induction resulting in relocation of the object to a tracheal or laryngeal site that causes airway obstruction. The need for a rapid sequence induction may be determined by the urgency of the situation, whether the child has recently ingested food and what the risk of airway compromise is relative to the usual fasting period, indexed by the age of the patient. There is not a particular advantage of one agent (inhaled versus intravenous) over another for anesthetic induction. However, one may consider the administration of atropine or glycopyrrolate to dry airway secretions, prevent bradycardia and to further reduce the risk of bronchoconstriction during airway manipulation.

After induction of anesthesia, the operating room table is usually tuned at a 90-degree angle from the anesthesiologist and a rigid bronchoscope is introduced with a ventilating sideport. This is a critical period of time as the airway is unsecured until the bronchoscope is in place—a smooth transition should be carefully planned. In general, the use of a total intravenous anesthetic at this point is wise, both to avoid operating room air pollution with anesthetic gases as the airway is intermittently open to the room during this process, and to maintain adequate anesthetic depth prior to instrumentation of the airway. If spontaneous ventilation is chosen, then topical airway anesthesia is critical to reduce the depth of anesthesia necessary to tolerate the bronchoscope placement and the optimize ventilation, oxygenation, and hemodynamic stability. If controlled ventilation is chosen, the periods of apnea necessary to remove the object may be short in younger children whose ability to oxygenate may be significantly impaired. Litman et al reviewed 94 cases of pediatric foreign body removal and did not find a significant advantage of one ventilatory technique over the other.[78] The anesthesiologist needs to be aware that retrieval of the object may involve one or more re-intubations if the object is larger than the diameter of the bronchoscope, necessitating the technique of securing the object with grasping forceps and then removal of the object by retracting the grasping forceps with the object and the bronchoscope at the same time.

Complications

One can anticipate the potential complication of partial or complete airway obstruction including the risk of prolonged apnea and potential hypoxia. However, depending on the length of time that the object has existed in the airway or bronchial tree, resultant localized irritation, secretion formation or even a postobstructive pneumonia may manifest with continued respiratory compromise, even after object removal. A more serious immediate complication can be pneumomediastinum and/or pneumothorax, which Burton reported to occur after 13% of foreign body removals.[79]

PEDIATRIC ANTERIOR MEDIASTINAL MASS

The anesthetic management for a patient presenting with an anterior mediastinal mass (AMM) is both complex and hazardous as respiratory and/or circulatory collapse may ensue during the course of the procedure, particularly during induction of anesthesia.[80] A thoughtful, staged approach to the perioperative care of these patients is essential.

Preoperative Assessment

Pediatric patients may present either for diagnosis or resection of an AMM. Common causes for an AMM in children include lymphoblastic lymphoma, Hodgkin disease, vascular malformations, neurogenic tumors, germ cell tumors, and bronchogenic cysts.

Symptoms may range from slight shortness of breath to significant dyspnea with stridor, associated with chest pain and superior vena cava syndrome. Symptoms may vary with position; however, the absence of symptoms does not exclude the possibility of cardiorespiratory collapse with anesthetic administration. Further, there is a poor relationship between clinical signs and size of tumor or tracheal compression on imaging studies.[81]

Preoperative evaluation should include chest radiography, CT, and possibly MRI or positron emission (PET) scanning. Assessment should include the presence and degree of tracheal compression, the tracheal cross-sectional area and the presence of bronchial compression. It may also be important to obtain an estimation of significant respiratory impingement through flow-volume studies (including peak expiratory flow rate) and significant vascular impingement through echocardiography. The degree of symptoms, size and location of the mass, and thoracic anatomical impingement determines the approach to obtaining a biopsy for tissue diagnosis or attempting resection (Figure 21–4).[80]

Preoperative measures may be taken to reduce the risk of a surgical procedure and anesthetic induction. Some have advocated for the preoperative use of steroids in the management of AMMs[81] as steroids may reduce the inflammatory reaction to the tumor as well as (perhaps) influence its size and vascularity. If feasible, a biopsy under local anesthesia and/or initiation of chemotherapy or limited radiation therapy may reduce the risk of a perioperative complication. Of note, the anterior Chamberlin procedure can be performed in a sitting, slightly sedated spontaneously breathing child under local anesthesia to obtain a tissue diagnosis (Figure 21–5).

Anesthetic Induction and Airway Management

After appropriate review of the imaging and functional studies, an anesthetic plan should be formulated including provisions for unintended airway and circulatory collapse. The availability of a rigid bronchoscope, the ability to easily move the OR table to effect positional changes and the availability of advanced circulatory support (ECMO) may be indicated for large and/or very symptomatic AMMs. Although a mask induction is often chosen to maintain spontaneous ventilation, one must ensure adequate intravenous access prior to establishment of a deep level of anesthesia (which may reduce respiratory muscle tone) and intubation. Other management strategies to consider include keeping the head of the bed elevated, considering a partial lateral decubitus position and using continuous positive airway pressure to maintain functional residual capacity.[80,82] One commonly utilized technique is to intubate the trachea without the use of muscle relaxants or positive pressure ventilation to optimize the transpulmonary pressure gradient

Assess anesthetic risk

Clinical assessment

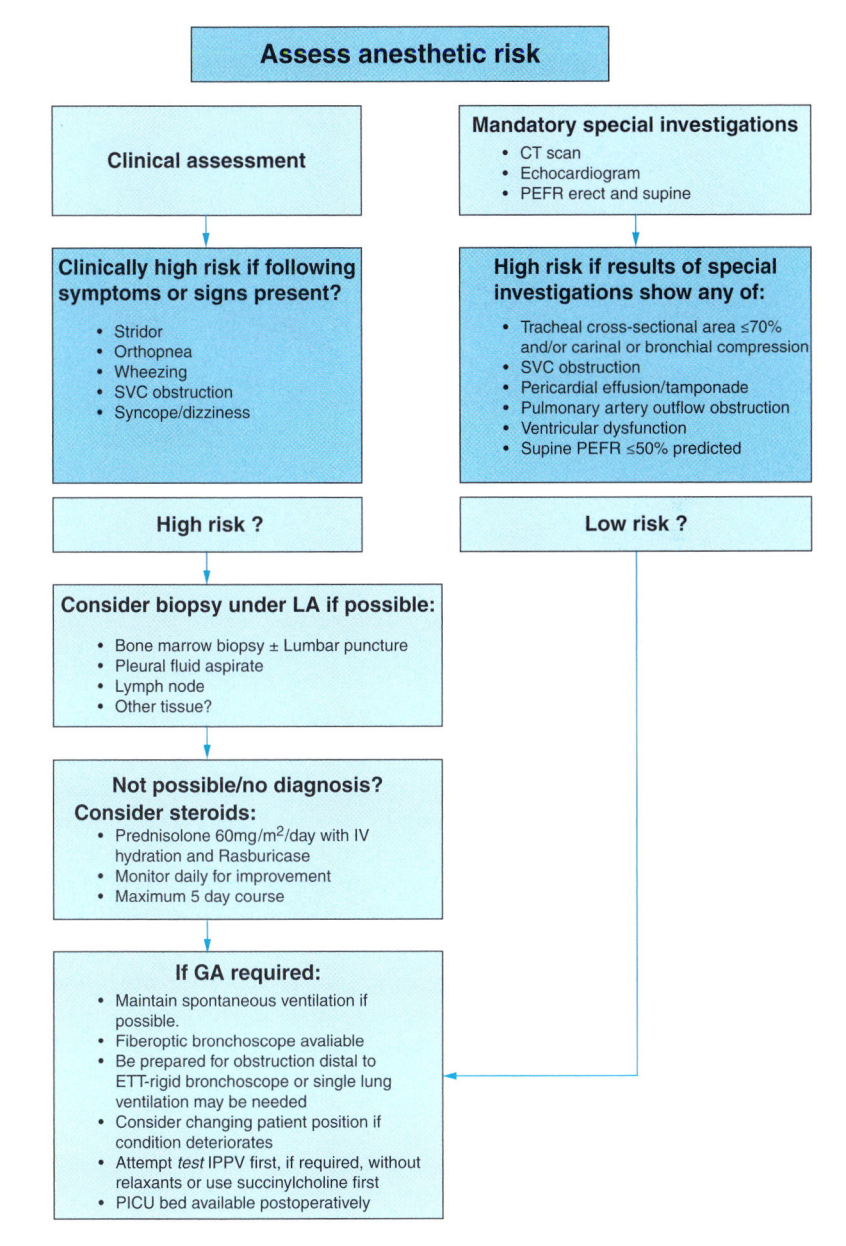

Mandatory special investigations
- CT scan
- Echocardiogram
- PEFR erect and supine

Clinically high risk if following symptoms or signs present?
- Stridor
- Orthopnea
- Wheezing
- SVC obstruction
- Syncope/dizziness

High risk if results of special investigations show any of:
- Tracheal cross-sectional area ≤70% and/or carinal or bronchial compression
- SVC obstruction
- Pericardial effusion/tamponade
- Pulmonary artery outflow obstruction
- Ventricular dysfunction
- Supine PEFR ≤50% predicted

High risk ?

Low risk ?

Consider biopsy under LA if possible:
- Bone marrow biopsy ± Lumbar puncture
- Pleural fluid aspirate
- Lymph node
- Other tissue?

Not possible/no diagnosis? Consider steroids:
- Prednisolone 60mg/m^2/day with IV hydration and Rasburicase
- Monitor daily for improvement
- Maximum 5 day course

If GA required:
- Maintain spontaneous ventilation if possible.
- Fiberoptic bronchoscope avaliable
- Be prepared for obstruction distal to ETT-rigid bronchoscope or single lung ventilation may be needed
- Consider changing patient position if condition deteriorates
- Attempt *test* IPPV first, if required, without relaxants or use succinylcholine first
- PICU bed available postoperatively

Figure 21-4. A suggested algorithm for the assessment of anesthetic risk and the subsequent management of an anterior mediastinal mass in a child. IPPV = intermittent positive pressure ventilation, PEFR = peak expiratory flow rate. (From: Hack HA, Wright NB, Wynn RF. The anaesthetic management of children with anterior mediastinal masses. *Anaesthesia.* 2008 Aug;63(8):837-846, reproduced with permission.)

AMM Location

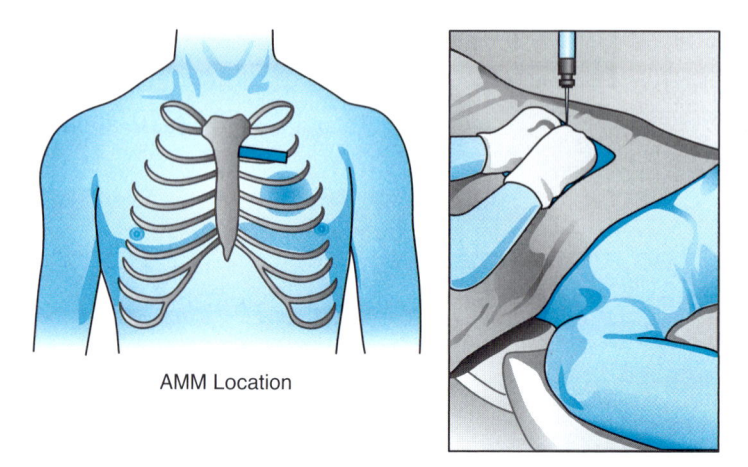

Figure 21–5. Chamberlin procedure under monitored anesthesia care with local infiltration.

and improve flow through the respiratory tree.[80] Using similar logic, the use of a laryngeal mask airway has been advocated.[80]

Perioperative Complications

Adult and pediatric patients are at significant risk for perioperative complications from mediastinal mass surgery. This is especially true in children with an immature and more cartilaginous airway. Lam et al found that several factors were associated with increased risk of respiratory compromise or failure: tracheal compression or displacement, superior vena cava and other vascular compression, anterior tumor location, preoperative diagnosis of lymphoma, pericardial effusion, and pleural effusion.[83,84] Postoperatively, patients may experience pulmonary edema, bleeding, respiratory failure and hypotension. The extent of the surgery and the intraoperative course will dictate postoperative decision making, including the need for ventilation and recovery in an intensive care unit.

SUMMARY

Thoracic surgery for pediatric patients is both challenging and rewarding. This chapter has focused on key points to guide management and care of these patients, using three representative conditions to illustrate the complexities of thoracic anesthesia in infants and children.

REFERENCES

1. Hammer GB. Pediatric thoracic anesthesia. *Anesth Analg.* 2001;92:1449-1464.
2. Adware L. Anatomy and assessment of the pediatric airway. *Pediatric Anesth.* 2009;19(Suppl 1):1-8.

3. Rolf N, Cote CJ. Frequency and severity of desaturation events during general anesthesia in children with and without upper respiratory infections. *J Clin Anesth.* 1992;4(3):200-203.
4. Rothenberg SS. Experience with thoracoscopic lobectomy in infants and children. *J Pediatr Surg.* 2003;38(1):102-104.
5. Mihalka J, Burrows FA, Burke RP, et al. One-lung ventilation during video-assisted thoracoscopic ligation of a thoracic duct in a three-year-old child. *J Cardiothorac Vasc Anesth.* 1994;8(5):559-562.
6. Baraka A. Right bevelled tube for selective left bronchial intubation in a child undergoing right thoracotomy. *Paediatr Anaesth.* 1996;6(6):487-489.
7. Lin WT, Cheng KC, Liu HP, et al. Alternation of one-lung and two-lung ventilations with the same single-lumen endobronchial tube during thoracoscopic surgery—a case report. *Acta Anaesthesiol Sin.* 1998;36(4):229-233.
8. Rehman M, Sherlekar S, Schwartz R, et al. One lung anaesthesia for video assisted thoracoscopic lung biopsy in a paediatric patient. *Paediatr Anaesth.* 1999;9(1):85-87.
9. Camci E, Tugrul M, Tugrul ST, et al. Techniques and complications of one-lung ventilation in children with suppurative lung disease: experience in 15 cases. *J Cardiothorac Vasc Anesth.* 2001;15(3):341-345.
10. Tobias JD. Variations on one-lung ventilation. *J Clin Anesth.* 2001;13(1):35-39.
11. Mohan VK, Darlong VM, Kashyap L, et al. Fiberoptic-guided Fogarty catheter placement using the same diaphragm of an adapter within the single-lumen tube in children. *Anesth Analg.* 2002;95(5):-1241-1242, table of contents.
12. Ho AC, Chung HS, Lu PP, et al. Facilitation of alternative one-lung and two-lung ventilation by use of an endotracheal tube exchanger for pediatric empyema during video-assisted thoracoscopy. *Surg Endosc.* 2004;18:1752.
13. Use T, Shimamoto H, Fukano T, et al. Single lung ventilation in a pediatric patient using a Fogarty catheter with a hollow center. *Masui.* 2004;53:69.
14. Choudhry DK. Single-lung ventilation in pediatric anesthesia. *Anesthesiol Clin North America.* 2005;23:693, ix.
15. Ho AC, Chen CY, Yang MW, et al. Use of the Arndt wire-guided endobronchial blocker to facilitate one-lung ventilation for pediatric empyema during video-assisted thoracoscopy. *Chang Gung Med J.* 2005;28:104.
16. Pawar DK, Marraro GA. One lung ventilation in infants and children: experience with Marraro double lumen tube. *Paediatr Anaesth.* 2005;15:204.
17. Wald SH, Mahajan A, Kaplan MB, et al. Experience with the Arndt paediatric bronchial blocker. *Br J Anaesth.* 2005;94:92.
18. Ho AM, Karmakar MK, Critchley LA, et al. Placing the tip of the endotracheal tube at the carina and passing the endobronchial blocker through the Murphy eye may reduce the risk of blocker retrograde dislodgement during one-lung anaesthesia in small children. *Br J Anaesth.* 2008;101:690.
19. Baraka A, Slim M, Dajani A, et al. One-lung ventilation of children during surgical excision of hydatid cysts of the lung. *Br J Anaesth.* 1982;54:523.
20. Ho CS, Huang CL. Comparison of double-lumen endobronchial versus single-lumen endotracheal tube anesthesia in bilateral thoracoscopic sympathectomy. *Acta Anaesthesiol Sin.* 1994;32:7.
21. Rowe R, Andropoulos D, Heard M, et al. Anesthetic management of pediatric patients undergoing thoracoscopy. *J Cardiothorac Vasc Anesth.* 1994;8:563.
22. Kubota H, Kubota Y, Toyoda Y, et al. Selective blind endobronchial intubation in children and adults. *Anesthesiology.* 1987;67:587.
23. Lammers CR, Hammer GB, Brodsky JB, et al. Failure to separate and isolate the lungs with an endotracheal tube positioned in the bronchus. *Anesth Analg.* 1997;85:946.
24. Cullum AR, English IC, Branthwaite MA. Endobronchial intubation in infancy. *Anaesthesia.* 1973;28:66.
25. Hammer GB, Manos SJ, Smith BM, et al. Single-lung ventilation in pediatric patients. *Anesthesiology.* 1996;84:1503.
26. Ginsberg RJ. New technique for one-lung anesthesia using an endobronchial blocker. *J Thorac Cardiovasc Surg.* 1981;82:542.
27. Hammer GB, Harrison TK, Vricella LA, et al. Single lung ventilation in children using a new paediatric bronchial blocker. *Paediatr Anaesth.* 2002;12:69.
27. Marciniak B, Fayoux P, Hebrard A, et al. Fluoroscopic guidance of Arndt endobronchial blocker placement for single-lung ventilation in small children. *Acta Anaesthesiol Scand.* 2008;52:1003.

28. Schmidt C, Rellensmann G, Van Aken H, et al. Single-lung ventilation for pulmonary lobe resection in a newborn. *Anesth Analg.* 2005;101:362, table of contents.
29. Borchardt RA, LaQuaglia MP, McDowall RH, et al. Bronchial injury during lung isolation in a pediatric patient. *Anesth Analg.* 1998;87:324.
30. Remolina C, Khan AU, Santiago TV, et al. Positional hypoxemia in unilateral lung disease. *N Engl J Med.* 1981;304:523.
31. Heaf DP, Helms P, Gordon I, et al. Postural effects on gas exchange in infants. *N Engl J Med.* 1983;308:1505.
32. Mansell A, Bryan C, Levison H. Airway closure in children. *J Appl Physiol.* 1972;33:711.
33. Hammer GB. Single-lung ventilation in infants and children. *Paediatr Anaesth.* 2004;14:98.
34. Wolf AR, Hughes D. Pain relief for infants undergoing abdominal surgery: comparison of infusions of i.v. morphine and extradural bupivacaine. *Br J Anaesth.* 1993;70:10.
35. Purcell-Jones G, Dormon F, Sumner E. The use of opioids in neonates. A retrospective study of 933 cases. *Anaesthesia.* 1987;42:1316.
36. Aspirot A, Puligandla PS, Bouchard S, et al. A contemporary evaluation of surgical outcome in neonates and infants undergoing lung resection. *J Pediatr Surg.* 2008;43:508.
37. Bosenberg AT, Bland BA, Schulte-Steinberg O, et al. Thoracic epidural anesthesia via caudal route in infants. *Anesthesiology.* 1988;69:265.
38. Valairucha S, Seefelder C, Houck CS. Thoracic epidural catheters placed by the caudal route in infants: the importance of radiographic confirmation. *Paediatr Anaesth.* 2002;12:424.
39. Tsui BC, Seal R, Koller J, et al. Thoracic epidural analgesia via the caudal approach in pediatric patients undergoing fundoplication using nerve stimulation guidance. *Anesth Analg.* 2001;93:1152, table of contents.
40. Tsui BC, Wagner A, Cave D, et al. Thoracic and lumbar epidural analgesia via the caudal approach using electrical stimulation guidance in pediatric patients: a review of 289 patients. *Anesthesiology.* 2004;100:683.
41. Chawathe MS, Jones RM, Gildersleve CD, et al. Detection of epidural catheters with ultrasound in children. *Paediatr Anaesth.* 2003;13:681.
42. Roberts SA, Galvez I: Ultrasound assessment of caudal catheter position in infants. *Paediatr Anaesth.* 2005;15:429.
43. Giaufre E, Dalens B, Gombert A. Epidemiology and morbidity of regional anesthesia in children: a one-year prospective survey of the French-Language Society of 44. Pediatric Anesthesiologists. *Anesth Analg.* 1996;83:904.
44. Willschke H, Marhofer P, Bosenberg A, et al. Epidural catheter placement in children: comparing a novel approach using ultrasound guidance and a standard loss-of-resistance technique. *Br J Anaesth.* 2006;97:200.
45. Golianu B, Hammer GB. Pain management for pediatric thoracic surgery. *Curr Opin Anaesthesiol.* 2005;18:13.
46. Lovstad RZ, Stoen R. Postoperative epidural analgesia in children after major orthopaedic surgery. A randomised study of the effect on PONV of two anaesthetic techniques: low and high dose i.v. fentanyl and epidural infusions with and without fentanyl. *Acta Anaesthesiol Scand.* 2001;45:482.
47. Berde CB. Convulsions associated with pediatric regional anesthesia. *Anesth Analg.* 1992;75:164.
48. Ganesh A, Adzick NS, Foster T, et al. Efficacy of addition of fentanyl to epidural bupivacaine on postoperative analgesia after thoracotomy for lung resection in infants. *Anesthesiology.* 2008;109:890.
49. Larsson BA, Lonnqvist PA, Olsson GL. Plasma concentrations of bupivacaine in neonates after continuous epidural infusion. *Anesth Analg.* 1997;84:501.
50. Luz G, Innerhofer P, Bachmann B, et al. Bupivacaine plasma concentrations during continuous epidural anesthesia in infants and children. *Anesth Analg.* 1996;82:231.
51. Luz G, Wieser C, Innerhofer P, et al. Free and total bupivacaine plasma concentrations after continuous epidural anaesthesia in infants and children. *Paediatr Anaesth.* 1998;8:473.
52. Bosenberg AT, Thomas J, Cronje L, et al. Pharmacokinetics and efficacy of ropivacaine for continuous epidural infusion in neonates and infants. *Paediatr Anaesth.* 2005;15:739.
53. Groban L, Deal DD, Vernon JC, et al. Cardiac resuscitation after incremental overdosage with lidocaine, bupivacaine, levobupivacaine, and ropivacaine in anesthetized dogs. *Anesth Analg.* 2001;92:37.

54. Mather LE, Chang DH. Cardiotoxicity with modern local anaesthetics: is there a safer choice? *Drugs.* 2001;61:333.
55. Ch'In KY, Tang MY. Congenital adenomatoid malformation of one lobe of a lung with general anasarca. *Arch Pathol (Chic).* 1949;48:221.
56. Laberge JM, Flageole H, Pugash D, et al. Outcome of the prenatally diagnosed congenital cystic adenomatoid lung malformation: a Canadian experience. *Fetal Diagn Ther.* 2001;16(3):178-186.
57. Cass DL, Crombleholme TM, Howell LJ, et al. Cystic lung lesions with systemic arterial blood supply: a hybrid of congenital cystic adenomatoid malformation and bronchopulmonary sequestration. *J Pediatr Surg.* 1997;32(7):986-990.
58. Hirose R, Suita S, Taguchi T, et al. Extralobar pulmonary sequestration mimicking cystic adenomatoid malformation in prenatal sonographic appearance and histological findings. *J Pediatr Surg.* 1995;30(9):1390-1393.
59. Adzick NS, Harrison MR, Glick PL, et al. Fetal cystic adenomatoid malformation: prenatal diagnosis and natural history. *J Pediatr Surg.* 1985;20(5):483-488.
60. Adzick NS: Management of fetal lung lesions. *Clin Perinatol.* 2009;36(2):363-376.
61. Benjamin DR, Cahill JL. Bronchioloalveolar carcinoma of the lung and congenital cystic adenomatoid malformation. *Am J Clin Pathol.* 1991;95(6):889-892.
62. d'Agostino S, Bonoldi E, Dante S, et al. Embryonal rhabdomyosarcoma of the lung arising in cystic adenomatoid malformation: case report and review of the literature. *J Pediatr Surg.* 1997;32(9):1381-1383.
63. Miniati DN, Chintagumpala M, Langston C, et al. Prenatal presentation and outcome of children with pleuropulmonary blastoma. *J Pediatr Surg.* 2006;41(1):66-71.
64. Murphy JJ, Blair GK, Fraser GC, et al. Rhabdomyosarcoma arising within congenital pulmonary cysts: report of three cases. *J Pediatr Surg.* 1992;27(10):1364-1367.
65. Ribet ME, Copin MC, Soots JG, et al. Bronchioloalveolar carcinoma and congenital cystic adenomatoid malformation. *Ann Thorac Surg.* 1995;60(4):1126-1128.
66. Hugh D, Cameron B. Anesthetic management of a neonate with a congenital cystic adenomatoid malformation and respiratory distress associated with gross mediastinal shift. *Paediatr Anaesth.* 2009;19(3):272-274.
67. Hata N, Wada T, Chiba T, et al. Three-dimensional volume rendering of fetal MR images for the diagnosis of congenital cystic adenomatoid malformation. *Acad Radiol.* 2003;10(3):309-312.
68. Williams HJ, Johnson KJ. Imaging of congenital cystic lung lesions. *Paediatr Respir Rev.* 2002;3(2):120-127.
69. Davenport M, Warne SA, Cacciaguerra S, et al. Current outcome of antenatally diagnosed cystic lung disease. *J Pediatr Surg.* 2004;39(4):549-556.
70. Laberge JM, Puligandla P, Flageole H. Asymptomatic congenital lung malformations. *Semin Pediatr Surg.* 2005;14(1):16-33.
71. Hancock BJ, Di Lorenzo M, Youssef S, et al. Childhood primary pulmonary neoplasms. *J Pediatr Surg.* 1993;28(9):1133-1336.
72. Adzick NS, Flake AW, Crombleholme TM. Management of congenital lung lesions. *Semin Pediatr Surg.* 2003;12(1):10-16.
73. Truitt AK, Carr SR, Cassese J, et al. Perinatal management of congenital cystic lung lesions in the age of minimally invasive surgery. *J Pediatr Surg.* 2006;41(5):893-896.
74. Tsai AY, Liechty KW, Hedrick HL, et al. Outcomes after postnatal resection of prenatally diagnosed asymptomatic cystic lung lesions. *J Pediatr Surg.* 2008;43(3):513-517.
75. http://emedicine.medscape.com/article/1001253. Accessesed May 31, 2011.
76. Eren S, Balci AE, Dikici B, Doblan M, Eren MS. Foreign body aspiration in children: experience of 1160 cases. *Ann Trop Paediatr Int Child Health.* 2003;23(1):31-37.
77. Zur KB, Litman RS. Pediatric airway foreign body retrieval: surgical and anesthetic perspectives. *Pediatr Anesth.* 2009;19(Suppl 1):109-117.
78. Litman RS, Ponnuri J, Trogan I. Anesthesia for tracheal or bronchial foreign body removal in children: an analysis of ninety-four cases. *Anesth Analg.* 2000;91(6):1389-1391.
79. Burton EM, Riggs W Jr, Kaufman RA, et al. Pneumomediastinum caused by foreign body aspiration in children. *Pediatr Radiol.* 1989;20(1-2):45-47.
80. Hammer GB. Anaesthetic management for the child with a mediastinal mass. *Pediatr Anesth.* 2004;14(1):95-97.
81. Hack HA, Wright NB, Wynn RF. The anaesthetic management of children with anterior mediastinal masses. *Anaesthesia.* 2008;63(8):837-846.

82. Rehder K. Anesthesia and the mechanics of respiration. In: Covino BG, Fozzard HA, Rehder K, et al, eds. *Effects of Anesthesia*. Bethesda, MD: American Physiological Society; 1985:91-106.
83. Lam JCM, Chui CH, Jacobsen AS, et al. When is a mediastinal mass critical in a child? An analysis of 29 patients. *Pediatr Surg Int*. 2004;20(3):180-184.
84. Huang YL, MD, Yang MC, Huang CH, et al. Rescue of cardiopulmonary collapse in anterior mediastinal tumor. *Pediatr Emer Care*. 2010;26(4):296-298.

PART 3

Postoperative Management of Thoracic Surgical Patients

CHAPTERS

22. Routine Postoperative Care of the Thoracic Surgical Patient 426
23. Respiratory, Renal, and Cardiovascular Postoperative Complications 440
24. Acute and Chronic Post-Thoracotomy Pain 467

Routine Postoperative Care of the Thoracic Surgical Patient

22

Christopher C.C. Hudson
Jordan K.C. Hudson
Steven E. Hill
Atilio Barbeito

Key Points

- Initial postoperative management of the thoracic surgical patient is best performed in an intermediate or high acuity area.
- These patients are generally at increased risk of respiratory complications, which carry a high mortality rate. Aggressive chest physiotherapy and early ambulation, together with meticulous attention to analgesia, fluid management, glycemic control and nutrition are key to a successful recovery.
- It is important that the treating team be familiar with the anatomy and physiology of the chest, and the management of the different chest drainage systems.

Clinical Vignette

The patient is a 64-year-old gentleman with severe COPD and an FEV_1 of 38% predicted who was found to have a 1.5-cm left upper lobe mass on a chest x-ray obtained during an evaluation for pneumonia. He underwent bronchoscopy, mediastinoscopy and thoracoscopic left upper lobectomy under general anesthesia. He is brought to the ICU awake and on oxygen by face mask. He is hemodynamically stable, having received a total of 800 mL of lactated ringer's solution and 400 mL of colloid solution intraoperatively. A thoracic epidural catheter at the level of T6-7 is in place that was bolused at the beginning of the case with hydromorphone 600 mcg. A 0.125% bupivacaine infusion with 10 mcg/mL of hydromorphone was started intraoperatively at 5 mL/h and continues to infuse.

The patient described in the vignette represents a common case scenario for patients undergoing pulmonary resection. While pulmonary resections are performed frequently in North America, this patient population represents a high morbidity group that merits special attention in the postoperative period. The increasing use of video-assisted thoracoscopic surgery (VATS) over the past

2 decades has led to decreased complications, but the overall goals and challenges of care in the thoracic surgery population remain.[1] In this chapter, we discuss the approach to routine postoperative care of the thoracic surgical patient. This will include risk stratification and initial assessment, pulmonary care and chest tube management, goals for fluid optimization, nutrition, glycemic control, and venous thromboembolism prophylaxis. Common respiratory, cardiovascular, and renal postoperative complications and their management have been discussed in Chapter 23. Analgesic strategies for thoracic surgical procedures will be covered in Chapter 24.

RISK STRATIFICATION

Optimal postoperative management of the thoracic surgical patient begins with a careful review of the patient's comorbidities and a clear understanding of the intraoperative course. It is useful to risk stratify these patients into low, intermediate and high risk categories using their predicted postoperative FEV_1 ($ppFEV_1$), and especially the predicted postoperative DLCO (ppDLCO). Patients in the high-risk category benefit the most from aggressive chest physiotherapy, judicious fluid management and optimal postoperative analgesia. If limited resources are available in the postoperative care unit (eg, only 1 respiratory therapist is available for 6-8 patients), they should be concentrated on the high-risk patients. For a more extensive discussion of risk stratification please refer to Chapter 9.

ASSESSMENT UPON ADMISSION

Thoracic surgical patients generally require an intermediate or high acuity area for recovery until their respiratory status and analgesia are optimized. Patients who require mechanical ventilation postoperatively are generally admitted to the intensive care unit. It is important that the providers caring for these patients be familiar with the management of chest tubes, epidural catheters, and respiratory equipment.

Upon admission to the recovery area, the admitting team must carefully examine the patient, paying particular attention to level of consciousness, analgesia, and respiratory status. The chest tubes need to be inspected and any obstruction ruled out, and the quantity and quality of the drainage noted. A portable chest x-ray is routinely obtained in the immediate postoperative period to confirm lung re-expansion and correct chest tube placement, and to rule out contralateral disease. A baseline ABG is also generally obtained to assess oxygenation and to rule out hypercarbia, which is common in the postoperative period and is usually mild and transient, but may manifest itself as hypertension and somnolence or agitation if severe. Other laboratory tests are obtained as indicated by the extent of the resection.

Hypertension should be treated with short acting intravenous antihypertensive medications only after hypercarbia, pain and a distended bladder have all been ruled out as the primary cause.

POSTOPERATIVE VENTILATORY SUPPORT

Not all patients will meet extubation criteria following thoracic surgery, and many will require a temporary period of noninvasive ventilatory support following extubation. In patients requiring invasive postoperative ventilation, the standard of care is to apply lung protective strategies according to ARDSNet guidelines unless contraindicated.[2] However, high PEEP should be avoided to minimize the risk of developing a bronchopleural fistula.

Noninvasive positive pressure ventilation (NIPPV) and continuous positive airway pressure (CPAP) are options for the management of patients requiring additional ventilatory support after extubation, who are able to protect their airways and are not at increased risk of aspiration. These strategies have been implemented successfully in patients following lung resection and lung transplant.[3-5] Noninvasive ventilation improves postoperative oxygenation and FEV_1 in patients with decreased preoperative FEV_1 and on those who used NIPPV or CPAP preoperatively.[4] Caution should be used in esophagectomy patients, as they may be at increased risk of pulmonary aspiration.

PULMONARY PHYSIOTHERAPY AND EARLY AMBULATION

Physiotherapeutic interventions are typically instituted on the first postoperative day, and may begin immediately after surgery if the patient is able to participate. Although prophylactic chest physiotherapy has been widely accepted, its routine use is of uncertain benefit.[6] Possible approaches include chest physiotherapy alone or in combination with incentive spirometry or noninvasive ventilation. Chest physiotherapy typically includes deep breathing exercises, airway clearance maneuvers, and early mobilization. Randomized controlled trials are currently underway to further evaluate the efficacy of various physiotherapy maneuvers in order to determine an evidence-based approach to postoperative care. In patients with acute respiratory failure after lung resection, chest physiotherapy combined with noninvasive ventilation reduces pulmonary complications, improves patient recovery, and reduces the need for intubation and invasive ventilation.[7]

When possible, early postoperative ambulation should be encouraged. Mobilization can begin as early as the first hour postoperatively, with staff accompaniment. A fast-track approach to rehabilitation consists of immediate postoperative extubation, early oral feeding, physiotherapy, and early removal of chest tubes, urinary catheters, and invasive lines. Appropriate patient selection is crucial, with low preoperative morbidity, adequate pain management, and avoidance of oversedation all being prerequisites. The fast-track approach has been shown to reduce postoperative complications and hospital length of stay after lobectomy.[8]

PNEUMONIA PREVENTION

Patients undergoing thoracic surgery are at increased risk of morbidity and mortality compared to the general surgical population.[9,10] Major respiratory complications, including pneumonia and respiratory failure are very common, occurring at an incidence of 13% in a recent review of the US data.[11] Pneumonia after lung resection has a mortality rate of 20% to 25%.[12] The most common causative organisms are community-acquired bacteria, notably Enterobacter, Streptococcus pneumoniae, Staphylococcus aureus, and Hemophilus influenzae. Risk factors include older age, cardiopulmonary comorbidities, smoking, worse pulmonary function, and more extensive surgical resections (pneumonectomy).[13] While most risk factors are not modifiable, preoperative smoking cessation, minimizing surgical and anesthetic duration, aggressive pulmonary physiotherapy, and fast-track rehabilitation may help to reduce the incidence of postoperative pneumonia.

CHEST TUBE MANAGEMENT

Chest tube management is a routine part of the postoperative care of thoracic surgical patients. Following lung resection, chest tubes are placed to allow closed drainage of air and fluid from the pleural space, permitting re-expansion of the remaining lung to fill the intrathoracic cavity. The tubes are attached to a drainage system that permits one-way drainage only. These systems have evolved from the single bottle version developed in the late 1800s to compact versions of the three-bottle system described by Howe in 1952. Traditional chest drainage devices are generally composed of three chambers: the collecting chamber, the water-seal chamber, and the suction control chamber (Figure 22–1). Newer chest drain models are now equipped with a one-way valve that replaces the traditional water seal bottle. This valve requires no water, and hence maintains the patient seal even if the unit is tipped over. Newer systems also incorporate a dry suction system, where the suction pressure level is controlled by a self-compensating regulator instead of a column of water. This provides several advantages over the wet system:

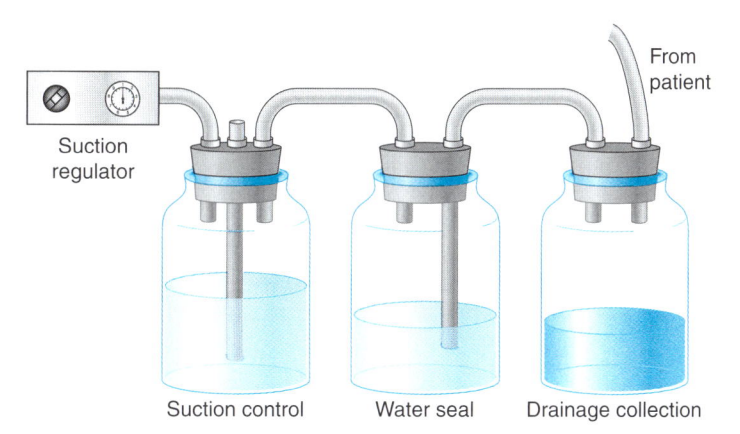

Figure 22–1. The traditional three-bottle system. Suction is applied to the system until it reaches the pressure that will draw ambient air into the open tube of the suction control bottle. At this point, the suction pressure will equal the height of the column of water in this bottle, and the suction level will be maintained regardless of the amount of additional suction applied, since this will only draw more air into the bottle.

It can achieve higher suction pressures; fluid does not evaporate; requires virtually no maintenance; and it has a quieter operation, since there is no continuous bubbling in the suction chamber. Newer devices also share several common features: automatic and manual high negative pressure relief valves, a positive pressure relief valve, sampling ports, serrated, tapered catheter connectors, and an air leak meter[14] (Figure 22–2).

The chest tubes and drainage system should be examined daily for patency, function, air leak, volume and character of drained fluid, and condition of the placement site. Chest tube drainage of less than 200 cc/d or 2 cc/kg/d is considered physiologic.[15,16] The character of chest tube fluid should gradually change from sanguineous to serous; purulent drainage is suggestive of empyema. Fluid oscillation in the water seal that is synchronous with patient respiration—known as "tidaling"—may be seen in the properly functioning chest tube and is a reflection of intrapleural pressure changes and a patent chest tube. These oscillations disappear once the lung is reinflated or if the chest tube is blocked or kinked. Blockages can be cleared by suction catheter aspiration, although this maneuver carries the risk of infection (empyema). "Stripping" refers to simultaneously occluding the tubing and pulling it away from the patient to produce a local suction effect.

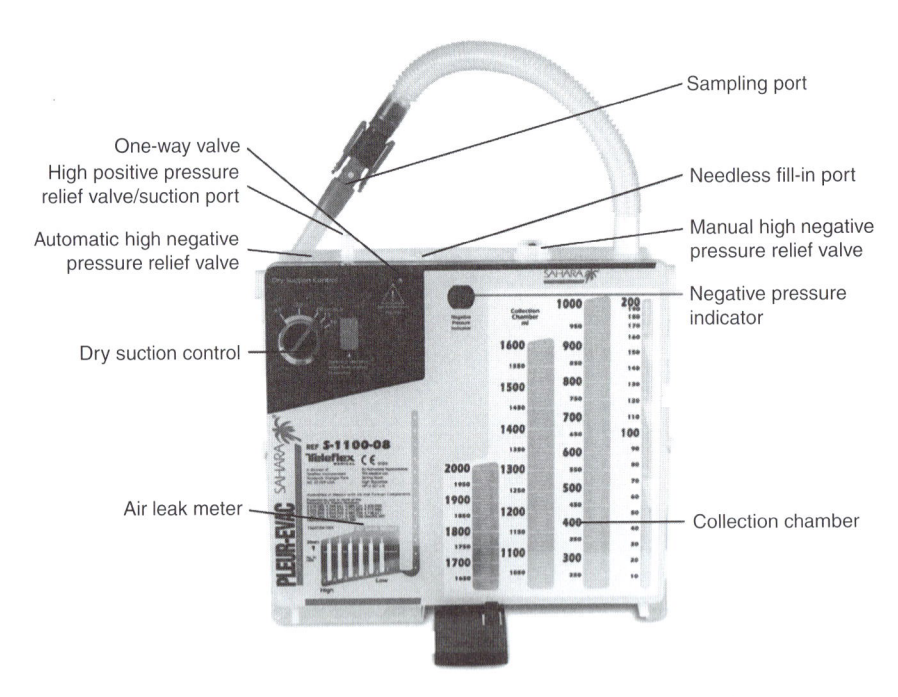

Figure 22–2. Components of a modern pleural drainage system. Note the one-way valve replacing the traditional water seal (second bottle in the three-bottle system) and the dry suction system replacing the traditional suction control bottle. (Reproduced with permission from Pleur-evac. Teleflex Medical).

Pressures of up to −400 cm water have been reported to result from this maneuver and it is therefore generally discouraged.[17]

Care must be exercised to ensure the connecting tubing is not allowed to droop below the top of the drainage system, since any fluid that accumulates in the loop prevents the suction applied to the drainage system to reach the pleura.[14] A chest tube should never be clamped, unless it is done temporarily to allow replacement of the collection system or with accidental disconnections.

Chest radiography should be performed early in the postoperative period to ensure proper chest tube placement and adequate lung re-expansion, but daily chest radiographs are otherwise not indicated in stable patients.[18]

Air Leaks

An air leak is defined as bubbling in the water-seal chamber after the air in the pleural space has been drained, and is termed "persistent" or "prolonged" if it persists beyond 4 to 7 days after chest tube insertion, or if it prolongs hospital stay.[19] Persistent air leaks occur in approximately 10% cases, and represent the most common pulmonary complication after lung resection surgery.[11] Most commonly, the leak is caused by inspired gas moving from denuded lung parenchyma into the pleural space, and onto the chest tube and collecting system with each respiratory effort or cough episode.

Factors that have been shown to predict a persistent air leak after lung resections are FEV_1% of less than 79%, a history of steroid use, male gender, preoperative radiotherapy or chemotherapy exposure, and lobectomy operations.[20,21]

In order to assess for an air leak, the patient should be asked to take 2 or 3 deep breaths and any bubbles consistently moving into the air leak reservoir should be noted. The patient should then be instructed to cough to rule out a forced expiratory air leak.

Air leaks have been classified according to their timing during the respiratory cycle (inspiratory [I], expiratory [E], forced expiratory [FE], or continuous [C]) and their extent (1, least severe, through 7, most severe, based on how many columns are filled with air bubbles upon observation of the air leak meter on the pleural drainage system)[22] (Figure 22–3). Digital air leak meters that allow a more precise quantification of air leaks are also available, and they have been shown to reduce hospital length of stay if used continuously during the postoperative period.[23]

While expiratory and forced expiratory air leaks are common following thoracic surgery, a large inspiratory or continuous air leak is concerning for large lung tissue disruptions, bronchopleural fistula, or a malfunctioning chest tube or drainage system. Small air leaks such as forced expiratory (FE) or low-volume expiratory (E1-E3) have in general a good prognosis and resolve within a few days with the use of water seal. Larger leaks may require surgical repair or discharge to home with a chest tube, flutter (Heimlich) one-way valve and collection system in place.[22]

Occasionally, the chest tube becomes dislodged or partially pulled outside of the pleural cavity, allowing one or more of its side-holes to entrain room air with

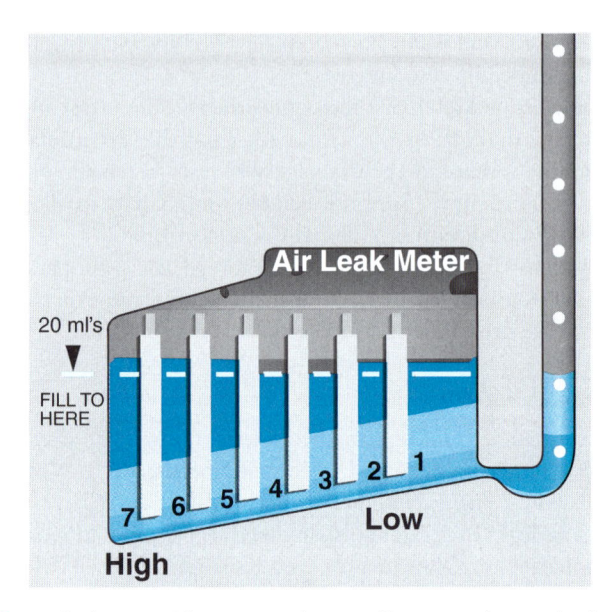

Figure 22–3. Air leak meter. The seven columns allow a semi-quantitative evaluation of air leaks at the bedside. (Reproduced with permission from Pleur-evac. Teleflex Medical).

each inspiratory effort in the spontaneously ventilated patient. This will similarly be signaled by continuous bubbling in the pleural drainage system.

Once air leak ceases, the chest tube output decreases to acceptable levels, and chest radiography demonstrates good lung expansion, chest tube removal can be considered. Despite misconceptions to the contrary, chest tubes can be safely removed at either end-inspiration or end-expiration.[24] In addition, removal of the chest tube can be safely performed while on suction, and protocols requiring weaning to water seal resulted in much longer chest tube duration and a greater number of chest radiographs.[25] Chest radiography is generally performed 1 to 3 hours after chest tube removal to look for significant pneumothorax. Two studies have demonstrated that this routine may be overly conservative in nonmechanically ventilated patients and suggested that chest radiography should be based on the individual's clinical signs and symptoms.[26,27]

Subcutaneous Emphysema

Subcutaneous emphysema is a common and troublesome complication after pulmonary resection, occurring in approximately 6% patients.[28] Air entering the pleural space is generally drained by the chest tube(s) and trapped into the pleural drainage system. Occasionally, the tube becomes obstructed by thrombus or a kink, or is inadvertently left clamped. This impedes the air in the pleura to escape and forces it to advance through the path of least resistance, dissecting through the recently surgically disrupted tissue planes into the subcutaneous fascia. Another mechanism for the development of subcutaneous emphysema is the adhesion of disrupted lung parenchyma onto the thoracotomy or thoracoscopy site, allowing the passage of air directly from the lung into the subcutaneous tissue through what is essentially a pulmonary alveolar-subcutaneous fistula.

Subcutaneous air in the chest wall is able to dissect through the soft tissue of the face, neck, chest, and shoulders, and may cause significant patient distress. Fortunately, more serious complications such as pneumomediastinum and pneumopericardium are exceedingly rare. Standard treatment of postoperative subcutaneous emphysema is to gradually increase the chest tube suction to higher pressures (20-40 cm of water). If this is unsuccessful, the insertion of a second chest tube, also placed to high suction, may alleviate the symptoms. In one-third of patients, such maneuvers will be unsuccessful—treatment options then include performing a small incision at the base of the neck or above the clavicle to allow air to escape, or simply waiting for the problem to resolve spontaneously over time. Early thoracoscopic pneumolysis and chest tube placement has been proposed as a management alternative and has been shown to reduce hospital stay in patients who develop this complication and do not respond to increased levels of chest tube suction.[28]

Balanced Drainage

Following pneumonectomy, the goals of pleural drainage differ from lesser lung resections. The pleural space rapidly becomes fluid-filled, and a careful balance between fluid accumulation and drainage needs to be maintained. Rapid fluid and/or air evacuation may lead to mediastinal shift toward the operative side, contralateral lung overinflation and potentially pulmonary edema, and even caval compression and a reduction in cardiac output. On the contrary, accumulation of air and fluid in the pneumonectomy space without drainage may cause mediastinal shift toward the nonoperative side, compromising lung function.[29] Therefore, a balanced approach to the management of intrathoracic volumes and pressures is necessary. The goal is to maintain the trachea in a midline position, classically accomplished by the careful drainage or injection of air into the operative side.[30] This is achieved by the use of "pneumonectomy" or "balanced drainage" systems commercially available today.[31-33] These systems are composed of three chambers: a collection chamber and two underwater valves for controlling both negative and positive pressures. They typically maintain pleural cavity pressure between +1 and −13 cm H_2O, thus avoiding large pressure differences and mediastinal shift. This technique also permits drainage and quantification of blood, as well as irrigation if deemed clinically necessary.

FLUID MANAGEMENT

Perioperative fluid management is an essential component of patient care especially with regards to thoracic surgery patients. In recent years, the optimal approach to fluid management has been controversial, due to a number of studies demonstrating adverse consequences of both liberal and restrictive fluid regimens.[34-37] Established doctrines such as third-spacing and fluid replacement algorithms based on deficits, maintenance, and losses are being increasingly challenged in favor of goal-directed individualized approaches.[38] It is clear that there are risks associated with both hypovolemia (organ hypoperfusion, systemic inflammatory response syndrome, and multi-organ failure) and hypervolemia (edema, ileus, nausea, pulmonary complications, and cardiac stress).[34-37,39]

The controversy of restrictive versus liberal fluid management has not materialized in thoracic surgery to the same extent as in other surgical populations due to the abundance of evidence that liberal fluid regimes result in poor outcomes following pulmonary surgery.[40-43] One of the most dire complications following lung resection, particularly pneumonectomy, is pulmonary edema. Post-pneumonectomy pulmonary edema, also known as post-lung resection pulmonary edema, noncardiogenic pulmonary edema, postoperative acute lung injury and postperfusion pulmonary edema is a severe form of acute lung injury that is associated with significant morbidity and mortality and has been partially linked to overzealous administration of fluids in the perioperative period (see Chapter 23).[41] In 1995, a landmark review article by Slinger summarized the existing knowledge of post-pneumonectomy pulmonary edema and proposed a goal-directed approach to the fluid management for thoracic surgery patients (Table 22–1).[44] Though there have been no randomized trials of goal-directed fluid management therapies in thoracic surgery patients, there is increasing evidence in other populations of the efficacy of this approach.[34,36,37,45-47]

PROPHYLACTIC ANTIBIOTICS

Prophylactic antibiotics should be administered one hour prior to skin incision and discontinued within 24 hours of the surgical end time. Current guidelines recommend the use of a first- or second-generation cephalosporin in patients undergoing thoracic surgery, with substitution of vancomycin or clindamycin in cephalosporin-allergic patients. It is important to note that although prophylactic antibiotics are administered to prevent surgical site infections, they will not necessarily be effective against other postoperative infectious complications. For example, although cefazolin is the most widely used prophylactic antibiotic for skin incision, a recent study demonstrated only 18% causative organisms for

Table 22–1. Goal-Directed Fluid Management for Thoracic Surgery

Assume that there is no "third space" in the thorax
No more than 20 cc/kg positive fluid balance in the first 24 h
Goal of >0.5 cc/kg/h urine output is excessive
If evidence of organ hypoperfusion exists, utilize invasive monitors to guide inotropic/fluid therapy rather then risk fluid overload

Adapted from Slinger.[44]

pneumonia were susceptible to cefazolin.[12] Bacterial resistance to antibiotics is an ever-present challenge affecting all areas of medicine, and new trials are necessary in order to update the existing guidelines.[48]

NUTRITION

Malnutrition in hospitalized patients is a very common condition affecting up to 50% surgical patients.[49] Furthermore, surgery induces a hyper-metabolic and catabolic state that further exacerbates nutritional deficiencies.[50] Malnutrition is not a benign process and can lead to numerous problems including increased mortality, infection, length of stay, and poor wound healing.[51,52] It is therefore essential that every effort should be made to optimize patients' nutritional status.

Nutrition should be initiated as early as possible in the postoperative period.[53-55] The European Society of Parenteral and Enteral Nutrition (ESPEN) published guidelines for both intensive care and surgical patients.[56,57] They recommend that enteral feeding (by mouth or feeding tube) be the preferred route, and that it be initiated within hours after the surgery. Furthermore, parenteral nutrition should be considered early in patients who are unable to receive and absorb adequate amounts of enteral feeds in the first postoperative week.

Two particularly unique populations are the esophagectomy and pneumonectomy patients. Pneumonectomy patients are extremely vulnerable to developing pneumonia, which is associated with a mortality rate of 20% to 30%.[58] It is essential to ensure that these patients are capable of swallowing and able to protect their airway prior to initiation of feeding.

Feeding following esophagectomy is particularly challenging due to the esophageal resection site.[59] Most surgeons allow a period of 5 to 7 days before enteral nutrition is introduced because of the delicate nature of the anastomosis and risk of leaks. Many times, a feeding jejunostomy is performed at the time of surgery to provide enteral nutrition. Transition to oral nutrition should be done judiciously following a clinical swallowing study and radiographic assessment to rule out esophageal leakage. In addition, esophagectomy patients have a reduced capacity to store food and therefore need to ingest small frequent meals in order to maintain adequate nutrition. Lastly, because these patients lack a gastroesophageal sphincter and are at risk of reflux and aspiration, it is recommended that they avoid lying flat, particularly 30 to 60 minutes after eating.

GLYCEMIC CONTROL

Increasing evidence suggests that in hospitalized patients, the presence of hyperglycemia is associated with poor clinical outcomes. This is true for diabetics and nondiabetics alike. Diabetes increases the risk of mortality, infection, metabolic derangements, and renal and cardiac complications.[60-63] In a landmark randomized controlled trial of more than 1500 surgical intensive care unit patients, Van den Berghe found that intensive insulin therapy (target blood glucose 80-110 mg/dL) significantly reduced mortality and morbidity compared to standard therapy (target blood glucose 180-200 mg/dL).[61] Regrettably, the results of this study have not been validated by subsequent trials and intensive insulin therapy has been linked to increased mortality and stroke due to hypoglycemia.[64-67]

This new conflicting data has resulted in the development of a new consensus statement on inpatient glycemic management.[68] For critically ill patients, insulin therapy should be initiated at a blood glucose level no greater than 180 mg/dL (10.0 mmol/L) and a target range of 140 to 180 mg/dL (7.8-10.0 mmol/L). Intravenous insulin infusions are the preferred method of administration and frequent glucose monitoring is essential to minimize hypoglycemia. For noncritically ill patients, the target glucose level should be less than 140 mg/dL, and blood glucose measurement can be performed more infrequently. Following lung resection surgery, most patients will be placed on a clear liquid diet and their diet advanced quickly. Sliding scale insulin coverage and resumption of their home oral and/or insulin regimen is generally sufficient to provide adequate glucose control in the postoperative period.

VENOUS THROMBOEMBOLISM PROPHYLAXIS

Cancer is a leading risk factor for venous thromboembolism, with the highest incidence found in hospitalized cancer patients receiving active therapy.[69] The use of anticoagulant medications, whether prophylactic or therapeutic, is frequently encountered in the thoracic surgery population and can complicate the management of neuraxial analgesia. In the absence of contraindications, the American College of Chest Physicians recommends using low molecular weight heparin, low-dose unfractionated heparin, or fondaparinux for routine thromboembolic prophylaxis of all patients undergoing major thoracic surgery.[70] In addition, early mobilization is strongly recommended, as well as utilization of graduated compression stockings and intermittent pneumatic leg compression devices.[70]

SUMMARY

While a relatively high-risk procedure, pulmonary resection is essential for curative management of lung cancer. With elevated postoperative morbidity and mortality, this patient population represents a group for which postoperative management has potential to markedly improve outcome. Attention to detail and utilization of a comprehensive approach to patient care as outlined in this chapter should benefit patients such as the one described in the vignette.

REFERENCES

1. Detterbeck F. Thoracoscopic versus open lobectomy debate: the pro argument. *GMS Thorac Surg Sci.* 2009;6:1-9.
2. Lytle FT, Brown DR. Appropriate ventilatory settings for thoracic surgery: intraoperative and postoperative. *Semin Cardiothorac Vasc Anesth.* 2008;12(2):97-108.
3. Aguilo R, Togores B, Pons S, Rubi M, Barbe F, Agusti AG. Noninvasive ventilatory support after lung resectional surgery. *Chest.* 1997;112(1):117-121.
4. Perrin C, Jullien V, Venissac N, et al. Prophylactic use of noninvasive ventilation in patients undergoing lung resectional surgery. *Respir Med.* 2007;101(7):1572-1578.

5. Antonelli M, Conti G. Noninvasive positive pressure ventilation as treatment for acute respiratory failure in critically ill patients. *Crit Care.* 2000;4(1):15-22.
6. Reeve JC, Nicol K, Stiller K, McPherson KM, Denehy L. Does physiotherapy reduce the incidence of postoperative complications in patients following pulmonary resection via thoracotomy? a protocol for a randomised controlled trial. *J Cardiothorac Surg.* 2008;3:48.
7. Freynet A, Falcoz PE. Does non-invasive ventilation associated with chest physiotherapy improve outcome after lung resection? *Interact Cardiovasc Thorac Surg.* 2008;7(6):1152-1154.
8. Das-Neves-Pereira JC, Bagan P, Coimbra-Israel AP, et al. Fast-track rehabilitation for lung cancer lobectomy: a five-year experience. *Eur J Cardiothorac Surg.* 2009;36(2):383-391; discussion 382-391.
9. Ramnath N, Demmy TL, Antun A, et al. Pneumonectomy for bronchogenic carcinoma: analysis of factors predicting survival. *Ann Thorac Surg.* 2007;83(5):1831-1836.
10. Nakahara K, Ohno K, Hashimoto J, et al. Prediction of postoperative respiratory failure in patients undergoing lung resection for lung cancer. *Ann Thorac Surg.* 1988;46(5):549-552.
11. Ferguson MK, Gaissert HA, Grab JD, Sheng S. Pulmonary complications after lung resection in the absence of chronic obstructive pulmonary disease: the predictive role of diffusing capacity. *J Thorac Cardiovasc Surg.* 2009;138(6):1297-1302.
12. Radu DM, Jaureguy F, Seguin A, et al. Postoperative pneumonia after major pulmonary resections: an unsolved problem in thoracic surgery. *Ann Thorac Surg.* 2007;84(5):1669-1673.
13. Algar FJ, Alvarez A, Salvatierra A, Baamonde C, Aranda JL, Lopez-Pujol FJ. Predicting pulmonary complications after pneumonectomy for lung cancer. *Eur J Cardiothorac Surg.* 2003;23(2):201-208.
14. Munnell ER. Thoracic drainage. *Ann Thorac Surg.* 1997;63(5):1497-1502.
15. Younes RN, Gross JL, Aguiar S, Haddad FJ, Deheinzelin D. When to remove a chest tube? A randomized study with subsequent prospective consecutive validation. *J Am Coll Surg.* 2002;195(5):658-662.
16. Davis JW, Mackersie RC, Hoyt DB, Garcia J. Randomized study of algorithms for discontinuing tube thoracostomy drainage. *J Am Coll Surg.* 1994;179(5):553-557.
17. Duncan C, Erickson R. Pressures associated with chest tube stripping. *Heart Lung.* 1982;11(2):166-171.
18. Silverstein DS, Livingston DH, Elcavage J, Kovar L, Kelly KM. The utility of routine daily chest radiography in the surgical intensive care unit. *J Trauma.* 1993;35(4):643-646.
19. Adebonojo SA. How prolonged is "prolonged air leak"? *Ann Thorac Surg.* 1995;59(2):549-550.
20. Brunelli A, Al Refai M, Muti M, Sabbatini A, Fianchini A. Pleural tent after upper lobectomy: a prospective randomized study. *Ann Thorac Surg.* 2000;69(6):1722-1724.
21. Cerfolio RJ, Bass CS, Pask AH, Katholi CR. Predictors and treatment of persistent air leaks. *Ann Thorac Surg.* 2002;73(6):1727-1730; discussion 1721-1730.
22. Cerfolio RJ, Bryant AS, Singh S, Bass CS, Bartolucci AA. The management of chest tubes in patients with a pneumothorax and an air leak after pulmonary resection. *Chest.* 2005;128(2):816-820.
23. Cerfolio RJ, Bryant AS. The benefits of continuous and digital air leak assessment after elective pulmonary resection: a prospective study. *Ann Thorac Surg.* 2008;86(2):396-401.
24. Bell RL, Ovadia P, Abdullah F, Spector S, Rabinovici R. Chest tube removal: end-inspiration or end-expiration? *J Trauma.* 2001;50(4):674-677.
25. Martino K, Merrit S, Boyakye K, et al. Prospective randomized trial of thoracostomy removal algorithms. *J Trauma.* 1999;46(3):369-371; discussion 363-372.
26. Pacanowski JP, Waack ML, Daley BJ, et al. Is routine roentgenography needed after closed tube thoracostomy removal? *J Trauma.* 2000;48(4):684-688.
27. Palesty JA, McKelvey AA, Dudrick SJ. The efficacy of x-rays after chest tube removal. *Am J Surg.* 2000;179(1):13-16.
28. Cerfolio RJ, Bryant AS, Maniscalco LM. Management of subcutaneous emphysema after pulmonary resection. *Ann Thorac Surg.* 2008;85(5):1759-1763; discussion 1755-1764.
29. Wolf AS, Jacobson FL, Tilleman TR, Colson Y, Richards WG, Sugarbaker DJ. Managing the pneumonectomy space after extrapleural pneumonectomy: postoperative intrathoracic pressure monitoring. *Eur J Cardiothorac Surg.* 2010;37(4):770-775.
30. Pezella AT, Conlan AA, Carroll GJ. Early management of the postpneumonectomy space. *Asian Cardiovasc Thorac Ann.* 2000;8:398-402.
31. Pecora DV, Cooper P. Pleural drainage following pneumonectomy: description of apparatus. *Surgery.* 1955;37(2):251-254.

32. Laforet EG, Boyd TF. Balanced drainage of the pneumonectomy space. *Surg Gynecol Obstet.* 1964;118:1051-1054.
33. Miller JI, Fleming WH, Hatcher CR Jr. Balanced drainage of the contaminated pneumonectomy space. *Ann Thorac Surg.* 1975;19(5):585-588.
34. Lobo DN, Bostock KA, Neal KR, Perkins AC, Rowlands BJ, Allison SP. Effect of salt and water balance on recovery of gastrointestinal function after elective colonic resection: a randomised controlled trial. *Lancet.* 2002;359(9320):1812-1818.
35. Nisanevich V, Felsenstein I, Almogy G, Weissman C, Einav S, Matot I. Effect of intraoperative fluid management on outcome after intraabdominal surgery. *Anesthesiology.* 2005;103(1):25-32.
36. Brandstrup B, Tonnesen H, Beier-Holgersen R, et al. Effects of intravenous fluid restriction on postoperative complications: comparison of two perioperative fluid regimens: a randomized assessor-blinded multicenter trial. *Ann Surg.* 2003;238(5):641-648.
37. Holte K, Kristensen BB, Valentiner L, Foss NB, Husted H, Kehlet H. Liberal versus restrictive fluid management in knee arthroplasty: a randomized, double-blind study. *Anesth Analg.* 2007;105(2):465-474.
38. Shires T, Williams J, Brown F. Acute change in extracellular fluids associated with major surgical procedures. *Ann Surg.* 1961;154:803-810.
39. Bellamy MC. Wet, dry or something else? *Br J Anaesth.* 2006;97(6):755-757.
40. Moller AM, Pedersen T, Svendsen PE, Engquist A. Perioperative risk factors in elective pneumonectomy: the impact of excess fluid balance. *Eur J Anaesthesiol.* 2002;19(1):57-62.
41. Zeldin RA, Normandin D, Landtwing D, Peters RM. Postpneumonectomy pulmonary edema. *J Thorac Cardiovasc Surg.* 1984;87(3):359-365.
42. Patel RL, Townsend ER, Fountain SW. Elective pneumonectomy: factors associated with morbidity and operative mortality. *Ann Thorac Surg.* 1992;54(1):84-88.
43. Verheijen-Breemhaar L, Bogaard JM, van den Berg B, Hilvering C. Postpneumonectomy pulmonary oedema. *Thorax.* 1988;43(4):323-326.
44. Slinger PD. Perioperative fluid management for thoracic surgery: the puzzle of postpneumonectomy pulmonary edema. *J Cardiothorac Vasc Anesth.* 1995;9(4):442-451.
45. Roche AM, Miller TE, Gan TJ. Goal-directed fluid management with trans-oesophageal Doppler. *Best Pract Res Clin Anaesthesiol.* 2009;23(3):327-334.
46. Lees N, Hamilton M, Rhodes A. Clinical review: goal-directed therapy in high risk surgical patients. *Crit Care.* 2009;13(5):231.
47. Rivers E, Nguyen B, Havstad S, et al. Early goal-directed therapy in the treatment of severe sepsis and septic shock. *N Engl J Med.* 2001;345(19):1368-1377.
48. Schussler O, Dermine H, Alifano M, et al. Should we change antibiotic prophylaxis for lung surgery? Postoperative pneumonia is the critical issue. *Ann Thorac Surg.* 2008;86(6):1727-1733.
49. Weinsier RL, Hunker EM, Krumdieck CL, Butterworth CE Jr. Hospital malnutrition. A prospective evaluation of general medical patients during the course of hospitalization. *Am J Clin Nutr.* 1979;32(2):418-426.
50. Kiyama T, Witte MB, Thornton FJ, Barbul A. The route of nutrition support affects the early phase of wound healing. *JPEN J Parenter Enteral Nutr.* 1998;22(5):276-279.
51. Santos JI. Nutrition, infection, and immunocompetence. *Infect Dis Clin North Am.* 1994;8(1):243-267.
52. Studley HO. Percentage of weight loss: a basic indicator of surgical risk in patients with chronic peptic ulcer. 1936. *Nutr Hosp.* 2001;16(4):141-143; discussion 140-141.
53. Moore FA, Feliciano DV, Andrassy RJ, et al. Early enteral feeding, compared with parenteral, reduces postoperative septic complications. The results of a meta-analysis. *Ann Surg.* 1992;216(2):172-183.
54. Artinian V, Krayem H, DiGiovine B. Effects of early enteral feeding on the outcome of critically ill mechanically ventilated medical patients. *Chest.* 2006;129(4):960-967.
55. Marik PE, Zaloga GP. Early enteral nutrition in acutely ill patients: a systematic review. *Crit Care Med.* 2001;29(12):2264-2270.
56. Weimann A, Braga M, Harsanyi L, et al. ESPEN guidelines on enteral nutrition: surgery including organ transplantation. *Clin Nutr.* 2006;25(2):224-244.
57. Kreymann KG, Berger MM, Deutz NE, et al. ESPEN guidelines on enteral nutrition: intensive care. *Clin Nutr.* 2006;25(2):210-223.

58. Schussler O, Alifano M, Dermine H, et al. Postoperative pneumonia after major lung resection. *Am J Respir Crit Care Med.* 2006;173(10):1161-1169.
59. Kight CE. Nutrition considerations in esophagectomy patients. *Nutr Clin Pract.* 2008;23(5):521-528.
60. Pomposelli JJ, Baxter JK III, Babineau TJ, et al. Early postoperative glucose control predicts nosocomial infection rate in diabetic patients. *JPEN J Parenter Enteral Nutr.* 1998;22(2):77-81.
61. van den Berghe G, Wouters P, Weekers F, et al. Intensive insulin therapy in the critically ill patients. *N Engl J Med.* 2001;345(19):1359-1367.
62. Gandhi GY, Nuttall GA, Abel MD, et al. Intraoperative hyperglycemia and perioperative outcomes in cardiac surgery patients. *Mayo Clin Proc.* 2005;80(7):862-866.
63. Ouattara A, Lecomte P, Le Manach Y, et al. Poor intraoperative blood glucose control is associated with a worsened hospital outcome after cardiac surgery in diabetic patients. *Anesthesiology.* 2005;103(4):687-694.
64. Van den Berghe G, Wilmer A, Hermans G, et al. Intensive insulin therapy in the medical ICU. *N Engl J Med.* 2006;354(5):449-461.
65. Brunkhorst FM, Engel C, Bloos F, et al. Intensive insulin therapy and pentastarch resuscitation in severe sepsis. *N Engl J Med.* 2008;358(2):125-139.
66. Preiser JC, Brunkhorst F. Tight glucose control and hypoglycemia. *Crit Care Med.* 2008;36(4):1391; author reply 1391-1392.
67. Finfer S, Delaney A. Tight glycemic control in critically ill adults. *JAMA.* 200827;300(8):963-965.
68. Moghissi ES, Korytkowski MT, DiNardo M, et al. American Association of Clinical Endocrinologists and American Diabetes Association consensus statement on inpatient glycemic control. *Diabetes Care.* 2009;32(6):1119-1131.
69. Khorana AA, Rao MV. Approaches to risk-stratifying cancer patients for venous thromboembolism. *Thromb Res.* 2007;120(Suppl 2):S41-S50.
70. Hirsh J, Guyatt G, Albers GW, Harrington R, Schunemann HJ, American College of Chest P. Antithrombotic and thrombolytic therapy: American College of Chest Physicians Evidence-Based Clinical Practice Guidelines (8th Edition). *Chest.* 2008;133(6 Suppl):110S-112S.

Respiratory, Renal, and Cardiovascular Postoperative Complications

23

Alessia Pedoto
David Amar

Key Points

1. Respiratory complications occur in 12% to 26% patients and account for the majority of morbidity and mortality following thoracic surgery. Postoperative predicted DLCO (ppDLCO) may be used to identify high-risk patients preoperatively. Prolonged air leak is the most common respiratory complication following thoracic surgery.
2. Renal complications following thoracic procedures are uncommon and usually occur in the setting of sepsis. Use of NSAIDs, dehydration, and preexisting renal disease are all predisposing factors. Pharmacologic therapy is generally not effective, and prevention continues to be the desired strategy.
3. Supraventricular arrhythmias are common after lung resection and are typically transient, but increase morbidity and hospital length of stay. Diltiazem appears to be effective in preventing postoperative atrial fibrillation.

Clinical Vignette

A 72-year-old man with long-standing smoking history underwent a thoracotomy and right pneumonectomy for nonsmall cell lung cancer and was admitted to the surgical ICU postoperatively. He has diet controlled diabetes mellitus type II and hypertension. Preoperative medications include lovastatin and lisinopril.

Pneumonectomy is one of the surgical curative options for nonsmall cell lung cancer (NSCLC).[1,2] It is usually considered for extensive tumors or for tumors located in specific anatomic areas, often as part of a multimodal approach combined with perioperative chemo[3] and radiation treatment.[4]

Despite strict selection criteria, improved surgical and anesthetic techniques, and enhanced postoperative care, patients like the one described in the clinical vignette still suffer significant postoperative complications following lung resection surgery. There is considerable variability in the reported mortality rates after pneumonectomy (5%-6%) which depend on the case volume of the hospital, the age of the patient, the side of surgery[4-7] and the use of induction chemotherapy.[3] Old age, poor nutritional status, current smoking, and coronary artery disease[8] are all well-known risks factors associated with an increased morbidity and mortality after lung resection. Respiratory complications are especially prevalent and a major contributor to morbidity in this patient population, who often exhibits preexisting pulmonary disease. The presence of COPD may increase the risk of developing bronchopleural fistulas and acute respiratory failure.[8] Additionally, predicted postoperative DLCO (ppDLCO) is the strongest predictor of increased operative mortality and respiratory morbidity, independently from the presence of COPD[9,10] (see Chapter 9). Unfortunately not all centers perform routine DLCO measurements, more so in the presence of normal spirometric measurements.

As a result of all the above, great effort should be tailored in preventing postoperative complications, since they are associated with an increase in ICU admission rates, hospital length of stay and mortality rates.[8] This chapter focuses on important respiratory, renal, and cardiovascular complications following thoracic surgery.

POD1: The patient's (from Clinical Vignette) oxygenation worsened and he was placed on 100% nonrebreather mask. His condition continued to deteriorate and was reintubated on the morning of POD2. His CXR showed diffuse pulmonary infiltrates on the left lung and normal postoperative changes in the right hemithorax.

RESPIRATORY COMPLICATIONS

Respiratory complications are common after pneumonectomy (especially right sided), and several risk factors have been suggested. They account for the majority of morbidity and mortality, despite an overall improvement in surgical and postoperative strategies.

Table 23-1 summarizes early complications after pneumonectomy, while Table 23-2 summarizes the common radiographic findings in these patients. Early respiratory complications are discussed here.

POSTPNEUMONECTOMY PULMONARY EDEMA

Postpneumonectomy pulmonary edema (PPPE) is characterized by a sudden onset of noncardiogenic pulmonary edema, which is fatal in more than 60% patients if not recognized. It occurs in 2% to 4% pneumonectomy cases, especially right-sided ones. The etiology is unknown and its clinical features are undistinguishable from the adult respiratory distress syndrome (ARDS).[11] A high index of suspicion is necessary for the diagnosis and cardiac failure, pneumonia, sepsis as well as bronchopleural fistula all need to be excluded. Pulmonary infiltrates on chest x-ray and respiratory distress on clinical exam are common diagnostic features.[11,12]

The onset of PPPE is usually within the first two postoperative days and can present with oliguria in patients with normal preoperative renal function.[11] Hypovolemia is usually present due to fluid restriction and possible sequestration of water into a "leaky" lung. Oliguria and pulmonary infiltrates on chest

Table 23–1. Incidence of Common Early Complications after Pneumonectomy[1,3,5,6,8,69,76]

	Incidence (in %)
Respiratory	**12-26**
Pneumonia	2.5-4
Bronchopleural fistula	0.3-2
Pulmonary edema	2-5
Empyema	0.3-1.1
Atelectasis	3-8
Prolonged air leak	2-10
Respiratory failure/ARDS	0.7-5
Cardiac	**10-14**
Supraventricular tachyarrhythmias	20
Sustained ventricular tachycardia/fibrillation	< 0.4
Nonsustained ventricular tachycardia	15
Bradyarrhythmias	0.1-0.4
Myocardial infarction	0.4-0.9
Cardiac herniation	Rare
Other	**3.9**
Deep venous thrombosis	0.5-1.5
Wound infection	0.3-1.3
Pulmonary embolism	0.4-1.1
Vocal cord paralysis	0.2-1.5

ARDS = adult respiratory distress syndrome

x-ray preceded the onset of dyspnea by an average of 23 hours in a small study.[13] Other signs included tachycardia, lung rales, and hypoxemia, and sometimes the presence of subcutaneous emphysema on the operative side.[12] Fever (>38°C) and leukocytosis can also be present. Hypoxemia is usually unresponsive to oxygen therapy or diuretics (including "renal dose" dopamine), and often requires endotracheal intubation within the first three days after surgery.[13] The treatment is largely supportive and includes diuretics, oxygen, mechanical ventilation, and fluid restriction.

The pathophysiology of PPPE is unclear, with several proposed mechanisms. *Volume overload* remains a very controversial explanation. Some of the landmark literature originated from animal studies, with variable results on the development of edema. Not all the fluid overloaded animals developed PPPE, and the timing between the clinical manifestation and the diagnosis made at the autopsy remains unclear.[12] In a series

Table 23–2. Radiographic Characteristics of Respiratory Complications[112]

	Pneumonia	Bronchopleural Fistula	ARDS/ALI	Pulmonary Edema	Empyema
CXR	Lobar consolidation or increased opacity	Failure of the space to fill Persistent PNX despite chest tube presence Progressive subcutaneous/mediastinal emphysema Filling of the remaining lung Sudden PNX/reappearance of air fluid level Decrease in air fluid level >1.5 cm <2 cm air fluid level + contralateral mediastinal shift	Increased opacity in the remaining lung	Kerley lines Peribronchial cuffs Ill-defined vessels	Filling of space with fluid Contralateral mediastinal shift Decreased air fluid space in pneumonectomy side New air fluid level in opacified space
CT	Useful in case of PNA related to BPF	Superior imaging technique to identify the fistula	Ground glass opacities Increased interlobar septa		

CXR = chest x-ray, CT = computerized tomography, PNA = pneumonia, PNX = pneumothorax, BPF = bronchopleural fistula, ARDS = adult respiratory distress syndrome, ALI = acute lung injury of 5 case reports,[13] PPPE developed in patients who were both eu- and hypovolemic, suggesting more complicated mechanisms.

An *increase in the alveolo-capillary membrane permeability* has been demonstrated by Waller et al[14] who measured the amount of radioisotopic tracer accumulation in lung tissue in patients who underwent pneumonectomy. The changes occurred within 5 hours of surgery. Proposed etiologic factors were neutrophil activation and an increase in pulmonary vascular resistance.[14]

Impaired lymphatic drainage has been suggested as another potential factor contributing to PPPE. Using a dog model, Little et al[15] showed that disruption of the lymphatic drainage was associated with PPPE. However, several other animal and human studies have failed to demonstrate a link between the two. Furthermore, the lung has a significant lymphatic drainage reserve, and further compensation can occur via pleural drainage.[11] It is therefore unlikely that lymphatic drainage impairment plays a major role in the development of PPPE.

One-lung ventilation (OLV) with high tidal volumes and hyperoxia has been linked to the damage of the alveolo-capillary membrane. Animal studies have shown that the production of reactive oxygen species associated with high peak airway pressure may cause injury of the alveolo-capillary membrane with an increase in pro-inflammatory cytokines, which may contribute to PPPE.[11] In humans, the use of large tidal volume (V_T) ventilation with increased peak inspiratory pressure (PIP >40 cm H_2O) can be associated with an increase in pulmonary vascular resistance and subsequent pulmonary hypertension.[11,16] An important lesson is learned form the ARDS data network on lung injury and high tidal volume.[17] A protective lung strategy includes tidal volumes of 3 to 4 cc/kg with OLV, peak inspiratory pressure less than 35 cm H_2O and plateau pressures less than 25 cm H_2O, with the potential need to accept permissive hypercapnia.

The pneumonectomy empty space can lead to mediastinal shift and *hyperinflation of the remaining lung* with consequent severe pulmonary hypertension, leading to respiratory distress and death.[11] Stabilization of the mediastinum in the midline using intermittent clamping of a water sealed chest tube or use of a balanced drainage system helps prevent this complication[12] (see Chapter 22).

A certain degree of right ventricular overload occurs after pneumonectomy, even in the absence of preoperative cardiac disease.[11] Patients who develop acute lung injury postoperatively exhibit an increase in mean pulmonary arterial pressures and right ventricular dilatation, and this is usually associated with a poor prognosis.[18] Although right ventricular dysfunction is unlikely to represent the main etiologic factor, it may contribute unfavorably to the course of PPPE.

Treatment for PPPE is mainly supportive, consisting of mechanical ventilation, fluid restriction and the use of diuretics. Steroid administration intraoperatively in the attempt to prevent PPPE remains controversial, with the majority of the trials done in the ICU setting in patients with ARDS. Cerfolio et al[19] designed a safety study on the role of methylprednisolone administered prior to clamping the pulmonary artery in patients undergoing pneumonectomy, and looked at the rate of complications. The 37 subjects who were treated with corticosteroids had a reduced incidence of PPPE/ARDS when compared to historical controls. However, the study was small, not randomized, and the definition of PPPE was very broad, with no mention of the degree of hypoxia and the amount of infiltrates on chest radiography. There was also no follow up on the potential long-term effects of steroids, making potential clinical recommendations difficult.

Given the grave prognosis and the lack of targeted interventions, it is imperative that the thoracic anesthesiologist be familiar with this complication and that he or she make every effort to minimize its occurrence. Suggested perioperative strategies include minimization of intraoperative volume replacement, the use vasopressors to treat intraoperative hypotension (as opposed to fluid boluses), the use of protective lung ventilation strategies, the administration of supplemental oxygen therapy in the postoperative period to reduce pulmonary vascular resistance, and the use of balanced drainage systems after pneumonectomy.

PNEUMONIA

Postoperative pneumonia still represents a major cause of morbidity and mortality after lung resection. The incidence is variable (2%-40%), depending on the population studied, the extent of surgery, and the type and timing of perioperative antibiotic prophylaxis.[20] Clinical diagnosis may be difficult, since hypoxia, fever, or an abnormal chest x-ray may be common findings in the postoperative period. Hypoventilation due to pain, as well as the inability to cough and clear secretions, is commonly associated with atelectasis and eventually postoperative pneumonia. Several independent risk factors have been proposed, such as COPD, FEV_1 <70%, age >75, induction chemotherapy, type of surgical resection (lobectomy and bilobectomy versus pneumonectomy), intraoperative bronchial colonization and male gender.[20,21] High tidal volumes and increased fluid administration are also contributing factors for pneumonia, as well as other postoperative respiratory complications such as ventilator induced lung injury and pulmonary embolism.[22] Postoperative pneumonia is associated with higher rates of re-intubation and noninvasive ventilation modalities, prolonged length of stay in the hospital and in the ICU and overall higher mortality rates (19%). It commonly occurs during the first postoperative week, with a peak on postoperative day four.[20,23] Lung resection is usually defined as a "clean–contaminated" procedure, due to the opening of the trachea and bronchi and migration of tracheobronchial contaminants, especially with bacterial strands that are resistant to common antibiotic prophylaxis.[20] Several studies[20,23] suggest that the most common causative micro-organisms are *Haemophilus influenzae* (41.7%), *Streptococcus pneumoniae* (25%), *Enterobacteriaceae* (8.7%), and *Pseudomonas* (25%) species. Despite recommended antibiotic prophylaxis, the incidence of postoperative pneumonia is still high, and no defined guidelines are available for noncardiac thoracic surgery.[23] First and second generation cephalosporins are commonly used in the United States to prevent wound infection, empyema, and pneumonia. While they are extremely efficacious against the former, controversial results exist for the latter.[23] In most of the cases the etiology for postoperative pneumonia favors gram negative microorganisms, which are susceptible to a broader coverage. Schussler et al[24] studied 455 patients who underwent major lung resection and noted a decrease in postoperative pneumonia after changing the antibiotic regimen from a second generation cephalosporin (cephamandole) to high-dose amoxicillin-clavulanate. The study was reflective of a clinical practice change, and it was neither prospective nor randomized, making the conclusions difficult to apply in the United States, where first generation cephalosporins still remain the recommended antibiotic of choice, with vancomycin or clindamycin as an alternative for β-lactamase allergic patients.[25] Current recommendations consist of a single dose antibiotic regimen at an appropriate dosage per body weight, with repeated administration intraoperatively if the wound is not closed after two half lives of the drug.[25] Temperature control, supplemental oxygen, and avoidance of hyperglycemia are all additional maneuvers suggested to decrease the incidence of postoperative infections;[25] however, their impact on postoperative pneumonia remains unclear.

BRONCHOPLEURAL FISTULA

Bronchopleural fistula (BPF) is defined as a communication between the bronchial lumen and the pleural space, and it can be confirmed via bronchoscopy, thoracotomy, or both.[26] It occurs most commonly after right pneumonectomy, probably due to the length of the remaining bronchial stump (longer on the right side), especially if not covered with a flap.[1,26] Its incidence is estimated to be from 0% to 9%, leading to a mortality rate of 16% to 23%. Local and systemic risks factors have been identified.[26] Local risk factors include bronchial invasion by the tumor, length of the stump, integrity of blood supply, preoperative radiation, stump closure technique (manual suturing vs stapling) and extent of the resection. Extensive lymph node dissection has also been suggested as a cause for BPF formation.[27] Systemic factors include patient age older than 70, male gender, diabetes, poor nutritional status, preoperative chemotherapy and underlying lung disease, COPD with low FEV_1 and DLCO, and the presence of empyema.[26] Common symptoms include cough, which may be productive and worsening when laying on the ipsilateral side of the fistula, or signs of infection if empyema is present. Conventional treatment consists of surgical repair with thoracoplasty and chest wall fenestration to allow drainage of the infected cavity and antibiotic irrigation.[28] However, this procedure is associated with high morbidity and mortality rates, especially in the elderly and frail, with many of these patients being unable to have their thoracic fenestration closed. Minimally invasive bronchoscopic approaches have been investigated in an attempt to avoid a repeat thoracotomy.[29] The studies published on this topic are mainly a summary of case reports, where the number of patients analyzed is still too small to allow any recommendations. Proposed procedures involve tracheo-endobronchial stent placement (mainly with metallic stents), fibrin glue occlusion, and scar tissue forming agents at the site of the fistula (Nd:YAG laser and sclerosing material). Fibrin glue use has been associated with 20% mortality, 35.6% rate of progression to surgical repair and 15.6% rate of chronic empyema. Better results seem to be achieved with synthetic glue, with a 67% resolution rate for the fistula and a survival rate of 83%. However, only 10% of the empyema seems to resolve with this technique.[29] In the majority of cases, serial CT scans or bronchoscopic follow up are required, with repeated treatment being frequently necessary. Overall, prevention still remains the best treatment for BPF, focusing on modifying the potential risk factors when possible. Please refer to Chapter 18 for an in-depth discussion of the anesthetic management of patients undergoing bronchopleural fistula repair.

ACUTE LUNG INJURY

Acute lung injury (ALI) without an obvious etiology has been described after major lung resection in 1% to 3% cases.[5,10] The incidence of ALI has significantly decreased in recent years, mainly due to an improvement in postoperative management and analgesic techniques. As a result, recent efforts have been directed toward understanding the pathophysiology and prevention of this serious complication.

According to the guidelines of the American-European Consensus Conference on ARDS, acute lung injury is defined as an acute onset of hypoxia with an abnormal PaO_2/FiO_2 ratio (usually <300) and radiographic infiltrates that are characteristic of pulmonary edema.[30] ALI can occur either in the early (day 0-3) or late (day 3-10) postoperative period.[31] The former is usually associated with PPPE, while the latter is associated with postoperative pneumonia or aspiration.

The strongest predictors for post-thoracotomy ALI seem to be related to patient characteristics (severe pulmonary disease, alcohol consumption) and perioperative medical care (extended resection, ventilator-induced lung injury and fluid overload).[10,32] Recent focus has been directed toward one-lung ventilation strategies, with the goal of avoiding alveolar hyperinflation, alveolar stretching, and enhanced release of proinflammatory mediators. A retrospective study on 146 patients who underwent pneumonectomy showed that high tidal volumes and peak airway pressures during one-lung ventilation were associated with an increased incidence of postoperative ALI/ARDS.[33] These findings were true both for healthy patients and those with decreased preoperative pulmonary compliance.[34] Several animal models have demonstrated an increased systemic inflammatory response in the lung when high tidal volumes and plateau airway pressures were used, leading to increased mortality.[35]

Overall, once post pneumonectomy ALI occurs, hospital length of stay is prolonged and in-hospital mortality increased.[10,33] Treatment is mainly supportive, focusing on mechanical ventilation with low tidal volumes (4-6 cc/kg predicted body weight), plateau airway pressures less than 30 cm H_2O, respiratory rates titrated to maintain pH between 7.3 and 7.45, and an appropriate FiO_2 and PEEP to achieve adequate oxygenation (O_2 saturations of 88%-95%).[35] As a consequence of the low minute ventilation, moderate hypercapnia may occur. This is usually well tolerated unless metabolic acidosis is also present, which may require an increase in respiratory rate and the use bicarbonate infusion. Recruitment maneuvers should be done intermittently and held for 30 seconds, as they may cause significant concomitant hypotension, limiting peak airway pressures to 35 cm H_2O. Prone positioning may be considered as a short-term rescue treatment in the ICU setting in case of persistent hypoxia despite high FiO_2 (>60%) and plateau pressures (>30 cm H_2O). In selected patients, oxygenation may improve. However, multiple studies have shown no effect on mortality, which still remains elevated.[35] The physiologic mechanisms by which the prone position may improve oxygenation are still unclear. Alveolar recruitment, redistribution of ventilation toward areas that have better perfusion, and elimination of cardiac compression by the lungs are suggested hypotheses.[35] Among the risks of prone positioning are dislodgment and occlusion of the endotracheal tube and pressure ulcers.[35]

Several randomized trials have shown a reduction in the duration of mechanical ventilation in patients who have been able to tolerate trials of spontaneous ventilation on a daily basis.[35] Patients who breathed unassisted for 30 to 120 minutes a day were able to be extubated earlier than those on pressure support or assist control ventilation. Ventilation with a T-piece, continuous positive airway pressure or 7 cm H_2O of pressure support may be used if patients meet certain criteria, such as PEEP less than 8 cm H_2O and FiO_2 less than 50%, hemodynamic stability and the ability to initiate respiratory efforts.[35] Moreover, trials of spontaneous ventilation paired with light sedation or wakeup periods are associated with earlier extubation rates, shorter ICU and hospital stay and decreased mortality rates.[36]

Several pharmacological interventions have been studied in addition to the protective lung ventilation strategies discussed above. However, the results are not too promising. Nitric oxide, prostaglandins and prostacyclins, surfactants, lisophylline, ketoconazole, and immuno-nutrition with fish oil have all been used successfully in animal models but have not shown the same positive results in clinical studies.[37] Novel strategies under investigation target the stimulation of proteins in the alveolar epithelium to enhance edema clearance, the proliferation of type 2 pneumocytes to repair damaged alveoli, and the use of anticytokine antibodies to target inflammatory mediators.[37]

The role of corticosteroids in ALI/ARDS patients is still controversial in terms of morbidity and mortality, especially when high doses are used (30 mg/kg/d of methylprednisolone or equivalent).[38] A meta-analysis of 5 cohort and 4 randomized controlled studies (a total of 648 subjects) favored the use of low dose methylprednisolone or equivalent (0.5-2.5 mg/kg/d) in the early stage of the disease, leading to a decreased mortality rate and improved morbidity.[39] Similar results were found when more than a 7-day course was investigated, even though the sample size analyzed was small.[38] Corticosteroid treatment needs to be initiated prior to the onset of the end-stage fibrosis, usually occurring within two weeks of diagnosis, and weaning should be gradual to prevent rebound inflammation. In the early phase, the disease is characterized by an intense inflammatory response, both generalized and local, with an increase in cytokines and chemokines, alveolar membrane disruption, and fibrogenesis.[38] An abnormal pathway in the proinflammatory response involving glucocorticoid receptors has been identified both in the systemic and pulmonary circulation, explaining a potential rationale for corticosteroid treatment.[38] A high index of suspicion for side effects is needed when steroids are used for a prolonged time, since nosocomial infections in the absence of fever and prolonged neuromuscular weakness may be quite common in the ICU setting.[38]

PROLONGED MECHANICAL VENTILATION AND THE NEED FOR TRACHEOSTOMY

Tracheostomy is usually performed in patients requiring prolonged mechanical ventilation or presenting with upper airway obstruction.[40,41] Despite being a procedure that is widely performed in ICU patients, the indications, timing and choice of technique remain controversial.[42] It seems that a consensus is reached only for mechanical ventilation longer than 3 weeks, as reported in a recent survey sent to several ICUs in France,[40] even though another French study suggested 7 days as optimal.[42] Some studies suggest an improved survival when tracheostomy is performed early, but the results are still controversial partly depending on patient risk factors such as age, neuromuscular status and COPD.[42]

Several advantages and disadvantages of tracheostomy were reported by the physicians responding to the aforementioned survey, the main advantage being easier weaning from the ventilator, better patient comfort and tracheal toileting, and the ability to take oral nutrition.

Among the complications of tracheostomy, tracheal injury and stomal infection were most commonly listed. See Table 23–3 for a summary of the indications, contraindications, and complications of tracheostomy. Tracheostomy can be performed surgically in the operating room, or percutaneously at the bedside in appropriate candidates. Percutaneous tracheostomy offers additional advantages, such as the fact that it is done at the bedside, eliminating the need for transport,

Table 23–3. Indications, Contraindications, and Complications of Tracheostomy[41,43,44]

Indications	Contraindications	Complications

Prolonged MV
Pulmonary toileting
Upper airway obstruction
Airway protection
	Absolute
	  Age <12 years
	Relative
	  Abnormal tracheal anatomy
	  Pulsatile blood vessels at the site
	  Active infection at the site
	  Thyroid mass/goiter
	  PEEP >15 cm H_2O
	  PLT <40.000
	  PT or PTT >1.5 of control values
	  Decreased neck extension
	  h/o difficult intubation
	  Previous tracheostomy
		Short term
		  Bleeding
		  Infection
		  Pneumothorax
		  Subcutaneous/mediastinal emphysema
		  Tracheal laceration
		Long term
		  Voice change
		  Tracheal stenosis
		  Tracheomalacia
		  Tracheo-innominate fistula
		  Trachea-esophageal fistula
		  Dysphagia/odynophagia
		  Chronic cough
		  Granuloma formation
		  Poor cosmesis
		  Persistent stoma

MV = mechanical ventilation, PEEP = positive end-expiratory pressure, PLT = platelet, PT = prothrombin time, PTT = partial thromboplastin time which can be labor intensive and risky, especially if the patient is unstable. By eliminating the need for operating room time and personnel, the overall costs of the procedure are significantly decreased.[43] In a survey of Dutch ICUs, the lack of operating room availability was listed in 9.1% cases as a reason for delaying tracheostomy, only preceded by the absence of a surgeon (11.4%).[44,45] This caused a delay of 2 to 3 days from the time the decision of performing a tracheostomy was made. The procedure is relatively contraindicated in patients with adverse anatomical conditions such as short, fat neck, or obesity an enlarged thyroid gland, an inability to extend the neck, including either documented or suspected cervical spine fracture, previous cervical spine surgery or tracheostomy, coagulopathy, and anticoagulation therapy. Ben Nun et al[46] reported a series of 157 patients who underwent percutaneous tracheostomy at the bedside, 58 of which had 1 or more relative contraindications. The incidence of short- and long-term complications for both percutaneous and surgical tracheostomy patients was similar, provided the procedure was performed by experienced personnel. The authors concluded that the only true contraindication for the percutaneous approach was the pediatric population because of the limited experience, agreeing with the majority of the experts in the field. A retrospective study conducted in Brazil showed similar results in terms of complications, when the procedure was performed by surgical residents supervised by a thoracic surgeon, and the patient population had no contraindications for the percutaneous approach.[47]

POD 2: Intravenous loop diuretics were administered on POD 1 with a modest response but his creatinine rose to 3.1 mg/dL. The diuretics were discontinued later.

RENAL COMPLICATIONS

Acute renal failure (ARF) after lung resection is an uncommon complication and usually occurs as a result of infection or sepsis.[48] Despite its low incidence (0.4%-1.0%),[5,48,49] it is associated with a 60% to 90% mortality rate.[45,48,50] Although the etiology is unclear, fluid restriction, sepsis, nephrotoxic agents, cardiogenic shock and tumor embolization have all been suggested as predisposing factors.[51] Kheterpal et al[49] in an observational study conducted on 75,952 patients undergoing noncardiac and nonvascular surgery found that age, male gender, diabetes mellitus, either on oral medications or insulin, acute heart failure, ascites, hypertension, and renal insufficiency were all associated with an increased risk of postoperative renal injury. Interestingly enough, low urinary output was not associated with ARF. This is in contrast with common clinical practice where a "good" urinary output is indicative of preserved renal function and a guide for fluid management. In a small study, Golledge et al[52] found that ARF significantly increased morbidity and mortality after thoracic surgery. Hospital length of stay was 50% longer and mortality 19% higher. They proposed similar risk factors to those described above. Systemic hypotension, which can occur with the use of epidural analgesia, was also suggested as another cause for ARF, especially if local anesthetics were used at high concentration or volume. In healthy subjects, thoracic epidural analgesia interferes with the renin-angiotensin-vasopressin system. Sharrock et al[53] in a retrospective study of 150 patients undergoing total hip replacement showed that hypotensive epidural anesthesia did not increase the incidence of postoperative ARF even in patients with preoperative renal disease. In that study, mean arterial pressure was kept at about 40 to 55 mm Hg for an average of 95 minutes, and low dose epinephrine infusion was used to maintain cardiac output. Patients with renal disease were rehydrated during surgery more liberally than the controls, and maybe this contributed to prevent long-term renal disease. As reassuring as these results may be, it must be kept in mind that this model does not completely apply to the thoracic population. Thoracic epidural analgesia is commonly used intraoperatively, but with lower concentrations of local anesthetic and with the goal of keeping the hemodynamics as close as possible to baseline. Rehydration is not used liberally, and average blood loss is usually less than 500 mL.

Renal failure is classified as oliguric (<400cc/d) or nonoliguric (>600 cc/d), the latter being easier to treat and associated with a better prognosis.[48,54] Other than supportive care, volume expansion and hemodialysis are the suggested treatments. However, volume expansion is poorly tolerated in the thoracic population, especially after pneumonectomy, due to the potential risk of pulmonary edema, and the use of diuretics can potentially cause harm, thus is not routinely recommended. Maintenance of tissue oxygenation, treatment of sepsis, nutritional support and some form of dialysis and filtration (continuous arteriovenous hemofiltration in case of volume overload, continuous arteriovenous hemodiafiltration for hyperkalemia, acidosis, or progressive azotemia) have also been suggested.[48]

Nonsteroidal anti-inflammatory drugs (NSAIDs) are usually used as an adjunct to intravenous narcotics or epidural analgesia in the postoperative period, and may potentially cause ARF due to their nonspecific inhibition of cyclooxygenase enzymes.[55] By decreasing prostaglandin production, NSAIDs decrease pain and inflammation, but may also cause hypertension, gastrointestinal hemorrhage and renal dysfunction. The analysis of the literature is inconclusive on the role of these medications on perioperative renal function. In patients without renal disease, NSAIDs may reduce creatinine clearance, as well as potassium and sodium elimination on postoperative day 1. However, no effect on urinary volume or need for hemodialysis has been described.[55-57] Preexisting renal disease as well as dehydration (or fluid restriction) may play a role in the development of renal insufficiency related to NSAID use, especially in patients with chronic renal failure, where residual function is prostaglandin dependent. When NSAIDs and aminoglycosides are administered together, there is an additive increased risk of developing ARF, even in the presence of normal preoperative renal function.[57] Cyclooxygenase (COX) inhibitors, especially COX_2, represent a potentially safer alternative to non specific NSAIDs, especially in the presence of preexisting renal dysfunction. However, a review of the literature has produced inconsistent results to be able to provide recommendations.[57] Moreover, these drugs are available only in the oral form in the United States, making their use difficult in the immediate postoperative period.

Several medications are still used for renal protection, however the data in the literature is extremely controversial in terms of whether they improve outcome (summary in Table 23–4).

Table 23–4. Possible Pharmacologic Treatment of Acute Renal Failure

	Dopamine[60]	Fenoldopam[61]	Loop Diuretics[62,63]	Dexmedetomidine[50]
Mechanism	D1, D2, D4	D1	Inhibition of Na-K-Cl channel	α_2-Agonist
"Renoprotective" Dose	2-3 mcg/kg/min	0.03-0.1 mcg/kg/min	Up to 200 mg in patients with renal insufficiency	0.5 mcg/kg/20 min then 0.4 mcg/kg/h
Urinary output	↑	↑	↑	↑
Serum creatinine	↑	↓		↓
Creatinine clearance	↑	↑		↑
Outcome	No difference		No difference	
Side effects	Ischemia: Myocardium Skin/limb	Compensatory tachycardia	Deafness tinnitus	Bradycardia Hypotension Rebound hypertension

Na-K-Cl = sodium-potassium-chloride

Low dose **dopamine** (2-5 mcg/kg/min) has been extensively used to improve renal perfusion and prevent or treat ARF. At this dose, dopamine activates the dopaminergic receptors D1, D2, and D4, promoting renal vasodilatation with a subsequent increase in renal perfusion and diuresis. While D1 receptors promote renal vasodilatation, D2 and α-receptors cause vasoconstriction, decrease glomerular filtration rate and sodium excretion. Selective D1 receptor activation may potentially be protective against acute tubular necrosis (ATN). However, there is a poor correlation between infusion rates and achieved plasma levels. Patients receiving renal dose dopamine often have activation of α- and β-receptors, leading to unwanted tachycardia, for example.[58] Despite the controversial results in the literature on the role of dopamine as a nephroprotective agent, several surveys in the ICU still confirm the popularity of this drug.[59] Lauschke et al[60] demonstrated that low dose dopamine neither prevents nor reverses ARF, and does not improve outcome. In critically ill patients, especially if older than 55 years of age, renal perfusion seems to deteriorate due to an increase in renal vascular resistance, which may be already increased at baseline and may be unaffected by dopamine infusion. A meta-analysis of 61 trials (3356 patients) using low-dose dopamine did not show any effect on mortality, need for renal replacement therapy and overall adverse events. Urinary output and creatinine clearance were increased during the first day of treatment, while serum creatinine levels were decreased. However, there was no clinical significance for patients with or at risk for ARF.[59] Tachyarrhythmias were reported as the most common adverse event, followed by myocardial, limb or cutaneous ischemia.

Fenoldopam, a selective postsynaptic D1 receptor agonist, has been used in critically ill patients with ARF as a nephroprotective agent at doses of 0.03 to 0.1 mg/kg/min. Fenoldopam increases blood flow to the renal cortex and to a greater extent to the outer medulla, and decreases oxygen demand in the thick ascending limb, the proximal convoluted tubule and the cortical collecting ducts by inhibiting sodium transport.[61] In the early stage of ARF, fenoldopam seems to produce a more significant reduction in creatinine in the first 3 days of infusion when compared to low-dose dopamine,[61] but does not affect the need for hemodialysis or mortality, except in patients with diabetes or after coronary artery bypass grafting.[58] The absence of β-effects has been associated with less arrhythmias, making this drug safer than dopamine when higher doses are needed.[45] Tachycardia may occur to compensate for rapid vasodilatation.

Loop diuretics such as furosemide or bumetanide can be used to convert oliguric to nonoliguric ARF, the latter having a better prognosis. However, several meta-analyses do not show a decrease in mortality in patients with ARF, despite a reduction in the oliguric period.[62,63] The requirement for hemodialysis, the number of dialysis sessions, the number of patients remaining oliguric despite the treatment and the length of hospital stay is also unchanged. Moreover, at higher doses (1-3.4 g/d), there is an increase in temporary deafness and tinnitus,[63] which may go undiagnosed if the patient is sedated and mechanically ventilated. Mehta et al[64] studied 552 critically ill patients with ARF who received either boluses or continuous infusion of loop diuretics alone or in combination with thiazide diuretics. They found a 68% increase in mortality, 77% increase in the odds of non recovery of renal function and an overall increase in hospital length of stay. They postulated that the increase in urinary output may have contributed to underestimate the severity of renal dysfunction, delaying proper treatment.

Dexmedetomidine is a selective α_2-agonist that has been shown, in a small study, to increase urinary output after thoracic procedures.[50] Binding of the α_2-receptors within the central nervous system causes a decrease in the sympathetic outflow and catecholamine level,[65] which is thought to cause less renal vasoconstriction. In a prospective randomized study of 28 patients undergoing lung resection, the use of dexmedetomidine as an adjunct to postoperative epidural analgesia was associated with increased urinary output, a decrease in serum creatinine and an improved creatinine clearance during the first four postoperative days.[50] Patients received a loading dose of 0.5 mcg/kg of medication over 20 minutes, followed by 0.4 mcg/kg/h continuous infusion for 24 hours. Proposed mechanisms were an improved glomerular function by decreasing circulating levels of norepinephrine, possibly a direct effect on the kidney (mainly seen in animal models) and an interference with the antidiuretic effect of arginine-vasopressin. Similar results were found in animal models of ARF from both ischemia-reperfusion injury[66] and after intravenous contrast injection.[67] In both cases, renal protection was more significant when the drug was started prior to the ischemic insult.

Sodium bicarbonate infusion has also been investigated as a possible protective strategy to prevent renal insufficiency. Medullary renal vasoconstriction with subsequent ischemia and oxidant/free radical injury are two proposed mechanisms leading to nephropathy. Bicarbonate infusion may reduce free radical production by increasing tubular pH.[68] However, a single-blinded randomized study conducted on 353 patients with stable renal disease undergoing coronary angiography showed that the use of sodium bicarbonate was not superior to the use of normal saline solutions to prevent contrast induced nephropathy.[68] Both estimated glomerular filtration rates and mortality at 30 days and 6 months were similar between the two groups.

POD3: The patient developed atrial fibrillation with rapid ventricular response. Vital signs: BP 80/40, HR 150, T 37.9, SpO_2 90% on FiO_2 60%. Medications included dopamine 3 mcg/kg/min, fentanyl 50 mcg/h and midazolam 1 mg/h.

CARDIAC COMPLICATIONS

Postoperative Arrhythmias

Supraventricular tachyarrhythmias affect about 18% to 20% patients undergoing noncardiac thoracic surgery.[69] The most important risk factors are age 60 years and older[70] and intrapericardial pneumonectomy.[8] Other markers associated with these arrhythmias are an elevated white blood cell count on post operative day one[71] and an elevated perioperative N-terminal-pro-B-type natriuretic peptide.[72] The most common rhythm disturbance is atrial fibrillation (AF), followed by supraventricular tachycardia (SVT), atrial flutter and premature ventricular contractions (PVCs). They are usually diagnosed on the second postoperative day and respond to pharmacological cardioversion.[70,73-75]

Sustained ventricular tachyarrhythmias are quite rare after lung resection.[69] A study conducted on 412 patients showed a 15% incidence of nonsustained ventricular tachycardia (≥3 beats) during the first 96 hours after major lung resection.[76] None of the patients with nonsustained ventricular tachycardia had hemodynamic instability that required treatment at any time, and the only preoperative risk factor identified was the presence of a left bundle branch block. There was no association with age, other clinical factors, or core temperature upon arrival to PACU. On multivariate analysis, there was an independent association between nonsustained ventricular tachycardia and postoperative atrial fibrillation (POAF). Proposed mechanisms for this observation included vagal withdrawal or irritation, and/or a surge in sympathetic activity. These findings differ from the cardiac surgical literature, where the presence of postoperative ventricular tachycardia is often associated with poor outcome.[69]

POAF can manifest either as an isolated complication or be associated with respiratory or infectious disease.[70] It is typically transient and reversible and seems to affect individuals with an electrophysiologic substrate for arrhythmias present before or as a result of surgery.[77] Despite the good prognosis, patients with POAF after thoracic surgery have a reported risk of 1.7% to develop cerebrovascular accidents.[69] This is mostly due to thromboembolism, which can occur within 24 to 48 hours from the onset of POAF. If sinus rhythm cannot be successfully restored within this time frame, anticoagulation should be considered, weighing the risk of postoperative bleeding.[69]

Several mechanisms have been proposed to explain POAF, but no consistent factors other than age have been proven. Aging per se has been associated with a remodeling of the atrial myocardium, with consequent changes in the sinoatrial and atrioventricular nodal conduction, as well as an increased sensitivity to catecholamine activity, especially after surgical trauma in the area.[69] By age 75, it appears that only 10% normal sinus nodal fibers are present.[78] Moreover, in the elderly, triggering of the inflammatory response, with activation of the complement and several proinflammatory cytokines has been suggested as responsible for POAF.[79] Amar et al[71] showed that in patients older than 60 years of age a doubling in white blood cells (WBC) count on post operative day 1 was associated with a threefold increase in the odds of developing POAF. The peak surge in WBC count paralleled the time of onset of POAF. They suggested that β_2-receptor activation could be responsible for this finding, probably secondary to an increase in catecholamine tone. An increase in sympathetic activity and high endogenous catecholamine levels have also been proposed in other studies.[71] The use of thoracic epidural analgesia had disappointing results on preventing POAF.[80] This may be due to the high individual variability of sympathetic blockade. Positive inotropic agents, such as dopamine, as well as anemia, fever, hypoglycemia, postoperative ischemia, and surgical complications represent other possible aggravating causes.[77] Stretching or inflammation of the pulmonary veins, as well as hilar manipulation and mediastinal shift have also been suggested as other contributing mechanisms.[73,81]

With rapid POAF, patients may exhibit dyspnea, palpitations, dizziness, syncope, respiratory distress, and hypotension. As is true for any type of arrhythmia, pulmonary embolism or myocardial ischemia and electrolyte abnormalities need to be excluded or corrected.[82] As part of the workup for new onset POAF, transthoracic echocardiography has been recommended by the American Heart Association guidelines to rule out any structural disease, if such information is not already available.[83]

Mortality seems to be increased in patients who develop arrhythmias, even though this is not the direct cause, except in the presence of heart failure or prolonged hypotension.[74] Hospital length of stay and overall costs are increased, suggesting the importance of prevention when possible.[70,84] In most cases, POAF resolves prior to hospital discharge and the great majority of these patients remain in sinus rhythm 6 weeks after surgery.[79]

Patients are considered at risk for postoperative supraventricular arrhythmias if they have two or more of the risk factors listed in Table 23–5, and if so, they may be started on pharmacological prophylaxis either preoperatively or in the immediate postoperative period.

Several regimens are available to prevent or treat atrial tachyarrhythmias. β-blockers have gained popularity as preventive medications due to their cardioprotective effects. The rationale for their use as prophylaxis is to counteract the

Table 23–5. Proposed Risk Factors for Supraventricular Tachyarrhythmias[69,70,74,77]

Preoperative	Intraoperative	Postoperative
Age >60	Right sided pneumonectomy	Increased WBC count on POD 1
Male gender	Intrapericardial procedure	
H/o paroxysmal AF		
Prolonged P wave duration		
Preoperative HR >72 bpm		
Elevated BNP level		

AF = atrial fibrillation, BNP = brain natriuretic peptide, bpm = beats per minute, h/o = history of, HR = heart rate, POD = postoperative day, WBC = white blood cell count

effects of the sympathetic predominance that occurs after surgery, which may enhance patient susceptibility to dysrhythmias. β-blockers inhibit intracellular calcium influx via second messenger systems and have a membrane stabilizing effect.[85] When used in the thoracic population, the respiratory side effects need to be taken into consideration as they may worsen pulmonary function in the postoperative period. Pulmonary edema has been described as a potential side effect after lung resection,[86] as well as hypotension and bradycardia. Moreover, in patients on chronic β-blockers, withdrawal may lead to rebound tachycardia.[87] The β-blocker length of stay study (BLOS) analyzed the effects of β-blockers administered after cardiac surgery as prophylactic agents in both naive patients and in those already taking β-blockers preoperatively. The goal was to prevent POAF, and possibly decrease the length of stay in the hospital and ICU. Despite a small decrease in the incidence of POAF in those patients already on β-blockers, an increased length of stay was observed in the very same group.[88] This was attributed to the development of adverse cardiac and pulmonary effects. Recently, the Perioperative Ischemic Evaluation (POISE) trial showed that aggressive β-blockade can reduce postoperative myocardial infarction and even POAF, but at the cost of an increase in mortality related to cerebrovascular events in patients who had hypotension and decreased cerebral perfusion.[89] These findings have been consistent with other trials using lower doses of β-blockers, and question the safety of this strategy.[90]

Sotalol is a class III antiarrhythmic with significant activity as a nonselective β-blocker and a potassium channel blocker. Potassium current blockade results in prolongation of both the action potential and the QT interval, which can predispose to ventricular dysrhythmias such as Torsades de Pointes.[87] This can occur at both therapeutic and toxic dosages.[85] Because of the renal excretion, its use is contraindicated in patients with a creatinine clearance less than 46 mL/min. As with other β-blockers, sotalol is effective in decreasing POAF, but does not reduce hospital length of stay or postoperative morbidity. Several studies have reported significant bradycardia that led to discontinuation of therapy.[77] Unfortunately, most of the literature on this medication comes from the cardiac surgical population rather than the thoracic one.[82]

The **calcium channel blockers** verapamil and diltiazem have been used for both prophylaxis and treatment of POAF. They directly block the L-type calcium channel, decreasing calcium entry in the cell. This causes a slowing of the sinoatrial automaticity and atrio-ventricular nodal conduction.[85] In addition, this class of drugs may reduce pulmonary vascular resistance and right ventricular pressure, making this an attractive option after major lung resection, where a potential increase in pulmonary arterial pressures may be present.[86] Hypotension, more frequent with verapamil, is one of the major side effects and one of the most common reasons to stop the medication. In the cardiac population, calcium channel blockers seem to cause a 40% decrease of postoperative myocardial infarction rates and 45% reduction of ischemia.[86] Amar et al[78] demonstrated that diltiazem is superior to digoxin when used to prevent supraventricular dysrhythmias, specifically POAF, in patients after intrapericardial or standard pneumonectomy. However, both drugs had equal effect on ventricular dysrhythmias, echocardiographic changes in right ventricular function and hospital length of stay. In the largest study to prevent POAF in thoracic surgical patients, diltiazem was shown to be safe and effective in reducing the rate of POAF by almost 50%.[84]

Prophylactic **digitalization** to prevent POAF is not a common practice nowadays, since there are no proven benefits and potential associated side effects.[91] At the present time, digoxin is not recommended in the postoperative period to prevent POAF.[91] In patients with chronic atrial fibrillation, digoxin does not seem to be able to restore normal sinus rhythm, and as a single agent it does not adequately control the ventricular response unless very high doses are used.[91] For this purpose, it is usually combined with β-blockers or calcium channel blockers[92] and it works better in cases of chronic atrial fibrillation and heart failure with systolic dysfunction.[91] Digitalis toxicity and the difficulty in assessing proper plasma levels are the main limiting factors for its use.[74] Moreover, several studies had demonstrated a superior effect of calcium channel blockers in preventing POAF, with less potential side effects.[78] Digoxin should be avoided in patients with renal insufficiency, electrolyte disturbances (hypokalemia, hypomagnesemia, and hypercalcemia), acute coronary syndromes and thyroid disorders. The main mechanism of action is by enhancing vagal activity, mainly on the atrioventricular node, thus decreasing ventricular response during atrial arrhythmias.[87] The sympathetic response is also inhibited in a way unrelated to the increase in cardiac output. Digoxin binds the sodium-potassium ATPase channel, mainly on the myocardium, blocking its transport.[92] This promotes an increase in intracellular calcium, which increases cardiac contractility.

Amiodarone is a multiple sodium-potassium-calcium channel blocker and a β-adrenergic inhibitor often used to maintain sinus rhythm after electrical cardioversion in the general population. It works best as prophylactic agent when administered 1 week prior to surgery;[93] however, the precise mechanism of action is unknown.[94] The calcium-potassium channel blockade causes an increase in the duration of the action potential and the refractory period in the cardiac tissue. Hypotension and bradycardia can be significant, especially in patients with congestive heart failure and left ventricular dysfunction, as well as QT prolongation.[81] Other side effects include hypo/hyperthyroidism, hepatic and neurotoxicity, and prolongation of warfarin half-life.[94] Pulmonary toxicity is, however, the main concern of amiodarone therapy after lung resection.[86] It can occur at lower dosages than the ones used in the general population, and can manifest as chronic interstitial pneumonitis, bronchiolitis obliterans, adult respiratory distress syndrome (ARDS) or a solitary lung mass.[81] In a very small prospective randomized study, Van Mieghem et al[95] examined the role of amiodarone prophylaxis on POAF after lung resection, comparing it to verapamil. No difference was observed between the two drugs in the interim analysis. However, the study had to be stopped prematurely due to an increased incidence of ARDS in the amiodarone group (7.4% in the patients who had a right pneumonectomy vs 1.6% for other types of lung resections). Mortality rates were also higher in the patients who received amiodarone. This occurred despite using standard intravenous regimens and having therapeutic plasma concentrations. Two mechanisms were proposed: an indirect one, by increasing inflammatory mediators, and a direct one, by causing direct damage to the cells and subsequent fibrosis. Independently from the etiology, they recommended to avoid amiodarone after lung resection. By surgically decreasing the amount of lung parenchyma available, standard doses of amiodarone can account for higher pulmonary concentrations of the drug, which may reach toxic levels. Later studies, when amiodarone was used for a short-time period, did not confirm an increased incidence of respiratory toxicity.[69] Overall, the efficacy of amiodarone in preventing POAF does not seem to be different from diltiazem.[69] The main indication for amiodarone as a treatment agent is for patients with POAF and pre-excitation conduction abnormalities, such as Wolf-Parkinson-White syndrome.[83]

Magnesium is indicated if hypomagnesemia exists. A randomized controlled study conducted in 200 patients to undergo cardiopulmonary bypass surgery showed a decreased incidence of POAF when magnesium sulfate was administered as a prophylactic drug.[96] However, several trials in the cardiac surgical population have given conflicting results on the benefits of magnesium and POAF prophylaxis, with the only agreement to maintain magnesium levels within normal values.[87] Except in patients with acute renal failure, magnesium has a relatively safe profile.

Statins, 3-hydroxy-3-methylglutaratyl coenzyme-A reductase inhibitors, have been shown to suppress electrical remodeling and prevent POAF in animal models.[81] They are powerful lipid lowering drugs, highly effective in preventing coronary artery disease. Studies conducted in hypercholesterolemic patients on statins undergoing coronary artery bypass grafting (CAGB) showed a decrease in postoperative major cardiac events.[97] When started 1 week prior to on pump CABG, they decreased the incidence of POAF, as well as hospital length stay.[77,98] This effect was potentiated if patients were also taking β-blockers.[98] One possible explanation seems to be related to their anti-inflammatory mechanism, and observational studies conducted in patients undergoing major lung resection have observed an increase in C-reactive protein and interleukin

6 in the postoperative period.[99] Preoperative use of statins was associated with a threefold decrease in the probability of developing POAF.[100]

Angiotensin-converting enzyme inhibitors (ACEIs) and angiotensin receptor blockers (ARBs) have been suggested to reduce the incidence of POAF, with the greatest effect on patients with heart failure and systolic left ventricular dysfunction, but not in patients with systemic hypertension.[101] They may also have a role in maintaining sinus rhythm after electrical cardioversion. Inhibition of the renin-angiotensin-aldosterone system seems to attenuate left atrial dilatation and fibrosis, and to contribute to slowing conduction in animal studies, all factors that can trigger and maintain re-entry circuits. These effects seem to be potentiated when β-blockers are used in conjunction in patients with chronic heart failure.[77] So far, the majority of the literature has focused on outcome in patients with chronic atrial fibrillation. When POAF is investigated, the results are controversial with both positive[77] and negative[102] findings.

Biatrial pacing and electrical cardioversion: Atrial pacing has been used as an alternative to pharmacological prophylaxis for POAF. There is a lot of controversy among the different pacing modalities and sites, current, rates and concurrent use of medications, with the majority of the studies conducted in the cardiac population after coronary surgery.[77] At the present time, the only recommended modality to prevent POAF is biatrial pacing.[103] Despite a 15% reduction in the incidence of POAF,[103] several technical difficulties can be encountered with this modality. Loss of sensing, diaphragmatic pacing and left ventricular pacing are some of them.[104] Most of the patients are paced at a rate of 80 to 90 or higher, depending on their intrinsic heart rate, and for a period of 3 to 5 days.[104]

Electrical cardioversion is used to treat atrial fibrillation in case of hemodynamic instability, and is successful in 67% to 94% cases.[81] Biphasic waveforms are more successful than monophasic, using a current around 100 to 200 J and in a synchronized mode. Higher energy can be used for patients with high body mass index, prolonged atrial fibrillation or left atrial enlargement. Bradycardia (more common in patients on antiarrhythmics prior to cardioversion), ventricular tachyarrhythmias (in case of shock applied during repolarization), hypotension, pulmonary edema (probably due to myocardial stunning) and embolism are all potential complications. Electrolytes should be checked and normalized before cardioversion. In case of digitalis toxicity and hypokalemia, cardioversion should be avoided due to the high incidence of ventricular fibrillation. In this setting, low currents and prophylactic lidocaine should be used. Since bradycardia can be profound up to the point of asystole, pacing capabilities should be readily available.[81]

Myocardial Ischemia

The postoperative period is one where significant physiologic changes such as decreases in pulmonary function, hypoxia, fluid shifts, electrolyte imbalances, right ventricular dysfunction, and fluctuations in pain occur. Myocardial ischemia can accompany these changes and is present as an electrocardiographic finding in 3.8% lung resection patients, while infarction can occur in 0.2% to 0.9% cases.[3,5,6] The incidence increases in patients with preoperative coronary artery disease and abnormal exercise testing. The highest risk is during the first 3 postoperative days, when a high degree of monitoring is suggested. The overall mortality ranges between 32% and 70%.[82]

It is estimated that 30% patients undergoing noncardiac surgery each year either have or are at risk for coronary artery disease.[105] Ideally, these patients should be identified preoperatively, so that appropriate preventive interventions can be delivered throughout the perioperative period. In this respect, beta blockade should be instituted around the time of surgery in patients with three or more risk factors for coronary ischemia or in those on chronic beta blocker therapy.[106] The risk of acute coronary syndrome is aggravated by the increased platelet adhesiveness and decreased fibrinolysis seen in the postoperative period. Furthermore, retrospective studies have shown that discontinuation of aspirin places patients at risk for myocardial infarction and stroke.[107,108] It is therefore recommended that aspirin therapy be continued throughout surgery in those patients who were taking aspirin preoperatively, except in very selected cases.[109]

Cardiac stents, especially drug eluting stents, represent a significant problem due to the prolonged need of anticoagulation. Stopping dual antiplatelet therapy (aspirin and clopidogrel) is associated with the risk of stent thrombosis, which may be significantly high, while continuing it leads to an increased risk of intra- and postoperative bleeding and precludes the possibility of using regional anesthetic techniques.[107] Duration of antiplatelet therapy is usually based on the type of stent: 4 to 6 weeks for bare metal stents, and 12 to 24 months for drug eluting ones. Patients with drug eluting stents are at higher risk of stent thrombosis, especially if the stent is long, at a bifurcation, if the revascularization is incomplete, or the patient has history of diabetes or heart failure.[108] A nonrandomized observational prospective study conducted in noncardiac surgery patients who had cardiac stents placed within a year from surgery[109] found that 44.7% patients suffered from cardiac complications postoperatively and 4.7% died. Dual antiplatelet therapy was stopped on average 3 days prior to surgery and substituted with intravenous unfractionated heparin or subcutaneous enoxaparin. Most of the complications occurred within the first 35 days from the stent placement and were cardiac in nature. Bleeding was not a significant variable. The recommendations for continuation of aspirin therapy mentioned above are especially important in this patient population. Clopidogrel should also be continued throughout surgery, or restarted as soon as possible after surgery if bleeding risk is high. In case stents are placed before surgery, bare metal stents are preferred due to their lower risk of thrombosis and the shorter duration of dual antiplatelet therapy. Of note, substitution of antiplatelet agents by an antithrombin such as heparin does not afford real protection against the risk of coronary or stent thrombosis.[109]

Heart Failure

Congestive heart failure can occur after major lung resection as a result of right- or left-sided dysfunction. Right heart failure can be secondary to changes either in contractility or afterload. Most of the studies that looked at changes in right ventricular function after lung resection were small, and found minor and transient differences when compared to the preoperative period. An increase in right ventricular end–diastolic volume was observed as a reversible finding during the first 2 postoperative days.[82] Moreover, pulmonary arterial pressures and pulmonary vascular resistance were mildly increased during the early postoperative period in another study done on 15 patients.[110] While postoperative changes in pulmonary arterial pressures, central venous pressures and pulmonary vascular resistance seem to be subtle at rest, they may become significant during exercise. Changes in right ventricular function are usually able to compensate for the former, but they may fail for the latter, leading to pulmonary hypertension.[82] Other possible causes of right ventricular failure, although rare, include pulmonary embolism and cardiac herniation (see below).

Left ventricular failure is usually a consequence of right heart dysfunction, either by decreasing left ventricular preload or by interatrial septal shifts.[82] Acute ischemia and valvular disease may also be contributing factors.

Cardiac herniation, a rare complication after pneumonectomy, may be responsible for both right and left heart failure. It occurs more commonly after intrapericardial pneumonectomy—right more often than left—and leads to a 50% mortality rate.[82] Herniation can be secondary to an incomplete closure of the pericardium or the breakdown of a pericardial patch.[111] One main contributing factor includes an increase in intrathoracic pressure, such as with coughing. Changes in position, with the operative side being dependent, positive pressure ventilation, rapid lung re-expansion or suction on the chest tube are also other possible causes. Symptoms depend on the side of the herniation. Right-sided cases present with superior vena cava syndrome due to kinking of the superior vena cava and decreased right ventricular filling, leading to hypotension, tachycardia and shock. Left-sided cases present with arrhythmias and myocardial ischemia leads to infarction, hypotension and ventricular fibrillation if untreated. This is due to less cardiac rotation, with myocardial compression from the pericardium. Clinical presentation and electrocardiographic findings are fairly nonspecific in suggesting the diagnosis, stressing the role of chest radiography and a high index of suspicion. Treatment is surgical, with repositioning of the heart and placement of a patch. In order to minimize hemodynamic instability, the patient should be kept on the lateral decubitus, with the operative side up.[111]

CONCLUSIONS

In the last few decades, a significant improvement in the surgical and anesthetic techniques has made pneumonectomy and major lung resection safer. The introduction of epidural analgesia, short acting anesthetics and minimally invasive surgical techniques have all contributed to decrease the incidence of postoperative complications. Fast track strategies and careful selection of patients undergoing lung resection procedures have also played an important role in postoperative and long-term outcome improvements. Better utilization of step down and acute postoperative care units have decreased the rate of ICU admissions, saving costs. Since the average age of patients requiring lung resection is increasing, anesthesiologists and surgeons will be facing more complex cases, due to the presence of multiple comorbidities. Careful preoperative workup, customizing the type of surgery as well as planning for in hospital and post discharge rehabilitation options will prove to be essential for decreasing complications and improving overall care for thoracic surgical patients.

REFERENCES

1. Alexiou C, Beggs D, Rogers ML, Beggs L, Asopa S, Salama FD. Pneumonectomy for non-small cell lung cancer: predictors of operative mortality and survival. *Eur J Cardiothorac Surg.* 2001;20(3):476-480.
2. Graham E. Indications for total pneumonectomy. *Chest.* 1944;10(2):87-94.
3. Martin J, Ginsberg RJ, Abolhoda A, et al. Morbidity and mortality after neoadjuvant therapy for lung cancer: the risks of right pneumonectomy. *Ann Thorac Surg.* 2001;72(4):1149-1154.
4. Van Schil PE. Surgery: therapeutic indications. *Cancer Radiother.* 2007;11(1-2):47-52.
5. Boffa DJ, Allen MS, Grab JD, Gaissert HA, Harpole DH, Wright CD. Data from The Society of Thoracic Surgeons General Thoracic Surgery database: the surgical management of primary lung tumors. *J Thorac Cardiovasc Surg.* 2008;135(2):247-254.
6. Allen MS, Darling GE, Pechet TT, et al. Morbidity and mortality of major pulmonary resections in patients with early-stage lung cancer: initial results of the randomized, prospective ACOSOG Z0030 trial. *Ann Thorac Surg.* 2006;81(3):1013-1019; discussion 1019-1020.
7. Strand TE, Rostad H, Damhuis RA, Norstein J. Risk factors for 30-day mortality after resection of lung cancer and prediction of their magnitude. *Thorax.* 2007;62(11):991-997.
8. Dancewicz M, Kowalewski J, Peplinski J. Factors associated with perioperative complications after pneumonectomy for primary carcinoma of the lung. *Interact Cardiovasc Thorac Surg.* 2006;5(2):97-100.
9. Ferguson MK, Vigneswaran WT. Diffusing capacity predicts morbidity after lung resection in patients without obstructive lung disease. *Ann Thorac Surg.* 2008;85(4):1158-1164; discussion 1155-1164.
10. Alam N, Park BJ, Wilton A, et al. Incidence and risk factors for lung injury after lung cancer resection. *Ann Thorac Surg.* 2007;84(4):1085-1091; discussion 1091.
11. Alvarez J. Post pneumonectomy pulmonary edema. In: Slinger, P, (ed). *Progress in Thoracic Anesthesia, SCA Monograph.* Lippincott Williams & Wilkins, Baltimore. Chapter 9. 2004:187-219.
12. Alvarez JM, Panda RK, Newman MA, Slinger P, Deslauriers J, Ferguson M. Postpneumonectomy pulmonary edema. *J Cardiothorac Vasc Anesth.* 2003;17(3):388-395.
13. Alvarez JM, Bairstow BM, Tang C, Newman MA. Post-lung resection pulmonary edema: a case for aggressive management. *J Cardiothorac Vasc Anesth.* 1998;12(2):199-205.
14. Waller DA, Keavey P, Woodfine L, Dark JH. Pulmonary endothelial permeability changes after major lung resection. *Ann Thor Surg.* 1996;61(5):1435-1440.
15. Little AG, Langmuir VK, Singer AH, Skinner DB. Hemodynamic pulmonary edema in dog lungs after contralateral pneumonectomy and mediastinal lymphatic interruption. *Lung.* 1984;162(3):139-145.
16. Van Der Werff YD, Van Der Houwen HK, Heijmans PJ, et al. Postpneumonectomy pulmonary edema. A retrospective analysis of incidence and possible risk factors. *Chest.* 1997;111(5):1278-1284.
17. Ventilation with lower tidal volumes as compared with traditional tidal volumes for acute lung injury and the acute respiratory distress syndrome. The Acute Respiratory Distress Syndrome Network. *N Engl J Med.* 2000;342(18):1301-1308.
18. Amar D, Burt ME, Roistacher N, Reinsel RA, Ginsberg RJ, Wilson RS. Value of perioperative Doppler echocardiography in patients undergoing major lung resection. *Ann Thorac Surg.* 1996;61(2):516-520.
19. Cerfolio RJ, Bryant AS, Thurber JS, Bass CS, Lell WA, Bartolucci AA. Intraoperative solumedrol helps prevent postpneumonectomy pulmonary edema. *Ann Thorac Surg.* 2003;76(4):1029-1033; discussion 1025-1033.
20. Schussler O, Alifano M, Dermine H, et al. Postoperative pneumonia after major lung resection. *Am J Respir Crit Care Med.* 2006;173(10):1161-1169.
21. Shiono S, Yoshida J, Nishimura M, et al. Risk factors of postoperative respiratory infections in lung cancer surgery. *J Thorac Oncol.* 2007;2(1):34-38.
22. Fernandez-Perez ER, Keegan MT, Brown DR, Hubmayr RD, Gajic O. Intraoperative tidal volume as a risk factor for respiratory failure after pneumonectomy. *Anesthesiology.* 2006;105(1):14-18.
23. Radu DM, Jaureguy F, Seguin A, et al. Postoperative pneumonia after major pulmonary resections: an unsolved problem in thoracic surgery. *Ann Thorac Surg.* 2007;84(5):1669-1673.
24. Schussler O, Dermine H, Alifano M, et al. Should we change antibiotic prophylaxis for lung surgery? postoperative pneumonia is the critical issue. *Ann Thorac Surg.* 2008;86(6):1727-1733.
25. Bratzler DW, Houck PM. Antimicrobial prophylaxis for surgery: an advisory statement from the National Surgical Infection Prevention Project. *Clin Infect Dis.* 2004;38(12):1706-1715.

26. Deschamps C, Bernard A, Nichols FC, III, et al. Empyema and bronchopleural fistula after pneumonectomy: factors affecting incidence. *Ann Thorac Surg.* 2001;72(1):243-247; discussion 248.
27. Darling GE, Abdurahman A, Yi QL, et al. Risk of a right pneumonectomy: role of bronchopleural fistula. *Ann Thorac Surg.* 2005;79(2):433-437.
28. Ng T, Ryder BA, Maziak DE, Shamji FM. Treatment of postpneumonectomy empyema with debridement followed by continuous antibiotic irrigation. *J Am Coll Surg.* 2008;206(3): 1178-1183.
29. West D, Togo A, Kirk A. Are bronchoscopic approaches to post-pneumonectomy bronchopleural fistula an effective alternative to repeat thoracotomy? *Interact Cardiovasc Thorac Surg.* 2007;6:547-550.
30. Bernard GR, Artigas A, Brigham KL, et al. The American-European Consensus Conference on ARDS. Definitions, mechanisms, relevant outcomes, and clinical trial coordination. *Am J Respir Crit Care Med.* 1994;149(3 Pt 1):818-824.
31. Slinger PD. Acute lung injury after pulmonary resection: more pieces of the puzzle. *Anesth Analg.* 2003;97(6):1555-1557.
32. Licker M, Fauconnet P, Villiger Y, Tschopp JM. Acute lung injury and outcomes after thoracic surgery. *Curr Opin Anaesthesiol.* 2009;22(1):61-67.
33. Jeon K, Yoon JW, Suh GY, et al. Risk factors for post-pneumonectomy acute lung injury/acute respiratory distress syndrome in primary lung cancer patients. *Anaesth Intensive Care.* 2009;37(1):14-19.
34. Schilling T, Kozian A, Huth C, et al. The pulmonary immune effects of mechanical ventilation in patients undergoing thoracic surgery. *Anesth Analg.* 2005;101(4):957-965, table of contents.
35. Girard TD, Bernard GR. Mechanical ventilation in ARDS: a state-of-the-art review. *Chest.* 2007;131(3):921-929.
36. Girard TD, Kress JP, Fuchs BD, et al. Efficacy and safety of a paired sedation and ventilator weaning protocol for mechanically ventilated patients in intensive care (Awakening and Breathing Controlled trial): a randomised controlled trial. *Lancet.* 2008;371(9607):126-134.
37. Jain R, DalNogare A. Pharmacological therapy for acute respiratory distress syndrome. *Mayo Clin Proc.* 2006;81(2):205-212.
38. Meduri GU, Marik PE, Chrousos GP, et al. Steroid treatment in ARDS: a critical appraisal of the ARDS network trial and the recent literature. *Intensive Care Med.* 2008;34(1):61-69.
39. Tang BM, Craig JC, Eslick GD, Seppelt I, McLean AS. Use of corticosteroids in acute lung injury and acute respiratory distress syndrome: a systematic review and meta-analysis. *Crit Care Med.* 2009;37(5):1594-1603.
40. Blot F, Melot C. Indications, timing, and techniques of tracheostomy in 152 French ICUs. *Chest.* 2005;127(4):1347-1352.
41. Pratt L. Tracheotomy: historical review. *Laryngoscope.* 2008;118:1597-1606.
42. Clec'h C, Alberti C, Vincent F, et al. Tracheostomy does not improve the outcome of patients requiring prolonged mechanical ventilation: a propensity study. *Crit Care Med.* 2007;35(1):132-138.
43. De Leyn P, Bedert L, Delcroix M, et al. Tracheotomy: clinical review and guidelines. *Eur J Cardiothorac Surg.* 2007;32(3):412-421.
44. Veelo D, Dongelmans D, Phoa K, Spronk P, Schultz M. Tracheostomy: current practice on timing, correction of coagulation disorders and peri-operative management—a postal survey in the Netherlands. *Acta Anesthesiol Scand* 2007;51:1231-1236.
45. Sear JW. Kidney dysfunction in the postoperative period. *Br J Anaesth.* 2005;95(1):20-32.
46. Ben Nun A, Altman E, Best LA. Extended indications for percutaneous tracheostomy. *Ann Thorac Surg.* 2005;80(4):1276-1279.
47. Perfeito J, Sterse da Mata C, Forte V, Carnaghi M, Tamura N, Leao L. Tracheostomy in the ICU: is it worthwhile? *J Brasileiro de Pneumologia.* 2007;33(6):687-690.
48. Urschel JD, Antkowiak JG, Takita H. Acute renal failure following pulmonary surgery. *J Cardiovasc Surg (Torino).* 1994;35(3):215-218.
49. Kheterpal S, Tremper KK, Heung M, et al. Development and validation of an acute kidney injury risk index for patients undergoing general surgery: results from a national data set. *Anesthesiology.* 2009;110(3):505-515.
50. Frumento RJ, Logginidou HG, Wahlander S, Wagener G, Playford HR, Sladen RN. Dexmedetomidine infusion is associated with enhanced renal function after thoracic surgery. *J Clin Anesth.* 2006;18(6): 422-426.

51. Karzai W, Schmidt J, Jung A, Kroger R, Clausner G, Presselt N. Delayed emergence and acute renal failure after pneumonectomy: tumor emboli complicating postoperative course. *J Cardiothorac Vasc Anesth.* 2009;23(2);219-222.
52. Golledge J, Goldstraw P. Renal impairment after thoracotomy: incidence, risk factors, and significance. *Ann Thorac Surg.* 1994;58(2):524-528.
53. Sharrock NE, Beksac B, Flynn E, Go G, Della Valle AG. Hypotensive epidural anaesthesia in patients with preoperative renal dysfunction undergoing total hip replacement. *Br J Anaesth.* 2006;96(2):207-212.
54. Lameire N, Vanholder R, Van Biesen W. Loop diuretics for patients with acute renal failure: helpful or harmful? *JAMA.* 2002;288(20):2599-2601.
55. Bainbridge D, Cheng DC, Martin JE, Novick R. NSAID-analgesia, pain control and morbidity in cardiothoracic surgery. *Can J Anaesth.* 2006;53(1):46-59.
56. Lee A, Cooper MG, Craig JC, Knight JF, Keneally JP. The effects of nonsteroidal anti-inflammatory drugs (NSAIDs) on postoperative renal function: a meta-analysis. *Anaesth Intensive Care.* 1999;27(6):574-580.
57. McCrory CR, Lindahl SG. Cyclooxygenase inhibition for postoperative analgesia. *Anesth Analg.* 2002;95(1):169-176.
58. Tumlin JA, Finkel KW, Murray PT, Samuels J, Cotsonis G, Shaw AD. Fenoldopam mesylate in early acute tubular necrosis: a randomized, double-blind, placebo-controlled clinical trial. *Am J Kidney Dis.* 2005;46(1):26-34.
59. Friedrich JO, Adhikari N, Herridge MS, Beyene J. Meta-analysis: low-dose dopamine increases urine output but does not prevent renal dysfunction or death. *Ann Intern Med.* 2005;142(7):510-524.
60. Lauschke A, Teichgraber UK, Frei U, Eckardt KU. "Low-dose" dopamine worsens renal perfusion in patients with acute renal failure. *Kidney Int.* 2006;69(9):1669-1674.
61. Brienza N, Malcangi V, Dalfino L, et al. A comparison between fenoldopam and low-dose dopamine in early renal dysfunction of critically ill patients. *Crit Care Med.* 2006;34(3):707-714.
62. Sampath S, Moran JL, Graham PL, Rockliff S, Bersten AD, Abrams KR. The efficacy of loop diuretics in acute renal failure: assessment using Bayesian evidence synthesis techniques. *Crit Care Med.* 2007;35(11):2516-2524.
63. Ho KM, Sheridan DJ. Meta-analysis of frusemide to prevent or treat acute renal failure. *BMJ.* 2006;333(7565):420.
64. Mehta RL, Pascual MT, Soroko S, Chertow GM. Diuretics, mortality, and nonrecovery of renal function in acute renal failure. *JAMA.* 2002;288(20):2547-2553.
65. Chrysostomou C, Schmitt CG. Dexmedetomidine: sedation, analgesia and beyond. *Expert Opin Drug Metab Toxicol.* 2008;4(5):619-627.
66. Sun P, Ma D, Hossain M, Sanders RD, Maze M. Dexmedetomidine provides renoprotection against renal ischaemia-reperfusion injury in mice. *Anesthesiology.* 2008;109:A420.
67. Billings FTt, Chen SW, Kim M, et al. Alpha-2-adrenergic agonists protect against radiocontrast-induced nephropathy in mice. *Am J Physiol Renal Physiol.* 2008;295(3):F741-F748.
68. Brar SS, Shen AY, Jorgensen MB, et al. Sodium bicarbonate vs sodium chloride for the prevention of contrast medium-induced nephropathy in patients undergoing coronary angiography: a randomized trial. *JAMA.* 2008;300(9):1038-1046.
69. Amar D. Prevention and management of perioperative arrhythmias in the thoracic surgical population. *Anesthesiol Clin.* 2008;26(2):325-335, vii.
70. Roselli EE, Murthy SC, Rice TW, et al. Atrial fibrillation complicating lung cancer resection. *J Thorac Cardiovasc Surg.* 2005;130(2):438-444.
71. Amar D, Goenka A, Zhang H, Park B, Thaler HT. Leukocytosis and increased risk of atrial fibrillation after general thoracic surgery. *Ann Thorac Surg.* 2006;82(3):1057-1061.
72. Cardinale D, Colombo A, Sandri MT, et al. Increased perioperative N-terminal pro-B-type natriuretic peptide levels predict atrial fibrillation after thoracic surgery for lung cancer. *Circulation.* 2007;115(11):1339-1344.
73. Vaporciyan AA, Correa AM, Rice DC, et al. Risk factors associated with atrial fibrillation after noncardiac thoracic surgery: analysis of 2588 patients. *J Thorac Cardiovasc Surg.* 2004;127(3):779-786.
74. Foroulis CN, Kotoulas C, Lachanas H, Lazopoulos G, Konstantinou M, Lioulias AG. Factors associated with cardiac rhythm disturbances in the early post-pneumonectomy period: a study on 259 pneumonectomies. *Eur J Cardiothorac Surg.* 2003;23(3):384-389.

75. Bobbio A, Caporale D, Internullo E, et al. Postoperative outcome of patients undergoing lung resection presenting with new-onset atrial fibrillation managed by amiodarone or diltiazem. *Eur J Cardiothorac Surg.* 2007;31(1):70-74.
76. Amar D, Zhang H, Roistacher N. The incidence and outcome of ventricular arrhythmias after noncardiac thoracic surgery. *Anesth Analg.* 2002;95(3):537-543, table of contents.
77. Mayson SE, Greenspon AJ, Adams S, et al. The changing face of postoperative atrial fibrillation prevention: a review of current medical therapy. *Cardiol Rev.* 2007;15(5):231-241.
78. Amar D, Roistacher N, Burt ME, et al. Effects of diltiazem versus digoxin on dysrhythmias and cardiac function after pneumonectomy. *Ann Thorac Surg.* 1997;63(5):1374-1381; discussion 1372-1381.
79. Amar D. Post-thoracotomy atrial fibrillation. *Cur Opin Anesthesiol.* 2007;20(1):43.
80. Ahn HJ, Sim WS, Shim YM, Kim JA. Thoracic epidural anesthesia does not improve the incidence of arrhythmias after transthoracic esophagectomy. *Eur J Cardiothorac Surg.* 2005;28(1):19-21.
81. Crawford TC, Oral H. Cardiac arrhythmias: management of atrial fibrillation in the critically ill patient. *Crit Care Clin.* 2007;23(4):855-872, vii.
82. Karamichalis JM, Putnam JB, Jr, Lambright ES. Cardiovascular complications after lung surgery. *Thorac Surg Clin.* 2006;16(3):253-260.
83. Fuster V, Ryden LE, Cannom DS, et al. ACC/AHA/ESC 2006 Guidelines for the Management of Patients with Atrial Fibrillation: a report of the American College of Cardiology/American Heart Association Task Force on Practice Guidelines and the European Society of Cardiology Committee for Practice Guidelines (Writing Committee to Revise the 2001 Guidelines for the Management of Patients With Atrial Fibrillation): developed in collaboration with the European Heart Rhythm Association and the Heart Rhythm Society. *Circulation.* 2006;114(7):e257-e354.
84. Amar D, Roistacher N, Rusch VW, et al. Effects of diltiazem prophylaxis on the incidence and clinical outcome of atrial arrhythmias after thoracic surgery. *J Thorac Cardiovasc Surg.* 2000;120(4):790-798.
85. DeWitt CR, Waksman JC. Pharmacology, pathophysiology and management of calcium channel blocker and beta-blocker toxicity. *Toxicol Rev.* 2004;23(4):223-238.
86. Sedrakyan A, Treasure T, Browne J, Krumholz H, Sharpin C, van der Meulen J. Pharmacologic prophylaxis for postoperative atrial tachyarrhythmia in general thoracic surgery: evidence from randomized clinical trials. *J Thorac Cardiovasc Surg.* 2005;129(5):997-1005.
87. Bradley D, Creswell LL, Hogue CW, Jr, Epstein AE, Prystowsky EN, Daoud EG. Pharmacologic prophylaxis: American College of Chest Physicians guidelines for the prevention and management of Postoperative atrial fibrillation after cardiac surgery. *Chest.* 2005;128(2 Suppl):39S-47S.
88. Connolly SJ, Cybulsky I, Lamy A, et al. Double-blind, placebo-controlled, randomized trial of prophylactic metoprolol for reduction of hospital length of stay after heart surgery: the beta-Blocker Length Of Stay (BLOS) study. *Am Heart J.* 2003;145(2):226-232.
89. Devereaux PJ, Yang H, Yusuf S, et al. Effects of extended-release metoprolol succinate in patients undergoing non-cardiac surgery (POISE trial): a randomised controlled trial. *Lancet.* 2008;371(9627):1839-1847.
90. Fleisher LA, Poldermans D. Perioperative beta blockade: where do we go from here? *Lancet.* 2008;371(9627):1813-1814.
91. Tamargo J, Delpon E, Caballero R. The safety of digoxin as a pharmacological treatment of atrial fibrillation. *Expert Opin Drug Saf.* 2006;5(3):453-467.
92. Gheorghiade M, Adams KF, Jr, Colucci WS. Digoxin in the management of cardiovascular disorders. *Circulation.* 2004;109(24):2959-2964.
93. Mitchell LB, Exner DV, Wyse DG, et al. Prophylactic oral amiodarone for the prevention of arrhythmias that begin early after revascularization, valve replacement, or repair: PAPABEAR: a randomized controlled trial. *JAMA.* 2005;294(24):3093-3100.
94. Zimetbaum P. Amiodarone for atrial fibrillation. *N Engl J Med.* 2007;356(9):935-941.
95. Van Mieghem W, Coolen L, Malysse I, et al. Amiodarone and the development of ARDS after lung surgery. *Chest.* 1994;105(6):1642-1645.
96. Toraman F, Karabulut EH, Alhan HC, et al. Magnesium infusion dramatically decreases the incidence of atrial fibrillation after coronary artery bypass grafting. *Ann Thorac Surg.* 2001;72(4):1256-1261; discussion 1252-1261.
97. Thielmann M, Neuhauser M, Marr A, et al. Lipid-lowering effect of preoperative statin therapy on postoperative major adverse cardiac events after coronary artery bypass surgery. *J Thorac Cardiovasc Surg.* 2007;134(5):1143-1149.

98. Patti G, Chello M, Candura D, et al. Randomized trial of atorvastatin for reduction of postoperative atrial fibrillation in patients undergoing cardiac surgery: results of the ARMYDA-3 (Atorvastatin for Reduction of MYocardial Dysrhythmia after cardiac surgery) study. *Circulation.* 2006;114(14):1455-1461.
99. Amar D, Zhang H, Park B, Heerdt PM, Fleisher M, Thaler HT. Inflammation and outcome after general thoracic surgery. *Eur J Cardiothorac Surg.* 2007;32(3):431-434.
100. Amar D, Zhang H, Heerdt PM, Park B, Fleisher M, Thaler HT. Statin use is associated with a reduction in atrial fibrillation after noncardiac thoracic surgery independent of C-reactive protein. *Chest.* 2005;128(5):3421-3427.
101. Healey JS, Baranchuk A, Crystal E, et al. Prevention of atrial fibrillation with angiotensin-converting enzyme inhibitors and angiotensin receptor blockers: a meta-analysis. *J Am Coll Cardiol.* 2005;45(11):1832-1839.
102. Coleman CI, Makanji S, Kluger J, White CM. Effect of angiotensin-converting enzyme inhibitors or angiotensin receptor blockers on the frequency of post-cardiothoracic surgery atrial fibrillation. *Ann Pharmacother.* 2007;41(3):433-437.
103. Maisel WH, Epstein AE. The role of cardiac pacing: American College of Chest Physicians guidelines for the prevention and management of postoperative atrial fibrillation after cardiac surgery. *Chest.* 2005;128(2 Suppl):36S-38S.
104. Dunning J, Treasure T, Versteegh M, Nashef SA. Guidelines on the prevention and management of de novo atrial fibrillation after cardiac and thoracic surgery. *Eur J Cardiothorac Surg.* 2006;30(6):852-872.
105. Hassan SA, Hlatky MA, Boothroyd DB, et al. Outcomes of noncardiac surgery after coronary bypass surgery or coronary angioplasty in the Bypass Angioplasty Revascularization Investigation (BARI). *Am J Med.* 2001;110(4):260-266.
106. Fleisher LA, Beckman JA, Brown KA, et al. ACC/AHA 2007 Guidelines on Perioperative Cardiovascular Evaluation and Care for Noncardiac Surgery: Executive Summary: A Report of the American College of Cardiology/American Heart Association Task Force on Practice Guidelines (Writing Committee to Revise the 2002 Guidelines on Perioperative Cardiovascular Evaluation for Noncardiac Surgery) Developed in Collaboration With the American Society of Echocardiography, American Society of Nuclear Cardiology, Heart Rhythm Society, Society of Cardiovascular Anesthesiologists, Society for Cardiovascular Angiography and Interventions, Society for Vascular Medicine and Biology, and Society for Vascular Surgery. *J Am Coll Cardiol.* 2007;50(17):1707-1732.
107. Collet JP, Himbet F, Steg PG. Myocardial infarction after aspirin cessation in stable coronary artery disease patients. *Int J Cardiol.* 2000;76(2-3):257-258.
108. Collet JP, Montalescot G, Blanchet B, et al. Impact of prior use or recent withdrawal of oral antiplatelet agents on acute coronary syndromes. *Circulation.* 2004;110(16):2361-2367.
109. Chassot PG, Delabays A, Spahn DR. Perioperative antiplatelet therapy: the case for continuing therapy in patients at risk of myocardial infarction. *Br J Anaesth.* 2007;99(3):316-328.
110. Reed CE, Spinale FG, Crawford FA, Jr. Effect of pulmonary resection on right ventricular function. *Ann Thorac Surg.* 1992;53(4):578-582.
111. Slinger P. Update on anesthetic management for pneumonectomy. *Curr Opin Anaesthesiol.* 2009;22(1):31-37.
112. Chae EJ, Seo JB, Kim SY, et al. Radiographic and CT findings of thoracic complications after pneumonectomy. *Radiographics.* 2006;26(5):1449-1468.

Acute and Chronic Post-Thoracotomy Pain

24

Srinivas Pyati
David R. Lindsay
Thomas Buchheit

Key Points

1. Without adequate analgesia, most patients would experience severe pain following thoracic surgery.
2. Epidural analgesia is widely practiced and has been shown to provide superior pain relief compared with systemic opioids.
3. Multimodal analgesic strategies improve overall outcomes including patient satisfaction.
4. Chronic post-thoracotomy pain (CPTP) is common and remains a challenging condition to treat. Further investigation into prevention of this syndrome is needed.

Clinical Vignette

The patient is a 64-year-old man who underwent a left thoracotomy and extrapleural pneumonectomy for mesothelioma. A mid-thoracic epidural catheter was placed preoperatively and used to deliver 0.6mg of hydromorphone prior to incision. Intraoperatively, no medications were administered through the epidural catheter to avoid sympathectomy and hemodynamic instability.

Upon the patient's arrival to the intensive care unit, an epidural infusion of bupivacaine 0.125% and hydromorphone 10 mcg/mL was initiated at 6 mL/h. The patient initially experienced 8/10 pain, requiring an epidural bolus of local anesthetic and an increase of the infusion rate. These adjustments resulted in reduction of his pain to 3/10. With improved analgesia, the patient was able to improve incentive spirometry performance, but he still continued to experience shoulder pain. He continued to do well with adequate pain control in the intensive care unit (pain score 3-5/10). His epidural was discontinued on postoperative day 3. He was discharged to home on postoperative day 5 with oral oxycodone as needed.

At his 2-month postoperative evaluation, the patient complained of significant chest wall pain localized to the thoracotomy incision. He described his pain as burning and aching.

The importance of postoperative pain management is well established.[1] Postoperative pain following thoracic procedures causes a reversible restrictive pattern of ventilation with a decrease in vital capacity (VC) and functional residual capacity (FRC), impaired cough, rapid, shallow breathing, and often retention of secretions. These physiologic changes are particularly significant in thoracic surgery patients with preexisting pulmonary comorbidities, and may result in atelectasis, hypoxemia, and respiratory failure.[2] Effective postoperative analgesia is of critical importance in these individuals. Nonetheless, effective treatment strategies for acute and chronic post-thoracotomy pain remain a significant challenge.[3,4]

The adverse effects of poor analgesia are not limited to the pulmonary system. Pain has been associated with increased myocardial oxygen demand, myocardial dysfunction, increased catecholamine release, poor glycemic control, deep vein thrombosis, and pulmonary embolism.[5,6] These complications of inadequate pain control have been shown to lead to increased mortality and morbidity, prolonged length of hospitalization, and increased cost of patient care.[7,8] In addition, several recent retrospective reviews suggest that a higher intensity of early (first week) postoperative pain is a risk factor for development of persistent pain.[9,10]

In this chapter, we will briefly review the mechanisms of thoracic pain. We will then discuss management strategies for acute postoperative pain and outline key concepts regarding chronic post-thoracotomy pain. The reader is referred to Chapter 6 for a more detailed discussion on the mechanisms of thoracic pain.

MECHANISMS OF PAIN

Nociceptive impulses from the thoracotomy incision, chest tube site, rib, muscle, and parietal pleural damage are transmitted along the intercostal nerves to the dorsal horn of the spinal cord. The autonomic nerves transmit noxious input from damaged visceral pleura. Pleural and bronchial manipulation may signal visceral pain through the afferent fibers of the vagus and phrenic nerves, which appear to be responsible for shoulder pain in some cases of acute and persistent pain.[11,12]

Tissue disruption triggers the release of inflammatory mediators such as prostaglandins, histamine, bradykinins, and potassium. These inflammatory mediators can directly activate nociceptors or enhance nociceptor activity. Furthermore, they cause a reduction in the pain threshold of the peripheral nerves. As a result, the severity of pain experienced by mechanical stimuli such as coughing or deep breathing may be intensified.[13] This process is known as peripheral sensitization. Continued nociceptive stimulation will cause hyperexcitability of the nerves in the dorsal horn and other central pain centers, a process known as central sensitization.[14] Central sensitization lowers the pain threshold of dorsal neurons and is associated with activation of NMDA receptors via substance P, calcitonin Gene Related Peptide (CGRP), and glutamate.[15] Additionally, ongoing nociceptive stimulation alters neural function, resulting in neuroplasticity within the central nervous system. Despite the healing of tissue injury and the absence of inflammation, some patients continue to experience pain via central mechanisms (Figure 24-1).

```
                    Tissue Trauma
                    /          \
        Phospholipase A2      Cytokines
               |              Interleukins-1 beta
        Activation of         TNF-alpha
        Arachidonic
        pathway
        (PG, LT, BK)
               |
        COX-1 and COX-2       Central
               |              Sensitization
        Nociceptor            (Wind up)
        activation
                              Nitric oxide/NMDA
               |              activation
        Peripheral → Facilitated → Release of pain → Neural
        Sensitization nociceptive  mediators        plasticity
               |      input       within dorsal    and
        Acute                     horn (PG,        amplification
        (physiological)           Kinases,         of pain
        pain                      Aspartate,       transmission
                                  Glutamate, CCK)
                                  Increased        Chronic
                                  sympathetic      (pathological)
                                  input in DRG     pain
```

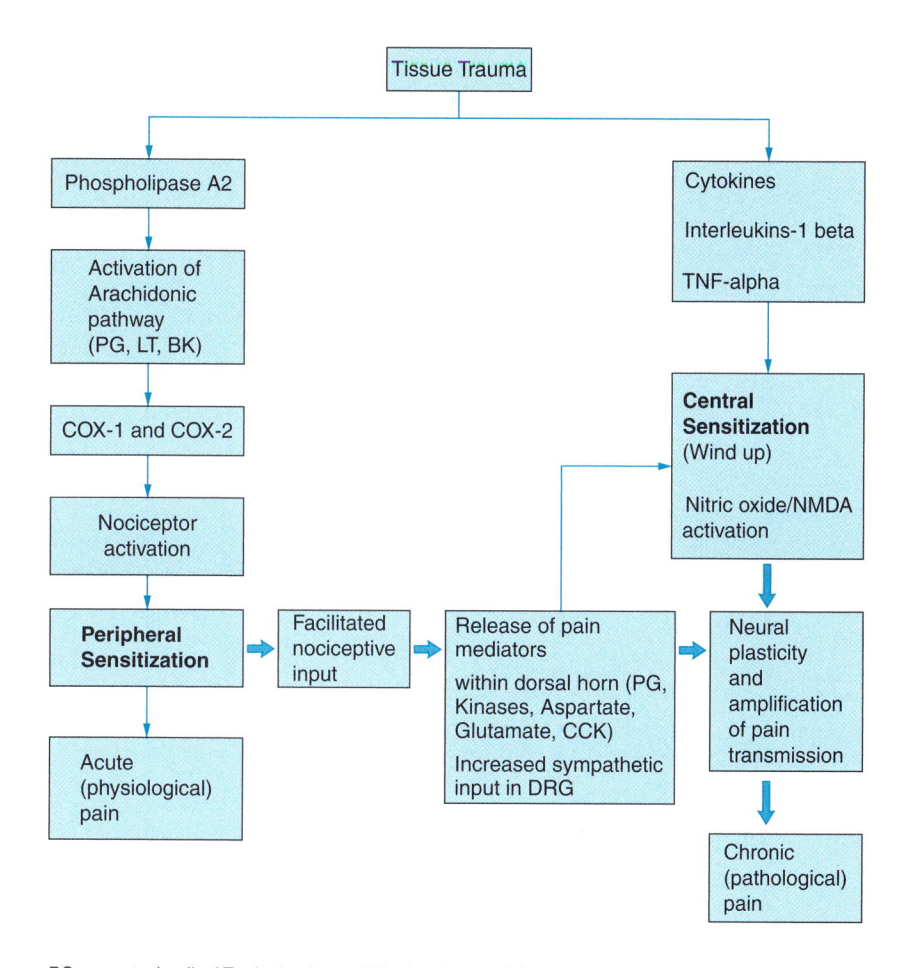

PG = prostaglandin, LT = leukotrienes, BK = bradykinin, COX = cyclooxygenase
CCK = cholecystokinin, DRG = dorsal root ganglia, TNF = tumor necrosis factor,
NMDA = N-methyl-D-aspartate

Figure 24–1. Mechanisms of acute and chronic pain. (Modified from Pyati S, Gan TJ. Perioperative pain management. *CNS Drugs*. 2007;21(13):185-211, with permission from Adis. © Springer International Publishing AG 2007. All rights reserved.)

MANAGEMENT OF ACUTE POST-THORACOTOMY PAIN

It is estimated that more than 70% patients undergoing thoracotomy experience moderate to severe pain,[16] even when a minimally invasive surgical approach is employed. Appropriate treatment of pain is necessary not only to prevent discomfort but also to prevent other negative sequelae. Despite effective management of somatic pain, some patients also complain of ipsilateral shoulder discomfort, occasionally severe in nature. The etiology of this visceral component of post-thoracotomy pain is suggested to be from contributions of the phrenic and vagus nerves.[17] The phrenic nerve supplies sensory branches to the diaphragmatic and mediastinal pleura and the pericardium. Although clinicians may have reservations about phrenic nerve infiltration and diminished pulmonary function, this does not appear to manifest clinically.[17,18] When evaluating patients before surgery, it is important to determine whether they have preexisting pain in the area of the proposed surgery, to document the intensity of such pain, and to note any preoperative narcotic use. The presence of preexisting pain may indicate greater difficulty in management of postoperative pain, necessitating a more aggressive analgesic approach. Pain assessment is often performed using the visual analogue scale (0-10) or another more sophisticated pain assessment tool, such as the brief pain inventory or McGill pain questionnaire.

Because of the involvement of multiple pain generators from the chest wall, viscera, and the parietal, diaphragmatic and mediastinal pleura, post-thoracotomy pain can be difficult to treat with a single analgesic modality. An ideal analgesic combination should reduce the intensity of movement-related pain, decrease the surgical stress response, and reduce the duration of hospitalization. Several techniques are employed to manage acute post-thoracotomy pain. For the purpose of this discussion, it is most convenient to treat each modality separately and to bear in mind that a multimodal analgesic approach is the most effective management strategy to control moderate to severe pain[19] (Figure 24-2). Multimodal strategies may include epidural analgesia, local

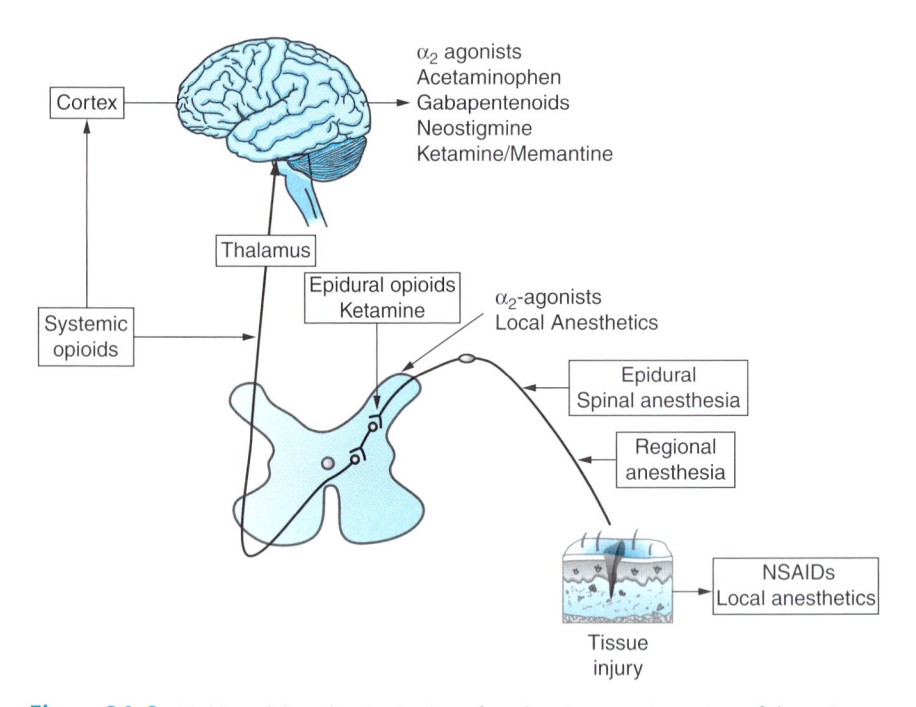

Figure 24–2. Multimodal analgesia. Action of analgesics at various sites of the pain pathway. (Modified from Pyati S, Gan TJ. Perioperative pain management. *CNS Drugs.* 2007;21(13):185-211, with permission from Adis. © Springer International Publishing AG 2007. All rights reserved.)

Table 24-1. Analgesic Options for Management of Acute Post-Thoracotomy Pain

I. Regional anesthesia techniques 　Thoracic epidural 　Paravertebral block 　Intercostal nerve block 　Interpleural block **II. Opioids** 　Patient-controlled analgesia (PCA) 　Epidurally administered opioids **III. Nonsteroidal anti-inflammatory drugs (NSAIDs)** **IV. Adjuvant analgesics** 　Acetaminophen 　Gabapentinoids (pregabalin/gabapentin) 　Tramadol 　Ketamine 　Alpha-2 adrenergic agonists (dexmedetomidine/clonidine)

anesthetic infiltration, opioids, nonsteroidal anti-inflammatory drugs (NSAIDs), and adjuvant medications (Table 24-1). Preoperative insertion of a thoracic epidural catheter is commonly performed to provide analgesia during the perioperative period. If an epidural catheter cannot be inserted, paravertebral blocks are the preferred analgesic technique. In a survey of post-thoracotomy pain management, approximately 80% respondents reported using epidural analgesia, with over 90% recommending a combination of a local anesthetic drug and opioids.[20]

Epidural Analgesia

Thoracic epidural catheterization is typically performed at mid-thoracic levels before induction of anesthesia. The paramedian approach to the epidural space is often the recommended technique because the obliquity of thoracic spinous processes makes the midline approach potentially difficult. Either a "loss of resistance" technique or "hanging drop" method may be used to identify the epidural space.

Most anesthesiologists are experienced with placement of lumbar epidural catheters using a "loss of resistance" technique. Although there are anatomic differences between the thoracic and lumbar spine, the fundamental technique of epidural space identification is consistent. Therefore, use of "loss of resistance" for placement of thoracic epidural catheters capitalizes on the anesthesiologist's technical experience and knowledge.

"Hanging drop" technique entails placing a small amount of saline in the hub of the epidural needle after the stylet has been withdrawn. Upon entering the epidural space, negative pressure causes the meniscus of the fluid to disappear into the hub of the epidural needle. There is debate about whether the negative pressure created with the "hanging drop" technique is secondary to negative intrathoracic pressure, tenting of the dura with needle advancement, or both. The authors find the "hanging drop" technique performed in the sitting position particularly useful when working with trainees: withdrawal of fluid into the hub of the epidural needle provides an unambiguous visual end-point for the supervising physician.

Thoracic epidural local anesthetic administration has been shown to reduce lower extremity motor block as compared with lumbar placement.[21] Additionally, given that the site of epidural needle/catheter placement determines the distribution pattern of neural blockade, there is a considerable theoretical advantage for thoracic catheter placement with a thoracic incision.[22,23] Common adverse effects and complications of epidural analgesia include dural puncture, post-dural puncture headache, excessive motor blockade, and unsuccessful placement. Uncommon complications include epidural abscess, nerve injury, epidural hematoma, and paraplegia. Epidural analgesia is generally contraindicated in patients who are anticoagulated, septic, or have evidence of infection at the intended site of epidural placement. Guidelines for the management of epidural analgesia in the setting of anticoagulation are included in Table 24-2. Thoracic epidural catheter placement is often considered to be significantly riskier than insertion at the lumbar spine level due to concerns for possible spinal cord injury; evidence does not support this perceived increased risk.[24,25]

Continuous infusion of local anesthetic and/or opioid into the epidural space is commonly used in the acute postoperative management of thoracic surgery patients. Compared with intravenous opioids, patients with epidural analgesia have superior

Table 24–2. Suggested Guidelines for Epidural Analgesia and Anticoagulation

Epidural may be placed 4 h after subcutaneous unfractionated heparin.
Heparin may not be given until 2 h after an epidural has been placed.
Heparin infusion should not be started until 12 h after insertion of an epidural (24 h if there was a bloody tap).
Catheter can be removed 4 h after stopping heparin if APTT is normal and platelet count is over 100,000.
An epidural catheter can be inserted/removed 12 h after the last dose of LMWH in a low-dose protocol. The next dose can be given 2 h after removing the catheter.
Needle insertion should be delayed for at least 24 h in patients receiving higher (treatment) doses of LMWH.
INR must be <1.5 before epidural is inserted or removed for patients on Coumadin (warfarin). Some practitioners recommend INR<1.2.
In the absence of other complications aspirin does not need to be stopped for insertion of epidurals.
Preoperatively stop clopidogrel for 7-10 days and ticlopidine for 14 days.
Caution should be exercised with platelet GP IIb/IIIa receptor inhibitors until platelet function is restored.
Allow 24 to 48 h for abciximab and 4 to 8 h with eptifibatide and tirofiban before needle insertion.

pain control, less respiratory depression, and fewer pulmonary complications.[26-28] In a comparative study of thoracic epidural analgesia versus systemic analgesia (PCA), there were well-demonstrated improvements in analgesia and quality of life in patients receiving epidurals.[29] Investigations have not shown a dramatic difference in analgesia between the thoracic and lumbar route when opioid alone is used for epidural administration.[30-32] Modest improvements in analgesic potency and clinical outcomes have been demonstrated with thoracic versus lumbar epidural administration of combined opioid and local anesthetic.[27,28] The procedure-specific postoperative pain management (PROSPECT) working group recommends thoracic epidural or paravertebral blocks as first-line analgesic methods.[33]

A wide variety of opioids have been used in epidural analgesic regimens. The hydrophilic opioids morphine and hydromorphone have been shown to have similar efficacy when compared to postoperative analgesia.[34] Hydromorphone has a favorable side effect profile with less respiratory depression, pruritus, and urinary retention when compared with morphine.[35] Thoracic epidural administration of the hydrophobic opioid fentanyl was initially considered to have the advantage of segmental spinal analgesia, as this phenomenon is present during bolus administration. However, during continuous administration the analgesic effect of epidural fentanyl appears largely due to systemic absorption.[36,37] The predominantly systemic distribution of epidural fentanyl infusion potentially makes this drug less desirable when other options are available. Nonetheless, patients with a history of pruritus, nausea, and other side effects with hydrophilic opioids such as morphine and hydromorphone may benefit from the choice of this lipophilic drug.[38]

Epidural administration of local anesthetic improves analgesia, but may produce sympathetic blockade, bradycardia, peripheral vasodilation, and hypotension. Sympathetic blockade is greater with thoracic epidural catheters than with lumbar epidural catheters,[39] although it rarely requires removal of the local anesthetic from the infusion. The combination of epidural local anesthetic and opioid is noted to provide superior analgesia and reduction of side effects when compared with either drug class alone.[40,41] Additionally, epidural local anesthetics have been shown to improve oxygenation and reduce pulmonary complications when compared with systemic analgesics (Table 24-3).[26]

Table 24–3. Drugs Used in Continuous Thoracic Epidural Analgesia

Bupivacaine 0.125%-0.25%	6-8 mL/h
Ropivacaine 0.2%	6-8 mL/h
Hydromorphone[a]	Bolus 0.4-0.8 mg followed by infusion (10-20 mcg/mL) at 6-8 mL/h
Morphine[a]	2-4 mg bolus followed by infusion (40-50 mcg/mL) at 6-8 mL/h
Fentanyl	2 to 10 mcg/mL

[a]Opioids can be used in combination with local anesthetics to obtain superior analgesia.

Table 24–4. Recommended Dosing Schedule for PCEA

Fentanyl 5 µg/mL + bupivacaine 0.125% (1.25 mg/mL) or
Hydromorphone 10 µg /mL + bupivacaine 0.125% (1.25 mg/mL)
PCEA protocol   Background 4-6 mL/h; 2-3 mL bolus; 20 min lockout

Patient controlled epidural analgesia (PCEA) has also been used in the delivery of thoracic epidural analgesia, and provides the ability to deliver effective analgesia with reduced opioid and local anesthetic doses.[21,42] The advent of PCEA offers the promise of improved analgesia and patient satisfaction.[43] PCEA has been shown to improve pain scores and cough as compared with continuous epidural analgesia and systemic analgesia.[44] It allows patients to control pain by administering a bolus dose of local anesthetic and opioid mixture according to their individual need, tailoring the drug requirements to their activity level.[45] A recent survey of PCEA with bupivacaine and hydromorphone demonstrated good analgesia without significant side effects in orthopedic patients.[46] Although the literature regarding PCEA use for thoracic surgery is more limited, the side effect profile seems comparable to that of the lumbar space.[47,48] The recommended dosing schedule for PCEA is included in Table 24-4.

In patients with poorly controlled pain, the use of clonidine may be considered. Epidural clonidine (0.2-0.5 µg/kg/h) may improve symptom control, especially in patients with preexisting chronic pain states.[49] Clonidine, an alpha-2 receptor agonist, has been found to provide analgesia, especially in neuropathic pain states.[50] It appears to have analgesic activity in the periphery, the spinal cord dorsal horn, and the brainstem. Clonidine's analgesic mechanism of action appears to predominantly involve spinal cholinergic activation and hyperpolarization of the primary afferent neuron.[49,51] While it may be quite effective in potentiating epidural opioid analgesia, dosing may be limited by bradycardia, hypotension, and sedation.[52]

Ketamine has also been used in the epidural space to potentiate the analgesic effect of opioids[53-55]; however, its safety in the neuraxis needs to be established prior to recommending it for clinical use. Current scientific evidence supports the use of ketamine as an intravenous infusion for patients with preoperative opioid tolerance. A loading dose of 0.5 mg/kg on induction of anesthesia and a continuous infusion of 10 µg/kg/min during surgery and terminated at wound closure has been shown to significantly reduce morphine consumption at 24 and 48 hours as well at 6 weeks postoperatively in this population.[56]

Thoracic Paravertebral Blockade

Paravertebral blockade (PVB) is an alternative analgesic technique to thoracic epidural placement. Studies comparing surgically placed paravertebral catheters with thoracic epidural catheters have demonstrated similar analgesic benefit after thoracic surgery with a better side effect profile with paravertebral catheterization.[57,58]

Research involving percutaneously placed paravertebral catheters has been more limited to date, although there appears to be a similar analgesic result when this approach is compared with the surgically performed approach.[59] The technique was first introduced in the early 1900s for analgesia following abdominal surgery; it was not until the 1970s that paravertebral blockade was commonly used for thoracotomies.[60] It is well suited for treating post-thoracotomy pain because of the unilateral action of the paravertebral blocks. While single-shot injections performed at multiple levels may provide adequate analgesia, given the limited duration of analgesia obtained, catheter placement and continuous infusion may be preferable.

ANATOMY AND TECHNIQUE

The thoracic paravertebral space (PVS) is a wedge-shaped space that lies on each side of the vertebral column (Figure 24-3). Paravertebral blockade involves injection of local anesthetic in the vicinity of each spinal nerve root within the paravertebral space, resulting in unilateral anesthesia for thoracic surgery. The PVS connects medially with the epidural space via the intervertebral foramen and laterally with

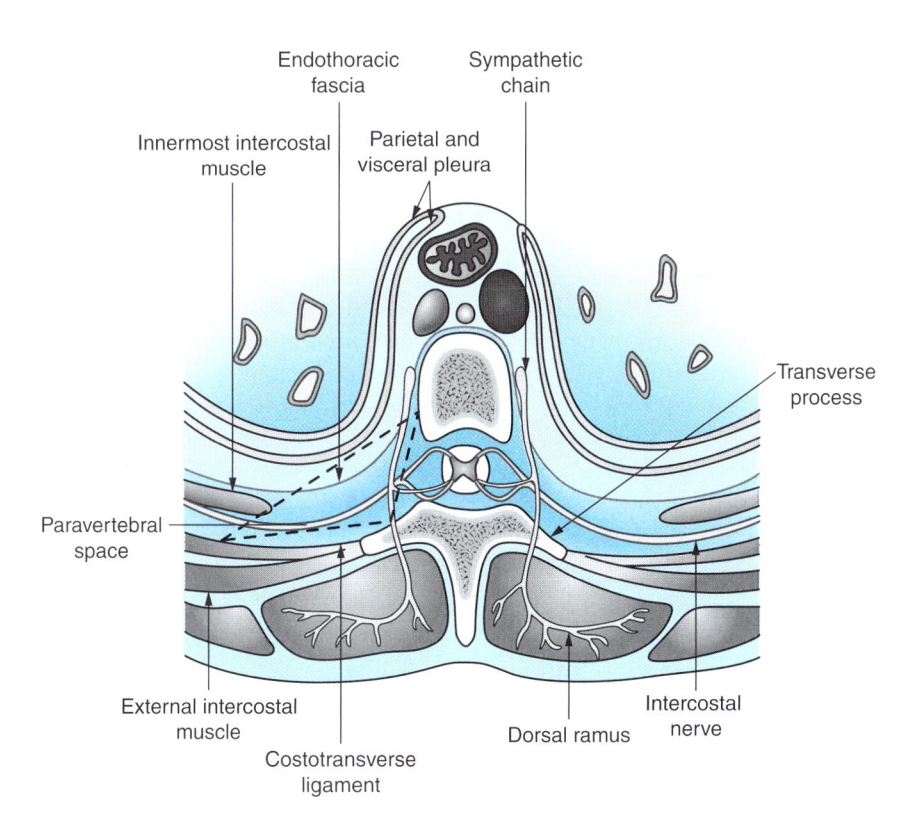

Figure 24-3. Transverse section of the thoracic spine depicting the boundaries, contents and structures surrounding the paravertebral space.

the intercostal space. The injectate may migrate to these spaces, but the magnitude of spread is unpredictable. On rare occasions, if the dural sleeve around the spinal nerve is inadvertently entered during the procedure, a subarachnoid injection may result. Injectate also frequently spreads both superiorly and inferiorly within the paravertebral space. While the spinal nerves course through the PVS as they exit the spinal canal, the sympathetic chain traverses the space anteriorly. The intercostal arteries, hemiazygos veins and lymphatics also pass through the PVS.

For thoracotomy, the levels blocked are usually between T4 and T9 when single-shot injection technique is used. Care must be exercised when counting the vertebrae before injection. Because of the steep angulations of the thoracic spinous processes, the tip of one spinous process corresponds to the transverse process and PVS of the vertebrae below (ie, T5 spinous process corresponds to T6 transverse process (Figure 24-4A and B). The thoracic transverse processes project laterally a mean distance of 3 cm from the midline. The needle should therefore be inserted 2½ cm lateral to the spinous process at each level. The mean depth from the skin to the PVS is 5.5 cm.

For single-shot injection, the sites are labeled, the skin cleansed, and a 20-gauge Tuohy needle is advanced, seeking contact with the transverse process. The needle is then withdrawn and redirected caudally, advancing about 1 cm further than the distance to the transverse process until a tactile "pop" is noted as the needle passes through the costotransverse ligament into the PVS. Alternatively, a nerve stimulation technique (0.5-0.6 mA) is used to identify contraction of intercostal muscles as a result of spinal nerve stimulation. Three to four milliliters of local anesthetic (eg, 0.5% ropivacaine with 1:400,000 epinephrine) are administered after careful aspiration. The total volume of local anesthetic injected should be kept below the toxic dose when multiple injections are performed.

Continuous PVB can be instituted either by threading a catheter through an epidural needle after an initial bolus dose of local anesthetic or by placement of a catheter under direct vision by the surgeon.[61] Various infusions have been used for paravertebral catheters; the reduced severity of sympathectomy often seen with the paravertebral technique may allow the use of more concentrated local anesthetics than are tolerable in the epidural space.[58]

The contraindications for PVB are similar to other regional anesthetic techniques and include local skin infection, coagulopathy, and hemodynamic instability.

Adverse Effects of PVB

The most common adverse event reported is technical failure. The published incidence of block failure ranges between 6% and 11%.[62,63] Block failure consists of inability to provide adequate analgesia. Unintentional vascular puncture can occur in PVBs and should be recognized before injection of local anesthetic. Other common side effects of PVBs are mild hypotension, hematoma, or pain at the site of injection. Unintentional pleural puncture and consequent pneumothorax can occur with deep insertion of the needle. Therefore, it is necessary to watch for aspiration of air and/or cough during needle insertion. In a small proportion of patients, epidural spread of injectate can occur.

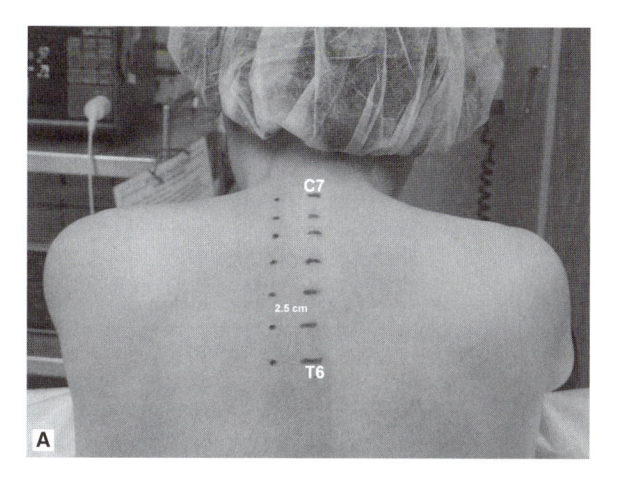

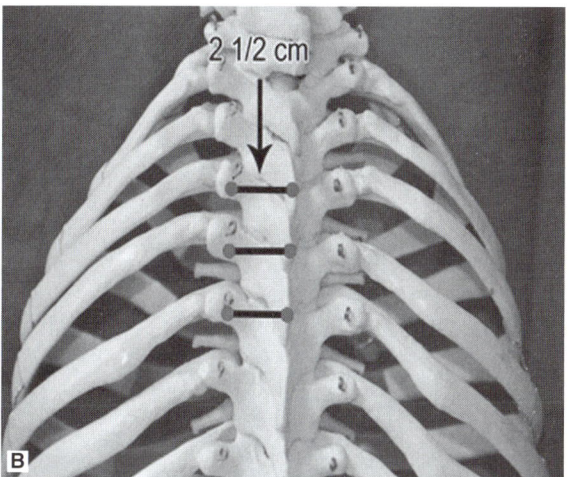

Figure 24–4. Landmarks for paravertebral block. **A**. Surface landmarks. The needle should be inserted 2½ cm lateral to the spinous process of each level to be blocked. **B**. Bony structure of the thoracic spine and ribcage. Note the steep angulations of the thoracic spinous processes. The tip of one spinous process corresponds to the transverse process and paravertebral space of the vertebra below. (Only part A reproduced with permission from Hadzic A: *The New York School of Regional Anesthesia Textbook of Regional Anesthesia and Acute Pain Management*. McGraw-Hill, Inc. 2007. Figure 43-6.)

Intercostal Nerve Blockade

Intercostal nerve blockade is another regional approach for analgesia following thoracotomy. It can be performed percutaneously prior to surgery or by the surgeon under direct vision prior to closure of the incision. Prior to surgery, the block can be administered as a single injection, multiple injections, or continuously via an indwelling intercostal catheter.[64] Due to the high levels of systemic vascular absorption, intercostal blockade achieves the highest blood levels of local anesthetic per volume injected of any block in the body. Therefore, particular attention must be given to the risk of local anesthetic toxicity. It is generally believed that intercostal blocks and catheters do not provide analgesia as effectively as thoracic epidural catheter infusions.[65] However, improved analgesia may be obtained when the catheter is placed under direct surgical exposure to cover several intercostal spaces.[66]

ANATOMY AND TECHNIQUE

The intercostal nerve is located in the neurovascular bundle at the lower border of each rib (Figure 24-5). The percutaneous block can be performed with the patient in the lateral, sitting, or prone position. The patient's ribs are palpated and the block is performed approximately 6 to 8 cm lateral to the spinous process. A small gauge needle, eg, (22-25 gauge) is inserted 2 to 4 mm beneath the inferior border

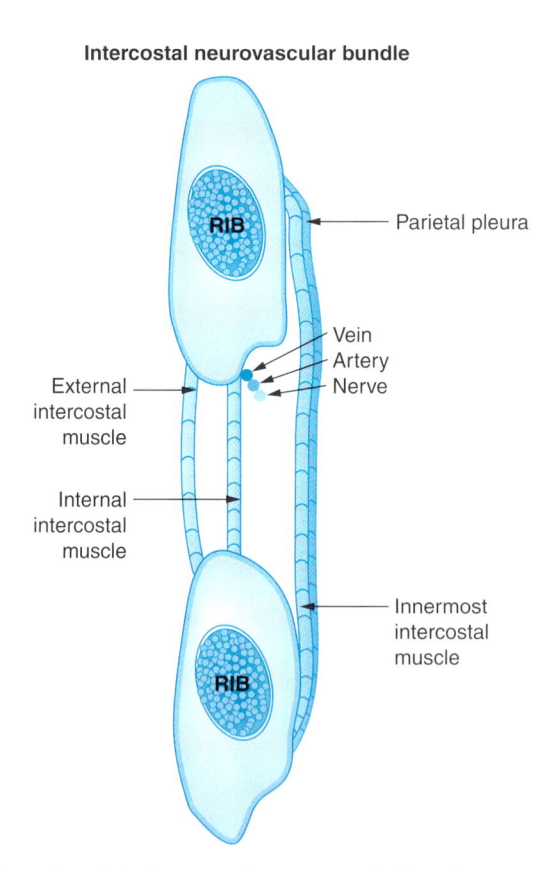

Figure 24–5. Location of the intercostal neurovascular bundle.

of the rib with a cephalic angle of 20 degrees in order to reach the subcostal groove. Following negative aspiration, 2 to 5 mL of local anesthetic is injected. Although pneumothorax is a potential complication, its incidence is rare despite the close proximity of the lung and pleura to the injection site.[67] With multiple injections, caution should be exercised not to exceed the total allowable local anesthetic volume.

Interpleural Block

Interpleural blockade is a technique wherein local anesthetic is injected between the parietal and visceral pleura, allowing local anesthetic to diffuse through the former to produce ipsilateral blockade of multiple thoracic dermatomes. This technique may be useful in patients for whom epidural analgesia is contraindicated or technically challenging. Although interpleural blockade has not been widely adopted by physicians, the proponents of this technique have demonstrated effective analgesia with a low incidence of complications; nonetheless, patients who undergo interpleural analgesia frequently require supplemental opioids.[68] In the treatment of post-thoracotomy pain, interpleural analgesia has been found to be inferior to other techniques such as epidural or paravertebral catheterization.[33]

The interpleural space is 10 to 20 microns in width, has a surface area of 2000 cm^2 in a 70-kg man, and a static volume of approximately 0.1 to 0.2 mL/kg.[69] Cadaver studies have demonstrated that interpleurally injected dye diffuses through the parietal pleura to the subpleural space and backwards to multiple intercostal nerves, and that the dye tends to pool in the interpleural paravertebral area.[69]

A significant amount of local anesthetic can be absorbed by the visceral pleura, offsetting the effectiveness of the drug administered in the interpleural space. The rapidity of absorption can be altered by the presence of inflammation, disease, or trauma to the thoracic cavity. While interpleural analgesia has been advocated after thoracotomy, satisfactory results are often elusive. Reasons why interpleural block may be ineffective for post-thoracotomy pain include uneven distribution of local anesthetic within the disrupted pleural cavity, loss of local anesthetic through chest tube drainage, and binding of local anesthetic to proteins in the surgical effusion.[70]

Technique

The key to successful interpleural block is identification of the interpleural space by detection of negative pressure. Negative interpleural pressure may be identified using different techniques: passive suction of an air- or fluid-filled syringe, a falling column of fluid, or by electronic devices.[71-74] It is recommended that the block be performed in the lateral position and the needle be inserted approximately 8 to 10 cm lateral from the dorsal midline.[75] Using sterile technique, the needle insertion site is infiltrated with local anesthetic. A Tuohy needle is placed into the interpleural space using one of the above referenced methods. A standard epidural catheter is then threaded approximately 5 to 10 cm into the interpleural space.

Analgesia has also been obtained by injecting 20 mL of 0.5% bupivacaine with epinephrine (5 μg/mL) every 8 hours into the pleural cavity using the chest drains in patients with tube thoracostomies for spontaneous pneumothorax. The duration of analgesia can last up to 4 hours.[76]

There are several contraindications to the use of this procedure, including the presence of pleural effusions, inflammation, fibrosis, bronchopleural fistula, and empyema. Complications related to interpleural block include pneumothorax, pleural effusion, Horner's syndrome and catheter-related problems such as displacement and loss. For a more extensive discussion of interpleural analgesia, the reader is directed to the 2-part review by Dravid et al.[70,75]

Multimodal Analgesia

Multimodal analgesia utilizes a combination of analgesics with different mechanisms of action. The use of local anesthetic infiltration, nonsteroidal anti-inflammatory agents, acetaminophen, and/or gabapentinoids has been demonstrated to reduce postoperative opioid consumption and opioid-related side-effects.[77-80] For patients with inadequate analgesia despite the use of a regional anesthetic technique, adjuvant analgesics should be considered. The multimodal approach may optimize analgesia and minimize the risks of sedation and respiratory depression.[81]

The ultimate goal of multimodal therapy is one of preventive analgesia—reducing perioperative pain sensitization with the intention of reducing the incidence or severity of acute and chronic pain states.[82] Although the longer-term benefits of prolonged local anesthetic nerve blockade have been questioned,[83,84] the use of systemic analgesics such as ketamine has been shown to improve pain scores and outcomes up to 6 months postoperatively.[85]

NSAIDs have demonstrated significant advantages in the perioperative period because of their opioid-sparing effects, but are not without their limitations and toxicities. Cyclooxygenase-2 (COX-2) selective inhibitors were developed with the hope to minimize the potential side-effects of non-selective NSAIDS.[86] COX-2 inhibitors have been shown to reduce the incidence of side effects such as gastrointestinal ulceration, bleeding tendencies and renal dysfunction that are common to nonspecific COX inhibition. Unfortunately, the reduction in gastrointestinal side effects has been associated with prothrombotic activity resulting in increased cardiac risk profile.[87-89]

Other drugs that have been used as part of a multimodal regimen include the alpha-2 agonists dexmedetomidine and clonidine. As discussed earlier, epidural clonidine is commonly used along with local anesthetics and/or opioids to improve the quality of analgesia.[90] Side effects such as bradycardia and hypotension can be minimized by carefully monitoring the dose. The more selective alpha-2 agonist dexmedetomidine[91] has analgesic activity at both spinal and supraspinal sites, and has been used as analgesic adjunct with minimal adverse effects.

CHRONIC POST-THORACOTOMY PAIN

Characteristics and Incidence

Thoracotomy, like amputation surgery, carries a high risk for the development of persistent postoperative pain. Chronic post-thoracotomy pain (CPTP) was first noted in 1944 during World War II in men who had undergone a thoracotomy for chest trauma.[92] Prior to the 1990s, CPTP was considered to be transient, lasting weeks to months, and was frequently attributed to recurrent malignant disease.[93] It was not until the 1991 that CPTP was described in the medical literature as a discrete entity, distinguishing it from disease recurrence.[94]

The International Association for the Study of Pain (IASP) defines CPTP as "chronic dysesthetic burning and aching pain that recurs or persists along a thoracotomy scar at least 2 months following a surgical procedure." It is generally considered a postoperative neuropathic pain. Other conditions causing thoracic pain, such as post-herpetic neuralgia, a thoracic herniated disc, or intercostal neuralgia from another source (ie, rib fracture, vertebral compression fracture) should be considered in the treatment plan, as the characteristics of pain are dependent upon the underlying pathophysiologic mechanisms. Patients in whom pain is caused by cancer usually present with costopleural syndrome of moderate to severe intensity. Pain in CPTP can be localized to the chest wall or along the scar and is usually associated with dysesthesia and allodynia in a segmental distribution. These symptoms are commonly exacerbated by temperature changes, touch, and shoulder motion. In a small group of patients, pain can be caused by a traumatic neuroma. This pain is burning and lancinating, with a positive Tinel's sign. CPTP patients, especially the elderly, may also display restriction in ipsilateral shoulder movement. The pain is oftentimes severe enough to limit daily functioning long after the procedure.[95] Some patients might even develop signs and symptoms of complex regional pain syndrome in the ipsilateral upper limb.

Etiology and Risk Factors

Patients who undergo a thoracotomy procedure often have postoperative pain accompanied by sensory loss in the distribution of the associated intercostal nerve, implying some degree of neural injury. The incidence of chronic postsurgical pain reported in the literature is anywhere from 5% to 70% depending on the type of surgery[13,15] (Table 24-5). Incidence of CPTP appears to be highly variable, but the literature reveals that up to 60% patients report persistent pain a month after surgery[33] and 30% to 50% patients have pain at 1 or 2 years. In a smaller percentage (3%-5%), this pain is severe in nature. However, true assessment of the impact of severe post-thoracotomy pain is difficult, as many patients do not seek medical help for their pain, declaring it only upon questioning.[96]

Apart from the surgical procedure itself, there are a number of other possible risk factors that have been elucidated for the development of CPTP. These include age, gender, genetics, severity of preoperative pain, type of surgery, a cancer diagnosis, radiation treatment, chemotherapy, and psychosocial factors. Additionally, patients with intense acute postoperative pain have an increased incidence and severity of CPTP, supporting the importance of the perioperative analgesic regimen in the prevention of chronic post-thoracotomy pain.[103] Katz et al[9] found that acute postoperative within the first 24 hours was the only factor that predicted the presence of long-term pain. This concept was further supported by a study of 250 thoracotomy patients demonstrating that severe acute pain was more likely to develop into persistent postoperative pain.[104]

Table 24-5. Incidence of Persistent Postoperative Pain after Various Surgical Procedures

Surgery	Percentage
Limb amputation[10]	60-80
Thoracic surgery[10]	25-60
Total hip arthroplasty[97]	30
Hysterectomy[98]	5-30
Cesarean section[99]	10
Breast surgery[10]	20-50
Hernia surgery[100]	10
Sternotomy[101]	28
Total knee arthroplasty[102]	35

PATIENT SUSCEPTIBILITY

Sensitivity to acute pain and its consequences varies between individuals and it has been recognized that genetic factors may contribute to pain perception. Female gender has also been associated with the risk of developing CPTP.[105,106] Several candidate genes have been identified, including polymorphism of catechol-o-methyltransferase (COMT) and genetic variants in the voltage gated sodium channels.[96] The exact role that these polymorphisms play in the predisposition to CPTP is unknown.

It is also well established that psychosocial conditions such as anxiety, depression, malignant disease, and social-economic conditions affect the perception of pain.[107] Preexisting chronic pain conditions have also been postulated to predispose patients to the development of CPTP. Keller et al found in their retrospective analysis that 52% users of preoperative analgesics developed CPTP, in contrast to only 5.5% patients who did not use them/preoperative analgesics.[3] Perttunen et al[95] reported an incidence of preoperative pain of 17% in a group of patients with CPTP, but they did not analyze preoperative pain as an independent risk factor.

SURGICAL FACTORS

The type of surgical intervention also plays a role in CPTP: patients undergoing more extensive surgical procedures (eg, pneumonectomy) are thought to be at higher risk of developing CPTP than those having less extensive procedures (eg, wedge resection). Using this rationale, the less invasive video-assisted thoracoscopic surgery (VATS) was thought to have the potential to reduce acute postoperative pain when compared to open thoracotomy. However, studies have demonstrated that there is no difference in the incidence of CPTP between VATS and open thoracotomy.[108-110] VATS is still likely to cause intercostal nerve injury secondary to trauma from trocar insertion and manipulation of instruments.

Rib retraction compresses the intercostal nerve; however, it is believed that closure and approximation of the ribs may be responsible for nerve injury and the development of CPTP. It is reasonable to expect that patients with an injured intercostal nerve would have higher postoperative pain levels and analgesic consumption, and a higher rate of CPTP. Current knowledge of surgical risk factors for CPTP is based entirely on nonrandomized trials and relatively low quality randomized data.[4]

Muscle-sparing thoracic incisions have also been used to attempt to decrease the incidence of postoperative pain and morbidity. A muscle sparing technique where the serratus anterior and latissimus dorsi muscles are retracted rather than incised was thought/theorized to reduce soft tissue injury and its consequences.[111] Unfortunately, this approach has not been shown to be superior to the traditional posterolateral incision.[112,113]

Management of Chronic Post-Thoracotomy Pain

Recurrence, progression, or metastasis of a malignant tumor should be ruled out prior to treatment. The management of most neuropathic pain is difficult and at times disappointing, emphasizing the importance of preventing this complication. Indeed, the initiation of a preoperative thoracic epidural regimen has been shown to reduce the incidence of CPTP.[114] This is consistent with the studies demonstrating an increased risk of CPTP with severe postoperative pain. Aggressive and multimodal analgesic regimens may decrease pain severity, analgesic consumption, and the cascade of neurophysiologic events that can lead to hyperalgesia and allodynia. Combinations of NSAIDs, opioid premedication, and regional anesthesia have been shown to be part of an effective regimen.[115,116]

Standard treatment of CPTP currently involves antineuropathic therapies such as anticonvulsants, tricyclic antidepressants, and consideration of neural blockade procedures such as intercostal and paravertebral blocks. In refractory cases, these treatments may be combined with complementary techniques such as cognitive behavioral therapy[117] and acupuncture.[118,119] NMDA receptor modulation with ketamine infusion may be a useful adjunct in conditions of allodynia, hyperalgesia and opioid tolerance (Table 24-6).

CONCLUSION

Although our current therapeutic armamentarium is growing, effective treatment of chronic post-thoracotomy pain remains a significant challenge. Indeed, it is best to prevent the cascade of neural sensitization in the perioperative period. Although the use of regional anesthesia and perineural catheters in the prevention of chronic pain following joint replacement has been disappointing to date,[83,84] there is evidence of decreased chronic pain following thoracotomy with preemptive epidural placement.[114] The difference in outcomes may lie in the stronger neuropathic nature of CPTP as compared with post-orthopedic surgery pain. In addition to significant physiologic and psychological consequences of untreated pain, inadequate pain relief can potentially increase the incidence of chronic

Table 24-6. Therapeutic Options for Chronic Post-Thoracotomy Pain (CPTP)

First line
Nonsteroid anti-inflammatory drugs (NSAIDs)
Tricyclic antidepressants
Antiepileptic drugs (AEDs)
Opioids
Topical capsaicin
Topical lidocaine
Transcutaneous nerve stimulation (TENS)
Nerve blocks (diagnostic or therapeutic)
Intercostal block
Paravertebral block
Thoracic epidurals
Sympathectomies
Cryoablation of intercostal nerves
Neuromodulation-spinal cord stimulation
Physical therapy
Acupuncture
Psychological modalities

persistent pain, mandating an aggressive approach to the acute treatment of the thoracic surgical patient. Preemptive thoracic epidural analgesia is considered the gold standard because it provides excellent analgesia and decreases pulmonary complications. When epidural analgesia is contraindicated, other pharmacological approaches combined with paravertebral block should be considered as part of an effective pain management strategy. In addition to regional anesthesia, multimodal techniques including COX-2 inhibitors, gabapentinoids, and acetaminophen should be considered in an effort to maximize analgesia and minimize side effects. In opioid tolerant patients, the NMDA antagonist ketamine may be helpful in the perioperative period.

Although there are medications, procedures, and psychological interventions that may improve the severity of chronic post-thoracotomy pain, results are frequently disappointing. Current knowledge suggests that aggressive management of acute pain may offer the best outcomes for patients undergoing thoracic surgery.

REFERENCES

1. Phillips DM. JCAHO pain management standards are unveiled. Joint Commission on Accreditation of Healthcare Organizations. *JAMA.* 2000;284(4):428-429.
2. Sabanathan S, Eng J, Mearns AJ. Alterations in respiratory mechanics following thoracotomy. *J Roy Coll of Surgeons Edinburgh.* 1990;35(3):144-150.

3. Keller S, Carp NZ, Levy MN, Rosen SM. Chronic post thoracotomy pain. *J Cardiovasc Surg.* 1994;35(6 Suppl 1):161-164.
4. Wildgaard K, Ravn J, Kehlet H. Chronic post-thoracotomy pain: a critical review of pathogenic mechanisms and strategies for prevention. *Eur J Cardiothorac Surg.* 2009;36:170-180.
5. Kruger M, McRae K. Pain management in cardiothoracic practice. *Surg Clin North Am.* 1999;79(2): 387-400.
6. Liu S, Carpenter RL, Neal JM. Epidural anesthesia and analgesia. Their role in postoperative outcome. *Anesthesiology.* 1995;82(6):1474-1506.
7. Power I, McCormack JG, Myles PS. Regional anaesthesia and pain management. *Anaesthesia.* 2010;65(Suppl 1):38-47.
8. Stadler M, Schlander M, Braeckman M, Nguyen T, Boogaerts JG. A cost-utility and cost-effectiveness analysis of an acute pain service. *J Clin Anesth.* 2004;16(3):159-167.
9. Katz J, Jackson M, Kavanagh BP, Sandler AN. Acute pain after thoracic surgery predicts long-term post-thoracotomy pain. *Clin J Pain.* 1996;12(1):50-55.
10. Perkins FM, Kehlet H. Chronic pain as an outcome of surgery. A review of predictive factors. *Anesthesiology.* 2000;93(4):1123-1133.
11. Li W, Lee RL, Lee TW, Ng CS. The impact of thoracic surgical access on early shoulder function: video-assisted thoracic surgery versus posterolateral thoracotomy. *Eur J Cardiothorac Surg.* 2003;23(3):390-396.
12. Steegers M, Snik DM, Verhagen AF, van der Drift MA, Wilder-Smith OH. Only half of the chronic pain after thoracic surgery shows a neuropathic component. *J Pain.* 2008;9(10):955-961.
13. Woolf C. Generation of acute pain: central mechanisms. *Br Med Bull.* 1991;47(3):523-533.
14. Pyati S, Gan TJ. Perioperative pain management. *CNS Drugs.* 2007;21(3):185-211.
15. Thompson S, King AE, Woolf CJ. Activity-dependent changes in rat ventral horn neurons in vitro: summation of prolonged afferent evoked postsynaptic depolarizations produce a d-2-amino-5-phosphonovaleric acid sensitive windup. *Eur J Neurosci.* 1990;2(7):638-649.
16. Gerner P. Postthoracotomy pain management problems. *Anesthesiol Clin.* 2008;26(2):355-367.
17. Martinez-Barenys C, Busquets J, de Castro PE, et al. Randomized double-blind comparison of phrenic nerve infiltration and suprascapular nerve block for ipsilateral shoulder pain after thoracic surgery. *Eur J Cardiothorac Surg.* 2011;40(1):106-112.
18. Danelli G, Berti M, Casati A, et al. Ipsilateral shoulder pain after thoracotomy surgery: a prospective, randomized, double-blind, placebo-controlled evaluation of the efficacy of infiltrating the phrenic nerve with 0.2% wt/vol ropivacaine. *Eur J Anaesthesiol.* 2007;24(7):596-601.
19. Muehling BM, Halter GL, Schelzig H, et al. Reduction of postoperative pulmonary complications after lung surgery using a fast track clinical pathway. *Eur J Cardiothorac Surg.* 2008;34(1):174-180.
20. Suwanchinda V, Suksompong, S, Prakanrattana, U, Udompunthurak, S. Epidural analgesia for pain relief in thoracic surgery. *J Med Assoc Thai.* 2000;83(4):358-363.
21. Liu S, Allen, HW, Olsson, GL. Patient-controlled epidural analgesia with bupivacaine and fentanyl on hospital wards: prospective experience with 1,030 surgical patients. *Anesthesiology.* 1998;88(3):688-695.
22. Visser WA, Lee RA, Gielen MJ. Factors influencing the distribution of neural blockade by local anesthetics in epidural anesthesia and a comparison of lumbar versus thoracic epidural anesthesia. *Anesth Analg.* 2008;107(2):708-721.
23. Visser WA, Liem TH, van Egmond J, Gielen MJ. Extension of sensory blockade after thoracic epidural administration of a test dose of lidocaine at three different levels. *Anesth Analg.* 1998;86(2):332-335.
24. Giebler R, Scherer RU, Peters J. Incidence of neurologic complications related to thoracic epidural catheterization. *Anesthesiology.* 1997;86(1):55-63.
25. Tanaka K, Watanabe R, Harada T, Dan K. Extensive application of epidural anesthesia and analgesia in a university hospital: incidence of complications related to technique. *Reg Anesth.* 1993;18(1):34-38.
26. Ballantyne JC, Carr DB, deFerranti S, et al. The comparative effects of postoperative analgesic therapies on pulmonary outcome: cumulative meta-analyses of randomized, controlled trials. *Anesth Analg.* 1998 86(3):598-612.
27. Hurford WE, Dutton RP, Alfille PH, Clement D, Wilson RS. Comparison of thoracic and lumbar epidural infusions of bupivacaine and fentanyl for post-thoracotomy analgesia. *J Cardiothorac Vasc Anesth.* 1993;7(5):521-525.

28. Kahn L, Baxter FJ, Dauphin A, et al. A comparison of thoracic and lumbar epidural techniques for post-thoracoabdominal esophagectomy analgesia. *Can J Anaesth*. 1999;46(5 Pt 1):415-422.
29. Ali M, Winter DC, Hanly AM, O'Hagan C, Keaveny J, Broe P. Prospective, randomized, controlled trial of thoracic epidural or patient-controlled opiate analgesia on perioperative quality of life. *Br J Anaesth*. 2010;104(3):292-297.
30. Guinard JP, Mavrocordatos P, Chiolero R, Carpenter RL. A randomized comparison of intravenous versus lumbar and thoracic epidural fentanyl for analgesia after thoracotomy. *Anesthesiology*. 1992;77(6):1108-1115.
31. Coe A, Sarginson R, Smith MW, Donnelly RJ, Russell GN. Pain following thoracotomy. A randomised, double-blind comparison of lumbar versus thoracic epidural fentanyl. *Anaesthesia*. 1991;46(11):918-921.
32. Larsen VH, Iversen AD, Christensen P, Andersen PK. Postoperative pain treatment after upper abdominal surgery with epidural morphine at thoracic or lumbar level. *Acta Anaesthesiol Scand*. 1985;29(6):566-571.
33. Joshi GP, Bonnet F, Shah R, et al. A systematic review of randomized trials evaluating regional techniques for postthoracotomy analgesia. *Anesth analg*. 2008;107(3):1026-1040.
34. Halpern SH, Arellano R, Preston R, et al. Epidural morphine vs hydromorphone in post-caesarean section patients. *Can J Anaesth*. 1996;43(6):595-598.
35. Goodarzi M. Comparison of epidural morphine, hydromorphone and fentanyl for postoperative pain control in children undergoing orthopaedic surgery. *Paediatr Anaesth*. 1999;9(5):419-422.
36. Ginosar Y, Riley ET, Angst MS. The site of action of epidural fentanyl in humans: the difference between infusion and bolus administration. *Anesth Analg*. 2003;97(5):1428-1438.
37. Glass PS, Estok P, Ginsberg B, Goldberg JS, Sladen RN. Use of patient-controlled analgesia to compare the efficacy of epidural to intravenous fentanyl administration. *Anesth Analg*. 1992;74(3):345-351.
38. White MJ, Berghausen EJ, Dumont SW, et al. Side effects during continuous epidural infusion of morphine and fentanyl. *Can J Anaesth*. 1992;39(6):576-582.
39. Kortgen A, Silomon M, Pape-Becker C, Buchinger H, Grundmann U, Bauer M. Thoracic but not lumbar epidural anaesthesia increases liver blood flow after major abdominal surgery. *Eur J Anaesthesiol*. 2009;26(2):111-116.
40. Wu CL, Cohen SR, Richman JM, et al. Efficacy of postoperative patient-controlled and continuous infusion epidural analgesia versus intravenous patient-controlled analgesia with opioids: a meta-analysis. *Anesthesiology*. 2005;103(5):1079-1088; quiz 1109-1010.
41. Kopacz D, Sharrock, NE, Allen, HW. A comparison of levobupivacaine 0.125%, fentanyl 4 microg/mL, or their combination for patient-controlled epidural analgesia after major orthopedic surgery. *Anesth Analg*. 1999;89(6):1497-1503.
42. van der Vyver M, Halpern S, Joseph G. Patient-controlled epidural analgesia versus continuous infusion for labour analgesia: a meta-analysis. *Br J Anaesth*. 2002;89(3):459-465.
43. Saeki H, Ishimura H, Higashi H, et al. Postoperative management using intensive patient-controlled epidural analgesia and early rehabilitation after an esophagectomy. *Surg Today*. 2009;39(6):476-480.
44. Kammoun W, Mestiri T, Miraoui W, et al. Patient controlled epidural analgesia: interest in thoracic surgery. *Tunis Med*. 2008;86(2):144-149.
45. Tan T, Wilson D, Walsh A, Hu P, Power C. Audit of a ward-based patient-controlled epidural analgesia service in Ireland. *Ir J Med Sci*. 2011;180(2):417-421.
46. Liu SS, Bieltz M, Wukovits B, John RS. Prospective survey of patient-controlled epidural analgesia with bupivacaine and hydromorphone in 3736 postoperative orthopedic patients. *Reg Anesth Pain Med*. 2010;35(4):351-354.
47. Valairucha S, Maboonvanon P, Napachoti T, Sirivanasandha B, Suraseranuvongse S. Cost-effectiveness of thoracic patient-controlled epidural analgesia using bupivacaine with fentanyl vs bupivacaine with morphine after thoracotomy and upper abdominal surgery. *J Med Assoc Thai*. 2005;88(7):921-927.
48. Ladak SS, Katznelson R, Muscat M, Sawhney M, Beattie WS, O'Leary G. Incidence of urinary retention in patients with thoracic patient-controlled epidural analgesia (TPCEA) undergoing thoracotomy. *Pain Manag Nurs*. 2009;10(2):94-98.
49. Eisenach JC, De Kock M, Klimscha W. alpha(2)-adrenergic agonists for regional anesthesia. A clinical review of clonidine (1984-1995). *Anesthesiology*. 1996;85(3):655-674.
50. Eisenach JC, DuPen S, Dubois M, Miguel R, Allin D. Epidural clonidine analgesia for intractable cancer pain. The Epidural Clonidine Study Group. *Pain*. 1995;61(3):391-399.

51. Lavand'homme PM, Eisenach JC. Perioperative administration of the alpha-2-adrenoceptor agonist clonidine at the site of nerve injury reduces the development of mechanical hypersensitivity and modulates local cytokine expression. *Pain.* 2003;105(1-2):247-254.
52. Curatolo M, Schnider, TW, Petersen-Felix, S, et al. A direct search procedure to optimize combinations of epidural bupivacaine, fentanyl, and clonidine for postoperative analgesia. *Anesthesiology.* 2000;92(2):325-337.
53. Wong CS, Liaw WJ, Tung CS, Su YF, Ho ST. Ketamine potentiates analgesic effect of morphine in postoperative epidural pain control. *Reg Anesth.* 1996;21(6):534-541.
54. Suzuki M, Haraguti S, Sugimoto K, Kikutani T, Shimada Y, Sakamoto A. Low-dose intravenous ketamine potentiates epidural analgesia after thoracotomy. *Anesthesiology.* 2006;105(1):111-119.
55. Subramaniam BS, Subramaniam K, Pawar DK, Sennaraj B. Preoperative epidural ketamine in combination with morphine does not have a clinically relevant intra- and postoperative opioid-sparing effect. *Anesth analg.* 2001;93(5):1321-1326.
56. Loftus RW, Yeager MP, Clark JA, et al. Intraoperative ketamine reduces perioperative opiate consumption in opiate-dependent patients with chronic back pain undergoing back surgery. *Anesthesiology.* 2010;113(3):639-646.
57. Gulbahar G, Kocer B, Muratli SN, et al. A comparison of epidural and paravertebral catheterisation techniques in post-thoracotomy pain management. *Eur J Cardiothorac Surg.* 2010;37(2):467-472.
58. Davies RG, Myles PS, Graham JM. A comparison of the analgesic efficacy and side-effects of paravertebral vs epidural blockade for thoracotomy—a systematic review and meta-analysis of randomized trials. *Br J Anaesth.* 2006;96(4):418-426.
59. Garutti I, Gonzalez-Aragoneses F, Biencinto MT, et al. Thoracic paravertebral block after thoracotomy: comparison of three different approaches. *Eur J Cardiothorac Surg.* 2009;35(5):829-832.
60. Eason M, Wyatt, R. Paravertebral thoracic block-a reappraisal. *Anaesthesia.* 1979;34(7):638-642.
61. Richardson J, Sabanathan S. Thoracic paravertebral analgesia. *Acta Anaesthesiol Scand.* 1995;39(8):1005-1015.
62. Pusch F, Freitag H, Weinstabl C, Obwegeser R, Huber E, Wildling E. Single-injection paravertebral block compared to general anaesthesia in breast surgery. *Acta Anaesthesiol Scand.* 1999;43(7):770-774.
63. Coveney E, Weltz, CR, Greengrass, R. Use of paravertebral block anesthesia in the surgical management of breast cancer: experience in 156 cases. *Ann Surg.* 1998;227(4):496-501.
64. Richardson J, Sabanathan S. Continuous intercostal bupivacaine. *Ann Thorac Surg.* 1993;56(3):596.
65. Debreceni G, Molnar Z, Szelig L, Molnar TF. Continuous epidural or intercostal analgesia following thoracotomy: a prospective randomized double-blind clinical trial. *Acta Anaesthesiol Scand.* 2003;47(9):1091-1095.
66. Luketich JD, Land SR, Sullivan EA, et al. Thoracic epidural versus intercostal nerve catheter plus patient-controlled analgesia: a randomized study. *Ann Thorac Surg.* 2005 Jun;79(6):1845-1849; discussion 1849-1850.
67. Moore D. Intercostal nerve block for postoperaive somatic pain following surgery of thorax and upper abdomen. *Br J Anaesth.* 1975;47(Suppl):284-286.
68. Bachmann-Mennenga B, Biscoping J, Kuhn DF, et al. Intercostal nerve block, interpleural analgesia, thoracic epidural block or systemic opioid application for pain relief after thoracotomy? *Eur J Cardio-Thorac Surg.* 1993;7(1):12-18.
69. McKenzie AG, Mathe S. Interpleural local anaesthesia: anatomical basis for mechanism of action. *Br J Anaesth.* 1996;76(2):297-299.
70. Dravid RM, Paul RE. Interpleural block - part 2. *Anaesthesia.* 2007;62(11):1143-1153.
71. Weston S, Clark I. Intrapleural catheter placement. *Anaesth Intensive Care.* 1990;18(1):140.
72. Ben-David B, Lee E. The falling column: a new technique for interpleural catheter placement. *Anesth Analg.* 1990;71(2):212.
73. Lee E, Ben-David B. Identification of the interpleural space. *Br J Anaesth.* 1991;67(130).
74. Kvalheim L, Reiestad, F. Interpleural catheter in the management of postoperative pain. *Anesthesiology.* 1984;61(A231).
75. Dravid RM, Paul RE. Interpleural block - part 1. *Anaesthesia.* 2007;62(10):1039-1049.
76. Engdahl O, Boe J, Sandstedt S. Interpleural bupivacaine for analgesia during chest drainage treatment for pneumothorax. A randomized double-blind study. *Acta Anaesthesiol Scand.* 1993;37(2):149-153.

77. Buvanendran A, Kroin JS. Multimodal analgesia for controlling acute postoperative pain. *Curr Opin Anaesthesiol.* 2009;22(5):588-593.
78. Buvanendran A, Kroin JS, Della Valle CJ, Kari M, Moric M, Tuman KJ. Perioperative oral pregabalin reduces chronic pain after total knee arthroplasty: a prospective, randomized, controlled trial. *Anesth Analg.* 2010;110(1):199-207.
79. Wenk M, Schug SA. Perioperative pain management after thoracotomy. *Curr Opin Anaesthesiol.* 2011;24(1):8-12.
80. Maund E, McDaid C, Rice S, Wright K, Jenkins B, Woolacott N. Paracetamol and selective and non-selective non-steroidal anti-inflammatory drugs for the reduction in morphine-related side-effects after major surgery: a systematic review. *Br J Anaesth.* 2011;106(3):292-297.
81. Memis D, Inal MT, Kavalci G, Sezer A, Sut N. Intravenous paracetamol reduced the use of opioids, extubation time, and opioid-related adverse effects after major surgery in intensive care unit. *J Crit Care.* 2010;25(3):458-462.
82. Pogatzki-Zahn EM, Zahn PK. From preemptive to preventive analgesia. *Curr Opin Anaesthesiol.* 2006;19(5):551-555.
83. Ilfeld BM, Ball ST, Gearen PF, et al. Health-related quality of life after hip arthroplasty with and without an extended-duration continuous posterior lumbar plexus nerve block: a prospective, 1-year follow-up of a randomized, triple-masked, placebo-controlled study. *Anesth Analg.* 2009;109(2):586-591.
84. Ilfeld BM, Meyer RS, Le LT, et al. Health-related quality of life after tricompartment knee arthroplasty with and without an extended-duration continuous femoral nerve block: a prospective, 1-year follow-up of a randomized, triple-masked, placebo-controlled study. *Anesth Analg.* 2009;108(4):1320-1325.
85. Remerand F, Le Tendre C, Baud A, et al. The early and delayed analgesic effects of ketamine after total hip arthroplasty: a prospective, randomized, controlled, double-blind study. *Anesth Analg.* 2009;109(6):1963-1971.
86. Goldstein JL, Eisen GM, Agrawal N, Stenson WF, Kent JD, Verburg KM. Reduced incidence of upper gastrointestinal ulcer complications with the COX-2 selective inhibitor, valdecoxib. *Aliment Pharmacol Ther.* 2004;20(5):527-538.
87. Trelle S, Reichenbach S, Wandel S, et al. Cardiovascular safety of non-steroidal anti-inflammatory drugs: network meta-analysis. *BMJ.* 2011;342:c7086.
88. Ross JS, Madigan D, Konstam MA, Egilman DS, Krumholz HM. Persistence of cardiovascular risk after rofecoxib discontinuation. *Arch Intern Med.* 2010;170(22):2035-2036.
89. Salinas G RU, Uretsky BF, Birnbaum Y. The cyclooxygenase 2 (COX-2) story: it's time to explain, not inflame. *J Cardiovasc Pharmacol Ther.* 2007;12(2):98-111.
90. El-Hennawy AM A-EA, Abd-Elmaksoud AM, El-Ozairy HS, Boulis SR. Addition of clonidine or dexmedetomidine to bupivacaine prolongs caudal analgesia in children. *Br J Anaesth.* 2009;103(2):268-274.
91. Congedo E, Sgreccia M, De Cosmo G. New drugs for epidural analgesia. *Curr Drug Targets.* 2009;10(8):696-706.
92. Blades B, Dugan, DJ. War wounds of the chest observed at the Thoracic Surgery Centre. *J Thorac Surg.* 1944;13:294-306.
93. Kanner R, Martini N. Nature and incidence of post-thoracotomy pain. *Proc Am Soc Clin Oncol.* 1982;1:152.
94. Dajczman E, Gordon A, Kreisman H, Wolkove N. Long-term postthoracotomy pain. *Chest.* 1991;99(2):270-274.
95. Perttunen K, Tasmuth T, Kalso E. Chronic pain after thoracic surgery: a follow-up study. *Acta Anaesthesiol Scand.* 1999;43(3):563-567.
96. Shaw A, Keefe FJ. Genetic and environmental determinants of postthoracotomy pain syndrome. *Curr Opin Anaesthesiol.* 2008;21(1):8-11.
97. Nikolajsen L, Brandsborg B, Lucht U, Jensen TS, Kehlet H. Chronic pain following total hip arthroplasty: a nationwide questionnaire study. *Acta Anaesthesiol Scand.* 2006;50(4):495-500.
98. Brandsborg B, Nikolajsen L, Kehlet H, Jensen TS. Chronic pain after hysterectomy. *Acta Anaesthesiol Scand.* 2008;52(3):327-331.
99. Nikolajsen L, Sorensen HC, Jensen TS, Kehlet H. Chronic pain following Caesarean section. *Acta Anaesthesiol Scand.* 2004;48(1):111-116.

100. Aasvang E, Kehlet H. Chronic postoperative pain: the case of inguinal herniorrhaphy. *Br J Anaesth.* 2005;95(1):69-76.
101. Meyerson J, Thelin S, Gordh T, Karlsten R. The incidence of chronic post-sternotomy pain after cardiac surgery—a prospective study. *Acta Anaesthesiol Scand.* 2001;45(8):940-944.
102. Puolakka PAE, Rorarius MGF, Roviola M, Puolakka TJS, Nordhausen K, Lindgren L. Persistent pain following knee arthroplasty. *Eur J Anaesthesiol.* 2010;27(5):455-460.
103. Yarnitsky D, Crispel Y, Eisenberg E, et al. Prediction of chronic post-operative pain: pre-operative DNIC testing identifies patients at risk. *Pain.* 2008;138(1):22-28.
104. Pluijms W, Steegers MA, Verhagen AF. Chronic post-thoracotomy pain: a retrospective study. *Acta Anaesthesiologica Scand.* 2006;50(7):804-808.
105. Ochroch E, Gottschalk A, Troxel AB, Farrar JT. Women suffer more short- and long-term pain than men after major thoracotomy. *Clin J Pain.* 2006;22(5):491-498.
106. Gotoda Y, Kambara N, Sakai T, Kishi Y, Kodama K, Koyama T. The morbidity, time course and predictive factors for persistent post-thoracotomy pain. *Eur J Pain.* 2001;5(1):89-96.
107. Taenzer P, Melzack R, Jeans ME. Influence of psychological factors on postoperative pain, mood and analgesic requirements. *Pain.* 1986;24(3):331-342.
108. Landreneau R, Mack MJ, Hazelrigg SR, et al. Prevalence of chronic pain after pulmonary resection by thoracotomy or video-assisted thoracic surgery. *J Thorac Cardiovasc Surg.* 1994;107(4):1079-1085.
109. Kirby T, Mack MJ, Landreneau RJ Rice, TW. Lobectomy—video-assisted thoracic surgery versus muscle-sparing thoracotomy. A randomized trial. *J Thorac Cardiovasc Surg.* 1995;109(5):997-1001.
110. Furrer M, Rechsteiner R, Eigenmann V, Signer C, Althaus U, Ris HB. Thoracotomy and thoracoscopy: postoperative pulmonary function, pain and chest wall complaints. *Eur J Cardiothorac Surg.* 1997;12(1):82-87.
111. Khan I, McManus KG, McCraith A, McGuigan JA. Muscle sparing thoracotomy: a biomechanical analysis confirms preservation of muscle strength but no improvement in wound discomfort. *Eur J Cardiothorac Surg.* 2000;18(6):656-661.
112. Ochroch E, Gottschalk A, Augoustides JG, Aukburg SJ, Kaiser LR, Shrager JB. Pain and physical function are similar following axillary, muscle-sparing vs posterolateral thoracotomy. *Chest.* 2005;128(4):2664-2670.
113. Landreneau R, Pigula F, Luketich et al. Acute and chronic morbidity differences between muscle-sparing and standard lateral thoracotomies. *J Thorac Cardiovasc Surg.* 1996;112(5):1346-1350.
114. Senturk M, Ozcan PE. The effects of three different analgesia techniques on long-term postthoracotomy pain. *Anesth Analg.* 2002;94(1):11-15.
115. Doyle E, Bowler GM. Pre-emptive effect of multimodal analgesia in thoracic surgery. *Br J Anaesth.* 1998;80(2):147-151.
116. Richardson J, Sabanathan S, Mearns AJ, Evans CS, Bembridge J, Fairbrass M. Efficacy of pre-emptive analgesia and continuous extrapleural intercostal nerve block on post-thoracotomy pain and pulmonary mechanics. *J Cardiovasc Surg.* 1994;35(3):219-228.
117. Naylor M, Naud S, Keefe FJ, Helzer JE. Therapeutic interactive voice response (TIVR) to reduce analgesic medication use for chronic pain management. *J Pain.* 2010;11(12):1410-1419.
118. Deng G, Rusch V, Vickers A, et al. Randomized controlled trial of a special acupuncture technique for pain after thoracotomy. *J Thorac Cardiovasc Surg.* 2008;136(6):1464-1649.
119. Vickers A, Rusch VW, Malhotra VT, Downey RJ, Cassileth BR. Acupuncture is a feasible treatment for post-thoracotomy pain: results of a prospective pilot trial. *BMC Anesthesiol.* 2006;3(6:5).

Index

NOTE: Page numbers followed by *f* and *t* denotes figures and tables, respectively.

A

ABCDE's (Breathing, Circulation, Disability, Exposure, Environment), 381
ACEIs. *See* angiotensin-converting enzyme inhibitors
active failures, 26, 26*f*, 39
acupuncture, 483
acute bronchopleural fistula (BPF), 344, 350-351
acute lung injury (ALI), 139-140, 250, 447-448
acute lung injury and adult respiratory distress syndrome (ALI/ARDS), 250-251, 448
acute pain, 102, 469*f*
acute postoperative pain, 102
acute post-thoracotomy pain, 467-484, 471*t*
acute renal failure, medications, 451-454, 452*t*
acute respiratory distress syndrome (ARDS), 139, 165, 351
adenocarcinoma, 322
   case vignette, 191
   mouse modeling, 122
adenoid cystic carcinoma of central airways, 212
adenosine triphosphate (ATP), 107
adrenal gland, metastases to, 165
advocacy, 34, 39
AF. *See* atrial fibrillation
age, pulmonary complications and, 68
air leak, 343, 431-432
   classification of, 431
   lung volume reduction surgery, 284, 284*f*
   severity assessment, 349
air leak meter, 431, 432*f*
airway
   anatomy, 128-130
   debridement, 203
   esophagectomy procedures, 331
   fire, 205-206
   malignancy, 202*t*, 206-207
   management
      laryngeal trauma, 392-393
      pediatric anterior mediastinal mass, 418, 420
      surgical, 393
   pericardial effusion, 318
   resistance, 47, 47*t*
   stenting, 207-210

airway injury, 393
   esophagectomy procedures, 332
   signs and symptoms, 392
airway obstruction, 231
   endobronchial laser, 201
   malignancy, 201-207, 202*t*
   spirometry, 223-224, 223*f*
   therapeutic procedures, 201-207, 202*t*
alarm
   auditory, 36
   monitors, 35-37
   visual, 37
ALI. *See* acute lung injury
ALI/ARDS. *See* acute lung injury and adult respiratory distress syndrome
almitrine, 57
alpha-2 agonists, 480
alveolar PCO_2 ventilation equation, 49, 50*f*
alveolar PO_2 (P_AO_2), 49
alveolar pressure. *See* plateau pressure
alveolar-arterial oxygen gradient (pA-aO_2), 293-294
alveolo-capillary membrane permeability, 444
ambulation, 428
American Society of Anesthesiologists Difficult Airway Guidelines, 39
amiodarone, 457-458
amoxicillin-clavulanate, high dose, 446
analgesia. *See also* epidural analgesia; thoracic epidural analgesia
   acute postoperative pain, 102
   continuous thoracic epidural analgesia, 473*t*
   delivery locations, 385-388, 386*f*
   intrapleural, 387
   lung resection, 252
   multimodal analgesia, 470, 470*f*, 480
   patient controlled epidural analgesia, 474, 474*t*
   postoperative, 19-20
   spinal/epidural, 242-243
   thoracic surgery-associated pain, 111
anastomosis stenosis, 209, 211*f*
anastomotic leaks, 335
anastomotic stricture, 335
anatomy
   airway, 128-130
   bronchopulmonary, 129-130, 129*f*
   chest wall, 127-128

anatomy (*Cont.*):
  esophagus, 130-131
  intercostal nerve blocks, 478*f*
  lungs, 128-130, 129*t*
  mediastinum, 131, 181-182, 182*f*, 218, 218*f*
  PVB, 475-476, 475*f*
  sternum, 127
  tracheal, 128-129
anesthesia. *See also* balanced anesthesia; general anesthesia; mediastinal masses; rigid bronchoscopy; single-lung anesthesia; thoracic anesthesia; tracheal insufflation anesthesia
  blood flow distribution and, 57, 60
  care errors, 27*t*
  endotracheal intubation, 6-11
  hypoxic pulmonary vasoconstriction, 294
  induction, 197-198
    hypotension, 246
    mediastinal masses, 230
  inhalational, 3
  maintenance, 247
  management, 227, 229-233
  mediastinal masses, 227, 229-233, 229*t*
  normal lung volumes and, 48-49
  post-esophagectomy patients, 336-337
  principles, 229*t*
  respiratory function and, 293-295, 295*t*
Anesthesia Crisis Resource Management, 39
anesthesia induction. *See specific surgical procedure for anesthesia induction*
anesthesia plan, 196-197, 263, 349. *See also specific surgical procedure for anesthesia plan*
anesthesiologists, 217-234
anesthetic
  delivery locations, 385-388, 386*f*
  induction, 245-246
    lung transplantation, 367-369
    pediatric anterior mediastinal mass, 418, 420
  intraoperative induction, 245-246
  pulmonary vascular function and, 64-65
  toxicity, 302
angiomas, 201, 202*t*
angiotensin-converting enzyme inhibitors (ACEIs), 459
anterior mediastinal mass. *See also* pediatrics
  perioperative
    complications, 221-222, 221*t*
    evaluation, 222-227
  signs and symptoms, 222-223
anterior mediastinotomy. *See* Chamberlain procedure

anthracyclines, 162
antibiotics, 3-4
  LT, 365-366, 375
  postoperative pneumonia, 446
anticoagulation
  guidelines for, 472, 472*t*
  therapy, 194-195
antineuropathic therapies, 483
aortic injury
  blunt, 380*f*
  CPB and, 400
aortic transection, 397-398
aortic valvular trauma, 394
APC. *See* argon plasma coagulation
apneic oxygenation, 53
ARDS. *See* acute respiratory distress syndrome
argon plasma coagulation (APC), 201, 205, 205*f*
Arndt blocker, 21, 90-92, 93*f*, 95*t*
arrhythmias, 455
arterial blood gas trends, 253
arterial carbon dioxide (P_aCO_2), 153, 288-289
arterial hypoxemia, 49
arterial oxygen desaturation, 247-248, 248*f*
arterial oxygenation (P_aO_2), 49, 153-154
  mixed venous oxygen content, 55-56, 56*f*
  positioning, 56-57, 58*f*
artery wedge pressures, 67
asbestos fiber, 256
ASD. *See* atrial septal defects
aspiration, 336-337, 336*f*, 374
aspirin, 194
assertion, 34
asthma/bronchospasm, 193
atelectasis, 293
ATP. *See* adenosine triphosphate
atrial fibrillation (AF), 265. *See also* postoperative atrial fibrillation
atrial septal defects (ASD), 312
atrial tachyarrhythmias, 455-456
auto-PEEP. *See* dynamic hyperinflation
autotransfusion techniques, 385
awake bronchoscopy, 177

B

balanced anesthesia, 247
ball valve induced barotrauma, 199
balloon blockade (of mainstem bronchus), 90
balloon bronchoplasty, 206
balloon-tipped catheters, 13
bare-metal stents (BMS), 159
barium swallow, 135-137, 136*f*
BCI. *See* blunt cardiac injury

benign airway stenosis, 201-207, 202*t*
benign chest tumors, 237-253
benzodiazepines, 65
beraprost, 67
beta blockers
    atrial tachyarrhythmias, 455-456
    perioperative myocardial ischemia, 159-160
biatrial pacing, 459
bilateral orthotopic lung transplantation (BOLT), 362
bilobectomy, 142-143
biologically variable ventilation (BVV), 60
biopsy
    cervical lymph node, 227
    CT-guided needle, 227
    transbronchial lung biopsy, 191, 375
bladder catheter placement, 244
blast injury, 380-381
    heart and, 393-396
blast overpressure, 380
blast wave, 380-381
bleeding
    FOB and, 176
    increased risk, 242
    massive, 173
    mediastinoscopy, 173, 186-187
bleomycin, 137, 162
blind method insertion technique, 86-87, 88*f*
blood. *See also* arterial blood gas trends
    deoxygenated, 49
    products, 244
    supply, 127-128
blood flow distribution, drug effects on, 57, 60
blood pressure monitoring, 246, 317
blunt cardiac injury (BCI), 380*f*, 393-396
blunt trauma, 379
    blunt aortic injury, 380*f*, 399-400
    blunt chest trauma, 388-389
blunt traumatic aortic injury (BTAI), 397*t*
BLVR. *See* bronchoscopic lung volume reduction
BMI. *See* body mass index
BMS. *See* bare-metal stents
BNP. *See* recombinant human B-type natriuretic peptide
body mass index (BMI), 287
BOLT. *See* bilateral orthotopic lung transplantation
bony metastasis, 165
BPF. *See* bronchopleural fistula
brachial plexus injury, 139
brachytherapy, 207
brain
    metastasis, 165-166
    nociceptive information, 104-105
Brauer's positive pressure technique, 5
breakthrough pain, 411
breath stacking. *See* dynamic hyperinflation
Breathing, Circulation, Disability, Exposure, Environment. *See* ABCDE's
bronchial blockers, 21
    advantages and disadvantages, 98*t*
    BPF, 346, 346*f*
    complications, 95-96
    history, 12-14
    independent, 90
        comparison of, 94
    lung isolation, 245-246
bronchial stump disruption, 343
bronchial tamponage technique, 13
bronchodilators, 165
bronchogenic carcinoma of left lung, surgical staging, 184
bronchopleural fistula (BPF), 446-447
    anesthetic problems, 349
    chapter summary, 356
    diagnosis, 346-347, 347*f*-348*f*, 349
    etiology, 343-344, 344*t*
    incidence, 343
    management, 350-355
        endoscopic, 352-354
        operative, 354-355
    pathophysiology, risk factors, types, 344-345, 345*f*
    presentation, 345-346, 346*f*
    prevention, 355-356
    prognosis, 355
    vignette and key points, 342-343
bronchopulmonary anatomy, 129-130, 129*f*
bronchoscopic lung volume reduction (BLVR), 285
bronchoscopy. *See also* awake bronchoscopy; fiberoptic bronchoscopy; flexible fiberoptic bronchoscopy; rigid bronchoscopy; therapeutic bronchoscopy
    anesthetic management, 177
    bronchopleural fistula, 350, 352-354
    case vignette and key points, 173
    under general anesthesia, 177-178
    preoperative assessment and monitoring, 177
    with transbronchial biopsy, 191
bronchospasm, 176
BTAI. *See* blunt traumatic aortic injury
bupivacaine
    epidural analgesic regimens, 473, 473*t*
    pediatrics, 410-411
BVV. *See* biologically variable ventilation

C

C fiber nociceptors, 103
CA^{2+}. *See* L-type calcium channels
CAD. *See* coronary artery disease
calcium channel blockers, 457
calcium-dependent vasoconstriction, 64
cancer. *See also* esophageal cancer; esophageal cancer staging; lung adenocarcinomas; lung cancer; malignancy; metastases; non-small cell lung cancer; small-cell lung cancer; tumor
    deep vein thrombosis, 166
    lung resection for, 237-253
    metabolic and paraneoplastic effects, 166-167
    therapy history, 150
cancer staging
    bronchogenic carcinoma of left lung, 184
    esophageal cancer classification system, 324-325, 324*t*
    NSCLC, 174
cancer stem cells, 123
CAO. *See* central airway obstruction
capnography, 18
carboplatin, 161-162
cardiac arrhythmias, 176
cardiac disease, 286-287
cardiac enzymes, 396
cardiac evaluation
    postoperative cardiac complications, 454-461
    preoperative non-cardiac surgery, 156, 158*f*
    summary recommendations, 161
    thoracic surgery, 156, 158*f*, 159-161
cardiac filling, 311
cardiac function assessment, 365
cardiac herniation, 461
    EPP and, 266-267, 267*f*
cardiac rupture, 393-394
cardiac stents, 460
cardiac tamponade, 310-312, 310*f*
cardiac trauma, 393-396
cardiopulmonary bypass (CPB), 231-232
    airway injuries, 393
    aortic injury, 400
    LT and, 371-372
cardiovascular postoperative complications, 440-461
care errors, 27*t*
carinal resection, 143
catheter
    balloon-tipped, 13
    bladder, 244
    Fogarty, 13-14, 407
    injection, 199
    pleural, 302
catheterization. *See also* pulmonary artery catheterization
    central venous, 70-71
    right heart, 70
    thoracic epidural, 471
CCAMs. *See* congenital cystic adenomatous malformations
cefazolin, 434-435
central airway disorders, multimodality approach, 212-214
central airway obstruction (CAO), 192
central airway tumors, 201, 202*t*, 203
central nervous system pain, 107
central nociceptive pathways, 104-106, 105*f*
central sensitization, 109-110
central venous access, 244
central venous catheterization, 70-71
central venous pressure (CVP), 70-71, 394
centrilobular emphysema, 276
cephalosporin, 434, 446
cervical anastomosis, 337
cervical lymph node biopsy, 227
cervical mediastinoscopy, 181, 184, 185*f*
CF. *See* cystic fibrosis
cGMP. *See* cyclic guanosine monophosphate
Chamberlain procedure (anterior mediastinotomy), 184-185, 418, 420*f*
Charlson score, 334-335
check-back, 34-35, 39
checklist
    perioperative tasks and, 29
    prompts, 28, 39
    Surgical Safety Checklist, 29, 29*f*
chemotherapeutic agents, 163
    with perioperative implications, 163*t*
    pulmonary toxicity and, 137, 138*t*, 164
    thoracic surgery, 137, 161
chemotherapy-induced pulmonary toxicity, 137, 138*t*, 164
chest cavity drainage, 350
chest drainage devices, 429-431, 429*f*, 430*f*
chest injury, 379
chest tube, 429-433, 429*f*
chest tube fluid, character of, 430
chest wall
    anatomy, 127-128
    blood supply to, 127-128
    extrathoracic muscles of, 128
    flail chest, 388-389
    lung resection closure, 252
    pleural space injuries, 385-388

chest x-ray. *See also* plain chest x-ray
   BPF, 346-347, 347f
   congenital heart disease, 364f
   malignant pleural mesothelioma, 257f
   pleural effusion, 132f
children. *See also* pediatrics
   foreign body in airway, 415-417, 415t
   LT indications, 359, 359f-360f
   mediastinal masses, 219t, 225, 229t
   OLV in, 408, 408t
chronic bronchopleural fistula (BPF), 344
   management, 351-352
   onset of, 345-346
chronic obstructive pulmonary disease (COPD), 441. *See also* severe chronic obstructive pulmonary disease
   anesthesia and, 293-294
   auto-PEEP, 59f
   characterizations, 275
   comorbid conditions with, 279
   flow-volume loops, 223f
   LT and, 359
   LVRS, 288-289, 291-293
   pathophysiology of, 275-276, 278-279
   PH and, 65, 69
   physiologic classification, 278f
   pulmonary rehabilitation, 164
   pulsus paradoxus and, 312
   therapeutic goals, 275
   two-lung and one-lung ventilation, 56f
chronic pain, 102
   mechanisms of, 469f
   nerve blocks, 111
   NSAIDS, 111
chronic post-thoracotomy pain (CPTP), 102, 467-484
   characteristics and incidence, 480-481
   conclusions, 483-484
   etiology and risk factors, 481-482
   key points and clinical vignette, 467
   management of, 483
chylothorax, 269, 335
cigarette smoking. *See also* smoking cessation; tobacco smoke
   lung tumors, 238, 239t
   PH and, 65
   physiologic effects, 291
   risks, 240-241
cisplatin (HIOC), 161-162, 269
C_L. *See* lung compliance
clindamycin, 434
clonidine, 474, 480
clopidogrel, 194-195, 460
CO_2 narcosis, 253

coagulation, 70
cognitive behavioral therapy, 483
Cohen flexitip endobronchial blocker
   characteristics of, 95t
   placement and positioning, 91-92, 94
combined heart lung transplantation, 363
commotio cordis, 395
communication tools/skills, 32, 33t, 34-35
compliance
   calculation, 46
   of respiratory system, 293
compression injury, 379
computed tomography (CT)
   BPF, 346-347, 347f-348f, 349
   diffuse mediastinal adenopathy, 133f
   esophageal cancer and, 322-323
   lung imaging, 132, 133f
   lungs, 132, 133f
   malignant pleural mesothelioma, 257, 258f
   mediastinal masses, 224-225, 225f
   mediastinum, 135
   pulmonary lesions and, 173
congenital cystic adenomatous malformations (CCAMs), 411
   characteristics of, 412, 412t
   classification of, by clinical or pathological criteria, 412, 413t
   monitoring, induction, maintenance, 414
   preoperative assessment, 413-414
   risks, 414-415
   surgery for, 412-413, 414
constrictive pericarditis, 316
continuous positive airway pressure (CPAP), 18-19, 248-250
continuous thoracic epidural analgesia, 473t
continuous thoracic paravertebral blockade (TPB), 387
COPD. *See* chronic obstructive pulmonary disease
cord medialization, 336
coronary artery disease (CAD), 286-287
coronary artery injuries, 395
coronary stents, 159
corticosteroids, 448
COX inhibitors. *See* cyclooxygenase inhibitors
COX-2 selective inhibitors. *See* cyclooxygenase-2 selective inhibitors
CPAP. *See* continuous positive airway pressure
CPB. *See* cardiopulmonary bypass
CPTP. *See* chronic post-thoracotomy pain
cryotherapy, 206
crystalloid administration, 140
CT. *See* computed tomography
CT-guided needle biopsy, 227

Cushing syndrome, 242
cutaneous injury, 108
CVP. *See* central venous pressure; elevated central venous pressure
cyclic guanosine monophosphate (cGMP), 74
cyclooxygenase (COX) inhibitors, 451
cyclooxygenase-2 (COX-2) selective inhibitors, 480
cystic fibrosis (CF), 359, 360*f*, 365
cytokines, 107

D

DECREASE trials, 160
deep vein thrombosis (DVT), 166
deferred tasks, 28, 40
DES. *See* drug-eluting stents
desflurane, 64-65
dexmedetomidine, 452*t*, 453, 480
diagnostic imaging modalities, 131-137. *See also specific imaging modality*
diaphragm length, after LVRS, 283
diaphragmatic injury, 390-391
diaphragmatic patch problems, 269
differential pressure breathing, 4-6
diffuse mediastinal adenopathy, 133*f*
diffusing capacity for carbon monoxide (DLCO), 153, 167, 282, 289
  perioperative risk, 154
  predicted postoperative DLCO, 441
digitalization, 457
direct energy transfer, 379
DLCO. *See* diffusing capacity for carbon monoxide
DLTs. *See* double-lumen endobronchial tubes; double-lumen endotracheal tubes
dobutamine
  hypotension, 77
  mechanism of action, 74
docetaxel, 162
dogs, thoracotomy, 4-5, 5*f*
dopamine, 452-453, 452*t*
Doppler tracing, pericardial tamponade and, 315, 315*f*
double-lumen endobronchial tubes (DLTs), 82-90
  advantages and disadvantages, 98*t*
  BPF, 351, 352, 355
  EPP, 263-264
  insertion technique, 86-87, 88*f*
  left-sided, 14, 15*f*, 83, 83*f*, 263
  lung collapse and, 245
  lung transplantation, 367-368
  placement choices, 83-84, 83*f*
  problems and complications, 87-88
  right-sided, 15, 84, 84*f*, 85*f*
double-lumen endotracheal tubes (DLTs), 21, 84, 85-86, 89*f*
  indications for, 84*f*
  pediatric thoracic surgery, 408
double-lung transplantation, 362
doxycycline, 122-123
drug-eluting stents (DES), 159
drugs. *See also* analgesia; anesthetic; chemotherapeutic agents; drug-eluting stents; narcotics; opioids
  blood flow distribution, 57, 60
  continuous thoracic epidural analgesia, 473*t*
  HPV, 57
  hypotension, 74
  hypoxic pulmonary vasoconstriction, 57
Dumon style silicone stent, 208*f*
DVT. *See* deep vein thrombosis
dynamic hyperinflation (breath stacking; auto-PEEP), 59-60, 59*f*, 74, 246
  COPD, 278-279
  detection of, 59*f*
dynamic respiratory system compliance, 46
dysphagia, 323
dyspnea, 442
dysrhythmias, 265-266

E

Eastern Cooperative Oncology Group (ECOG) performance status, 261-262, 261*t*
Easton-Lambert syndrome, 166
EBUS. *See* endobronchial ultrasound
echocardiography, 71-72
  BCI and, 395-396
  drainage guidance through, 308
  mediastinal masses, 226
ECMO
  LT and, 373
  pediatric anterior mediastinal mass, 418, 420
ECOG performance status. *See* Eastern Cooperative Oncology Group performance status
EEG. *See* electrocardiogram
EGFR. *See* epidural growth factor receptor
electrical cardioversion, 459
electrocardiogram (EEG), 312-313
electrocautery
  airway obstruction, 201
  tumor mass and, 203-204, 204*f*
elevated central venous pressure (CVP), 313, 394
emergency carts, checklist prompts, 39

EMLA cream, 227
emphysema, 276, 276f-277f, 282
empyema
 chronic bronchopleural fistula, 351
 EPP, 268
endobronchial blocker. *See also Cohen flexitip endobronchial blocker*
 DLT and, 90
 pediatric thoracic surgery, 407
endobronchial laser, 201
endobronchial ultrasound (EBUS), 174
endoscopic mucosal resection, 326
endotracheal intubation
 anesthesia and, 6-11
 history, 6-8, 7f
endotracheal tube
 with detachable inflatable cuff, 10, 10f
 development of, 9-11, 10f
 Mallinckrodt right-sided double-lumen endotracheal tube, 84, 85f
 OLV in children, 408, 408t
 single-lumen, 13
 univent endotracheal tube, 94-95
end-stage pulmonary disease, 359
enflurane, 64-65
enhanced-blast explosive pattern, 381
epidural analgesia, 19-20, 70, 471-474. *See also* continuous thoracic epidural analgesia
 coagulation and, 70
 guidelines for, 472, 472t
 HPV and, 65
epidural analgesic regimens, 473, 473t
epidural growth factor receptor (EGFR), 117, 118f
epiglottis, 404, 405f
epinephrine, 74, 75t
EPP. *See* extrapleural pneumonectomy
ERV. *See* expiratory reserve volume
esophageal cancer
 clinical presentation and workup, 323-324
 endoscopic mucosal resection, 326
 epidemiology, 323
 esophagectomy and, 322-323
 gastroesophageal reflux disease, 322
 induction chemotherapy, 326
 operations, 322-337
 photodynamic therapy, 326
 postoperative radiation, 326
 surgery, 325-326, 325t
 surgical treatment and survival, 325-326, 325t
 survival, 325-326, 325t
 upper GI endoscopy, 323

esophageal cancer staging
 classification system, 324-325, 324t
 T stage definition, 325f
esophageal diagnostic modalities, 135-137, 136f
esophageal pathology, 135-137, 136f
esophageal resection, 143-144, 144t
esophagectomy. *See also* Ivor Lewis esophagectomy; left thoracoabdominal esophagectomy; post-esophagectomy patients; three-incision esophagectomy; transhiatal esophagectomy
 advantages and disadvantages of, 328t
 airway, ventilation, and extubation, 331
 anastomotic complications, 335
 anesthetic management for, 330
 chylothorax and, 335
 fluid management, 331-332
 general considerations, 330-331
 immediate and long-term outcomes, 333-334
 intraoperative complications, 332
 morbidity following, 334-335, 334t
 mortality, 322-323, 333-334
 pain management, 333
 respiratory complications, 335
 techniques of, 325-328, 327t
 vocal cord paralysis, 336
esophagogastrectomy, 143
esophagus anatomy, 130-131
ET receptor blockers, 68
exercise
 capacity, 290-291, 290f
 testing, 155-156
expiratory reserve volume (ERV), 48
extended cervical mediastinoscopy, 185-186, 185f
extrapleural pneumonectomy (EPP), 143, 255-271
 anesthetic management, 262-264, 262t
  planning, 263
  thoracic epidural anesthesia, 263
 cardiac complications, 265-267, 267f
 complications, 264-269, 270t
 conclusions, 270-271
 dissection phase of, 264
 history, 255-256
 intraoperative management, 263-264
 key points, 255
 mortality of, 256, 256t, 265t
 MPM, 258-259
 patient selection criteria, 261-262, 261t
 respiratory complications, 267-268, 268t
 steps in, 259-260, 260f
 thromboembolic complications, 268-269

extrathoracic muscles of chest wall, 128
extubation. *See also* tracheal extubation
    esophagectomy procedures, 331
    LVRS, 300, 300*t*
    pericardial effusion procedure, 319

F

FAST exam. *See* focused assessment with sonography for trauma exam
FDG-PET, malignant lesions, 132, 133*f*, 134*f*, 135*f*
Fell-O'Dwyer laryngeal tube, 6-8, 7*f*
fenoldopam, 452*t*, 453
fentanyl
    epidural analgesic regimens, 473, 473*t*
    lung transplantation, 368
    pediatrics, 410
FEV_1. *See* forced expiratory volume in one second
fever, 176
fiberoptic bronchoscope, 16, 86-87
fiberoptic bronchoscopy, 86-87
fire, airway, 205-206
5-KTP laser, angiomas, 201, 202*t*
flail chest, 388-389
flexible fiberoptic bronchoscopy (FOB), 174
    bleeding, 176
    under general anesthesia, 177-178
    indications for, 174, 175*t*
    lung cancer and, 174
    mediastinal masses, 225*f*, 226
    procedural complications, 175-176
flow-volume loops, 155, 223*f*
fluid management, 139-140. *See also* volume overload; volume replacement
    esophagectomy, 331-332
    pericardial space, 313, 313*f*
    restrictive *versus* liberal, 434
    thoracic surgical patient, 433-434, 434*t*
fluvastatin, 160
FOB. *See* flexible fiberoptic bronchoscopy
focused assessment with sonography for trauma (FAST) exam, 394
Fogarty catheters, 13-14, 407
forced expiratory volume in one second (FEV_1), 152
    impaired pulmonary function and, 242*f*
    lung volume reduction surgery and, 288-289
    after LVRS, 282
forced vital capacity (FVC), 282
foreign body in airway
    anesthetic induction, 416-417
    children, 415-417, 415*t*
    complications, 417
    tracheobronchial tree with, 416*f*

FRC. *See* functional residual capacity
Frenckner spiropulsator, 16-17, 17*f*
Fuji uniblocker
    characteristics of, 95*t*
    placement and positioning, 95*t*
functional residual capacity (FRC), 48-49, 48*f*
FVC. *See* forced vital capacity

G

gamma-amino-butyric acid (GABA), 108
gas exchange
    pH manipulation and, 57, 60
    thoracic surgery and, 153
gas transport, 198-199
gastroesophageal reflux disease (GERD), 322
gemcitabine, 162
general anesthesia
    alternatives, 11-12
    bronchoscopy, 177-178
    history of, 3-4
    induction and maintenance, 295-297
    lung volume reduction surgery, 295-297
    LVRS, 295-297
    respiratory system compliance, 293
genomics, 120-121
GERD. *See* gastroesophageal reflux disease
glossary of terms, 39-40
glutamate receptor N-methyl-D-aspartate (NMDA), 107
    receptor modulation with ketamine infusion, 483
glycemic control, 435-436
glycine, 108
great vessel trauma, 397-400

H

halothane, 64-65
handoffs, 34-35, 40
hanging drop technique, 471-472
head trauma, 193-194
healthcare systems, latent conditions, 26-27, 27*t*
heart
    blast injury, 393-396
    blunt injury, 380*f*
heart failure, 460-461
heat therapy, 201
hemodynamic collapse, 317
hemodynamic stabilization, 399
hemorrhage
    esophagectomy procedures, 332
    laser and, 203
    with lung surgery, 244
    mediastinoscopy, 140-141

hemorrhagic shock, 385
hemothorax, 384-385
heparin prophylaxis, 166-167
Her-2-neu, tumor survival, 118*f*
high-frequency jet ventilation (HFJV), 19, 179-180
high-resolution computer tomography (HRCT), 289
high-velocity injury, 379
HIOC. *See* cisplatin
Hodgkin lymphoma, 225*f*, 226
Horner syndrome, 220, 238
HPV. *See* hypoxic pulmonary vasoconstriction
HRas, 116
HRCT. *See* high-resolution computer tomography
human factors, 25-41
human factors engineering, 28, 40
hybrid silicone stents, 209, 211*f*
hybrid stents, 209-210, 211*f*
hydromorphone, 473, 473*t*
hyperalgesia, 109-110
hypercapnia, 288, 298
hyperglycemia, 435
hyperthermia, 296
hyponatremia, lung cancer and, 242
hypoperfusion, 331-332
hypotension, 143, 297
  with anesthesia induction, 246
  dobutamine, 77
  drugs for, 74
  EPP, 264
  following LT, 374
  intraoperative, 72-73, 73*t*, 274
  pericardial effusion and, 319
  phenylephrine, 72
hypovolemia, 331-332
hypoxemia, 38, 49
  causes, 248
  FOB and, 175-176
  PPPE, 442
  rigid bronchoscopy, 194
hypoxemia-associated OLV, 162-163
  response algorithm, 249*f*
  sources of, 248-250
hypoxia, 52-53. *See also* hypoxic pulmonary vasoconstriction
  trauma and, 381
  treatment cognitive aid, 31*t*-32*t*
hypoxic pulmonary vasoconstriction (HPV), 52-53, 294
  drugs and, 57
  pathways involved, 54*f*, 63-65, 64*f*
hysteresis, 47*t*

I
ICNB. *See* intercostal nerve blocks
ICP. *See* intracranial pressure
iloprost, 67, 75*t*
imaging
  diagnostic imaging modalities, 131-137
  NETT and, 289-291
  pediatric thoracic surgery, 406
immunodeficiency disorders, 359
immunosuppression, 374-375
immunosuppressive induction, 365-366
impaired pulmonary function, extubation criteria and, 252-253
IMRT. *See* intensity-modulated radiation therapy
induction. *See specific surgical procedure and anesthesia procedure*
induction chemotherapy, 326
infant epiglottis, 404, 405*f*
infection
  bronchopleural fistula, 350
  chronic bronchopleural fistula, 351
  pediatric upper respiratory, 406
  pleural cavity, 4
inflammatory soup, 106
inhalational agents, 64-65
inhalational anesthesia, 3
inhalation-based maintenance strategies, 247
inhaled nitric oxide (iNO)
  intracellular mechanism of, 75-76
  lung transplantation, 370, 373
inhibitory neurotransmitters, 108
injection catheter, 199
injuries, life-threatening, 381, 382*t*
iNO. *See* inhaled nitric oxide
inotrope, 370
inspired air:oxygen ratios, 250
inspired oxygen fraction, 56*f*
insulin therapy, 435-436
integrated PET/CT studies, 134, 134*f*
intensity-modulated radiation therapy (IMRT)
  mesothelioma, 269-270
  MPM, 258
intercostal nerve blocks (ICNB), 302, 477-478
  anatomy and, 478*f*
  rib fracture pain, 386, 386*f*
intercostal nerves, 103
intercostal neurovascular bundle, 478-479, 478*f*
interpleural block technique, 479-480
intracranial pressure (ICP), elevated, 193-194
intrapleural analgesia (IPA), 387
intra-thoracic procedures, 294

intrathoracic surgery classification, 156
IPA. *See* intrapleural analgesia
isoflurane, 64-65, 368
Ivor Lewis esophagectomy, 143, 144*t*, 328*t*, 329*f*, 330

J
jet ventilation, 179*f*, 180. *See also* high-frequency jet ventilation
  complications, 200
  components needed, 199*f*
  gas transport, 198-199
  rigid bronchoscopy, 197, 198-200

K
ketamine, 317, 474
ketorolac tromethamine (Toradol), 301
KRas, 116

L
Lambert-Easton myasthenic syndrome, 241-242
laminae, 103
  distribution, 104*f*
  primary afferent innervation to, 104*f*
laryngeal trauma, 391-393
laryngoscopy history, 9
LAS system. *See* Lung Allocation Score system
laser. *See also* Nd-YAG laser
  central airway tumors, 201, 202*t*, 203
  hemorrhage and, 203
  LVRS and, 281
latent conditions, 26-27, 26*f*, 40
latent conditions in healthcare systems, 26-27, 27*t*
leadership, 40
left thoracoabdominal esophagectomy, 328*t*, 329*f*, 330
left ventricular failure, 461
living donor lung transplantation, 362-363, 363*t*
lobectomy, 142
loop diuretics, 450, 452*t*, 453
low-molecular-weight heparin, 166-167
LT. *See* lung transplantation
L-type calcium channels (Ca^{2+}), 63-65, 64*f*
lungs
  anatomy, 128-130
  CT imaging, 132, 133*f*
  diagnostic imaging modalities, 131-132, 132*f*, 133*f*
  elastic effects and, 45-46, 48
  lobar and segmental anatomy, 129*t*
  PET imaging, 132, 133*f*, 134*f*, 135*f*
  resistive effects and, 47

lung adenocarcinomas, 116
Lung Allocation Score (LAS) system, 361
lung cancer, 20
  anesthetic plan
    anesthesia emergence and recovery, 251-253
    anesthesia maintenance, 246-251
    intraoperative anesthesia induction, 245-246
    preinduction, 243-244
  biology of, 116-123
  FOB, 174
  hyponatremia, 242
  metastasis, 165
  mouse modeling, 121-123
  p53 abnormalities and, 118, 119*f*
  paraneoplastic syndromes, 241-242
  preoperative preparation, 68-70
  symptoms, 238
  syndrome of inappropriate anti-diuretic hormone secretion, 166
lung collapse, 53-55, 55*f*
  distal lung collapse, 90
  double-lumen endobronchial tube, 245
  following lung separation, 97
lung compliance (C$_L$), 46
lung deflation, 298
lung isolation
  BPF, 354
  bronchial blockers, 245-246
  DLT and, 263-264
  postoperative pain control, 167
lung resection, 237-253
  acute lung injury, 447-448
  air leaks, 431-432
  analgesia, 252
  anesthetic plan
    anesthesia emergence and recovery, 251-253
    anesthesia maintenance, 246-251
    intraoperative anesthesia induction, 245-246
  case vignette, 237
  heart failure, 460-461
  key points, 237
  lung tumor classification, 238, 239*t*
  patient positioning, 246
  preoperative assessment, 157*f*, 240-243
  procedure planning, 239-240
  renal complications after, 450-454
  respiratory failure, 251
  summary, 461
  surgical risks, 139-140
  thoracotomy, 240

thoracotomy complication rates, 241*t*
tidal volume, 250
VATS, 240
lung separation
  lung collapse following, 97
  techniques, 82-98
  tracheostomized patient, 96-97
lung transplantation (LT), 358-376. *See also* bilateral orthotopic lung transplantation; post-transplant bronchial stenosis
  anesthesia after, 375-376, 375*t*
  antibiotics, 365-366, 375
  background, 359, 361
  bilateral lung transplantation, 362
  case study, 212-213
  children, 359, 359*f*-360*f*
  combined heart lung transplantation, 363
  COPD, 359
  ECMO, 373
  extracorporeal assistance, 372*t*
  indications for, 359, 359*f*-360*f*
  intraoperative
    management, 367-372
    monitors, 366, 366*t*
  key points and case vignette, 358
  living donor lung transplantation, 362-363, 363*t*
  postoperative management, 372-375
  preoperative evaluation and preparation, 364-366
  preoperative risk assessment, 365
  pulmonary vasodilators, 370
  recipient qualifications, 361
  single-lung transplantation, 359*f*, 361-362
lung tumor
  cigarette smoking, 238, 239*t*
  classification of, 238, 239*t*
  lung resection classification, 238, 239*t*
  types, 238-239
lung tumor-related hormone effects, 242
lung volume reduction surgery (LVRS), 20, 274-302
  air leak, 284, 284*f*
  candidacy determination criteria, 291, 292*t*
  cardiac complications, 284-285, 284*f*
  clinical evaluation, 286-287
  clinical vignette, 275
  extubation after, 300*t*
  general anesthesia, 295-297
  key points, 274
  outcome and complications, 283-285
  pain management, 301-302
  patient selection, 285-286
  perioperative management, 293-295

physiologic variables, 287-289
physiological effects of, 282-283, 283*t*
preoperative
  assessment, 285-286
  preparation, 291-293
pulmonary complications, 284
respiratory function after, 282-283
summary, 302
surgical approach, 280-282, 280*f*
surgical techniques for, 279-280
survival, 289-291, 290*f*
lung volumes
  normal, 48-49
  subdivision of, 48*f*
lung-protective ventilatory strategy, 298
LVRS. *See* lung volume reduction surgery
lymph nodes. *See also* Mountain-Dressler lymph node map
  cancer staging, 324-325, 324*t*
  malignant, 137
  station 3A, 183*f*
lymphatic drainage, 444
lymphomas, 219

M
magnesium, 458
magnetic resonance imaging (MRI), 225
malignancy. *See also* malignant pleural mesothelioma; non-small cell lung cancer; small-cell lung cancer
  airway obstruction, 201-207, 202*t*
  FDG-PET, 132, 133*f*, 134*f*, 135*f*
malignant pleural mesothelioma (MPM), 256
  chest x-ray of, 257*f*
  CT scan, 257, 258*f*
  treatment of, 257-259
Mallinckrodt right-sided double-lumen endotracheal tube, 84, 85*f*
malnutrition, 435
MARS trial (Mesothelioma and Radical Surgery trial), 259
maximal oxygen consumption (VO_2max), 155-156
maximum voluntary ventilation (MVV), 151-152
McGill pain questionnaire, 470
McKeown esophageal resection, 143, 144*t*, 145
mean pulmonary arterial pressure (mPAP), 65
mechanical ventilation
  intraoperative, 16
  lung transplantation, 369
  spontaneous ventilation and, 448
  tracheostomy and, 449-450
  weaning, 374

median sternotomy, 280-281
mediastinal masses
  airway management, 230-231
  anesthesia
    induction, 230
    management, 227, 229-233
    principles, 229*t*
  anesthesiologists and, 217-234
  cardiopulmonary bypass, 231-232
  case vignette, 217
  in children, 219*t*
  clinical aspects of, 218-220
  complications, 231
  intraoperative complications
    children, 229*t*
    incidence, 228*t*
  key points, 217
  pathology of, 218-219
  perioperative approach, 232-233, 232*f*
  perioperative complications, 226-227
  radiographic evaluation, 224-225
  signs and symptoms, 219-220, 220*t*
  surgery, 220
mediastinal tumor, nerve involvement, 220
mediastinoscopy
  case vignette, 173
  cervical, 181, 184, 185*f*
  indications, 181
  NSCLC and, 140-141
  postoperative care, 188
  surgical complications, 186-188, 187*t*
mediastinum, 185
  anatomy, 131, 181-182, 182*f*, 218, 218*f*
  imaging, 135
  video-assisted thoracoscopic surgery, 185
medical errors, 34, 37-38
medications. *See also* drugs
  acute renal failure, 451-454, 452*t*
  errors, 37-38
  perioperative respiratory, 165
  pulmonary hypertension, 77
  for renal protection, 451, 452
  respiratory, perioperative, 165
mesothelioma. *See also* malignant pleural mesothelioma
  trimodality therapy, 269-270
Mesothelioma and Radical Surgery trial. *See* MARS trial
metastases, 165. *See also* tumor-node-metastasis classification system
metastatic disease, 324-325, 324*t*
  pulmonary resection and, 165-166
methylene blue, 346
microRNA, 117

MIE esophageal resection. *See* minimally invasive esophagogastrectomy esophageal resection
milrinone, 74, 75*t*, 77
minimally invasive esophagogastrectomy (MIE) esophageal resection, 143-145, 144*t*, 333-334
minimally invasive techniques, 20
minute ventilation, 49, 50*f*
mistake, 40
mixed venous oxygen content, 55-56, 56*f*
modified McKeown approach. *See* three-incision esophagectomy
modified rapid-sequence induction, 367
monitors
  and alarms, 35-37
  bronchoscopy, 177
  CCAMs resection, 414
  intraoperative, 17-18
  lung transplantation, 366, 366*t*
  patient status, 35-37
  pericardial effusion, 317
  rigid bronchoscopy, 179-180
morphine, 302, 473, 473*t*
mortality
  esophagectomy, 322-323, 333-334
  LVRS, 283-284
motor vehicle crash (MVC), 379
  BCI and, 393
  thoracic injury, 397-398
motorcycle crashes, 397-398
Mountain-Dressler lymph node map, 182, 183*f*
mouse modeling, 121-123
mPAP. *See* mean pulmonary arterial pressure
MPM. *See* malignant pleural mesothelioma
MR cells. *See* multi-receptive cells
MRI. *See* magnetic resonance imaging
Muller's handgrip, 4
multimodal analgesia, 470, 470*f*, 480
multi-receptive (MR) cells, 103-104
muscle relaxants, 245, 296
mutual support, 34, 40
MVC. *See* motor vehicle crash
MVV. *See* maximum voluntary ventilation
myasthenia gravis, 166
myocardial filling, 311
myocardial ischemia, 459-460
  EPP and, 266
  perioperative, 159-160

N
NANC systems, 47
narcotics, 368

National Emphysema Treatment Trial
(NETT), 280-281
  imaging and, 289-291
  LVRS and, 284-285
  operative mortality and, 286
  study, 288
Nd-YAG laser
  LVRS and, 281
  tumor and, 201
negative pressure chamber, 4-5, 5f
nerve blocks, 111
nerve growth factor (NGF), 107
nesiritide, 77
NETT. See National Emphysema Treatment Trial
neuraxial injection, 243-244
neuraxial opioids, 19-20
neuroaxial procedure guidelines, 243
neuroendocrine tumors, 242
neurokinin A, 108
neurons of central nervous system, 111
neuropathic pain, 102, 110-111
neuropeptides, 106
NGF. See nerve growth factor
nicardipine, 370
nitinol stents, 209
nitric oxide (NO), 57, 75t
  generation, 47
  pain and, 107
nitroglycerin, 370
NMDA. See glutamate receptor N-methyl-D-aspartate
NO. See nitric oxide
nociceptive information, 104-105
nociceptive specific (NS) neurons, 103, 104f
nociceptive stimulation, 468, 469f
nociceptive system, persistent activation of, 102
nociceptors, 103
nondependent arm, brachial plexus injury, 139, 139t
nondependent lung deflation, 53-55, 55f
nonmalignant disease surgery, 20
non-small cell lung cancer (NSCLC)
  mediastinoscopy, 140-141
  pneumonectomy, 440-441
  staging, 174
  tumor suppressor gene p16, 120
nonsteroidal anti-inflammatory drugs (NSAIDs), 480
  chronic pain, 111
  LVRS, 301
  renal dysfunction and, 451
norepinephrine, 74

normothermia, 140, 297, 368
NRas, 116
NS neurons. See nociceptive specific neurons
NSAIDs. See nonsteroidal anti-inflammatory drugs
NSCLC. See non-small cell lung cancer

O

obesity, 322
OLV. See one-lung ventilation
oncogenes, 116, 118f
one-lung ventilation (OLV), 2-3. See also pediatrics
  chronic obstructive pulmonary disease, 56f
  early, 12-14, 16
  EPP, 264
  hemodynamic changes, 55
  oxygenation during, 55-57
  oxygenation improvements, 18-19
  pediatric thoracic surgery, 406, 407
  pericardial effusion and, 319
  physiology, 45-61, 55f
  PPPE and, 444
  severe COPD and, 297-299
  summary of, 61
  three-incision esophagectomy, 328-329, 329f
open pneumothorax, 383-384
operating room, time-outs, 39
opioids
  epidural analgesic regimens, 473, 473t
  HPV and, 65
  intravenous, 296
  neuraxial, 19-20
  pediatrics, 410
  pericardial effusion and, 319
oxygenation, for one-lung ventilation, 18-19, 55-57

P

pA-aO$_2$. See alveolar-arterial oxygen gradient
PAC. See pulmonary artery catheterization
paclitaxel, 162
P$_a$CO$_2$. See arterial carbon dioxide
pain. See also chronic pain; chronic post-thoracotomy pain; pediatrics; rib fracture pain
  acute pain, 102, 469f
  acute postoperative, 102
  acute post-thoracotomy pain, 467-484, 471t
  adenosine triphosphate, 107
  brain areas and, 104-105
  breakthrough pain, 411

pain (*Cont.*):
   central nervous system pain, 107
   central neural mechanisms, 103-106
   mechanisms of, 102-111, 468
   neurochemistry of, 106-108, 106*f*
   neuropathic pain, 102, 110-111
   nitric oxide, 107
pain management. *See also* McGill pain questionnaire
   esophagectomy, 333
   LT and, 374
   lung isolation and, 167
   LVRS, 301-302
   pediatric thoracic surgery, 409
   poor, 468
   postoperative, 468
   postoperative analgesia, 19-20
   rib fractures, 385*t*
panlobular emphysema, 276, 277*f*
P_AO_2. *See* alveolar PO_2
P_aO_2. *See* arterial oxygenation
paraneoplastic syndromes, 241-242
paravertebral blockade, 19-20, 302
   landmarks, 477*f*
patient
   positioning
      BPF, 354
      lung resection, 246
      lung transplantation, 368
      LVRS and, 281-282
      normal lung volumes and, 48-49
      OLV, 56-57
      during thoracic surgery, 139*t*
   safety
      case vignette, 39
      thoracic anesthesia, 25-41
   selection, LVRS, 285-286
   status, monitoring and alarms, 35-37
patient controlled epidural analgesia (PCEA), 474
   dosing schedule, 474*t*
PCEA. *See* patient controlled epidural analgesia
P/D. *See* pleurectomy/decortication
peak airway pressure, 46
pediatrics
   anterior mediastinal mass
      anesthetic induction and airway management, 418, 420
      anesthetic risk assessment algorithm, 419*f*
      anterior Chamberlain procedure, 418, 420*f*
      perioperative complications, 420
      preoperative assessment, 417
   bupivacaine, 410-411

local anesthetic infusion, 410
one-lung intubation, 406
one-lung ventilation
   endotracheal tube selection, 408, 408*t*
   principles of, 408-409
TEA, 409-411
thoracic surgery, 403-420
   anatomic differences, 404, 405*f*
   conditions necessitating, 404
   double-lumen endotracheal tubes, 408
   imaging, 406
   key points and clinical vignette, 403
   one-lung ventilation, 406
   overview of, 404, 406-411
   pain management, 409
   preoperative assessment, 404, 406
   summary of, 420
   upper respiratory infections, 406
PEEP. *See* positive end-expiratory pressure
pendelluft, 3
penetrating thoracic trauma, 397*t*
penetrating trauma, 379
perforation of major vessel, 203
pericardial drainage procedures, summary for, 320
pericardial effusion, 318
   anesthetic considerations, 316-319, 318*f*
   diagnosis, 312-316
   echocardiography, 313, 313*f*, 314*f*
   pre-induction invasive arterial blood pressure monitoring, 317
   surgical management, 316
pericardial perfusion
   etiologies and associated pathophysiology, 309-310, 309*t*
   thoracoscopy, 308
pericardial pressure-volume curves, 310*f*
pericardial space, fluid in, 313, 313*f*
pericardial tamponade, 315
   diagnosis, 312-316
   inspiration, 315-316, 315*f*
pericardial window procedures, 308-320
pericardiectomy, constrictive pericarditis, 316
pericarditis, 309-310, 309*t*
perioperative cardiac complications, 68
perioperative tracheobronchial compression, with inability to ventilate, 221
peripheral neural mechanisms, 103
permissive hypercapnia, 246
PET imaging, 132, 133*f*, 134*f*, 135*f*
PET/CT fusion studies, 134, 135*f*
PGD. *See* pulmonary graft dysfunction
PGI_2. *See* prostacyclin
PH. *See* pulmonary hypertension

pH manipulation, 57, 60
phenylephrine, 72
photodynamic therapy, 206-207, 326
physical trauma, thoracic surgery, 102
physiologic dead space, 49, 50f
plain chest x-ray
    aortic transection, 397-398
    mediastinal masses, 224
plateau pressure (alveolar pressure), 46, 47f
pleiotropic effects, 160
pleural catheters, 302
pleural cavity, infection and, 4
pleural drainage, 433
pleural effusion
    chest x-ray, 132f
    MPM and, 257
pleural space injuries
    chest wall, 385-388
    hemothorax, 384-385
    open pneumothorax, 383-384
    pneumothorax, 382-383
pleurectomy/decortication (P/D), 258-259
pneumomediastinum, 203
pneumonectomy, 142-143. *See also* post-pneumonectomy pulmonary edema
    common complications after, 442t
    NSCLC and, 440-441
    respiratory complications, 441
pneumonia
    air leak, 284, 284f
    lung volume reduction surgery, 284
    postoperative, 445-446
    prevention, 428-429
pneumothorax, 3-4, 140, 297. *See also* open pneumothorax
    anesthetic considerations, 383
    BPF, 349
    clinical signs and symptoms, 382
    FOB and, 176
    management, 383
    mediastinoscopy, 187
    pleural space injuries, 382-383
POAF. *See* postoperative atrial fibrillation
POISE trial, 160
positive end-expiratory pressure (PEEP), 18-19, 74
    chronic bronchopleural fistula, 351
    hypoxemia with OLV, 248-250
    LVRS, 295-296
positive pressure chamber, 5, 197
positive pressure ventilation
    normal lung volumes and, 48-49
    pericardial effusion, 318-319
post thoracotomy, 467

post-esophagectomy patients, 336-337, 336f
postoperative atrial fibrillation (POAF), 454-455
    ACEIs, 459
    calcium channel blockers, 457
    digitalization, 457
    statins, 458-459
postoperative pain control, 167
post-pneumonectomy pulmonary edema (PPPE), 441-445
    prognosis, 445
    treatment, 444-445
post-transplant bronchial stenosis, 213
ppo-FEV$_1$. *See* predicted postoperative FEV$_1$
PPPE. *See* post-pneumonectomy pulmonary edema
predicted postoperative FEV$_1$ (ppo-FEV$_1$), 152, 153f
pre-induction invasive arterial blood pressure monitoring, 317
preoxygenation, 245
pressure-volume relationship, 46, 47f
primary hyperalgesia, 109
primary lung cancer, 238
primary survey, life-threatening injuries and, 381, 382t
procedure violations, 26, 26f
propofol
    HPV and, 65
    TIVA and, 296
PROSPECT group, 473
prospective memory, 28-30
prostacyclin (PGI$_2$, Epoprostenol, Flolan), 67
    continuous aerosol delivery protocol, 76-77, 76t
proximal descending aorta, 398f
pseudodiaphragm, 391
P$_{tP}$. *See* transpulmonary pressure
pulmonary arteriolar vasoconstriction, 52-53
pulmonary arteriolar vasodilation, 52-53
pulmonary artery
    clamping, 369-370
    unclamping and reperfusion, 370-371
pulmonary artery catheterization (PAC), 71-72
    BCI, 396
    hypotension diagnosis with, 73t
    LVRS, 295-296
pulmonary circulation, 50-51
pulmonary circulation pressure-flow relationships, 51-52
    gravitational effect, 52
pulmonary contusion, 389-390

506 / Index

pulmonary edema, 373
pulmonary embolism, 268-269
pulmonary function, impaired, 242*f*
pulmonary function tests, 150
    COPD diagnosis, 278
    lung volume reduction surgery, 287-288
pulmonary gas exchange, 49-50
pulmonary graft dysfunction (PGD), 373
pulmonary hypertension (PH), 65
    COPD, 279
    determination of presence, 69
    initial management, 75*t*
    intraoperative, initial management of, 74-75
    LT, 365, 370
    LVRS, 287
    perioperative
        care, 70-72
        management, 63-78
    postoperative, recovery, 77-78
    preoperative
        management, 67-68
        preparation, 68-70
    supportive medications, 77
    thoracic surgery and, induction and maintenance, 72
    WHO classification of, 65, 66*t*
pulmonary laceration, 390
pulmonary lesions, 173
pulmonary morbidity, 287
pulmonary perfusion, 51-52
pulmonary physiology, normal, 63-65
pulmonary physiotherapy, 428
pulmonary rehabilitation, 69, 164
pulmonary resection, 141
    effects of, 66-67
    indications, 151
    metastatic disease and, 165-166
pulmonary restrictive syndrome, 294
pulmonary toxicity, chemotherapeutic agents, 137, 138*t*, 164
pulmonary vascular disease, 359
pulmonary vascular dynamics, 66-67
pulmonary vasodilators, 75-77, 370
pulmonary venous thromboembolism, 166
pulmonary ventilation, elastic effects and, 45-46, 48
pulse oximetry, 18
pulsus paradoxus, 311, 312*t*, 315, 315*f*
    right ventricular hypertrophy, 312
PVB. *See* thoracic paravertebral blockade
PVS. *See* thoracic paravertebral space

R

radiation, 161, 163
    pneumonia, 137, 164
    postoperative, 326
    therapy, 137
radiofrequency ablation, 326
radiographic evaluation, mediastinal masses, 224-225, 225*f*
rapid-sequence induction, 367
Ras, 116-117
recombinant human B-type natriuretic peptide (BNP), 77
regional nerve blocks, 319
remifentanil, 296
renal complications, postoperative, 450-454
renal failure, 451
renal postoperative complications, 440
rescue analgesic medication, pediatric breakthrough pain, 411
respiratory acidosis, 298
respiratory complications, radiographic characteristics, 443*t*
respiratory evaluation, summary recommendations, 156
respiratory events, 38-39
respiratory failure
    after lung resection, 251
    postoperative, 300-301, 373
respiratory function
    anesthesia effects on, 293-295, 295*t*
    evaluation, 151-156
    after lung volume reduction surgery, 282-283
respiratory medications, perioperative, 165
respiratory postoperative complications, 440-450
restrictive lung disease, 359, 360*f*
resuscitative thoracotomy, 381-382
rib
    retraction, 483
    stabilization, 389
rib fracture, 385-388, 387
rib fracture pain, 385-388, 386*f*
    adverse effects of, 385-386, 385*t*
    anesthetic/analgesic solutions, 385-388, 386*f*
right heart catheterization, 70
right heart failure, 370
right radial artery cannulation, 173
right ventricular ejection fraction (RVEF), 66
right ventricular end diastolic volume (RVEDV), 66
right ventricular (RV) failure, 266
right ventricular hypertrophy (RVH), 312
right ventricular impairment, 160-161

right ventricular vascular dynamics, 66-67
right-sided double-lumen endotracheal tube
  indications for, 84, 84f, 85f
  positioning, 89f
  sizing of, 85-86
rigid bronchoscopy
  anesthesia, 196-198
  anesthesia management, 179-180
  complications, 178
  emergence, 181
  equipment, 179f, 195
  hypoxemia, 194
  indications, 178, 179t, 192, 192t, 193
  induction and maintenance, 180
  insertion, 195-196, 196f
  jet ventilation, 197, 198-200
  key points, 191
  monitoring, 179-180
  patient selection, 193-195
  positive pressure chamber, 197
  procedure risks and complications, 195
  Sanders jet ventilator, 197
  thrombocytopenia, 195
  ventilation, 180-181
ropivacaine, 411
RV failure. See right ventricular failure
RVEDV. See right ventricular end diastolic volume
RVEF. See right ventricular ejection fraction
RVH. See right ventricular hypertrophy

S
Sanders jet ventilator, 197
Sauerbruch, E. F., 4-55f
SBAR (situation, background, assessment, recommendation), 34-35, 40
second gas effect, 49
secondary hyperalgesia, 109
segmentectomy, 141-142
self-expanding metal stents, 209
sensitization, 109
sensory spinal neurons, classes of, 103, 104f
septal injuries, 394-395
severe chronic obstructive pulmonary disease, 297-299
sevoflurane, 64-65
shared mental model, 34, 40
Sheridan right-sided double-lumen endotracheal tube, 84, 85f
SIADH. See syndrome of inappropriate anti-diuretic hormone secretion
sign out, 29-30
Silbroncho left-sided double-lumen endotracheal tube, 84, 85f

sildenafil, 68
silicone stents, 207, 208f, 209
simple pneumothorax, 382
single-lung anesthesia, 247-248
sinus tachycardia, unexplained, 395
situation, background, assessment, recommendation. See SBAR
situation awareness, 34
sleeve resections, 142-143
sliding scale insulin coverage, 436
slip, 34
small-cell lung cancer, metabolic and paraneoplastic effects, 166-167
smoking cessation, 164-165, 287
sodium bicarbonate infusion, 452t, 454
sodium nitroprusside, 370
solitary pulmonary nodule (SPN), 174
somatosensory system, 108
somatostatin (SST), 107
sotalol, 456
spinal cord
  laminae distribution, 104f
  neurochemical mediators in, 108f
spirometry, 167
  airway obstruction, 223-224, 223f
  thoracic surgery and, 152-153
split lung function tests, 154
SPN. See solitary pulmonary nodule
spontaneous assisted ventilation, 196
spontaneous ventilation, 448
squamous cell carcinoma, 323
SST. See somatostatin
standard fire precautions, 39
staples, 281
static respiratory system compliance, 46, 47f
statins, 160, 458-459
stent grafts, 400
stents, 22
  airway, 207-210
  BMS, 159
  coronary, 159, 460
  drug-eluting stents, 159
  hybrid stents, 209-210, 211f
  nitinol stents, 209
  placement, 210
  self-expanding metal stents, 209
  silicone stents, 207, 208f, 209
  types of, 207-210
sternum anatomy, 127
steroids
  pediatric anterior mediastinal mass, 417
  PPPE and, 445
  systemic, 293
stripping, 430-431

stroke, 187
stroke volume (SV), changes, 311
subacute cerebellar degeneration, 241
subcutaneous emphysema, 432-433
sublobar resections, 141-142
substance P, 108
sufentanil, 368
superior vena cava syndrome
    (SVC syndrome), 233, 234, 234*t*
supraventricular tachyarrhythmias, 454, 456*t*
surgery. *See also* lung volume reduction
        surgery; pediatrics; thoracic surgery;
        unilateral video-assisted thoracoscopic
        surgery; video-assisted thoracoscopic
        surgery
  airway management, 393
  approach, 151
  blunt aortic injury, 399-400
  congenital cystic adenomatous
        malformations, 412-413, 414
  esophageal cancer, 325-326, 325*t*
  with lung surgery, 244
  lung volume reduction surgery, 288-289,
        295-297
  mediastinal masses, 220
  nonmalignant disease, 20
  pericardial effusion, 316
  preoperative non-cardiac surgery, 156
  thoracic surgical patient, 433-434, 434*t*
Surgical Safety Checklist, 29, 29*f*
survival
  epidural growth factor receptor, 118*f*
  esophageal cancer, 325-326, 325*t*
  lung volume reduction surgery, 289-291,
        290*f*
  LVRS and, 289-291, 290*f*
  tumor and, 118*f*
SV. *See* stroke volume
SVC syndrome. *See* superior vena cava
        syndrome
Swiss cheese model of system accidents,
        26, 26*f*
syndrome of inappropriate anti-diuretic
        hormone secretion (SIADH), 166
systemic syndromes, 220
systolic blood pressure, 246

T
tachycardia, 312-313
tamponade, 313
TBA. *See* transbronchial needle aspiration
TDR. *See* traumatic diaphragmatic rupture
TEA. *See* thoracic epidural analgesia
teamwork, 32, 33*t*, 34-35, 39

TEE. *See* transesophageal echocardiograph
tension pneumothorax, 90, 297, 382-383
therapeutic bronchoscopy, 191-192
  conclusion, 214
  key points, 191
thoracentesis, 227
thoracic anesthesia
  algorithm, 30
  current scope of, 20-22
  history and scope, early years, 2-6
  history and scope of, 2-22
  patient safety, 25-41
thoracic aortic injury
  blunt trauma and, 397*t*
  factors associated, 397*t*
thoracic compliance, measurement of, 46, 47*f*
thoracic duct ligation, 335
thoracic epidural analgesia (TEA). *See also*
        continuous thoracic epidural analgesia
  esophagectomy procedures, 333
  extrapleural pneumonectomy, 263
  LVRS, 301
  pediatrics, 409-411
  rib fracture, 387
thoracic epidural catheterization, 471
thoracic paravertebral blockade (PVB),
        474-475
  adverse effects, 476
  anatomy and technique, 475-476, 475*f*
thoracic paravertebral space (PVS), 475, 475*f*
thoracic surgery, 2-6, 127-145, 151,
        426-427. *See also* pediatrics
  advances in, 11
  cardiac evaluation, 156, 158*f*, 159-161
  chemotherapeutic agents, 137, 161
  fluid management, 433-434, 434*t*
  gas exchange, 153
  induction and maintenance, pulmonary
        hypertension and, 72
  management guidelines, 137-140
  pain in, 102-111
  patient positions during, 139*t*
  physical trauma, 102
  preoperative evaluation and, conclusions
        on, 167
  preoperative risk stratification, 150-167
    key points and case vignette, 150
  procedures, 140-145
  pulmonary hypertension, 72
thoracic surgical patient
  cardiac complications, 454-461
  chest tube management, 429-433, 429*f*
  fluid management, 433-434, 434*t*
  glycemic control, 435-436

Index / 509

nutrition, 435
pneumonia prevention, 428-429
postoperative care of, 426-436
postoperative ventilatory support, 428
prophylactic antibiotics, 434-435
pulmonary physiotherapy and ambulation, 428
recovery area admission, 427
summary, 436
venous thromboembolism prophylaxis, 436
ventilatory support, 428
thoracic trauma
management, 378-400
triage and initial management, 381-400
thoracoscopy
pericardial effusion drainage, 319
pericardial perfusion and, 308
thoracostomy tube, 354
thoracotomy
on dogs, 4-5, 5*f*
lung resection, 240, 241*t*
three-compartment lung model, 293
three-incision esophagectomy (modified McKeown approach), 328-329, 328*t*, 329*f*
thrombocytopenia, 195
tidal volume, 250
tidaling, 430
time-outs, 29-30, 29*f*, 39
tissue
injury, 106-108, 106*f*
trauma, 468, 469*f*
TIVA-based maintenance strategies. *See* total intravenous anesthetic-based maintenance strategies
TMN classification system. *See* tumor-node-metastasis classification system
tobacco smoke, 275
Toradol. *See* Ketorolac tromethamine
Torsades de Pointes, 456
total intravenous anesthetic-based maintenance strategies (TIVA-based maintenance strategies), 247, 295-296
total ventilation, 49
toxicity
anesthetic, 302
chemotherapeutic agents, 137, 138*t*, 164
TPB. *See* continuous thoracic paravertebral blockade
tracheal anatomy, 128-129
tracheal extubation, 251, 274
tracheal insufflation, 8-9
tracheal insufflation anesthesia, 9
tracheal intubation, 245

tracheal re-intubation, 300-301
tracheal resection, 143
tracheal stenosis, 200
tracheobronchial anastomosis, 343
tracheobronchial trauma, 391-393
tracheobronchial tree, foreign body in airway, 416*f*
tracheostomy
indications, contraindications, complications, 449*t*
lung separation in, 96-97
mechanical ventilation and, 449-450
transbronchial lung biopsies, 191, 375
transbronchial needle aspiration (TBA), 174
transesophageal echocardiograph (TEE), 35
BCI, 396
extrapleural pneumonectomy, 263
intraoperative, 370-371
LT and, 371
LVRS, 295-296
pericardial effusion and, 313, 313*f*, 314*f*
perioperative hemodynamic measurement and, 71
transhiatal esophagectomy, 328*t*, 329, 329*f*
transplantation. *See* bilateral orthotopic lung transplantation; combined heart lung transplantation; living donor lung transplantation; lung transplantation
transpulmonary pressure (P_{tP}), 46
trans-thoracic echocardiography (TTE), 69
trauma, 378
bronchopleural fistula, 350
rib fractures, 385-388
traumatic diaphragmatic rupture (TDR), 390-391
treprostinil, 67
trimodality therapy, 269-270
TTE. *See* trans-thoracic echocardiography
tumor. *See also* lung tumor
benign chest tumors, 237-253
central airway tumors, 201, 202*t*, 203
electrocautery, 203-204, 204*f*
mediastinal tumor, 220
nd-YAG laser, 201
neuroendocrine tumors, 242
NSCLC, 120
suppressor gene p16, 119-120
suppressor gene p53, 117-118
suppressors, 117-120
survival, 118*f*
tumor-node-metastasis (TMN) classification system, 324-325, 324*t*
two-lung ventilation, 56*f*

U

unilateral video-assisted thoracoscopic surgery (VATS), 281
univent endotracheal tube, 94-95, 297
universal differential pressure chamber, 5-6
upper GI endoscopy, esophageal cancer and, 323

V

valvular injuries, 394
vancomycin, 434
vasodilators, 57
  pulmonary vasodilators, 75-77, 370
  vasodilatory shock, 77
vasopressin, 74, 77
vasopressors, 77
VATS. *See* unilateral video-assisted thoracoscopic surgery; video-assisted thoracoscopic surgery
venous thromboembolism prophylaxis, 436
ventilation. *See also* jet ventilation; mechanical ventilation; one-lung ventilation; pediatrics; positive pressure ventilation
  alveolar PCO_2 ventilation equation, 49, 50f
  biologically variable ventilation, 60
  esophagectomy, 331
  high-frequency jet ventilation, 19, 179-180
  intraoperative mechanical ventilation, 16
  maximum voluntary ventilation, 151-152
  mechanical effects, 59-60, 59f
  minute ventilation, 49
  myocardial filling and, 311
  pattern of, 60
  pericardial effusion, 318
  pulmonary gas exchange and, 49-50
  spontaneous assisted ventilation, 196
  spontaneous ventilation, 448
  strategies, 197
  total ventilation, 49
  two-lung and one-lung ventilation, 56f
ventilation-perfusion scans (V/Q scan), 134-135, 154
video-assisted thoracoscopic surgery (VATS), 20-21
  lung resection, 240, 241t
  LVRS and, 280-281
  of mediastinum, 185, 186
  pericardial effusion, 316-319
  pleural space injuries, 384-385
  thoracic surgery and, 151, 426-427
violation, 34
vital lung capacity, 223-224, 223f
VO_2max. *See* maximal oxygen consumption
vocal cords
  dysfunction, 268
  paralysis, 336
volume overload, 442, 444
volume replacement, LT and, 374
V/Q scan. *See* ventilation-perfusion scans

W

WDR cells. *See* wide-dynamic range cells
wedge resection, 141-142
weight loss, 323
WHO classification. *See* World Health Organization classification
wide-dynamic range (WDR) cells, 103-104
World Health Organization classification (WHO classification), pulmonary hypertension, 65, 66t
written treatment algorithms, 30